Sixth Edition

Kelsey's Midwifery & Women's Health Nurse Practitioner
Certification Review Guide

Jamille Nagtalon-Ramos,
EdD, WHNP-BC, FAANP
Assistant Professor
School of Nursing – Camden
Rutgers University
Camden, NJ
and
Women's Health Nurse Practitioner
Department of Obstetrics & Gynecology
Pennsylvania Hospital
Philadelphia, PA

Melicia Escobar,
DNP, CNM, WHNP-BC, FACNM
Assistant Professor & Program Director
NM/WHNP & WHNP Programs
Georgetown University School of Nursing
Washington, DC
and
Certified Nurse-Midwife
Department of Obstetrics and Gynecology
Jefferson Einstein Montgomery
East Norriton, PA

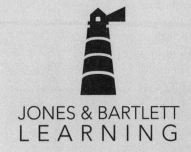

JONES & BARTLETT
LEARNING

T0295289

World Headquarters
Jones & Bartlett Learning
25 Mall Road
Burlington, MA 01803
978-443-5000
info@jblearning.com
www.jblearning.com

Jones & Bartlett Learning books and products are available through most bookstores and online booksellers. To contact Jones & Bartlett Learning directly, call 800-832-0034, fax 978-443-8000, or visit our website, www.jblearning.com.

28462-1

Production Credits

Senior Director, Content Production and Delivery: Christine Emerton
Product Manager: Melissa Kleeman Moy
Senior Outsourcing Specialist: Carol Brewer Guerrero
Content Strategist: Karan Rana
Content Coordinator: Samantha Gillespie
Manager, Intellectual Properties and Content Production: Kristen Rogers
Content Production Manager: Eliza Lewis
Senior Digital Project Specialist: Angela Dooley
Director, Marketing: Andrea DeFronzo
Senior Product Marketing Manager: Lindsay White
Procurement Manager: Wendy Kilborn
Media Development Editor: Faith Brosnan
Rights Specialist: Robin Silverman
Content Vendor: MPS Limited
Composition and Project Management: S4Carlisle Publishing Services
Text and Cover Design: MPS Limited
Cover Image (Title Page, Part Opener, Chapter Opener): © Jasmin Merdan/Moment/Getty Images
Printing and Binding: Sheridan Michigan

Library of Congress Cataloging-in-Publication Data
Library of Congress Cataloging-in-Publication Data unavailable at time of printing.

LCCN: 2024020009

6048

Printed in the United States of America
28 27 26 25 24   10 9 8 7 6 5 4 3 2 1

Dedication

This book is a labor of love dedicated to our women's health nurse practitioner (WHNP) and midwifery students—past, present, and future. Your unwavering commitment to learning fuels us to continue updating this book. In honor of Dr. Beth Kelsey, the visionary who conceived of this wonderful resource, we proudly rename this text: Kelsey's *Midwifery & Women's Health Nurse Practitioner Certification Review Guide, Sixth Edition.* For more than three decades, Dr. Kelsey's certification review books and her work as an educator and journal editor have guided thousands of WHNPs and midwives. We are honored to continue Dr. Kelsey's work guiding future WHNPs and midwives well in their studies.

To all our WHNP and midwifery colleagues, thank you for your dedication to the important work that you do.

A special thanks to our editorial assistant, Erin Finch, for your diligent support; to our graduate student assistants, Samantha Noblejas, and Dr. Kendra Faucett, for working hard to improve the online question bank; and to each of our contributors for your time and effort coauthoring and editing the sixth edition with us. We are grateful to our reviewers, students, and colleagues for all your feedback.

—Jamille and Melicia

This book would not have been possible without the loving support of my husband Reg and my children, Leo, Leilani, and Leah. Leo and Leilani, I am proud of you for carrying the nursing tradition and being our family's fourth generation of nurses (no pressure, Leah!). Bean and Luna, thank you for unlimited snuggles while I wrote. I appreciate my colleagues at Rutgers and Penn Medicine, my sister Brooke, family, and friends for showing me kindness and grace during the writing and editing process. Salamat. We are grateful to my WHNP and midwifery colleagues for your continued support. I enjoy meeting and receiving messages from students who enthusiastically share where they've brought this book as their trusted companion to study beyond the classroom—to parks, waiting rooms, vacations, and even honeymoons! We love your dedication. You inspire us to continue making this book better with each new edition.

Thank you, Beth, for the wonderful opportunity to be your writing partner for three editions of the book. What an honor it was when you asked me to join you in this endeavor over a decade ago. I am so lucky to have you as a mentor and a friend.

Melicia, I am so thankful to you for agreeing to work with me on the latest edition of the book. Thank you, my friend, for your organizational skills, kind support, and being the ultimate cheerleader to get us to the finish line!

—Jamille

I am so grateful: To Beth Kelsey, who, with Jamille Nagtalon-Ramos, welcomed me into this important editorial project and placed your trust in me to carry on your legacy in this text. To my in-home support team, Eric, Mona, and Opal—for your endless support, patience, understanding, and space that you create for me to take on meaningful, professional projects; I love you. To my dad, Fredy Escobar, for providing Colombian comfort food to fuel me. To my sister Mia, for your care and good humor. To my midwife and WHNP community for the fellowship. To my Georgetown students, graduates, and colleagues—you inspire my passion for developing a more inclusive curriculum and resources. And finally, to Jamille, for always seeing me, for your grace, partnership, friendship, and mentorship.
I look forward to continued collaboration.

—Melicia

Brief Contents

Contents

CHAPTER 1 Strategies for Studying and Test Taking 1

Jamille Nagtalon-Ramos
Melicia Escobar

CHAPTER 2 Health Assessment and Diagnostic Tests 8

Beth M. Kelsey
Komkwuan P. Paruchabutr

CHAPTER 3 Primary Care 38

Heather C. Quaile
Komkwuan P. Paruchabutr
Beth M. Kelsey

CHAPTER 4   Gynecologic, Reproductive, Sexual, and Menopause Health 150

Beth M. Kelsey
Sandi Tenfelde
Signey Olson

CHAPTER 5   Gynecologic, Reproductive, and Sexual Disorders 201

Beth M. Kelsey
Heather C. Quaile
Signey Olson

CHAPTER 6 Prenatal Care and Assessment of Fetal Well-Being 252

Jamille Nagtalon-Ramos
Melicia Escobar

CHAPTER 7 Complex Pregnancy Care 282

Jamille Nagtalon-Ramos
Melicia Escobar

CHAPTER 12 Professional Practice Issues **420**

Beth M. Kelsey
Kathryn Trotter

Preface

A comprehensive review is essential for those preparing to take the midwifery (American Midwifery Certification Board [AMCB]) examination or the women's health nurse practitioner (WHNP) certification (National Certification Corporation [NCC]) examination. *Midwifery & Women's Health Nurse Practitioner Certification Review Guide, Sixth Edition* was developed for both nursing specialties because of the many commonalities they share in providing health care for individuals throughout their lifespan. A diverse group of experts in the field of primary care and sexual and reproductive health combined their expertise to create a valuable resource that will assist WHNPs and midwives in their pursuit of success on their respective certification examinations. Multiple resources have been utilized to ensure the integrity of this text so that it is representative of the content that both specialties may encounter during the examination process. Additionally, great care has been taken to include inclusive language throughout the text to echo what readers have experienced in key textbooks and will encounter on the board examinations. Similarly, when referencing literature, the study populations cited were described accordingly.

When preparing for certification examinations, many nurses find that reviewing an extensive body of scientific knowledge requires a very difficult search of many sources that must be synthesized to provide a review base for the examination. This review guide aims to provide a succinct yet comprehensive review of the core material.

This guide is organized to first provide the reader with test-taking and study strategies (Chapter 1, *Strategies for Studying and Test Taking*). This prerequisite for success in the certification examination arena should not be overlooked. The major content is then provided in Chapter 2, *Health Assessment and Diagnostic Tests*; Chapter 3, *Primary Care*; Chapter 4, *Gynecologic, Reproductive, Sexual, and Menopause Health*; Chapter 5, *Complex Gynecologic, Reproductive, and Sexual Care*; Chapter 6, *Prenatal Care and Assessment of Fetal Well-Being*; Chapter 7, *Complex Pregnancy Care*; Chapter 8, *Intrapartum*; Chapter 9, *Postpartum and Lactation*; Chapter 10, *Midwifery Care of the Newborn*; Chapter 11, *Principles of Pharmacology*; and Chapter 12, *Professional Practice Issues*. A diverse group of WHNPs and midwives across various identities and clinic perspectives have reviewed the chapters in this sixth edition to provide feedback and recommendations. New and revised content reflects this review.

Test questions are included at the end of each chapter and in the Navigate TestPrep. New and revised questions are intended to provide the reader with test-taking practice and represent those found on the certification examinations. The correct answers with rationales are also provided. A bibliography is included at the end of each chapter for those who wish to conduct a more detailed review of specific content.

It is assumed that readers of this review guide have completed a course of study in either a WHNP and/or midwifery program. This text is not intended to be a basic learning tool. Readers should be aware that practice guidelines, diagnostic criteria and tests, treatment, and management recommendations and protocols are always evolving. The information provided in this review guide was current at the time the guide went to print.

Exam Blueprints

The American Midwifery Certification Board (AMCB) is the certifying body for certified nurse-midwives (CNMs) and certified midwives (CMs), and the National Certification Corporation (NCC) is the certifying body for WHNPs.

The content of the certification examinations and the percentages for each area of content are based on periodic job analysis surveys of practitioners, with AMCB focusing on CNMs and CMs and NCC focusing on WHNPs. Both NCC and AMCB use a rigorous process to ensure that test questions reflect current evidence-based practice and that the questions are constructed using psychometric test construction principles. AMCB and NCC exam blueprints are provided here.

AMCB Exam Blueprint

Antepartum: 21%	
Intrapartum: 21%	
Postpartum: 18%	
Newborn: 10%	
Well-woman/gynecology: 19%	
Women's health/primary care: 11%	

Note that approximately two-thirds of the content for each area is devoted to "*normal* phenomena," while the remaining one-third covers deviations from normal. Similarly, two-thirds of each content area will test clinical judgment while one-third will test knowledge.

Data from American Midwifery Certification Board. (2024). *AMCB certification exam candidate handbook: Nurse-midwifery and midwifery.* https://www.amcbmidwife.org/docs/default-source/default-document -library/candidate-handbook-march-1-2024.pdf?sfvrsn=374e46bd_0

NCC Exam Blueprint

Assessment, Diagnostic Testing and Interpretation: 12%

Primary care: 13%

Gynecologic and Reproductive Health: 33%

Obstetrics: 29%

Pharmacology: 10%

Professional issues: 3%

Note that care of male patients including physical examination, management of sexually transmitted diseases, and infertility are a part of the WHNP scope and will be included on examination.

Data from National Certification Corporation. (2024). *2024 Candidate guide: Women's health nurse practitioner WHNP-BC®*. https://www.nccwebsite.org/content/documents/cms/whnp-candidate_guide.pdf

Exam Content Outlines

Both AMCB and NCC provide exam content outlines. In preparing the sixth edition of *Kelsey's Midwifery & Women's Health Nurse Practitioner Certification Review Guide*, the coeditors used a crosswalk of the AMCB content outline and NCC content outline to assess the content of the previous edition of the review guide. Revisions have been made to cover the topics in the 2024 certification exam content outlines more comprehensively.

Because content outlines are updated regularly, the reader is encouraged to visit the AMCB or NCC websites for the most current information. The AMCB website is http://www.amcbmidwife.org, and the NCC website is http://www.nccwebsite.org.

Walkthrough

New to the **Kelsey's Midwifery & Women's Health Nurse Practitioner Certification Review Guide, Sixth Edition**

This book is a comprehensive review designed to help midwives and women's health nurse practitioners prepare for their certification exams. Based on the American Midwifery Certification Board (AMCB) and the National Certification Corporation (NCC) test blueprints.

- Extensive use of **lists** to organize information and help students understand and retain the main points better.

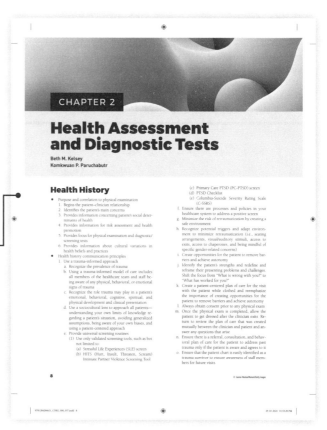

- Use of **tables** to make difficult material more manageable and easily understood.

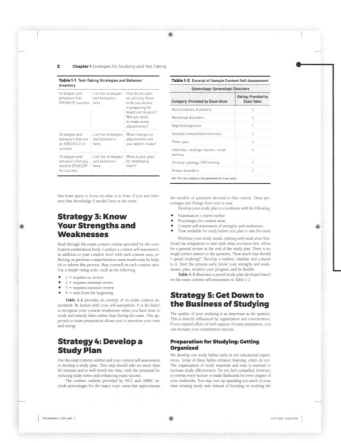

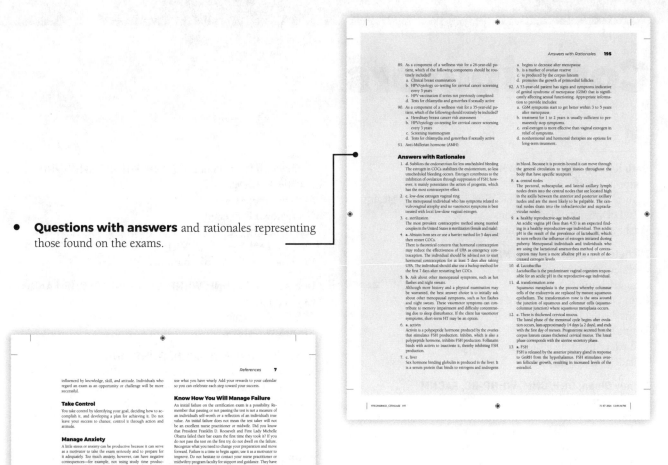

- **Questions with answers** and rationales representing those found on the exams.

- **Bibliography:** *Bibliographies* provide a list of additional resources to help readers better understand the material. New references have been included to reflect the current research in the field.

Online Resources

Included with each new purchase of this text:

- Navigate eBook
- Test Prep: Certified Nurse Midwife (CNM)
- Test Prep: Women's Health Nurse Practitioner (WHNP)

Contributors

Beth Kelsey, EdD, APRN, WHNP-BC, FAANP
Editor-in-Chief
Clinical Journal for Nurse Practitioners in Women's Health
NPWH Director of Publications
Washington, District of Columbia

Michele J. LaMarr-Suggs, MSN, CNM
Certified Nurse Midwife
Obstetrics and Gynecology
Penn OBGYN and Midwifery Care
Pennsylvania Hospital Philadelphia, Pennsylvania
Adjunct Professor
Midwifery Institute at Jefferson University
Philadelphia, Pennsylvania

Signey Olson, DNP, CNM, WHNP-BC, FACNM
Nurse Practitioner
Signey Olson Health, LLC
Washington, District of Columbia
Assistant Professor
Georgetown University
Washington, District of Columbia

Komkwuan P. Paruchabutr, DNP, FNP-BC, WHNP-BC, CNM, FACNM
Assistant Professor
Georgetown University
President, The National Association of Nurse Practitioners in Women's Health (NPWH)
Washington, District of Columbia

Heather Quaile, DNP, WHNP-BC, AFN-C, CSC, IF, FAANP
CEO/Founder
The SHOW Center
Kennesaw, Georgia

Sandi Tenfelde, PhD, APRN, WHNP-BC
Associate Professor and Director of the Women's Health/ Gender Related Nurse Practitioner Program
Marcella Niehoff School of Nursing
Loyola University Chicago
Maywood, Illinois

Kathryn Trotter, DNP, CNM, FNP-BC, FAANP, FAAN
Associate Professor
Duke University School of Nursing
Director, Women's Health NP major
Durham, North Carolina

Reviewers

Alexander Aguiar, APRN, CNM, C-EFM
Full-scope midwife
AdventHealth Orlando
Orlando, Florida

Kathryn Atkin, DNP, WHNP-BC, ANP-BC
Assistant Professor
Georgetown University
Washington, District of Columbia

Lauren Baeringer
University of Alabama at Birmingham
Birmingham, Alabama

Rebecca C. Bagley, DNP, CNM, FACNM
Clinical Associate Professor
Nurse-Midwifery Program Director
East Carolina University
Greenville, North Carolina

Casey Benchimol, MSN, WHGRNP-BC AGPCNP-C
WHGRNP Standing Faculty
University of Pennsylvania School of Nursing
Philadelphia, Pennsylvania

Melissa Black
East Carolina University
Greenville, North Carolina

Julie Blumenfeld, DNP, CNM, FACNM, FAAN
Program Director, Nurse-Midwifery and Dual Women's
    Health/Nurse-Midwifery
Clinical Assistant Professor, School of Nursing
Rutgers, The State University of New Jersey
Newark, New Jersey

Sara Brown
Frontier Nursing University
Hyden, Kentucky

Jatolloa M. Davis, MSN, CNM, WHNP-BC
Certified Nurse Midwife
Thomas Jefferson University Hospital
Philadelphia, Pennsylvania

Rachel Dennis
Georgetown University
Washington, District of Columbia

Amber M. DePra, CNM, MSN
Provider and Clinical Instructor
University of Pittsburgh Medical Center (UPMC)
Farrell, Pennsylvania

Hadja Diallo, MSN, CNM, WHNP
Certified Nurse Midwife
Penn Medicine
Philadelphia, Pennsylvania

CE Durfee, CNM, ARNP, CLC
Perinatal Nurse Practitioner
Maternal-Fetal Medicine Specialists of Puget Sound
Seattle, Washington

Cari Erickson
Case Western Reserve
Cleveland, Ohio

Kendra Faucett, DNP, CNM, APRN, CNE, FACNM
Nurse-Midwifery Specialty Director, Assistant Professor
Vanderbilt School of Nursing
Nashville, Tennessee

Matilda Field, MSN, CNM
Vancouver Clinic
Vancouver, Washington

Jolene Frame, MSN, WHNP
Exceptional Care for Women
Colorado Springs, Colorado

Martha Hardin
Frontier Nursing University
Hyden, Kentucky

Holly Harner, PhD, MBA, MPH, RN, WHCNP-BC, FAAN
Afaf I. Meleis Director for the Center for Global Women's
    Health
Director, Women's Health Gender-Related Nurse Practitioner
    Track
Practice Professor of Women's Health
Penn Nursing
University of Pennsylvania
Philadelphia, Pennsylvania

**Aimee Chism Holland, DNP, WHNP-BC, FNP-C,
    FAANP, FAAN**
Professor & Associate Dean for Graduate Clinical Education
University of Alabama at Birmingham School of Nursing
South, Birmingham, Alabama

Laura Masimore
Georgetown University
Washington, District of Columbia

Chaia McAdams, DNP, CNM, WHNP-BC
Lieutenant Commander
United States Navy Nurse Corps
United States Naval Hospital
Okinawa, Japan

Shawana S. Moore, DNP, APRN, WHNP-BC, PNAP, FAAN
Associate Professor, Clinical Track
Nell Hodgson Woodruff School of Nursing
Emory University
Atlanta, Georgia

Elizabeth G. Muñoz, DNP, CNM, FACNM
Assistant Director, Nursing Midwifery Pathway
Assistant Professor of Nursing
University of Alabama at Birmingham
Birmingham, Alabama

Shaunna Parker, APRN, WHNP-BC
Instructor in Nursing
Vanderbilt University School of Nursing
Nashville, Tennessee

Amy Riley
University of Cincinnati
Cincinnati, Ohio

Sherri Sellers, DNP, APRN, WHNP-BC
Clinical Assistant Professor
University of Missouri-Kansas City
Kansas City, Missouri

Ellen Chaney Solis, DNP, CNM, FACNM
Teaching Professor and Track Lead: Nurse-Midwifery Track,
    Women's Health CNS Track and Graduate Certificate in
    Sexual and Reproductive Health
University of Washington School of Nursing
Seattle, Washington

Beth Steinfeld, DNP
Boro Park OB/GYN
Brooklyn, New York

April Verta, MSN
Private Practice Midwife
Joyful Heart Midwifery and Women's Healthcare
Leesburg, Indiana

Jessica Wahler, DNP, CNM, WHNP-BC
Midwife/Women's Health NP
Monmouth Medical Center
Long Branch, New Jersey

Kelly Caramore Walker, DNP, CNM, FACNM
Assistant Dean Evaluations and Outcomes
Clinical Associate Professor
Stony Brook University School of Nursing
Stony Brook, New York

Aimee White
Frontier Nursing University
Hyden, Kentucky

Angela Wright
Texas Woman's University
Denton, Texas

Student Feedback

This book is a valuable study tool for any student preparing for their WHNP/CNM boards. I actually bought this during my GYN course, and it has helped break down all the relevant and important information necessary to survive any midwifery program. The review book has helpful practice questions that best represent boards and test a student's knowledge. I wish there were more books like this to supplement WHNP/CNM education!

—Cindy W., MSN, CNM, WHNP-BC

I was pleased with this review guide and wish there were more just like it. Personally, I am most successful when I am testing my knowledge, so this book was truly my best tool for review. The practice questions and rationales included all the salient points that we learned during the WHNP/CNM program. The assessments would direct me to my weaker content areas while giving me the resources to strengthen my understanding. I am excited for future students who will be getting a new edition. I will likely buy it for my own review as a new midwife.

—Elise J.D., MSN, CNM, WHNP-BC

I must have taken hundreds of pages of notes throughout my WHNP courses, but when it came time to study for my boards, this review book was the sole guide I used. It created a comprehensive outline of the core subjects we need to have a complete grasp on, and I just sorted them in order of what I needed to review the most to the least. Studied the guide once through and passed my boards on the first try! The content in this book is gold.

—Erika L., MSN, WHNP-BC

I worked my way through *Midwifery & Women's Health Nurse Practitioner Certification Review Guide, Fourth Edition* during my program, and when it came time to take my Boards, I reviewed the sections and questions, completed the online question bank, and felt prepared. When I did not understand a question, I would return to the review book. I used no outside study materials and felt pleasantly surprised by how prepared I felt. This book provides a systematic approach to the daunting task of multiple topics. It helped me hone in on what was important and not get lost in a study abyss. Overall, I would recommend this book to anyone preparing for the WHNP/Midwifery boards. My entire cohort used this book, and we all passed the boards on our first try!

—Alexis P., MSN, WHNP-BC

This review guide provided a condensed yet comprehensive review of exam topics and made studying for my WHNP boards easy and efficient. The online assessment allowed me to take numerous practice tests that identified areas to focus my studying and prepared me for test day.

—Liz F., MSN, WHNP-BC

To be honest, aside from *Contraceptive Technology*, it was the only other reference I used to study for the boards. I must've combed through it cover to cover, three to four times in preparation. I also used the online access code that came with it as well to get a sense of what the question structure/setup would be like when I actually sat down to take the exam. It provided a good foundation/base content and also covered a wide range of potential topics that could be tested. I believe it's also what got me through the primary care portion of the exam with a passing score.

—Gena W., MSN, WHNP-BC

I personally used the Kelsey–Nagtalon-Ramos book throughout my master's education and found it to be concise where it needed to be and expansive where it needed to be. We received so much information throughout our education, and having the Red Book (third edition) at our side to help us organize and study effectively was incredibly valuable. I can unreservedly recommend using this book to study during school and for the certification examinations thereafter.

—Noura A.Q., MSN, CNM, WHNP-BC

The Midwifery and Women's Health Nurse Practitioner Certification Review Guide was all I needed to help me pass the NCC WHNP board exam with confidence. I had used other review guides that did not prepare me as well as this one had. I read this book cover to cover, answered all of the questions, reviewed all the ones I got wrong, reviewed the topics I wasn't confident in, took the test, and passed with a score of "very strong" in all categories. I highly recommend this book!

—Jacinth Alano, DNP, MSN, WHNP-BC

I used this guide as my main study tool outside of class for both completing my master's degree and passing my AMCB and NCC board exams. I significantly increased my ability to retain knowledge when I started reviewing each section in conjunction with topics in my classes and using the practice questions before exams. I often brought the book to clinicals so I could review difficult topics whenever I had down time. It was helpful to have a concise, yet comprehensive, review to guide my studies and prepare for boards!

—Gabrielle G., MS, CNM, WHNP-BC

As an older student, the Midwifery & WHNP Certification Review Guide was invaluable to both my WHNP certification and my postgraduate CNM certification. I never realized that I needed to learn to break down the exam questions in order to best answer those questions. This review guide was comprehensive without being overly wordy. I honestly don't think I would have passed my boards without this awesome guide.

—LaTasha L., WHNP-BC, CNM

CHAPTER 1

Strategies for Studying and Test Taking

Jamille Nagtalon-Ramos
Melicia Escobar

In preparing for your certification examination, understanding your current study and test-taking strategies is an important step in deciding where you may benefit from adjusting them, as they are very important to success. Preparing yourself to be a successful test taker is just as important as studying for the test and is well worth the time and attention it may take. The primary goal of this chapter is to assist potential test takers in knowing how to study for and take a certification exam. You should use the strategies described to best meet your individualized study and test-taking needs.

Strategy 1: Know Yourself

Over years of test taking, each of us has developed certain study and testing behaviors–some of which promote and others that may present obstacles to success. Take control of your preparation for your certification exam by first identifying study and test-taking behaviors that will likely serve you, recognizing behaviors that require change, and developing new skills to improve your study and test-taking abilities.

Flavell (1979) conceived of the term "metacognition," which means "thinking about your own thinking." Take the time now to think about how you think and process information. Use metacognition to help you become more purposefully aware of the best way you think and learn and to determine problems/difficulties you may encounter (e.g., time management, easily distracted) (McGuire et al., 2018). Being proactive in seeking solutions to these problems/difficulties will help you course correct and develop better study strategies that work for you.

Take 20–30 minutes and complete **Table 1-1** Test-taking Strategies and Behavior Inventory. Feel free to strategize with peers or educators invested in your success.

Strategy 2: Know the Content to Study

The National Certification Corporation (NCC) is the certifying body for women's health nurse practitioners (WHNPs), and the American Midwifery Certification Board (AMCB) is the certifying body for certified nurse–midwives (CNMs) and certified midwives (CMs). Both the NCC and the AMCB provide content outlines and information on examination content development on their websites. The website for NCC is http://www.nccwebsite.org, and the website for AMCB is http://www.amcbmidwife.org.

The content of these certification examinations and the percentages for each area of content are based on periodic job analysis surveys of practitioners, with NCC focusing on WHNPs and AMCB focusing on CNMs and CMs. NCC and AMCB use a rigorous process to ensure that test questions reflect current evidence-based practice and are constructed using psychometric test construction principles.

Both NCC and AMCB offer lists of study resources that include textbooks and other widely used reference books in their candidate handbooks. These lists are not meant to be inclusive; they are meant to provide you with examples of resources you might consider, along with the textbooks you have from your WHNP and/or midwifery programs. Although you may want to use various resources, do not overload yourself with too many articles and books to review. Trying to cover all of them will be very time consuming, overwhelming, anxiety provoking, and likely redundant in the information you need for the examination.

As you begin a practice exam or the actual board certification exam, it is valuable to do a "brain dump." This practice involves quickly writing down top-of-mind knowledge (e.g., concepts, terms, definitions, images, etc.) so that you can free

Table 1-1 Test-Taking Strategies and Behavior Inventory

Strategies and behaviors that PROMOTE success	List the strategies and behaviors here.	How do you plan on utilizing these to be successful in preparing for board certification? Will you need to make some adjustments?
Strategies and behaviors that are an OBSTACLE to success	List the strategies and behaviors here.	What changes or adjustments will you need to make?
Strategies and behaviors that you need to DEVELOP for success	List the strategies and behaviors here.	What is your plan for developing them?

Table 1-2 Excerpt of Sample Content Self-Assessment

Gynecology: Gynecologic Disorders	
Category: Provided by Exam Giver	**Rating: Provided by Exam Taker**
Abnormalities of puberty	3
Menstrual disorders	3
Vaginitis/vaginosis	1
Sexually transmitted infections	2
Pelvic pain	3
Infertility—etiologic factors, initial workup	4
Cervical cytology, HPV testing	2
Breast disorders	2

Note. This is not a complete or fully representative list of exam content.

that brain space to focus on what is in front of you and reference that knowledge if needed later in the exam.

Strategy 3: Know Your Strengths and Weaknesses

Read through the exam content outline provided by the certification examination body. Conduct a content self-assessment. In addition to your comfort level with each content area, reflecting on previous comprehensive exam results may be helpful to inform this process. Rate yourself on each content area. Use a simple rating scale, such as the following:

- 1 = requires no review
- 2 = requires minimal review
- 3 = requires intensive review
- 4 = start from the beginning

Table 1-2 provides an excerpt of an exam content assessment. Be honest with your self-assessment. It is far better to recognize your content weaknesses when you have time to study and remedy them rather than during the exam. This approach to exam preparation allows you to prioritize your time and energy.

Strategy 4: Develop a Study Plan

Use the exam content outline and your content self-assessment to develop a study plan. This step should take no more than 60 minutes and is well worth the time, with the potential for reducing study stress and enhancing exam success.

The content outlines provided by NCC and AMBC include percentages for the major topic areas that approximate

the number of questions devoted to that content. These percentages can change from year to year.

Develop your study plan to coordinate with the following:

- Examination content outline
- Percentages for content areas
- Content self-assessment of strengths and weaknesses
- Time available for study before you plan to take the exam

Prioritize your study needs, starting with weak areas first. Avoid the temptation to start with what you know best. Allow for a general review at the end of the study plan. There is no single correct answer to the question, "How much time should I spend studying?" Develop a realistic timeline and commit to it. Start the process early, know your strengths and weaknesses, plan, monitor your progress, and be flexible.

Table 1-3 illustrates a partial study plan developed based on the exam content self-assessment in Table 1-2.

Strategy 5: Get Down to the Business of Studying

The quality of your studying is as important as the quantity. This is directly influenced by organization and concentration. If you expend effort on both aspects of exam preparation, you can increase your examination success.

Preparation for Studying: Getting Organized

We develop our study habits early in our educational experiences. Some of these habits enhance learning; others do not. The organization of study materials and time is essential to increase study effectiveness. Do not feel compelled, however, to rewrite every lecture or make flashcards for every chapter of your textbooks. You may end up spending too much of your time creating study aids instead of focusing on studying the

Table 1-3 Sample Study Plan: Gynecologic Disorders Content

Study Day	Date	Content	Resources	Time
1		Infertility—etiologic factors, initial workup Rating 4	Chapter 7 Textbook A Chapter 14 Textbook B Class notes	6:00–7:30 p.m.
		Abnormalities of puberty Rating 3	Chapter 3 Textbook A Class notes	7:30–8:30 p.m.
2		Menstrual disorders Rating 3	Chapter 4 Textbook A Class notes	6:00–7:00 p.m.
		Pelvic pain Rating 3	Chapter 5 Textbook A Class notes	7:00–8:00 p.m.
3		Sexually transmitted infections Rating 2	Chapter 6 Textbook A Class notes CDC STD Treatment Guidelines	6:00–7:00 p.m.
		Cervical cytology, HPV testing Rating 2	Class notes ASCCP Guideline Algorithms	7:00–8:00 p.m.

content. Organization decreases frustration, allows for easy resumption of study, and increases concentrated study time.

Create Your Own Study Space

Select a study area that is yours alone, free from distractions, comfortable, and well-lit. If you have young children, consider asking family, friends, and trusted neighbors for help with childcare. The ventilation and room temperature should be comfortable because a cold room makes concentrating difficult, and a warm room may make you sleepy. You should leave your study materials in your study space. The basic premise of a study space is that it facilitates a mindset that you are there to study. When you interrupt your study, it is best to leave your materials just as they are. Do not close books or put away notes because you will have to relocate them when you resume study, which wastes your study time.

Spatial learners may benefit from relocating when studying. For example, consider studying *listeria* in the living room or *herpes* on a **h**ammock. Studying in different places/locations may help you recall the information in relation to where you were studying.

Identify Your Peak Study Times and Maximize Them

Study in short bursts. Each of us has our own biological clock that dictates when we are at our peak during the day. If you are a morning person, you are generally active and alert early in the day, slowing down and becoming drowsy by evening. If you are an evening person, you do not completely wake up until late morning and hit your peak in the afternoon and evening. Each person generally has several peaks during the day. It is best to study when your alertness is at its peak.

Spread Out Study Time and Give Your Brain Breaks

Studying is more effective when spread out over a longer period. This concept, called "distributed effort" or "spaced studying" (Susser & McCabe, 2013), is the opposite of cramming. In addition to spreading study time over several days or weeks, you need to give your brain rests during any one study period. The best approach to breaks is to plan them and give yourself a conscious break. This approach eliminates the daydreaming or wandering-thought approach to breaks that many of us use. Getting up, leaving the study area, and doing something nonstudy-related for longer breaks is better. For shorter breaks of 5 minutes or so, leave your desk, gaze out the window, or do some stretching exercises. When your brain says to give it a rest, accommodate it! You will learn more with less stress.

Focus on Major Concepts and Facts

Study the correct content. It is easy to become bogged down in the detail of the content you are studying. A better approach is to focus on the major concepts. Leave the details, the suppositions, and the anecdotal experience at the door of your study area. Concentrate on the major textbook facts and concepts that revolve around the subject matter being tested.

Use Your Study Plan Wisely

Your study plan is meant to be a guide, not a rigid schedule. You should take your time studying. Do not rush through the content to remain on schedule. Occasionally, study plans need revision. If you take more or less time than planned, readjust the plan for the time gained or lost. The plan can guide you, but you must go at your own pace.

Study Actively

Active study techniques have been shown to strengthen neural connections and improve the ability to remember materials being studied. Three techniques for active study are recitation, visualization, and association (Hopper, 2016).

- *Recitation:* When you recite something in your own words, you pay more attention to it and get immediate feedback. If you can explain something in your own words out loud, you understand it. Also, when you hear something, you use a different part of your brain than when you read it. Having a study partner or group can facilitate the use of recitation if you ask each other questions and answer out loud.

- *Visualization:* Try to visualize the concepts you are studying in some way, such as by imagining a patient—either someone you have met or a fictional person—with a specific condition. Use illustrations and pictures from textbooks as you study. Take notes or make flashcards to promote visualization. Convert connected information into a visual graph (e.g., pie chart, other type of chart, concept map). Color coding may help with organizing your notes. One strategy we have implemented with students is using the following colors: red ink for medications (Red Med), blue ink for important terms you need to know to better understand concepts (Blues Clues), and purple ink for patient education (Purple Patient Teaching).

- *Association:* You can remember new information more efficiently if you link that information to something you already know. Ask yourself: If I were to put this in a computer (brain) file, does a similar or related file already exist so that I don't have to create a new one? Alternatively, perhaps try associating the information you are learning with a story. Tell the story out loud to a friend or a family member. This creative exercise will prompt and challenge you to apply what you learned beyond just repetition (McGuire et al., 2018).

Use your individual study quirks. Some people stand, others walk around, and some play background music. Whatever helps you to concentrate and study better is what you should use.

Use Study Aids

Although there is no substitute for individual studying, several resources, if available, are useful in facilitating learning. One study aid already discussed is the detailed content outline provided by NCC and AMCB. Reviewing courses and books such as this one can provide an effective means of organizing or summarizing your individual study. They generally provide the content parameters, the major concepts of the content you need to know, an opportunity to clarify not-well-understood content, and a review of known material. Question-and-answer resources provide test-taking practice and are most helpful when answer rationales are included to reinforce the correct information. Study groups are an excellent resource for summarizing and refining content. They provide an opportunity for thinking through your knowledge base, with the advantage of hearing another person's point of view. Each of these study aids increases understanding of content and, when used correctly, increases the effectiveness of knowledge application.

Consider Joining a Study Group

A study group can be valuable for creating accountability, collaboration around complex content, reinforcement of concepts, and sharing strategies. Small study groups of 5–6 participants help maintain the focus and engagement of all group members. The following considerations are useful in planning for efficient and productive group work:

- What will be the goal for each session? Determine what content area(s) or concepts will be reviewed.

- How are participants expected to prepare? Set clear expectations about what each group member should review or prepare to discuss and any review questions that should be completed.

- What will be the agenda for your study session to help meet your goal? Plan what activities will occur during your study session (e.g., complete a practice exam, review a practice exam, quiz each other, teach each other, clarify muddy points, create a study tool, etc.).

- What are the study group agreements that will promote engagement? Setting a positive and shame-free tone for group time can help encourage participation and ensure all group members are moving forward. Participants should feel comfortable asking questions or seeking clarification at any point. Disagreement can be the basis for clarification and deeper understanding. Perfectionism can undermine progress: describe concepts in your own words to the best of your ability, without fear of being correct.

Know When to Quit

When your concentration ebbs, you should stop studying. It is unproductive and frustrating to force yourself to study. A far better strategy is to rest or unwind and resume later in the day. Avoid studying outside your morning or afternoon concentration peaks and focus your study energy on the right time of day or evening.

Strategy 6: Become Testwise

Purpose of a Test Question

Test questions are developed to examine different cognitive domains: knowledge, comprehension, application, analysis, synthesis, and evaluation. You will most likely see questions on the certification exam in the knowledge, comprehension, application, and analysis domains. A knowledge question requires the test taker to recall a fact; comprehension questions require the test taker to understand the meaning of the fact; application questions require the test taker to be able to apply knowledge in a concrete situation; and analysis questions require the test taker to break down information and identify parts, relationships, and organization (Wittman-Price et al., 2018).

When taking a test, you want to know whether you are being asked to remember or use that fact. Here is an example of a knowledge question:

Recurrent *herpes genitalis* is most effectively treated with:

- A. *suppressive antiviral therapy to reduce viral shedding.*
- B. mRNA vaccination to prevent similar infections.
- C. topical acyclovir to limit the spread on the skin.
- D. a steroid taper to address inflammation.

To answer this question correctly, you must retrieve memorized facts. Understanding the fact, knowing why it is important, and analyzing what should be done with the fact are not needed.

An example of a question that tests comprehension is:

A 24-year-old patient presents with a complaint of itching and pain in her genital area that started 2 days ago, along with pain on urination. Physical examination reveals bilateral inguinal lymphadenopathy, vulvar edema with multiple vesicles and ulcerated lesions, and a large amount of watery vaginal discharge. Which of the following is the most likely diagnosis?

A. *Genital herpes*
B. Genital warts
C. Syphilis
D. Trichomoniasis

To answer this question correctly, you must retrieve several facts about the signs and symptoms of *herpes genitalis* and understand that, when put together, the findings are likely indicative of herpes rather than some other diagnosis.

An example of an application question is:

A 24-year-old patient reports a history of herpes diagnosis 6 months ago and asks if there is anything the patient can do to deal with recurrent outbreaks. There have been two recurrences since the initial occurrence. Which of the following is the most appropriate information to address this patient's question?

A. Comfort measures and topical acyclovir are the best approaches to managing recurrences.
B. The patient can be assured that greater than two recurrences annually is unlikely.
C. *The patient can consider either episodic therapy for recurrences or suppressive therapy with acyclovir.*
D. Suppressive medication is not recommended for someone who has fewer than four recurrences a year.

To answer this question correctly, you must know and comprehend facts about herpes recurrences and suppression and apply this information to a patient's situation. You must think through each answer and decide its relevance and importance to the situation.

An example of an analysis question is:

A 24-year-old patient reports having had a sex partner for the past year who has a history of *herpes genitalis*. The clinician orders a herpes type-specific serologic test. The results show HSV-1 positive and HSV-2 negative. The accurate interpretation of these results is that the patient:

A. has acquired a herpes infection from the sex partner.
B. has acquired another viral infection from the sex partner.
C. does not have the herpes virus type that causes genital herpes infection.
D. *may or may not have acquired a herpes infection from the partner.*

To answer this question correctly, you must be able to break down the information about the type-specific serologic test results and identify the parts and relationships with the information you have about the patient and the partner.

Question Format

Most standardized tests, such as those used for nursing licensure and certification, rely on multiple-choice questions (MCQs) with three or four answer options, from which you are required to select the one best answer. While MCQs are not the only way to assess knowledge and competence, the NCC and AMCB certification exams use MCQs with either three or four answer options, respectively (AMCB, 2024; NCC, 2024. Board certification relies on successful test taking. Successful test taking depends on both content knowledge *and* test-taking skills. If you cannot impart your knowledge through the vehicle used for its conveyance—that is, the MCQ—your test-taking success is in jeopardy.

Components of MCQs

MCQs include two basic components: a stem and a set of answer options. The stem presents information needed by the test taker to select an answer. It may be short, consisting of just a phrase or a sentence or two, or it can be a paragraph in length. When the stem is more than a phrase or sentence, it usually includes a separate interrogatory question or statement that poses the question to be answered. The interrogatory question or statement helps to direct the test taker's thinking.

The answer options present three or four possible responses to the question. The correct option is called the *keyed response*, and all other options are called *distractors* (Sefcik et al., 2013). The keyed response may be the only correct answer or the best answer. Higher-level questions usually have a best answer along with distractor options that may be partially correct or that may not address all the data presented in the question stem.

Knowing the components of a test question helps you sift through the information presented and focus on the question's intent. Always focus on the information in the stem and, more specifically, what the interrogatory question or statement is asking. Avoid reading elements into the question that are not specifically included in the stem and options (**Table 1-4**).

Practice, Practice, Practice

Taking practice tests can improve performance. Although they can assist in evaluating your knowledge, their primary benefit is improving your test-taking skills. You should use practice tests to evaluate your thinking process; your ability to read,

Table 1-4 Anatomy of a Test Question

Stem	A patient using the contraceptive vaginal ring (NuvaRing) removes the ring during sex and forgets to reinsert it, realizing this 2 days later.
Interrogatory statement	If this is week 1 or 2 for this ring, the patient should be advised to:
Options	a. discard this ring and insert a new one immediately. b. discard this ring, wait for withdrawal bleed, and insert a new ring. c. reinsert this ring with no backup needed. d. *reinsert this ring and use a backup method for 7 days.*

understand, and interpret questions; and your skills in completing the mechanics of the test.

Exam resources, including sample questions for the NCC and AMCB exams, are available in the examination content information provided in this text. The questions at the end of each chapter and the separate online test questions provide you with approximately 1,600 MCQs. The answers to the questions are provided along with rationales.

Strategy 7: Apply Basic Rules of Standardized Test-Taking

Read All Directions Carefully

Be sure that you have completed all the information needed to register for the exam and that you have all the required documents and personal identification. Know what you are permitted to have in the testing area and what is not permitted. It is helpful to list everything you need for admission to the examination and the permitted items you want to have with you during the exam.

The Night Before the Test

Follow your regular routine the night before a test. Eat familiar foods. Avoid the temptation to cram all night. If possible, do not change or initiate any new medications. Go to bed at your regular time.

The Day of the Test

Be prepared for exam day. It is important to familiarize yourself with the test site, the building, the parking, and the travel route before the exam day. If the exam is online at home, familiarize yourself with the testing software and ensure your computer hardware and software are fully functional and updated. Ensure that you have a power source and a stable internet connection. Prepare your testing space to limit distractions and for any 360-degree room scan you will be required to obtain before the exam. Plan for uninterrupted time during the examination.

On exam day, allow yourself plenty of time to arrive at the site and get settled; plan to get there 30 minutes before your scheduled exam time. Wear comfortable clothes and have a good breakfast that morning. Know whether you will be able to have food or drink in the exam area or will be able to have them available for a short break.

Know what to do if you experience electronic issues or other difficulties during the examination. In addition to addressing the issue at the test site (e.g., student distractions), you should notify the certifying board should any problems arise.

Use Your Time Wisely and Effectively

Most standardized, computer-delivered exams have a digital clock on the computer indicating how much time you have

remaining. This feature may be turned off and on during the exam if you find it creates anxiety for you. Know the number of questions on the exam and the total time you have to complete the exam. For example, if there are 175 questions and you have 3 hours to complete the exam, you have approximately 1 minute per question. If there are 175 questions and you have 4 hours to complete the exam, you have approximately 1½ minutes per question. Many questions will likely take you less than 1 minute to answer. Skip or make an educated guess on difficult questions, and mark and return to them later.

Identify keywords in the stem before looking at the options for each question. Confine your thinking to the information provided.

Read and consider all options. Be systematic and use problem-solving techniques. Relate options to the question and balance them against each other. Eliminate answers you know are wrong and focus on the remaining most likely correct responses.

Answer all the questions on the exam. Currently, the NCC and AMCB certification examination scores are based only on the total number of correct answers selected. This means that you are not further penalized for an incorrect answer. So, answer all the test questions, even if you are only guessing. Unlike the National Council Licensure Examination (NCLEX), the AMCB and NCC exams are not adaptive. Both exams have a total of 175 questions, respectively, including embedded pretest items. These pretest items are questions undergoing validation and do not count toward the final score. The NCC exam contains 25 of these pretest items. AMCB does not specify the number of pretest items in the midwifery exam (AMCB, 2024; NCC, 2024).

Go back to questions you were not able to answer on the first pass through the test. Subsequent questions may have provided information helpful in answering previous questions, or you may have become less anxious and more objective by the end of the test.

However, avoid second-guessing answer choices you have already made. Your first response is likely the best. If you tend to second-guess your responses, review only those questions you could not answer on the first pass through the exam. Computer-based exams allow you to mark questions that you may want to address later in the exam.

Do not change an answer without a good reason. Good reasons might be realizing you misread the question the first time or running across information in later questions that either jogs your memory or gives you a better idea of the correct answer (McGuire et al., 2018).

Strategy 8: Psych Yourself Up

Adopt an "I Can" Attitude

Believing you can succeed is the key to success. Self-belief inspires and gives you the power to achieve your goals. The road to your goal will be much easier with a success-oriented attitude. This "I can" attitude must permeate all your test-taking efforts, from studying and improving your test-taking skills to completing the exam. Think positively. Performance is influenced by knowledge, skill, *and* attitude. Individuals who regard an exam as an opportunity or challenge will be more successful.

Take Control

You take control by identifying your goal, deciding how to accomplish it, and developing a plan for achieving it. Do not leave your success to chance; control it through action and attitude.

Manage Anxiety

A little stress or anxiety can be productive because it can serve as a motivator to take the exam seriously and to prepare for it adequately. Too much anxiety, however, can have negative consequences—for example, not using study time productively; misreading questions; changing answers from right to wrong; and developing physical symptoms, such as diarrhea, nausea, and palpitations.

Active anxiety-control strategies include relaxation techniques (i.e., guided imagery, meditation), stress management, attention to wellness behaviors (i.e., healthy eating, adequate sleep, regular exercise), combining individual review with review in small study groups for social support and increased confidence, completing practice questions, preparing well in advance, and taking the time to review all the processes on examination day (McGuire et al., 2018).

For persons with severe test anxiety, interventions, such as cognitive therapy, systematic desensitization, study skills counseling, and biofeedback, have all been used with some success. Techniques derived from these approaches can influence the results achieved by changing attitudes and approaches to test taking, thereby reducing anxiety.

Persevere, Persevere, Persevere!

Endurance must underlie all your efforts. Call forth those reserve energies when you have had all you think you can take. Rely on yourself and your support systems to help you maintain a sense of direction and keep your goal in the forefront.

Reward Yourself

Reward yourself during your exam preparation and once the exam has been completed. You alone hold the key to success; use what you have wisely. Add your rewards to your calendar so you can celebrate each step toward your success.

Know How You Will Manage Failure

An initial failure on the certification exam is a possibility. Remember that passing or not passing the test is not a measure of an individual's self-worth or a reflection of an individual's true value. An initial failure does not mean the test taker will not be an excellent nurse practitioner or midwife. Did you know that President Franklin D. Roosevelt and First Lady Michelle Obama failed their bar exam the first time they took it? If you do not pass the test on the first try, do not dwell on the failure. Recognize what you need to change your preparation and move forward. Failure is a time to begin again; use it as a motivator to improve. Do not hesitate to contact your nurse practitioner or midwifery program faculty for support and guidance. They have a vested interest in your success and entry into the profession.

Accommodations

The NCC and AMCB offer accommodations per the American Disabilities Act (ADA). Test takers must identify their needs for accommodation when submitting their applications to take their respective exams.

Summary

This chapter provided concepts, strategies, and techniques for improving study and test-taking skills. Your first task in improving your performance is knowing yourself: how you study and how you take a test. You should use your strengths and remedy the weaknesses. Next, you need to organize your study time and concentrate on using your strengths and new and improved skills to be successful. Create a study space, develop a plan of action, and then implement that plan during your periods of peak concentration. Before taking the exam, make sure you understand the components of a test question, can identify keywords and phrases, and practice. Apply the test-taking rules during the exam process.

Finally, believe in yourself, your knowledge, and your talent. If you are sitting for a board certification exam, you have worked hard and successfully completed a rigorous course of study. Believing you can accomplish your goal makes it more likely that you will.

Bibliography

American Midwifery Certification Board. (2024). *AMBC certification exam candidate handbook nurse-midwifery and midwifery*. American Midwifery Certification Board, Inc.

Flavell, J. H. (1979). Metacognition and cognitive monitoring: A new area of cognitive-developmental inquiry. *The American Psychologist, 34*(10), 906–911. https://doi.org/10.1037/0003-066X.34.10.906

Hopper, C. N. (2016). *Practicing college learning strategies* (7th ed.). Cengage Learning.

McGuire, S. Y., McGuire, S., & McDaniel M. (2018). Teach yourself how to learn: Strategies you can use to ace any course at any level (1st ed.). Stylus.

National Certification Corporation. (2024). *2024 Candidate guide: Women's health nurse practitioner WHNP-BC®*. National Certification Corporation.

Sefcik, D. Bice, G., & Prerost, F. (2013). *How to study for standardized tests*. Jones & Bartlett Learning.

Susser, J. A. & McCabe, J. (2013). From the lab to the dorm room: Metacognitive awareness and use of spaced study. *Instructional Science, 41*, 345–363.

Wittman-Price, R., Godshall, M., & Wilson, L. (2018). *Certified nurse educator (CNE) review manual* (3rd ed.). Springer.

CHAPTER 2

Health Assessment and Diagnostic Tests

Beth M. Kelsey
Komkwuan P. Paruchabutr

Health History

- Purpose and correlation to physical examination
  1. Begins the patient–clinician relationship
  2. Identifies the patient's main concerns
  3. Provides information concerning patient's social determinants of health
  4. Provides information for risk assessment and health promotion
  5. Provides focus for physical examination and diagnostic/screening tests
  6. Provides information about cultural variations in health beliefs and practices
- Health history communication principles
  1. Use a trauma-informed approach
     a. Recognize the prevalence of trauma
     b. Using a trauma-informed model of care includes all members of the healthcare team and staff being aware of any physical, behavioral, or emotional signs of trauma
     c. Recognize the role trauma may play in a patient's emotional, behavioral, cognitive, spiritual, and physical development and clinical presentation
     d. Use a sociocultural lens to approach all patients—understanding your own limits of knowledge regarding a patient's situation, avoiding generalized assumptions, being aware of your own biases, and using a patient-centered approach
     e. Provide universal screening routines
        (1) Use only validated screening tools, such as but not limited to:
           (a) Stressful Life Experiences (SLE) screen
           (b) HITS (Hurt, Insult, Threaten, Scream) Intimate Partner Violence Screening Tool
           (c) Primary Care PTSD (PC-PTSD) screen
           (d) PTSD Checklist
           (e) Columbia-Suicide Severity Rating Scale (C-SSRS)
     f. Ensure there are processes and policies in your healthcare system to address a positive screen
     g. Minimize the risk of retraumatization by creating a safe environment
     h. Recognize potential triggers and adapt environment to minimize retraumatization (i.e., seating arrangements, visual/auditory stimuli, access to exits, access to chaperones, and being mindful of specific gender-related concerns)
     i. Create opportunities for the patient to remove barriers and achieve autonomy
     j. Identify the patient's strengths and redefine and reframe their presenting problems and challenges. Shift the focus from "What is wrong with you?" to "What has worked for you?"
     k. Create a patient-centered plan of care for the visit with the patient while clothed and reemphasize the importance of creating opportunities for the patient to remove barriers and achieve autonomy
     l. Always obtain consent prior to any physical exam
     m. Once the physical exam is completed, allow the patient to get dressed after the clinician exits. Return to review the plan of care that was created mutually between the clinician and patient and answer any questions that arise
     n. Ensure there is a referral, consultation, and behavioral plan of care for the patient to address past trauma only if the patient is aware and agrees to it
     o. Ensure that the patient chart is easily identified as a trauma survivor to ensure awareness of staff members for future visits

p. Recognize the patient may require a longer appointment time and ensure adequate time for future appointments

2. Use inclusive language—"partner" or "spouse" instead of "boyfriend" or "husband"; patient-identified pronouns; options on forms regarding gender to include transgender and "other," with an option to write in gender identity

3. Assess health literacy—the degree to which an individual can obtain, process, and understand basic health information and services needed to make health decisions; use appropriate written and graphic materials, patient navigators, trained medical interpreters

4. Use active listening—start with open-ended questions, focus on what is being said, reflect on what is heard to confirm mutual understanding, and allow silence for the patient to have time to express thoughts and feelings

5. Address sensitive issues in a nonjudgmental, respectful manner; ensure confidentiality

- Components of the health history
  1. Reason for visit/chief concern—brief statement in patient's own words of reason for seeking health care
  2. Presenting problem/illness—chronological account of problem(s) for which patient is seeking care
     a. Description of principal symptoms should include *OLD-CARTS* mnemonic:
        (1) *Onset*
        (2) *Location*
        (3) *Duration*
        (4) *Characteristics*
        (5) *Aggravating/Associated factors*
        (6) *Relieving factors*
        (7) *Temporal factors*
        (8) *Severity*
     b. Include pertinent negatives in symptom descriptions; when a symptom suggests that an abnormality may exist or develop in that area, include documentation of the absence of symptoms that may help eliminate some of the possibilities
     c. Describe the impact of illness/problem on the patient's usual lifestyle
     d. Summarize current health status and health promotion/disease prevention needs if the patient has no presenting problem
  3. Health history
     a. General state of health as the patient perceives it
     b. Childhood illnesses
     c. Trauma history
     d. Major adult illnesses
     e. Psychiatric illnesses
     f. Accidents/injuries
     g. Surgeries/other hospitalizations
     h. Blood transfusions—dates and number of units
  4. Current health status
     a. Current medications—prescription, over-the-counter, herbal; review medications prescribed by all clinicians the patient sees for care (medication reconciliation)
     b. Allergies—name of allergen, type of reaction

c. Tobacco, vaping, marijuana, alcohol, substances (e.g., paint fumes), prescription drugs taken as other than the intended use, illicit drugs—type, amount, frequency

d. Nutrition—24-hour diet recall, recent weight changes, eating disorders, special diet

e. Screening tests—dates and results

f. Immunizations—dates

g. Sleep patterns

h. Exercise/leisure activities

i. Environmental/occupational hazards

j. Use of safety measures—safety belts, smoke detectors

k. Disabilities—functional assessment, if indicated

5. Family health history—provides information about possible genetic, familial, and environmental associations with the patient's health
   a. Age and health or age and cause of death of immediate family members—parents, siblings, children, spouse/significant other
   b. Specific conditions to ask about—heart disease, hypertension, stroke, diabetes, cancer, epilepsy, kidney disease, thyroid disease, asthma, arthritis, blood diseases, tuberculosis, alcohol or other substance use disorders, allergies, congenital anomalies, mental illness, genetic disorders
   c. Include targeted genetic/familial risk assessment for hereditary breast and ovarian cancer syndrome as well as other hereditary cancer syndromes
   d. Indicate if the patient is adopted and does not know the family health history

6. Psychosocial history
   a. Living situation
   b. Access to care
   c. Support system
   d. Intimate-partner violence/domestic violence
   e. Stressors and coping mechanisms
   f. Religious/spiritual/cultural practices and preferences
   g. Outlook on present and future
   h. Special issues to address with adolescent patients include *HEADSS*: *Home, Education, Activities, Drugs, Sex, Suicide*
   i. Cultural assessment considerations
   j. Military status
      (1) Avoid making generalizing assumptions and imposing stereotypes
      (2) Cultural/ethnic identification—place of birth, length of time in country
      (3) Communication—language spoken, use of nonverbal communication, use of silence
      (4) Space—degree of comfort with distance between self and others, degree of comfort with touching by others
      (5) Social organization—family structure and roles, influence of religion/spirituality
      (6) Time—past-, present-, or future-oriented; view of time—clock-oriented or social-oriented
      (7) Environmental control—internal or external locus of control, belief in supernatural forces

(8) Use of culturally based healing practices or remedies

7. Obstetric history—may include in a separate section, health history, or review of systems—includes all pregnancies regardless of outcome
   a. Gravidity—total number of pregnancies including a current pregnancy
   b. Parity—total number of pregnancies reaching 20 weeks or greater gestation
      (1) Include term, preterm, and stillbirth deliveries
      (2) Include the length of each pregnancy; type of delivery; weight and sex of infant; length of labor; complications during prenatal, intrapartum, or postpartum periods; infant complications; cause of stillbirth, if known
         (a) Ectopic pregnancies—treatment provided
         (b) Abortions—spontaneous and induced
         (c) GTPAL—Gravida, Term, Preterm, Abortion, Living children is a commonly used method of obstetric history notation
         (d) Any infertility evaluation and treatment
         (e) Other children: Stepchildren, fostered, adopted

8. Menstrual history—may be included in a separate section or in a review of systems
   a. Age at menarche, regularity, frequency, duration, and amount of bleeding
   b. Date of last normal menstrual period
   c. Use of pads, tampons, douching
   d. Abnormal uterine bleeding
   e. Premenstrual symptoms
   f. Dysmenorrhea
   g. Perimenopausal symptoms
   h. Age at menopause, use of hormone therapy, postmenopausal bleeding

9. Sexual history/contraceptive use—may be included in a separate section, under current health status, or in a review of systems
   a. Age at first sexual intercourse—consensual/nonconsensual
   b. History of sexual abuse or sexual assault
   c. Sexual orientation
   d. Gender identity
   e. Current sexual relationship(s)
   f. Frequency of sexual intercourse
   g. Satisfaction or concerns with sexual relationship(s)
   h. Dyspareunia, orgasmic, or libido problems

10. Sexually transmitted infection (STI)/human immunodeficiency virus (HIV) infection risk assessment
    a. Total number of sexual partners in the past 3 months
    b. Types of sexual contact—vaginal, oral, and/or anal
    c. Use of condoms or other barrier methods
    d. Previous history of STIs
    e. Use of injection drugs or sex with a partner who has used injection drugs
    f. Sex while under the influence of alcohol and/or drugs
    g. Previous testing for HIV

11. Current and future desire for pregnancy

12. Contraceptive use
    a. Establish if pregnancy is not a concern—hysterectomy, sterilization, not sexually active, only sexually active with nonsperm-producing partners, menopausal
    b. Current method, length of time used, satisfaction, problems, or concerns
    c. Previous methods used, when, length of time used, satisfaction, problems or concerns, the reason for discontinuation

- Review of systems—used to assess common symptoms for each major body system to avoid missing any potential or existing problems; special focus for gynecologic and reproductive health includes:
  1. Endocrine
     a. Amenorrhea or infrequent menses
     b. Heavy or prolonged menstrual bleeding
     c. Premenstrual symptoms
     d. Difficulty becoming pregnant
     e. Heat/cold intolerance
     f. Excessive hair growth or hair loss
     g. Recent weight change
     h. Hot flashes
  2. Genitourinary
     a. Painful periods
     b. Abnormal vaginal discharge
     c. Pain with sex
     d. Pain with urination, blood in urine, frequent urination
     e. Unintended urine leaking, leaking urine with cough or lifting, urgency to urinate
     f. Postmenopausal bleeding
  3. Breasts—pain, lumps/masses, nipple discharge

Concluding question—Is there anything else I need to know about your health so I can provide you with the best health care?

- Risk factor identification
  1. Consider prevalence (existing level of disease) and incidence (rate of new disease) in the general population and in your patient population
  2. Determine risks specific to the patient related to the following:
     a. Age
     b. Family health/genetics history
     c. Lifestyle behaviors—e.g., smoking, poor nutrition, low physical activity, risky sexual behavior, alcohol and other substance misuse
     d. Living conditions—e.g., inadequate housing, violence, toxins, exposure to communicable diseases
     e. Experiences of discrimination and bias related to social and structural inequities—e.g., race, ethnicity, gender, sexual orientation, immigration status, weight bias
     f. Employment conditions—e.g., unemployed, low income, occupational hazards, military service-related physical and mental health issues
     g. Military service—Currently serving or veteran, deployment locations, role, related physical/mental issues

h. Inadequate access to or use of preventive health care—e.g., lack of transportation, inability to access transportation, childcare issues
i. Experience of human trafficking

See the section on Psychosocial Problems in Chapter 3, Primary Care, for information on human trafficking

- Problem-oriented medical record—organized sequence of recording information using SOAP format
  1. SOAP format

     S—subjective information obtained during history. When writing the history, use terms such as "reports," "endorses," or "describes" rather than "complains of."

     O—objective information obtained through physical examination and laboratory/diagnostic test results

     A—assessment of objective and subjective data to determine a diagnosis with rationale or a prioritized differential diagnosis

     P—plan to include diagnostic tests, therapeutic treatment regimen, patient education, referrals, and date for reevaluation
  2. Problem list—list each identified existing or potential problem and indicate both the onset and resolution date
  3. Progress notes—use SOAP format for information documented at follow-up visits

Physical Examination

- Purpose and correlation to health history
  1. Findings may indicate a need for further health history information
  2. Takes into account normal physical variations of different age and racial/ethnic groups
- Techniques of examination
  1. Inspection—observation using sight and smell
     a. Takes place throughout the history and physical examination
     b. Includes general survey and body system-specific observations
  2. Auscultation—use of hearing, usually with a stethoscope, to listen to sounds produced by the body
     a. Diaphragm is best for high-pitched sounds (e.g., S_1, S_2 heart sounds)
     b. Bell is best for low-pitched sounds (e.g., large blood vessels)
  3. Percussion—use of light, brisk tapping on body surfaces to produce vibrations in relation to the density of underlying tissue and/or to elicit tenderness
     a. Provides information about the size, shape, location, and density of underlying organs or tissue
     b. Percussion sounds are distinguished by intensity (soft–loud), pitch (high–low), and quality
     c. Tympany—loud, high-pitched, drum-like sound (e.g., gastric bubble, gas-filled bowel)
     d. Hyperresonance—very loud, low-pitched, boom-like sound (e.g., lungs with emphysema)
     e. Resonance—loud, low-pitched, hollow sound (e.g., healthy lungs)

f. Dull—soft to moderate, moderate-pitched, thud-like sound (e.g., liver, heart)
g. Flat—soft, high-pitched sound, very dull (e.g., muscle, bone)
  4. Palpation—use of hands and fingers to gather information about body tissues and organs through touch
     a. Finger pads, palmar surface of fingers, ulnar surface of fingers/hands, and dorsal surface of hands are used
     b. Light palpation—about 1 cm in depth, used to identify muscular resistance, areas of tenderness, and large masses or areas of distention
     c. Deep palpation—about 4 cm in depth, used to delineate organs and to identify less obvious masses
- Physical examination
  1. General appearance—posture, dress, grooming, personal hygiene, body or breath odors, facial expression
  2. Anthropometric measurements
     a. Height and weight

        Body mass index (BMI) provides measurement of total body fat; weight (kg)/height (m^2); tables available to calculate BMI based on the individual's height and weight
        (1) Underweight—BMI less than 18.5
        (2) Normal weight—BMI 18.5–24.9
        (3) Overweight—BMI 25–29.9
        (4) Obesity—BMI 30–39.9
        (5) Extreme obesity—BMI 40 or greater
     b. Waist circumference
        (1) Provides measurement of abdominal fat as an independent prediction of risk for type 2 diabetes, dyslipidemia, hypertension, and cardiovascular disease in individuals with a BMI between 25 and 39.9 (overweight and obesity)
        (2) Has little added value in disease risk prediction in individuals with BMI 40 or greater (extreme obesity)
        (3) Measure with a horizontal mark at the uppermost lateral border of the right iliac crest and cross with a vertical mark at the midaxillary line; place tape measure at the cross and measure in a horizontal plane around the abdomen while the patient is standing
        (4) In adult females, increased relative risk is indicated at greater than 35 in. (88 cm)
  3. Skin, hair, and nails
     a. Skin—color, texture, temperature, turgor, moisture, lesions, tattoos, piercings
     b. Hair—color, distribution, quantity, texture
     c. Nails—color, shape, thickness
     d. Skin lesion characteristics—size, shape, color, texture, elevation, exudate, location, and distribution
        (1) Primary lesions—occur as an initial, spontaneous reaction to an internal or external stimulus (macule, papule, plaque, pustule, vesicle, wheal)
        (2) Secondary lesions—result from later evolution or trauma to a primary lesion (ulcer, fissure, lichenification, crust, scar)

e. ABCDEs of malignant melanoma—*Asymmetry*, *Borders* irregular, *Color* blue/black or variegated, *Diameter* greater than 6 mm, *Elevation*

4. Head, eyes, ears, nose, and throat
   a. Head and neck
      (1) Skull and scalp—no masses or tenderness
      (2) Facial features—symmetrical, without swelling, without involuntary movements (tics)
      (3) Trachea—midline
      (4) Thyroid—no masses or tenderness, rises symmetrically with swallowing
      (5) Neck—full range of motion (ROM) without pain
      (6) Lymph nodes
         (a) Preauricular, postauricular, occipital, tonsillar, submandibular, submental, superficial cervical, posterior and deep cervical chains, supraclavicular
         (b) Normal findings—less than 1 cm in size, nontender, mobile, soft, and discrete
      (7) Sample deviations from normal
         (a) Enlarged, smooth, soft, nontender thyroid—goiter
         (b) Single thyroid nodule—cyst, benign tumor, malignant tumor
   b. Eyes
      (1) Visual acuity
         (a) Snellen chart for central vision; normal 20/20
         (b) Rosenbaum card or newspaper for near vision
         (c) Impaired near vision—presbyopia
         (d) Impaired far vision—myopia
      (2) Peripheral vision—estimated with visual fields by confrontation test
      (3) External eye structures—eyebrows equal; lids without lag or ptosis; lacrimal apparatus without exudate, swelling, or excess tearing; conjunctiva clear with small blood vessels and no exudate; sclera white or buff colored
      (4) Eyeball structures
         (a) Cornea and lenses—no opacities or lesions
         (b) Pupils—*Pupils Equal, Round, React to Light, and Accommodate* (PERRLA)
      (5) Extraocular muscle (EOM) function—symmetrical movement through the six cardinal fields of gaze without lid lag or nystagmus
      (6) Ophthalmoscopic examination—red reflex present with no clouding or opacities; optic disc yellow to pink color with distinct margins; arterioles light red and two-thirds of the diameter of veins with bright light reflex; veins dark red and larger than arterioles with no light reflex; no venous tapering at the arteriole–venous (AV) crossings
      (7) Sample deviations from normal
         (a) Opacity of lens—cataracts
         (b) Dysconjugate gaze—diseases, injuries, or lesions affecting cranial nerves III, IV, VI
         (c) Nystagmus—cerebellar system disorders, vestibular disorders, drug toxicity
         (d) Lid lag—exophthalmos, hyperthyroidism
         (e) Papilledema—increased intracranial pressure
         (f) AV nicking—hypertension
         (g) Retinal hemorrhages and exudates—diabetes, hypertension
   c. Ears
      (1) Hearing evaluation
         (a) Whispered voice—able to hear softly whispered words in each ear at 1–2 ft
         (b) Weber test—tests for lateralization of sound through bone conduction; normally hear sound equally in both ears
         (c) Rinne test—compares bone and air conduction of sound; normally air-conducted (AC) sound is heard for twice as long as bone-conducted (BC) sound (AC:BC = 2:1)
         (d) Weber and Rinne tests may help in differentiating conductive and sensorineural hearing loss
         (e) Precision, test–retest reproducibility, and accuracy of Weber and Rinne tests have been questioned
      (2) External ears—symmetrical; no inflammation, lesions, nodules, or drainage
      (3) Tragus tenderness may indicate otitis externa; mastoid process tenderness may indicate otitis media
      (4) Otoscopic examination
         (a) External canal—no discharge, inflammation, lesions, or foreign bodies; varied amount, color, and consistency of cerumen
         (b) Tympanic membrane—intact, pearly gray, translucent, with cone of light at 5 o'clock position in the right ear and at the 7 o'clock position in the left ear; umbo and handle of malleus visible; no bulging or retraction
      (5) Sample deviations from normal
         (a) Conductive hearing loss—sound transmission impaired through external or middle ear; exudate/swelling, perforated eardrum
         (b) Sensorineural hearing loss—defect in inner ear distorting sound; loud noise exposure, aging, acoustic neuroma
   d. Nose and sinuses
      (1) Nasal mucosa pinkish red; septum midline
      (2) Frontal and maxillary sinuses nontender
   e. Mouth and oropharynx
      (1) Mouth—lips, gums, tongue, mucous membranes all pink, moist, without lesions or inflammation; teeth—none missing, free from caries or breakage
      (2) Oropharynx—tonsils, posterior wall of pharynx without lesions or inflammation

(3) Sample deviations from normal
    (a) White patch (leukoplakia) on the side or underside of the tongue—possible squamous cell carcinoma
    (b) Pharynx erythematous, tonsils 3+, white exudate, enlarged and tender anterior cervical nodes—probable streptococcal pharyngitis

5. Respiratory system
  a. Chest symmetrical, anterior–posterior diameter less than transverse diameter; respiratory rate 16–20 breaths/min, rhythm regular; no rib retraction or use of accessory muscles; no cyanosis or clubbing of fingers
  b. Anterior and posterior respiratory expansion—symmetrical movement when the patient inhales deeply
  c. Tactile fremitus (palpable vibration of chest wall that results from speech or other verbalizations)—decreased with emphysema, asthma, pleural effusion; increased with lobar pneumonia, pulmonary edema
  d. Percussion—resonant throughout lung fields
  e. Auscultation—vesicular over most of lung fields; bronchovesicular near main bronchus and bronchial over trachea
    (1) Adventitious sounds—see **Table 2-1**
    (2) Transmitted voice sounds/vocal resonance—normally voice sounds are muffled or indistinct when auscultating the chest; louder or more distinct voice sounds (e.g., bronchophony, egophony, whispered pectoriloquy indicate fluid or a solid mass in lungs)

6. Cardiovascular system
  a. Blood pressure (BP)—less than 120/80 mm Hg; pulse—60 to 90 beats per minute (bpm), regular, not bounding or thready
  b. Heart
    (1) Apical impulse—fourth to fifth left intercostal space (ICS) medial to the midclavicular line (MCL), no lifts or thrills
    (2) Auscultation at second right ICS; second, third, fourth, and fifth left ICS at the sternal border; and fifth left ICS at the MCL (**Figure 2-1**)
      (a) Assess rate and rhythm
      (b) Identify S_1 and S_2 at each site using the diaphragm endpiece of the stethoscope—S_1 occurs at the start of systole, heard best at the apex (tapered inferior tip of heart, left fifth ICS 7–9 cm lateral to midsternal line); S_2 occurs at the start of diastole, heard best at the base (superior aspect of heart, right and left second ICS next to sternum)
      (c) Identify extra heart sounds at each site—see **Table 2-2**
      (d) Murmurs—note timing, duration, pitch, intensity, pattern, quality, location, radiation, respiratory phase variations

Table 2-1 Adventitious Breath Sounds

Breath Sound	Characteristics	Cause
Crackles	Fine crackles—heard during inspiration; high pitch, crackling or popping, short duration Course crackles—heard during inspiration, may be present during expiration; low pitch, loud, bubbling or gurgling, longer duration Crackles usually don't disappear with coughing	Air flowing by fluid—pneumonia, bronchitis, early heart failure
Rhonchi	Heard during inspiration and expiration Low pitch, loud, sounds like a snore, tend to disappear after coughing	Air passing over solid or thick secretions in large airways—bronchitis, pneumonia
Wheezes	Heard during inspiration and/or expiration High pitch, continuous, louder during expiration, sounds like a squeak	Air flowing through constricted passageways—asthma, chronic emphysema
Pleural friction rub	Heard during inspiration or expiration Dry, rubbing, grating	Inflammation of pleural tissue—pleuritis, pericarditis

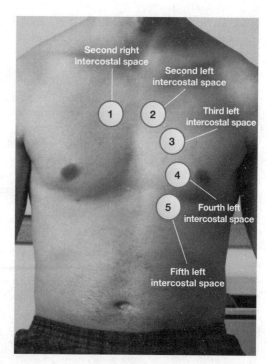

Figure 2-1 Five traditional auscultatory areas and related valves

Table 2-2 Examples of Extra Heart Sounds

Heart Sound	Location	Characteristics	Causes
Physiologic split S_2	Base; heard best with diaphragm	Heard during inspiration	Normal finding, S_2 actually two sounds that merge during expiration
Fixed split S_2	Base; heard best with diaphragm	Heard during inspiration and expiration	Delayed closure of pulmonic valve caused by atrial septal defect, right ventricular failure
Increased S_3 (ventricular gallop)	Apex; heard best with bell	Early diastole, low pitched, increased on inspiration	May be normal finding in young adults and in late pregnancy Rapid ventricular filling caused by decreased myocardial contractility, heart failure, volume overload
Increased S_4 (atrial gallop)	Apex; heard best with bell	Late diastole, low pitched, increased on inspiration	May be normal finding in well-trained athletes and older adults Forceful atrial ejection into distended ventricle caused by aortic stenosis, hypertensive heart disease, cardiomyopathy
Physiologic murmur	Second to fourth left ICS between left sternal border and apex	Mid-systole, little radiation, grades 1–3, soft to medium pitched, usually disappears or decreases on sitting	Normal finding, common in pregnancy
Murmur of mitral stenosis	Apex; heard best with bell	Early to late diastole, no radiation, grades 1–4, low pitched	Narrowed mitral valve restricts forward flow, forceful ejection into ventricle
Systolic click	Apex; heard best with diaphragm	Mid- to late systole, high pitched, increased with inspiration	Mitral valve prolapse
Pericardial friction rub	Variable, usually best in third ICS to left of sternum; heard best with diaphragm	Grating sound heard throughout cardiac cycle, high pitched, little radiation	Pericarditis

   c. Neck vessels
     (1) No jugular venous distention
     (2) Carotid arteries—strong, symmetrical, no bruits
   d. Extremities (peripheral arteries)
     (1) No erythema, pallor, or cyanosis; no edema or varicosities; skin warm; capillary refill time less than 2 seconds; normal hair distribution; no muscle atrophy
     (2) Pulses strong and symmetrical—brachial, radial, femoral, dorsalis pedis, posterior tibial
     (3) Lymph nodes less than 1 cm, nontender, mobile, soft, and discrete—axillary, epitrochlear, inguinal
 7. Abdomen
   a. Symmetrical, no lesions or masses; no visible pulsations or peristalsis
   b. Auscultation—active bowel sounds; no vascular bruits or friction rubs
   c. No guarding, tenderness, or masses on palpation
   d. Liver border—edge smooth, sharp, nontender; no more than 2 cm below right costal margin
   e. Spleen and kidneys—usually not palpable
   f. Aorta—slightly left of the midline in the upper abdomen; less than 3 cm width
   g. Percussion—tympany is the predominant tone; dullness over organs or any masses

   h. Liver span—normally 6–12 cm at the right MCL
   i. Splenic dullness—sixth to tenth ICS just posterior to the midaxillary line on the left side
   j. No tenderness on fist percussion over the costovertebral angle; costovertebral angle tenderness (CVAT) may indicate a kidney problem
   k. Special maneuvers/signs used to evaluate acute abdominal pain
     (1) Possible peritonitis—guarding, rigidity, rebound tenderness
     (2) Possible appendicitis
       (a) McBurney's point—localized tenderness right lower quadrant
       (b) Rovsing's sign—referred rebound tenderness, pain in the right lower quadrant when left-sided pressure is applied and then quickly withdrawn
       (c) Psoas and obturator signs—irritation of the right psoas or obturator muscles by inflamed appendix, maneuvers cause increased abdominal pain
     (3) Possible cholecystitis—Murphy's sign: a sharp increase in tenderness and sudden stop in inspiratory effort with upward pressure under the right costal margin while the patient takes deep breath

(4) Other red flags suggesting serious pathology with acute abdominal pain include absent bowel sounds and signs of shock
8. Musculoskeletal system
    a. No gross deformities; body aligned, extremities symmetrical, normal spinal curvature, no involuntary movements
    b. Muscle mass and strength equal bilaterally; full ROM without pain
    c. No inflammation, nodules, swelling, crepitus, or tenderness of joints
9. Neurologic system
    a. Cranial nerves (CN)—CN II through XII routinely tested, CN I tested if an abnormality is suspected (**Table 2-3**)
    b. Cerebellar function—smooth coordinated gait, able to walk heel to toe, balance maintained with eyes closed (Romberg test), rapid rhythmic alternating movements smooth and coordinated
    c. Sensory function—able to identify superficial pain and touch, able to identify vibration on bony prominences and passive position change of fingers and toes, normal response to discriminatory sensation tests, all findings symmetrical
    d. Deep tendon reflexes—brisk and symmetrical (biceps, brachioradialis, triceps, patellar, Achilles)
10. Mental status
    a. Physical appearance and behavior—well groomed, emotional status appropriate to situation, makes eye contact, posture erect
    b. Cognitive abilities—alert and oriented, able to reason, recent and remote memory intact, able to follow directions
    c. Emotional stability—no signs of depression or anxiety, logical thought processes, no perceptual disturbances
    d. Speech and language skills—normal voice quality and articulation, coherent, able to follow simple instructions
    e. Mini Mental Status Examination (MMSE)—standardized screening tool used for mental status assessment

Table 2-3 Cranial Nerves Function and Tests

Number	Name	Type	Function	Test
I	Olfactory	Sensory	Smell	Test ability to identify familiar odors
II	Optic	Sensory	Vision	Test visual acuity, peripheral vision, inspect optic discs
III	Oculomotor	Motor	Most extraocular movement (EOM), pupil constriction, upper eyelid elevation	Observe for PERRLA, EOM function, and ptosis
IV	Trochlear	Motor	Downward internal rotation of eye	Observe for EOM function
V	Trigeminal	Sensory/Motor	Transmission of stimuli from face and head; mastication and lateral jaw movements	Test for sharp/dull and light touch sensation on forehead, cheeks, and chin; palpate strength of temporal and masseter muscles
VI	Abducens	Motor	Lateral movement of the eye	Observe for EOM function
VII	Facial	Sensory/Motor	Taste on anterior two-thirds of tongue; facial muscle movement, including muscles of expression	Observe for any weakness, asymmetry, or abnormal movements of face
VIII	Acoustic	Sensory	Hearing	Assess auditory acuity
IX	Glossopharyngeal	Sensory/Motor	Taste on posterior one-third of tongue; movement of pharynx	Observe ability to swallow, symmetry of movement of soft palate and uvula when patient says, "Ah," gag reflex, any abnormal voice quality
X	Vagus	Sensory/Motor	Sensations in pharynx and larynx; movement of palate, larynx, and pharynx	Same as for CN IX
XI	Spinal accessory	Motor	Shoulder movement, head rotation	Observe and palpate strength and symmetry of trapezius and sternocleidomastoid muscles
XII	Hypoglossal	Motor	Tongue movement	Observe tongue for any deviation, asymmetry, abnormal movement

f. Depression screening tools—Patient Health Questionnaire (PHQ), Geriatric Depression Scale, Edinburgh Postnatal Depression Scale (EPDS)

- Detailed female reproductive examination
  1. Breasts
     a. The female breast extends from the second to the sixth ribs and from the sternal border to the midaxillary line
     b. Inspect breasts with patient in sitting position and hands above the head, pushing against hips, and leaning forward; view breasts from all sides to assess for symmetry and skin changes
        (1) Tanner sexual maturity rating in adolescent
        (2) Skin—smooth, color uniform, no erythema, masses, retraction, dimpling, or thickening
        (3) Symmetry—breast shape or contour is symmetrical; some difference in size of breasts and areola is common and usually normal
        (4) Nipples—pointing in the same direction, no retraction or discharge, no scaling; long-standing nipple inversion is usually a normal variation
     c. Palpate axillary, supraclavicular, and infraclavicular lymph nodes with the patient in a sitting position and arms relaxed at the sides
     d. Palpate breasts with the patient lying down, arm above head, a small pillow under shoulder/lower back on the side being examined, if needed, to provide even breast tissue distribution
        (1) Include the entire area from the midaxillary line, across the inframammary ridge and fifth/sixth rib, up the lateral edge of the sternum, across the clavicle, back to the midaxillary line
        (2) Palpate using finger pads of the middle three fingers with overlapping dime-shaped circular motions in a vertical strip pattern over the entire area including nipples; do not squeeze nipples unless the patient indicates having spontaneous nipple discharge (**Figure 2-2**)
        (3) Palpate each area of breast tissue using three levels of pressure—light, medium, and deep (**Figure 2-3**)

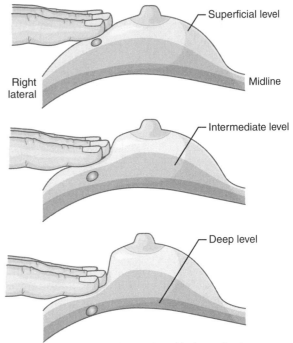

Apply pressure in a circular motion with the pads of your fingers to increasing levels, making three circles: superficial, intermediate, and deep pressure.

Figure 2-3 Palpation of breast tissue to three different levels of pressure.

        (4) Follow the same procedures for a patient with implants because correctly placed implants are located behind breast tissue
        (5) Include palpation of the chest wall, skin, and incision area in patients with mastectomy
        (6) Breast tissue—consistency varies from soft fat to firmer glandular tissue; physiologic nodularity may be present; there may be a firm ridge of compressed tissue under the lower edge of the breasts
        (7) Describe any palpable mass or lymph nodes in terms of location according to a clock face as the examiner faces the patient—size, shape, mobility, consistency, delimitation, and tenderness
        (8) Describe any nipple discharge in terms of whether spontaneous/not spontaneous, bilateral/unilateral, single or multiple ducts, color, and consistency
  2. Pelvic examination
     a. Pelvic examination can trigger anxiety, fear, or post-traumatic stress disorder symptoms in individuals with a history of sexual abuse or prior experience with painful or insensitive care
     b. Trauma-informed care during the pelvic examination uses strategies to allow patients to maintain control (e.g., obtain permission; adapt positioning, use of stirrups, use of speculum, specimen collection techniques for comfort; explain steps of exam in advance; touch thigh gently before touching genitals; use gentle technique; monitor comfort throughout exam)

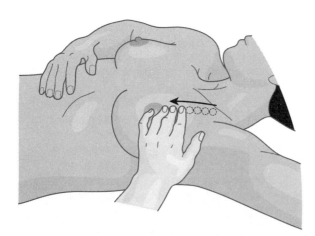

Figure 2-2 Palpation technique for clinical breast examination.

c. Prepare equipment/supplies prior to the examination
d. Conduct pelvic examination with attention to preventing contamination of equipment, such as examination lights and lubricant containers
e. Positioning—patient lying supine with head and shoulders elevated, lithotomy position, arms relaxed at the side or across the abdomen, buttocks extending slightly beyond the edge of the table, draped from mid-abdomen to knees, drape depressed between knees to allow eye contact
f. Inspection and palpation of external structures—mons pubis, labia majora and minora, clitoris, urethral meatus, vaginal introitus, paraurethral (Skene's) glands, Bartholin's glands, perineum
   (1) Tanner sexual maturity rating in adolescent
   (2) Mons pubis—pubic hair inverted triangular pattern, skin smooth with uniform color
   (3) Labia majora—may be gaping or closed and dry or moist, tissue soft and homogenous, covered with hair after puberty
   (4) Labia minora—moist and dark pink, tissue soft and homogenous
   (5) Clitoris—approximately 2 cm or less in length and 0.5 cm in diameter
   (6) Urethral meatus—irregular opening or slit
   (7) Vaginal introitus—thin vertical slit or large orifice, irregular edges from hymenal remnants, moist
   (8) Skene's and Bartholin's glands—opening of Skene's glands just posterior to and on each side of the urethral meatus; the opening of Bartholin's glands located posteriorly on each side of the vaginal orifice and not usually visible
   (9) Perineum—consists of tissue between introitus and anus; smooth; may have episiotomy scar
   (10) Note the presence of any abnormal hair distribution, discoloration, erythema, swelling, atrophy, lesions, masses, discharge, malodor, fistulas, tenderness
g. Pelvic floor muscles—form a supportive sling for pelvic contents and functional sphincters for vagina, urethra, and rectum; able to constrict introitus around examining fingers, snug compression of examining fingers for 3 or more seconds is full strength; assess for anterior or posterior bulging of vaginal walls, incontinence, or protrusion of cervix or uterus when patient bears down
h. Inspection of internal structures—speculum examination
   (1) Choose speculum type and size that facilitate visualization while minimizing discomfort
      (a) Pederson speculum—straight sided; pediatric, narrow, and regular sizes
      (b) Graves speculum—duck-billed shape; may be used when lax vaginal musculature or submucosal fat impedes visualization; small, average, and large sizes
   (2) Vaginal walls—pink, rugated, homogenous; may have thin, clear/cloudy, odorless discharge
   (3) Cervix—midline, smooth, round, pink, about 2.5 cm in diameter; protrudes 1–3 cm into the vagina; points posteriorly with an anteverted uterus, anteriorly with a retroverted uterus, horizontally with a midposition uterus; nabothian cysts may be present; os small and round (nulliparous); may be oval, slit-like, or stellate, if parous; may have an area of darker red epithelial tissue around os if squamocolumnar junction is on ectocervix
   (4) Note the presence of discoloration; erythema; swelling; atrophy; friable tissue; lesions; masses; discharge that is profuse, malodorous, thick, curdy, frothy, gray, green, yellow, or adherent to vaginal walls
i. Palpation of internal structures—bimanual examination
   (1) Vaginal walls—smooth, nontender
   (2) Cervix—smooth, firm, mobile, nontender, about 2.5 cm in diameter; protrudes 1–3 cm into the vagina
   (3) Uterus—smooth, rounded contour, firm, mobile, nontender; 5.5–8 cm long and pear shaped in nulliparous female; may be 2–3 cm larger in parous female; position anteverted, anteflexed, midplane, retroverted, or retroflexed (**Figure 2-4**)
   (4) Adnexa—fallopian tubes nonpalpable; ovaries ovoid, smooth, firm, mobile, slightly tender; size during reproductive years 3 cm × 2 cm × 1 cm
   (5) Note the presence of enlargements, masses, irregular surfaces, consistency other than firm, deviation of positions, immobility, tenderness
j. Rectovaginal examination
   (1) Purpose—palpate retroverted/retroflexed uterus; assess pelvic pathology; not recommended for colorectal cancer screening
   (2) Repeat the maneuvers of the bimanual examination with the index finger in the vagina and the middle finger in the rectum
   (3) Rectum—smooth, nontender without masses; firm anal sphincter tone
   (4) Rectovaginal septum—smooth, intact, nontender, without masses
k. See Chapter 5, *Gynecologic, Reproductive, and Sexual Disorders*, for descriptions of deviations from normal pelvic exam findings
- Male-focused reproductive health assessment
  1. Health history
     a. Reason for the visit and any presenting problems/illness
     b. Review of health history, current health status, family health history, and psychosocial history as appropriate for the reason for the visit
     c. Review of systems—endocrine, genitourinary
     d. Sexual health history
        (1) Age at first intercourse—consensual/nonconsensual
        (2) History of sexual abuse or sexual assault
        (3) Sexual orientation

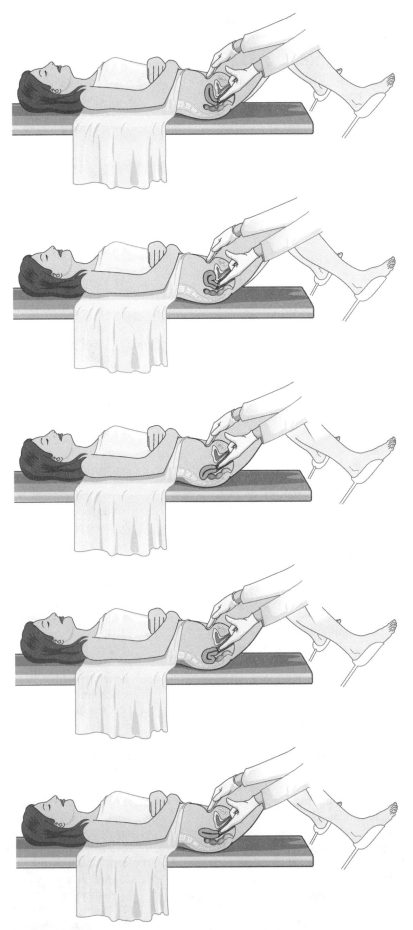

Figure 2-4 Variations in uterine positions.

    (4) Gender identity

    (5) Current sexual relationship(s)—frequency of sexual intercourse; satisfaction or concerns with sexual relationship(s); libido; ability to achieve and sustain erection; ability to achieve orgasm; dyspareunia

    (6) STI/HIV risk assessment—total number of sexual partners and number in past 3 months; types of sexual contact (vaginal, oral, anal); use of condoms; previous history of STIs; use of injection drugs or sex with a partner who uses injection drugs; sex while under the influence of drugs and/or alcohol; previous testing for HIV

    (7) Contraceptive use by female partner(s) or self if not desiring pregnancy

    (8) Fertility/infertility concerns

    (9) Any current penile discharge, lesions, scrotal swelling, or pain

2. Physical examination

  a. Tanner sexual maturity rating in adolescent

  b. Pubic hair—skin smooth with uniform color, hair course in triangular pattern pointing toward umbilicus

  c. Penis—skin smooth without hair, no lesions, no tenderness; prepuce (foreskin), if present, retracts easily; may have some smegma under prepuce; glans penis without lesions or erythema; urethral meatus on ventral surface at tip of glans penis, without lesions or erythema

  d. Scrotum—loose, wrinkled skin with darker pigment than the rest of the body; no lesions; may appear asymmetrical with one testis, usually the left testis, lower than the other

  e. Testes—oval, smooth, rubbery, move freely when palpated, sensitive to pressure but not tender

  f. Epididymis—posterolateral surface of testes, comma shaped, smooth, softer than testes, nontender

  g. Spermatic cords—starts at lower end of epididymis and extends to external inguinal ring; smooth; nontender

  h. Prostate gland—surrounds urethra at bladder neck; heart shaped, approximately 4 × 3 × 2 cm, smooth, rubbery, nontender

  i. Perianal area—skin smooth with no lesions or inflammation, anus moist, sphincter closed

  j. Examples of deviations from normal

    (1) Hypospadias—congenital displacement of urethral meatus to the inferior surface of the penis

    (2) Peyronie's disease—palpable nontender, hard plaques just beneath the skin, usually along the dorsum of the penis; may have crooked, painful erections

    (3) Varicocele—varicose veins of the spermatic cord, usually on the left, feels like a "bag of worms" separate from the testes; may be associated with infertility

    (4) Acute epididymitis—acutely inflamed, tender, swollen epididymis; scrotum may be reddened; most common cause is chlamydia infection

    (5) Torsion of spermatic cord—twisting of the testicle on its spermatic cord; acutely painful, tender, swollen organ retracted upward in scrotum; scrotum red and edematous; most common in adolescents; surgical emergency

• Older adults

1. Aging—the process of becoming older; genetically determined and environmentally modulated

2. Anatomic and physiologic changes with aging/potential clinical implications (not all inclusive)

  a. Skin

    (1) Thinner, decreased elasticity, cell regeneration slower; sebaceous and sweat gland activity decreases: dry skin, pruritus, increased risk of skin infection, decreased wound healing

    (2) Cutaneous sun exposure damage contributes to an increase in skin changes—wrinkles; irregular pigmentation; solar lentigines (brown/age spots); telangiectasia; cherry angiomas; seborrheic keratosis; and actinic keratosis, which are premalignant sun-induced growths

  b. Eyes—decreased tear production, pupils smaller, lens stiffens: dry eyes, decreased near vision, decreased adaptation to darkness

  c. Ears—atrophy of auditory neurons; increased cerumen; sclerosis of tympanic membrane: sensorineural hearing loss (high frequency first), conductive hearing loss

  d. Mouth, nose, and teeth—decreased number of taste buds, atrophy of salivary glands, gingival tissue less elastic, softening of teeth, decrease in olfactory neurons: decreased appetite, dry mouth, loss of teeth, difficulty chewing

  e. Thorax and lungs—rib cage less mobile, decreased strength of expiratory muscles, alveoli less elastic: decreased ability to clear lungs with less efficient cough; decreased ventilation at lung bases; decreased reserve for response to exercise, stress, or disease

  f. Heart—left ventricular wall thickens, myocardium becomes less elastic, fibrosis and sclerosis of heart valves and within conduction system (SA node), stroke volume decreases, heart rate slows, but resting heart rate not significantly influenced; cardiac output during exercise declines with less efficient response to increased oxygen demand and longer recovery time to baseline, irregular heart rhythms, mild ECG changes

  g. Peripheral vascular system—aorta and large arteries stiffen: rise in systolic blood pressure, tendency toward orthostatic hypotension

  h. Gastrointestinal (GI) system—decreased motility of intestines, decreased secretion of digestive enzymes and protective mucus in the intestinal tract, decrease in liver size and hepatic blood flow: constipation, indigestion, decreased ability to metabolize some drugs and alcohol, increased risk of stomach ulcers and GI bleeding with long-acting nonsteroidal anti-inflammatory drugs (NSAIDs)

  i. Musculoskeletal system—bone demineralization, decreased muscle mass and strength, decreased

ROM, joint and cartilage erosion: decreased bone density, decreased agility and endurance, gait disturbances, increased risk for falls

   j. Neurologic system—general decrease in brain volume and cerebral blood flow, decrease in velocity of nerve impulse conduction, diminished sensory perceptions of touch and pain stimuli, motor responses slow: slower reaction time, possible decreased response to pain, decrease in coordination and balance

   k. Genitourinary—vulvovaginal atrophy, ovarian atrophy, decreased bladder capacity and tone; urethral carbuncles common, dyspareunia; ovaries usually not palpable; urinary frequency, urgency, incontinence; pelvic prolapse

3. Cognitive changes
   a. Definitions/characteristics
     (1) Cognition is multidimensional, including mental functions involved in attention, thinking, understanding, learning, remembering, solving problems, and making decisions
     (2) Cognitive aging is inherent in all humans as they age; highly dynamic process with variability within and between individuals
     (3) Some cognitive domains may not change, some decline, and some may actually improve
     (4) Factors that may influence cognitive aging include genetics, education, environment, culture, chronic medical conditions, physical activity, and other health behaviors
     (5) Cognitive aging is not a neurologic or psychiatric disease
   b. Abnormal (pathologic) causes of cognitive changes
     (1) Dementia (the most common form is Alzheimer's disease)—insidious onset; slowly progressive; persistent; recent memory and new learning especially impaired; changes in speech, mood, thought processes, judgment; behavior may become inappropriate; may have delusions and/or hallucinations; may have fragmented sleep
     (2) Delirium (may be caused by infection, toxins, medications, withdrawal from alcohol or other substances, trauma, neurologic or neoplastic disorders)—sudden onset; fluctuating with lucid intervals, worse at night; lasts hours to weeks; immediate and recent memory impaired; changes in alertness, attention, speech, mood, thought processes, judgment; may be agitated or somnolent; may have delusions and/or hallucinations; disrupted sleep
     (3) Depression—may have some cognitive symptoms along with depressed mood, such as the inability to think or concentrate, indecisiveness, psychomotor agitation, or retardation; individuals with a diagnosis of dementia may also have clinical depression
     (4) MMSE—screens for dementia, although not definitive; may be used to detect the progression of dementia

Diagnostic Studies/ Laboratory Tests

- Complete blood count (CBC) with differential
  1. Red blood cell (RBC) count—measurement of RBCs per cubic millimeter of blood
     a. Normal findings (adult female)—4.2 to 5.4 million/mm^3
     b. Potential causes of low values include hemorrhage, hemolysis, dietary deficiencies, hemoglobinopathies, bone marrow failure, chronic illness, medications
     c. Potential causes of high values include dehydration, diseases causing chronic hypoxia, such as congenital heart disease, polycythemia vera, medications
  2. Hematocrit (Hct)/hemoglobin (Hgb)—rapid indirect measurement of RBC count
     a. Hct—percentage of total blood volume that is made up of RBCs
        (1) Normal findings (nonpregnant adult female)—37%–47%
        (2) Normal findings (pregnant adult female)—33% or greater in first and third trimesters, 32% or greater in second trimester
     b. Hgb—measurement of total Hgb (which carries oxygen) in the blood
        (1) Normal findings (nonpregnant adult female)—12 to 16 g/dL
        (2) Normal findings (pregnant adult female)—11 g/dL or greater in first and third trimesters, 10.5 g/dL or greater in second trimester; adjustment in values for Black women—10.2 g/dL in first and third trimesters, 9.7 g/dL in second trimester
     c. Potential causes of low values include anemia, hemoglobinopathies, cirrhosis, hemorrhage, dietary deficiency, bone marrow failure, renal disease, chronic illness, some cancers
     d. Potential causes of high values include erythrocytosis, polycythemia vera, severe dehydration, and severe chronic obstructive pulmonary disease. Exogenous use of testosterone
     e. Heavy smokers and individuals living at higher elevations may also have higher Hgb levels
  3. RBC indices—provide information about the size, weight, and Hgb concentration of RBCs; useful in classifying anemias
     a. Mean corpuscular volume (MCV)—average volume or size of a single RBC
        (1) Normal finding—80 to 95 mm^3, normocytic
        (2) Microcytic/abnormally small—seen with iron-deficiency anemia and thalassemia
        (3) Macrocytic/abnormally large—seen with megaloblastic anemias, such as vitamin B deficiency and folic acid deficiency
     b. Mean corpuscular hemoglobin (MCH)—average amount or weight of Hgb within an RBC
        (1) Normal finding—27 to 31 pg/cell

(2) Causes for abnormalities same as for MCV

  c. Mean corpuscular hemoglobin concentration (MCHC)—average concentration or percentage of Hgb within a single RBC

    (1) Normal finding—32 to 36 g/dL, normochromic

    (2) Decreased concentration or hypochromic—seen with iron-deficiency anemia and thalassemia

4. White blood cell (WBC) count with differential—provides information useful in evaluating individuals with infection, neoplasm, allergy, or immunosuppression (**Table 2-4**)

5. Peripheral blood smear—microscopic examination of smear of peripheral blood to examine RBCs, platelets, and leukocytes

- Blood clotting studies

1. Used as part of an investigation of a possible bleeding disorder or thrombotic episode

2. Includes platelet count, prothrombin time (PT), partial thromboplastin time (PTT), coagulation factors

3. Platelet count

  a. Normal finding (adult)—150,000 to 400,000/mm^3

  b. Potential causes of low count (thrombocytopenia) include autoimmune disorders, cirrhosis, sepsis, hypersplenism, hemorrhage, leukemia, cancer chemotherapy, viral infection, some medications

  c. Potential causes of high count (thrombocytosis) include some malignant disorders, polycythemia vera, rheumatoid arthritis, myeloproliferative disease

4. PT and PTT

  a. Used to evaluate how well coagulation factors in coagulation cascade work together

  b. Measures the number of seconds it takes for a clot to form in a blood sample after reagents are added; prolonged results indicate that blood clotting is taking longer than normal

  c. Conditions that may cause a prolonged PT with normal PTT include, but are not limited to, liver disease, vitamin K deficiency, chronic low-grade disseminated intravascular coagulation (DIC), defective factor VII, anticoagulation drug (warfarin) therapy

  d. Conditions that may cause a normal PT with prolonged PTT include, but are not limited to, decreased/defective factor VIII, IX, XI, XII; von Willebrand disease; the presence of systemic lupus erythematosus (SLE) anticoagulant

Table 2-4 White Blood Cell (WBC) Count with Differential

Normal Values (Adult)	Low Values: Potential Causes	High Values: Potential Causes
Total WBC count 5,000–10,000/mm^3	Bone marrow suppression Autoimmune disorders Immunosuppressive disorders Overwhelming infection Cancer that spreads to bone marrow	Dehydration Infection Inflammatory conditions Some malignancies May be elevated in late pregnancy and during labor Traumatic injury
Neutrophils 30%–70%	Bone marrow suppression Autoimmune disorders Immunosuppressive disorders Overwhelming infection Cancer that spreads to bone marrow	Acute bacterial infection Inflammation or tissue necrosis Some malignancies Cushing syndrome Increased immature forms (band and stabs) sometimes called shift to left with ongoing acute bacterial infection
Basophils 0%–3%	Occasional low number is usually not medically significant	Hypersensitivity reaction Chronic inflammatory disorders Some leukemias Uremia
Eosinophils 0%–5%	Occasional low number is usually not medically significant	Allergic reaction Parasitic infections Chronic inflammatory disorders Some malignancies Addison's disease
Lymphocytes 15%–40%	Autoimmune disorders Debilitating illness Immunodeficiency syndromes Some malignancies Corticosteroids	Acute viral infections Chronic bacterial infections Chronic inflammatory disorders Some malignancies
Monocytes 2%–8%	Chronic diseases—rare	Chronic infections Recovery phase of infections Some malignancies

e. Conditions that may cause both prolonged PT and PTT include, but are not limited to, decreased or defective factor I, II, V, X; severe liver disease; acute DIC, warfarin overdose

f. PT and PTT do not provide specific information on the cause of blood clotting abnormality; further testing for specific coagulation factor deficiency or defect may be indicated, as well as tests for other underlying conditions

5. Comprehensive metabolic panel (CMP)

a. Provides information on the status of metabolism; monitors status of known conditions and kidney- or liver-related side effects of medication

b. Fasting for 10–12 hours may be needed depending on the reason for ordering CMP

c. CMP includes glucose, calcium, albumin, total protein, electrolytes (sodium, potassium, CO_2, chloride), kidney tests (blood urea nitrogen [BUN], creatinine), liver tests (ALP, ALT, AST, bilirubin)

d. Abnormal test results are usually followed up with specific tests to confirm or rule out a suspected diagnosis

- Blood glucose—used for diagnosis and evaluation of diabetes mellitus

1. Fasting glucose

a. No caloric intake for at least 8 hours

b. Normal finding (adult)—less than 100 mg/dL

c. Impaired fasting glucose—100 to 125 mg/dL

d. Diagnostic for diabetes—126 mg/dL or greater

2. Two-hour postload glucose during oral glucose tolerance test (OGTT)

a. Sample obtained 2 hours after a glucose load containing the equivalent of 75 g of glucose dissolved in water

b. Normal finding—less than 140 mg/dL

c. Impaired glucose tolerance—140 to 199 mg/dL

d. Diagnostic for diabetes—200 mg/dL or greater

3. American Diabetes Association (ADA) criteria for the diagnosis of diabetes mellitus with blood glucose tests

a. Classic symptoms of hyperglycemia plus random nonfasting glucose concentration of 200 mg/dL or greater

b. Fasting glucose of 126 mg/dL or greater

c. Two-hour postglucose of 200 mg/dL or greater

d. Repeat testing on a subsequent day to confirm the diagnosis

4. HbA_{1c} or A_{1c}

a. May be used for the diagnosis of diabetes

b. Threshold for diagnosis of diabetes is 6.5% or greater; prediabetes is 5.7%–6.4%

c. Gold standard for measurement of long-term (previous 60–90 days) glycemic control in individuals with diabetes

d. Reliable tool for evaluating the need for drug therapy and monitoring the effectiveness of therapy

e. Good diabetic control—less than 7%

- Lipid profile

1. Determines risk for coronary heart disease and evaluation of hyperlipidemia

2. Includes total cholesterol, triglycerides, high-density lipoproteins (HDLs), and low-density lipoproteins (LDLs)

3. Fast for 12–14 hours prior to obtaining a sample

4. Total cholesterol normal level (adult)—less than 200 mg/dL; may be elevated in pregnancy

5. Triglycerides normal finding (adult female)—35 to 135 mg/dL; may be elevated in pregnancy

6. HDL—removes cholesterol from peripheral tissues and transports it to the liver for excretion

a. Normal level (adult)—40 mg/dL or greater

b. Low levels associated with increased risk for heart and peripheral vascular disease

7. LDL—cholesterol carried by LDL can be deposited into peripheral tissues

a. Normal finding (adult)—less than 130 mg/dL

b. High levels associated with increased risk for heart and peripheral vascular disease

- Renal function tests

1. BUN—indirect measure of renal and liver function

a. Normal finding (adult)—10 to 20 mg/dL

b. Increased levels—hypovolemia, dehydration, reduced cardiac function, GI bleeding, starvation, sepsis, renal disease

c. Decreased levels—liver failure, malnutrition, nephrotic syndrome

2. Serum creatinine—indirect measure of renal function

a. Normal finding (adult female)—0.5 to 1.1 mg/dL

b. Increased levels—renal disorders, dehydration

c. Decreased levels—debilitation and decreased muscle mass

3. Creatinine clearance—calculated from serum and 24-hour urine creatinine levels to determine the rate at which kidneys are clearing creatinine from the blood, reflecting glomerular filtration rate (GFR)

a. Normal finding—serum creatinine (adult female), 0.5–1.1 mg/dL; 24-hour urine creatinine, 500–2000 mg; GFR determined with an equation that considers age, sex, and race

b. Increased levels—increased muscle mass, exercise, pregnancy, high dietary meat intake, some medications

c. Decreased levels—impaired renal function, reduced renal blood flow, heart failure, shock, some medications

4. Urine protein/creatinine (PC) ratio

a. Helps evaluate kidney function when significant and persistent protein is found on urinalysis

b. Random urine sample

c. Approaches accuracy of a 24-hour urine sample when both protein and creatinine are measured

d. Persistent and/or increased amounts of protein in urine may indicate kidney damage or disease; also associated with other diseases/conditions (e.g., preeclampsia, diabetes, multiple myeloma, other)

- Thyroid function studies

1. Thyroid-stimulating hormone (TSH)—used to diagnose hyperthyroidism and primary hypothyroidism, differentiate primary from secondary hypothyroidism, and monitor thyroid replacement or suppression therapy

a. Normal finding (adult)—0.4 to 4.12 mU/mL

b. Increased levels—seen with primary hypothyroidism and thyroiditis

c. Decreased levels—seen with secondary hypothyroidism, hyperthyroidism, suppressive doses of thyroid medication

d. Upper limit of normal may be higher in older adults

e. Upper limits during pregnancy are lower and based on trimester—2.5 to 3.5 mU/mL

2. Free thyroxine (FT$_4$)—used in diagnosing thyroid disease

a. Normal finding (adult female)—0.58 to 1.64 ng/dL

b. Increased levels—hyperthyroidism and acute thyroiditis

c. Decreased levels—hypothyroidism

3. Total thyroxine (T$_4$)

a. Normal finding (adult female)—4.5 to 12.0 µg/dL

b. Measurement affected by increases in thyroxine-binding globulin (TBG)

c. Causes of increased TBG include pregnancy, oral contraceptive use, and estrogen therapy

4. Antithyroid peroxidase antibodies (anti-TPO)—used in differential diagnosis of thyroid disorders associated with autoimmune disease

a. Normal finding—negative antithyroid antibodies

b. Positive antithyroid antibodies—Graves' disease; Hashimoto's thyroiditis

- Liver function studies

1. Bilirubin

a. Normal findings (adult)—total bilirubin 0.3–1.0 mg/dL; direct (conjugated) bilirubin 0.1–0.3 mg/dL; indirect (unconjugated) bilirubin 0.2 to 0.8 mg/dL

b. Elevated direct bilirubin level—occurs with gallstones and obstruction of the extrahepatic duct

c. Elevated indirect bilirubin level—seen with hepatocellular dysfunction (hepatitis, cirrhosis) and hemolytic anemias

2. Albumin

a. Normal finding (adult)—3.5 to 5.0 g/dL

b. Increased levels—dehydration

c. Decreased levels—seen with liver disease, malabsorption syndromes, nephropathies, severe burns, malnutrition, and inflammatory disease

3. Liver enzymes

a. Alkaline phosphatase (ALP)

(1) Normal finding—30 to 120 U/L

(2) Elevated levels—liver disease, bone disease, and myocardial infarction

b. Aspartate aminotransferase (AST), alanine aminotransferase (ALT), lactic dehydrogenase (LDH)

(1) Normal findings—AST 0–35 U/L, ALT 4–36 U/L, LDH 100–190 U/L

(2) Useful in differentiating causes for ALP elevation

c. Gamma-glutamyl transpeptidase (GGT)

(1) Normal finding—8–38 U/L

(2) Elevated levels with liver disease, myocardial infarction, pancreatic disease, and heavy or chronic alcohol use

- Fecal occult blood testing

1. Evaluation of GI conditions that may cause GI bleeding

2. Positive test—may indicate GI cancer or polyps, peptic ulcer disease, inflammatory or ischemic bowel disease, GI trauma, bleeding caused by medications

3. Guaiac-based fecal occult blood test

a. Requires stool sample from 3 separate bowel movements

b. Low sensitivity if specimen obtained during a digital rectal exam

4. Several interfering factors can cause false positives or negatives

a. Red meat and some raw fruits and vegetables, if consumed within 3 days prior to or during the test period, or nonsteroidal anti-inflammatory drugs 7 days prior to testing can result in a false positive

b. Large amounts of vitamin C consumed within 3 days prior to or during the test period can result in a false negative

(1) Fecal immunochemical test

c. only requires one stool sample

d. High sensitivity

e. No drug or dietary restrictions are required prior to testing

5. Positive tests require further evaluation with sigmoidoscopy, colonoscopy, or barium enema

- Blood type and Rh factor

1. Used to determine blood type prior to donating or receiving blood and to determine blood type in a pregnant individual

2. Blood types are grouped according to the presence or absence of antigens A, B, and Rh on RBCs

3. Individuals without a particular antigen may develop antibodies to that antigen if exposed through blood transfusion or fetal–maternal/parental blood mixing

4. Blood type O negative is the universal donor because no antigens on RBCs

5. Indirect Coombs test/antibody screen is used to screen for the presence of any circulating antibodies against RBCs during pregnancy and to monitor antibody titers if a pregnant person is Rh negative

6. Direct Coombs test—test done on newborn's cord blood if a birthing person is Rh negative and the infant is Rh positive to determine if the infant has antibodies on RBCs that could cause hemolysis

- Sickle cell screening (Sickle Cell Prep, SICKLEDEX®)

1. Used to screen for sickle cell disease and trait

2. Positive test—presence of Hgb S indicates sickle cell disease or trait

3. Hgb electrophoresis is the definitive test to be performed if the screening test is positive; identifies Hgb type and quantity

- Autoantibodies/antinuclear antibodies (ANA)

1. Test used as part of the diagnostic workup for SLE and other connective tissue autoimmune disorders, such as scleroderma, rheumatoid arthritis, Sjögren's syndrome

2. Positive ANA found in 95% of individuals with SLE; titer may be negative early in the disease

3. Test results must be correlated with other criteria for the particular autoimmune disease
4. Antinuclear antibody subtypes may be used to aid in diagnosis—anti-dsDNA and anti-Sm are highly specific to SLE but have variable sensitivity
5. Higher titers indicate more active disease; lower titers associated with effective treatment

- Pregnancy test
  1. Used to detect human chorionic gonadotropin (hCG) in blood/urine
  2. Urine hCG tests
     a. Highly sensitive urine tests provide accurate qualitative (positive/negative) results with hCG levels as low as 5–50 mIU/mL
     b. May detect pregnancy as early as 28 days from last menstrual period
     c. First-morning urine is best, as it will be the most concentrated
     d. Cross-reactions with other hormones are not a problem with highly sensitive urine tests
  3. Serum hCG radioimmunoassay (RIA) or immunometric assay
     a. Provides level of hCG (quantitative); not any advantage for use as qualitative (positive/negative) test over highly sensitive urine tests in most situations
     b. Single level useful in conjunction with ultrasound if concern about ectopic pregnancy—should be able to visualize intrauterine pregnancy when level is 1500–2000 mIU/mL
     c. Serial testing of serum hCG allows for following the rise or fall of levels—assists in diagnosis of ectopic pregnancy, evolving spontaneous abortion, possible retained products of conception, surveillance for persistent trophoblastic proliferation after uterine evacuation of hydatidiform mole

- Reproductive hormone studies
  1. Used to evaluate and monitor treatment of infertility; assist in differential diagnosis of gonadal dysfunction; assist in diagnosis of certain neoplasms
  2. Levels fluctuate throughout the menstrual cycle in reproductive-age individuals and may be affected using hormonal contraception
  3. Results should be correlated with the individual's age and clinical presentation
  4. Estradiol (E$_2$)
     a. Increased—adrenal tumor, estrogen-producing tumor, hepatic cirrhosis, hyperthyroidism
     b. Decreased—postmenopause, primary hypogonadism (e.g., Turner's syndrome, gonadal radiation exposure), secondary/central hypogonadism (pituitary/hypothalamic disorders)
  5. Progesterone
     a. Increased—pregnancy, ovulation, progesterone-secreting ovarian tumor or cyst, congenital adrenal hyperplasia, hydatidiform mole
     b. Decreased—primary or secondary/central hypogonadism, threatened abortion, fetal demise, preeclampsia, short luteal phase syndrome
  6. Follicle-stimulating hormone (FSH)

a. Increased—postmenopause, gonadotropin-secreting pituitary tumor, primary hypogonadism
b. Decreased secondary/central hypogonadism
  7. Luteinizing hormone
     a. Increased—postmenopause, gonadotropin-secreting pituitary tumor, primary hypogonadism
     b. Decreased secondary/central hypogonadism

- Urinalysis—dipstick and/or microscopic evaluation of urine
  1. Includes evaluation of appearance, color, odor, pH, protein, specific gravity, leukocyte esterase, nitrites, ketones, crystals, casts, glucose, WBCs, and RBCs
  2. Obtain midstream clean-catch specimen so culture can be performed if urinalysis indicates infection
  3. Normal findings
     a. No nitrites, ketones, crystals, casts, or glucose
     b. Clear, amber yellow, aromatic
     c. pH 4.6–8.0
     d. Protein 0–8 mg/dL
     e. Specific gravity (adult)—1.005 to 1.030
     f. Leukocyte esterase negative
     g. WBCs 0–4 per high-power field (HPF)
     h. RBCs at 2 or less

- Urine culture
  1. Used for diagnosis of urinary tract infection (UTI) and antimicrobial susceptibility testing of causative organisms
  2. Specimen obtained from mid-stream clean catch urine, sometimes obtained via sterile catheter
  3. Positive culture indicates UTI
     a. Typically considered positive with the presence of a single type of bacteria at 100,000 colony-forming units (CFU)/mL
     b. Lower CFU/mL of 1000 or greater may be used to indicate infection when UTI symptoms are present
     c. Growth of several different types of bacteria is likely due to the contamination of the specimen
  4. Susceptibility testing identifies antimicrobials that are likely to be effective for the identified bacteria
  5. See Chapter 3, *Primary Care*, for more information on UTIs

- Vaginal microscopy/wet mount/pH/amine test
  1. Used to aid in detection of organisms responsible for symptoms of vaginal infections through evaluation of vaginal discharge
  2. Obtain specimen (vaginal discharge/secretions) from lateral vaginal walls—avoid contamination with cervical secretions
  3. pH test—place a strip of pH litmus paper directly on the wall of the vagina or place discharge from a collection swab on the strip
  4. Prepare the initial slide with a drop of saline and a drop of discharge
  5. Alternative procedure—place the swab used to collect the specimen into a test tube containing less than 1 mL of saline and stir gently; place a drop of the mixture onto a slide
  6. Place a cover slip over the solution on the slide, followed by an immediate examination under a microscope at both low (10×) and high (40×) power; scan

thoroughly for clue cells, motile trichomonads, WBCs; delays of more than 10 minutes reduce the chance of visualizing motile trichomonads

7. Prepare second slide with vaginal discharge specimen and 10% potassium hydroxide (KOH) to facilitate visualization of yeast buds and pseudohyphae
8. Addition of KOH may be used to detect the presence of amines (whiff test)
9. Health history and pelvic examination findings are essential to correlate with wet mount, pH, and whiff test findings for diagnosis
10. Other in-office point-of-care tests used for vaginal infection diagnosis—vaginal fluid sialidase test positive with bacterial vaginosis (BV), rapid antigen test positive with *Trichomonas vaginalis*
11. In-office diagnostic test findings—normal, BV, *Trichomonas vaginalis*, vulvovaginal candidiasis (VVC) (**Table 2-5**)
12. Additional tests for vaginal infection diagnosis
    a. Nucleic acid amplification tests (NAAT)—CDC-recommended test for *Trichomonas vaginalis*
    b. Culture
       (1) Yeast culture may be useful when wet mount is negative but symptoms, discharge, or other signs suggestive of VVC are present; can help confirm the diagnosis and identify species of yeast when recurrent or persistent signs/symptoms are present
       (2) Culture for *Trichomonas vaginalis* is available; less sensitive and more expensive than NAAT
       (3) Culture for BV is not recommended; no bacteria are specific for BV
13. See Chapter 5, *Gynecologic, Reproductive, and Sexual Disorders*, for detailed information on assessment and management of vaginal infections
- Tests for STIs
  1. Health history and pelvic examination findings are essential to correlate with test findings for diagnosis
  2. Tests for screening and diagnosis of STIs—see **Table 2-6**
  3. See Chapter 5, *Gynecologic, Reproductive, and Sexual Disorders*, for detailed information on assessment and management of STIs
- HIV
  1. Window period—time between HIV exposure and an accurate test result
  2. Nucleic acid tests (NATs)—detect HIV RNA; 50% have detectable plasma RNA within 12 days
  3. Antibody tests—detect HIV IgM and/or IgG antibodies; on average antibodies are detectable by 21–28 days; HIV antibodies are detectable in 95% of individuals within 6 months of exposure
  4. HIV-1 p24 antigen test—detects HIV-1 antigen; detectable at 15 days, peaks at 25–30 days, then declines with antibody development
  5. Combined HIV antibody and p24 antigen test detects HIV p24 antigen as well as IgM and IgG antibodies
  6. Confirm reactive tests with IgG HIV type 1 and 2 antibody differential supplemental assay

Table 2-5 In-Office Diagnostic Test Findings: Normal, Bacterial Vaginosis, *Trichomonas vaginalis*, and Vulvovaginal Candidiasis

Condition	In-Office Diagnostic Test Findings
Normal	■ Vaginal pH 3.8–4.5 ■ Whiff test negative ■ Wet mount: epithelial cells, few or no WBCs, lactobacilli present
Bacterial vaginosis	■ Vaginal pH > 4.5 ■ Whiff test positive ■ Wet mount: >20% of epithelial cells are clue cells, 0–1 WBCs per epithelial cell, lactobacilli reduced or absent ■ Point-of-care vaginal fluid sialidase test positive
Trichomonas vaginalis	■ Vaginal pH > 4.5 ■ Whiff test negative or positive ■ Wet mount: motile trichomonads, >1 WBC per epithelial cell, lactobacilli reduced or absent ■ Point-of-care rapid antigen test positive
Vulvovaginal candidiasis (VVC)	■ Vaginal pH ≤ 4.5* ■ Whiff test negative ■ Wet mount: hyphae/spores (best seen after KOH applied), > 1 WBC per epithelial cell, lactobacilli present

*When VVC and a concomitant BV or *T. vaginalis* infection occur, the vaginal pH may be greater than 4.5.

7. See Chapter 3, *Primary Care*, for detailed information on the diagnosis and management of HIV
- Other infectious disease tests
  1. Rubella (German measles)
     a. Hemagglutination inhibition (HAI) test—used to detect immunity to rubella and to diagnose rubella infection
        (1) Titer of 1:10 or greater indicates immunity to rubella
        (2) High titers (1:64 or greater) may indicate current rubella infection
     b. Rubella IgM antibody titer—used if a pregnant person has a rash suspected to be from rubella; if titer is positive, a recent infection has occurred; IgM antibodies appear 1–2 days after onset of rash and disappear 5–6 weeks after infection
  2. Hepatitis B (HBV) tests
     a. Hepatitis B surface antigen (HBsAg)—rises before the onset of clinical symptoms, peaks during the first week of symptoms, and returns to normal by the time jaundice subsides
        (1) Indicates active HBV infection—individual is infectious
        (2) Individual is considered a carrier if HBsAg persists

Table 2-6 Tests for Diagnosis of Sexually Transmitted Infections

STI/Causative Organism	Screening/Diagnostic Tests
Chlamydia/*Chlamydia trachomatis*	■ Nucleic acid amplification test (NAAT)—test recommended by Centers for Disease Control and Prevention (CDC) ■ NAAT provides option of testing with urine, vaginal (clinician or patient obtained), or endocervical sample; some approved for liquid-based cytology specimens; few approved for rectal or oropharyngeal specimens
Gonorrhea/*Neisseria gonorrhoeae*	■ NAAT provides same testing ability as with *chlamydia* ■ Culture with antimicrobial sensitivity testing should be used with suspected or documented treatment failure

Syphilis/*Treponema pallidum*	■ Dark field microscopy examination and direct fluorescent antibody tests of lesion exudate or tissue are definitive methods of diagnosing early syphilis
	■ Serology—provides for presumptive diagnosis
	  1. Nontreponemal tests (nonspecific)—Venereal Disease Research Laboratories (VDRL), rapid plasma reagin (RPR)
	    a. Become positive 1–2 weeks past chancre
	    b. Reported as nonreactive or reactive
	    c. Reactive test also reported quantitatively as titer
	    d. False positives associated with mononucleosis, collagen vascular disease, and some other medical conditions; usually see low titer 1:8
	    e. Reactive nontreponemal tests must be confirmed with a treponemal test
	    f. Titers also used for follow-up after treatment
	    g. Usually become nonreactive with time after successful treatment
	  2. Treponemal tests (specific)—fluorescent treponemal antibody absorption test (FTA-ABS), treponema pallidum immobilization test (TPI)
	    a. Reported as positive or negative; not quantitative
	    b. Usually remain positive indefinitely after treatment

Genital herpes/herpes simplex virus (HSV)	■ Tissue culture and polymerase chain reaction (PCR) are the CDC-recommended tests for patients presenting with genital lesions
	  1. PCR assays are more sensitive than tissue culture
	  2. Sensitivity varies with stage of infection—highest if sample comes from vesicular lesion
	■ Type-specific serologic tests—serum; detect presence of HSV-1 and HSV-2 antibodies; may take 4–12 weeks for seroconversion; useful if history is suggestive of HSV but no current lesions, negative culture of lesions but suspect HSV infection, partner with known HSV infection, or patient with HIV infection

Chancroid/*Haemophilus ducreyi*	■ Culture—specimen obtained from lesion or bubo, difficult to isolate ■ Gram stain—gram negative or chains
Trichomoniasis/*Trichomonas vaginalis*	■ NAAT—test recommended by CDC ■ NAAT provides option of testing with urine, vaginal (clinician or patient obtained); some approved for liquid-based cytology specimens ■ Several NAAT assays test for N. gonorrhoeae, C. trachomatis, and T. vaginalis on the same sample ■ See Table 2-4
Mycoplasma genitalium	NAAT approved for use with urine, urethral, endocervical, and vaginal swab samples Culture not recommended as *M. genitalium* is extremely slow-growing organism

   b. Hepatitis B surface antibody (HBsAb)—appears 4 weeks after the disappearance of surface antigen
     (1) Indicates the end of an acute infectious phase and signifies immunity to subsequent infection
     (2) Also used to denote immunity after administration of HBV vaccine
   c. Hepatitis B core antibody (HBcAb)—indicates a past infection; chronic hepatitis

   d. Hepatitis B e-antigen (HBeAg)—seen with acute infection; indicates infectivity
   e. Hepatitis B e-antibody (HBeAb)—seen with convalescence; indicates decreased infectivity
 3. Hepatitis C (HCV) tests
   a. HCV antibody assay (rapid fingerstick/venipuncture blood test or laboratory test)
   b. Follow reactive antibody test with HCV RNA test; positive HCV RNA test indicates current HCV

infection; negative HCV RNA test indicates either past resolved HCV infection or false HCV antibody positivity

4. Tuberculosis (TB) tests
   a. Usually positive within 6–8 weeks after infection
   b. Does not indicate whether the infection is active or dormant
   c. Interpretation of purified protein derivative (PPD) skin test results—measure area of induration, not erythema
      (1) High-risk population: 5 mm induration or greater
      (2) Moderate-risk population: 10 mm induration or greater
      (3) General population: 15 mm induration or greater
   d. Once a positive reaction, usually persists for life
   e. False-negative PPD test may result from incorrect administration (must be intradermal), administration after recent live virus vaccination, or immunosuppression
   f. False-positive PPD test may result if the individual had prior immunization with the bacillus Calmette–Guérin (BCG) vaccine
   g. PPD test is contraindicated if history of BCG vaccination or active TB because severe local reaction can occur
   h. TB blood test (interferon-gamma release assay [IRGA]) measures how the immune system reacts to bacteria causing TB; result reported as positive or negative; preferred method for a person who has had BCG vaccination or will have trouble returning in 48–72 hours to read PPD skin test

5. Cytomegalovirus (CMV) antibody test
   a. Used to diagnose current, past, or reactivated CMV infection
   b. Indicated for pregnant or immunocompromised person if exposure is suspected or has flu-like symptoms that suggest a CMV infection
   c. IgM antibodies can be detected within a week or two after an initial exposure, usually decline and fall below detectable levels after a few months, levels rise again if latent CMV is reactivated
   d. IgG antibodies are produced several weeks after the initial CMV infection and provide protection from getting another primary infection; levels stabilize as infection resolves but remain detectable for the rest of life

6. Toxoplasmosis antibody test
   a. Used to diagnose current or past infection with *Toxoplasma gondii*
   b. Indicated for pregnant or immune-compromised individuals if exposure is suspected or have flu-like symptoms
   c. IgM antibodies can be detected within a week or two after an initial exposure; usually decline and fall below detectable levels after a few months
   d. IgG antibodies are produced several weeks after the initial infection and provide long-term protection; levels stabilize as infection resolves but remain detectable for the rest of life

- Strep throat test
   1. Determines if pharyngitis is caused by group A beta-hemolytic streptococci (GABHS)
   2. Indicated in adults with pharyngitis who meet two or more of the following criteria: fever, lack of cough, tonsillar exudates, tender anterior cervical adenopathy
   3. Specimen obtained with sterile swab rubbed against back of throat and tonsils
   4. Rapid streptococcal antigen test—positive test indicates presence of GABHS, negative test indicates individual probably does not have GABHS infection but more likely has a viral infection; 5%–15% of adult pharyngitis cases are caused by GABHS
   5. Throat culture not recommended for routine evaluation of adult pharyngitis or confirmation of a negative rapid antigen test
   6. Throat culture useful if other pathogens (e.g., gonococcus) are being considered
   7. See Chapter 3, *Primary Care*, for more information on pharyngitis

- Skin/wound culture
   1. Identifies organisms causing infection through superficial breaks in skin or involving deeper tissues
   2. Indicated if skin/wound is tender, red, swollen, draining fluid or pus, or slow to heal or is accompanied by fever
   3. Specimen obtained with sterile swab from cells or pus from the site of suspected infection; may include aspiration of fluid with syringe
   4. Specimen placed on appropriate nutrient media; if fungal infection is suspected, may require separate type of media
   5. Identifies type of pathogenic organism; includes susceptibility testing to identify antimicrobials that are likely to be effective against identified organism
   6. A Gram stain is often also performed to provide a more rapid preliminary result while culture is pending

- Cervical cytology and human papillomavirus (HPV) test
   1. Screening technique for detection of precancerous and early cancerous lesions of the uterine cervix
   2. Instruct patient to avoid douching, intercourse, and use of vaginal creams for 48 hours prior to the test
   3. Avoid scheduling when on menses
   4. Speculum may be lubricated with water prior to insertion
   5. Entire squamocolumnar junction (transformation zone) must be sampled with a spatula/broom device to avoid false negatives related to the sampling technique
   6. Endocervical sampling must be obtained with a broom device/endocervical brush
   7. Spatula—insert longer end into cervical os, press and rotate spatula 360°
   8. Endocervical brush—insert so bristles are fully in cervical os, rotate brush 180°
   9. Broom device—insert central bristles in the endocervical canal so that shorter bristles fully contact the ectocervix, push gently and rotate in a clockwise direction 5 times
   10. If slide preparation of specimen is used, rapid cytologic fixative application is essential to avoid air-drying artifact

11. HPV DNA testing can be performed on specimens transferred in aqueous solution
12. See Chapter 3, *Primary Care*, for cervical cancer screening recommendations and Chapter 5, *Gynecologic, Reproductive, and Sexual Disorders*, for information on management of abnormal results

- Colposcopy
  1. Used to inspect vagina, cervix, and/or vulva using a binocular microscope; detects lesions/abnormalities that may be biopsied for histologic examination; also used in anogenital examination to identify injuries from sexual assault
  2. Vagina and/or cervix—position speculum and colposcope for adequate visualization
  3. Swab cervix/vagina to remove secretions; wash cervix/vagina with 2% acetic acid to allow for easier identification of abnormalities
  4. Look for areas of abnormalities—aceto-white areas, abnormal vascular patterns (e.g., punctation, mosaic pattern, "corkscrew vessels"), leukoplakia visible before application of acetic acid
  5. Biopsy any abnormal areas
  6. Apply pressure to the biopsy site(s) with a large swab to stop bleeding
  7. Apply silver nitrate or Monsel's solution if bleeding continues

- Vulvar biopsy
  1. Used to sample areas of vulva that appear abnormal for diagnostic purposes; use on lesions smaller than 0.5 cm
  2. Use good lighting, magnifying lens, or colposcope; application of 5% acetic acid can enhance the identification of abnormal areas
  3. Identify vulvar lesion(s) to biopsy and inject local anesthetic
  4. Cleanse the area with an antiseptic solution or iodine-soaked swabs
  5. Place punch biopsy instrument over site and rotate several times with downward pressure to obtain specimen
  6. Elevate specimen from skin with forceps and incise at base with scissors
  7. Place specimen in histologic solution for transport to lab
  8. Control bleeding—pressure, silver nitrate, Monsel's solution
  9. Instruct patient to call if any redness, increasing discomfort, malodorous or bloody drainage, fever

- Endometrial biopsy
  1. Used to evaluate abnormal bleeding (perimenopause, postmenopause); rule out/confirm endometritis; determine endometrial response to progesterone in infertile individuals suspected to have luteal-phase defect
  2. If pregnancy is a possibility, time to avoid potential disruption of implantation
  3. Inform patient that there may be cramping while biopsy instrument is in uterus; may take NSAID 30–60 minutes before procedure and/or use topical anesthesia on cervix

  4. Perform bimanual examination—determine uterine position and size
  5. Insert appropriate-size speculum; evaluate cervix and vagina for any signs of infection—do not proceed if suspect infection
  6. Cleanse ectocervix and vagina with antiseptic
  7. May manually curve tip of endometrial pipelle while in sterile package to accommodate uterine curvature
  8. Apply tenaculum to stabilize cervix/straighten uterus, as needed, if anteflexed or retroflexed, remove tenaculum after pipelle is inserted
  9. Gently pass endometrial pipelle through cervix up to fundus
  10. Pull back rapidly on the piston as far as it will go to create suction; rotate the pipelle 360 degrees, moving from the fundus down to the internal cervical os and repeating 3 or 4 times
  11. Transfer contents of pipelle into histologic solution for transport to lab
  12. Have the patient remain supine for a few minutes until any pain or dizziness passes, and observe for vasovagal response
  13. Provide perineal pad, may use NSAIDs for cramping; advise to return if severe cramping, heavy bleeding, bleeding lasting longer than 2 days, foul-smelling discharge

- Breast biopsy
  1. Used to determine whether breast mass found on examination or through imaging contains benign or malignant cells
  2. Fine-needle aspiration—obtains fluid/cells from breast mass
     a. Cleanse the area with antiseptic; local anesthesia usually not required
     b. Secure breast mass with one hand; introduce a 20- or 22-gauge needle attached to a 10- to 20-mL syringe
     c. Withdraw all fluid from the cyst and prepare a slide of specimen if the fluid is not clear
     d. If no fluid obtained, the mass is likely solid; pass the needle through the mass several times with suction to obtain a cellular specimen, then prepare the slide
     e. Apply firm pressure over site for 5–10 minutes to prevent a hematoma
  3. Tissue biopsy—leads to a definitive diagnosis, with histologic findings providing the foundation for a treatment plan
     a. Wire-guided excisional biopsy—wire placed percutaneously in the vicinity of abnormality by the radiologist; needle may be placed over the wire for better localization; surgeon uses the wire to guide the removal of abnormal tissue
     b. Stereotactic core needle biopsy—patient placed prone on table with breast in dependent position; breast imaged to localize lesion; core biopsy needle advanced into lesion; cores of tissue obtained for evaluation

- Genetic testing
  1. Identifies changes in chromosomes, genes, or proteins
  2. Genes—basic unit of heredity passed from parents to offspring; consist of segments of DNA arranged along a chromosome; humans have about 23,000 genes

3. Chromosomes—found in the nucleus of the cell; contain genes; normal human cell contains 46 chromosomes in pairs; 22 pairs are autosomes, and one pair is the sex chromosomes

4. Karyotype—individual's collection of chromosomes; also lab technique used to produce an image of an individual's chromosomes and look for abnormal numbers or structures—for example, trisomy 21, or Down syndrome, in which individual has three copies of chromosome 21 instead of two copies

5. Gene mutation—change in DNA sequence
   a. Somatic mutation—acquired; occurs after conception; DNA copying mistake during cell division or exposure to ionizing radiation, chemicals, or viruses during gestation or later in life
   b. Germ cell mutation—inherited; occurs during conception; present in egg or sperm cells of parent

6. Genetic marker—DNA sequence with known physical location on a chromosome; can help link inherited disease with the responsible genes; several genetic markers are associated with increased risk of breast cancer

7. Purposes of genetic testing
   a. Susceptibility testing—determines whether an individual carries a genetic variation that increases the potential risk for developing a condition (e.g., *BRCA* 1 or 2); not every person with the variant will develop the condition
   b. Predictive testing—determines whether an individual carries genetic variation associated with the later development of a genetic disorder (e.g., Huntington's disease); a person with the variant will eventually develop the disorder
   c. Carrier screening—determines whether an asymptomatic individual has a variant within a gene associated with a particular disorder (e.g., sickle cell disease, cystic fibrosis disease); may be part of prepregnancy or prenatal screening; expanded carrier screening evaluates individual's carrier state for multiple conditions simultaneously and regardless of ethnicity

8. Basic principles of genetic testing
   a. Respect patient autonomy and confidentiality; testing is voluntary
   b. Provide information in a clear, objective, nondirective fashion
   c. Inform about protections and limitations of the Genetic Information Discrimination Act (GINA)—illegal for health insurers to require results/use to make decisions about coverage, rates; illegal to discriminate against employees or applicants because of genetic information; does not apply to life, long-term, or disability insurance
   d. If testing reveals a significant variant with heritable potential, encourage the patient to inform relatives of the results
   e. Offer screening to reproductive partner if patient is identified as carrier of specific condition

9. Pattern of inheritance of genetic conditions caused by mutations in a single gene depends on the gene involved (**Table 2-7**)

Table 2-7 Inheritance Patterns

Inheritance Pattern	Description	Examples
Autosomal dominant	<ul><li>Only one mutated copy of gene in each cell needed</li><li>Usually have one affected parent</li><li>Each offspring has 50% chance of inheriting abnormal gene and having condition and 50% chance of not being affected</li></ul>	Huntington's disease, *BRCA1/BRCA2* mutations, Lynch syndrome
Autosomal recessive	<ul><li>Two mutated copies of gene present needed to have disease</li><li>Usually have unaffected parents (carriers—each has single copy of mutated gene)</li><li>If both parents are carriers, offspring has 50% chance of being a carrier, 25% chance of having disease, 25% chance of being unaffected</li></ul>	Cystic fibrosis, sickle cell anemia
X-linked dominant	<ul><li>Mutation in genes on X chromosome</li><li>Females more frequently affected than males</li><li>Males cannot pass trait to sons</li><li>If female is affected, both male and female offspring have 50% chance of inheriting the disorder</li></ul>	Fragile X syndrome
X-linked recessive	<ul><li>Mutation in genes on X chromosome</li><li>Males more frequently affected than females</li><li>Males cannot pass trait to sons</li><li>Female offspring (XX) need to inherit affected X chromosome from both parents as carriers to have the condition</li><li>Males (XY) need to inherit only the affected X chromosome from female to have the condition</li></ul>	Hemophilia

10. Other disorders may be caused by a combination of effects of multiple genes or by interactions between genes and the environment—heart disease, diabetes, schizophrenia, certain types of cancer

Imaging Studies

- Pelvic ultrasonography
  1. Use of high-frequency sound waves to evaluate internal pelvic organs/structures for diagnostic purposes
     a. Distinguish between solid and cystic pelvic masses
     b. Confirm viability and location of gestation/products of conception
     c. Determine endometrial thickness
     d. Evaluate the size/location of uterine myomas
     e. Evaluate adnexal masses/fullness
     f. Evaluate fetal growth
     g. Detect fetal anomalies/abnormalities
  2. Transabdominal pelvic ultrasound—use if pelvic structures to be examined extend into abdomen; instruct patient to have full bladder; pass transducer over tissue/organs to be examined
  3. Transvaginal ultrasound—better resolution than transabdominal ultrasound; instruct patient to empty bladder, use vaginal probe placed in sterile sheath (glove, condom)
- Mammography
  1. Radiographic examination of the breast to determine the presence of small cancerous, precancerous, and benign lesions; screening and diagnostic use
  2. Digital mammography—detectors convert X-rays into electric signals, produce images that can be seen on a computer screen; most centers now use digital mammography
  3. Digital mammography and conventional film mammography are similar in overall inability to detect breast cancer
  4. Digital mammography may offer better detection in individuals who are premenopausal, perimenopausal, and/or have dense breast tissue
  5. Tomosynthesis/three-dimensional (3D) mammography—modification of digital mammography providing images as thin slices; FDA approved for screening
  6. Mammographic findings standardized terminology—Breast Imaging Reporting and Data System (BI-RADS): six assessment categories (0–5) provide an overall assessment of the likelihood that findings represent a malignancy
  7. Instruct patient to avoid use of any underarm deodorant spray or powder prior to procedure

8. Typically, two views are taken of each breast for screening mammogram
9. Target specific area with multiple views and magnifications if a suspicious lesion found on clinical breast examination or screening mammogram—diagnostic mammogram
10. Referral and/or biopsy recommended on any clinically suspicious lesion regardless of mammography results
11. See Chapter 3, *Primary Care*, for mammography screening recommendations

- Breast ultrasound
  1. Use of high-frequency sound waves as adjunct to mammography to assist in diagnosis of breast disease; not a screening tool
  2. Helpful in differentiating cystic from solid masses
  3. May be used as a guide for needle aspiration, needle core biopsy, and localization procedures
  4. Handheld, real-time, high-frequency probe passed over tissue to be examined
- Bone densitometry/bone density testing
  1. Used for screening, diagnosis and monitoring treatment of osteopenia and osteoporosis
  2. T-score used to compare bone density in postmenopausal individuals to same-sex young adult reference population
     a. Normal—bone mineral density (BMD) within 1 standard deviation (SD) of young normal adult; T-score greater than −1
     b. Osteopenia—BMD between 1 and 2.5 SD below that of young normal adult; T-score between −1 and −2.5
     c. Osteoporosis—BMD 2.5 SD or more below that of young normal adult; T-score at or less than −2.5
  3. Z-score used to compare bone density in individual to age-, sex, and ethnicity-matched reference population; may be used in evaluation for secondary causes of osteoporosis
  4. Procedure for dual-energy X-ray absorptiometry (DEXA) scan—most-used technique, low radiation exposure
     a. Patient lies supine while imager passes over body
     b. Process takes 10–15 minutes
     c. Computer calculates the density of the patient's bones
     d. Image/regions scanned for osteoporosis diagnosis—hip, spine, radius; use of other sites, such as heel or finger, may predict fracture risk but cannot be used for diagnosis
     e. See Chapter 3, *Primary Care*, for bone density screening guidelines and more information on osteoporosis

Questions

Select the best answer.

1. A 17-year-old patient presents at the clinic with the following reason for seeking care: "I have been sick for 3 days. I feel sick to my stomach and have diarrhea." Which of the following would be most appropriate to document as their reason for their visit/chief complaint?
   a. Flulike symptoms
   b. GI distress
   c. "I feel sick to my stomach and have diarrhea."
   d. Possible pregnancy, needs further evaluation

2. Which of the following would be considered a subjective assessment finding to be placed in the S section of SOAP format charting?
   a. Motile trichomonads
   b. Mucopurulent discharge
   c. *Tichomoniasis vaginitis*
   d. Vaginal itching

3. Which of the following includes a pertinent negative that needs to be documented?
   a. 16-year-old patient who has never been sexually active; no history of STIs
   b. 25-year-old patient with abdominal pain; no nausea, vomiting, or diarrhea
   c. 40-year-old patient with depression; past history of suicidal attempt
   d. 60-year-old patient with stress incontinence; no breast mass or nipple discharge

4. Appropriate information in the review of systems section of the health history would include:
   a. alert, cooperative, well groomed.
   b. had measles and chickenpox as a child.
   c. occasional loss of urine with coughing.
   d. walks 2 miles a day for exercise.

5. Which of the following would most appropriately be documented in the A section of SOAP charting format?
   a. CBC ordered
   b. Patient states that she would like to quit smoking.
   c. Medication instructions provided
   d. Mucopurulent cervicitis

6. The bell of the stethoscope should be used when listening for:
   a. bowel sounds.
   b. carotid bruits.
   c. lung sounds.
   d. S_1 and S_2 heart sounds.

7. Evaluation of EOM movement includes:
   a. ophthalmoscopic examination.
   b. PERRLA evaluation.
   c. the six cardinal fields of gaze.
   d. visual fields by confrontation.

8. The adventitious lung sound most associated with asthma is:
   a. crackles.
   b. pleural rub.
   c. rhonchi.
   d. wheezes.

9. When auscultating lung sounds, the normal finding over most of the lung fields is:
   a. bronchial.
   b. resonant.
   c. tympanic.
   d. vesicular.

10. Increased tactile fremitus would be an expected finding in a patient with:
    a. asthma.
    b. emphysema.
    c. lobar pneumonia.
    d. pleural effusion.

11. The sound heard over the cardiac area if the patient has pericarditis is mostly likely to be a(n):
    a. diastolic murmur.
    b. fixed split S_2.
    c. friction rub.
    d. increased S_4.

12. Which of the following is an abnormal abdominal examination finding in an adult?
    a. Abdominal aorta 2.5 cm in width
    b. Liver border nonpalpable
    c. Liver span 8 cm at the right MCL
    d. Splenic dullness at the left anterior axillary line

13. One of the cranial nerves for which you would test both motor and sensory function is:
    a. CN II—optic nerve.
    b. CN V—trigeminal nerve.
    c. CN VI—abducens nerve.
    d. CN XI—spinal accessory nerve.

14. A patient with an Hgb of 10.2 g/dL and RBC indices indicating both microcytosis and hypochromia most likely has:
    a. folic acid deficiency.
    b. iron deficiency.
    c. severe dehydration.
    d. vitamin B_{12} deficiency.

15. A patient with an increased WBC count related to infectious hepatitis would most likely have an elevated level of:
    a. basophils.
    b. eosinophils.
    c. lymphocytes.
    d. neutrophils.

16. Expected thyroid function test findings with primary hypothyroidism include:
    a. decreased TSH and decreased FT_4.
    b. decreased TSH and increased FT_4.
    c. increased TSH and decreased FT_4.
    d. increased TSH and increased FT_4.

17. A pregnant patient presents with a recent-onset rash. Which of the following laboratory results would be reassuring that this is not likely rubella?
    a. HAI titer of 1:10 at their initial visit 1 month earlier
    b. HAI titer of 1:128 at the current visit
    c. Increased IgG antibody levels at the current visit
    d. Increased IgM antibody levels at the current visit

18. A patient who had HBV 6 months ago currently has no symptoms but has a positive test for HBsAg. This most likely indicates that she:
    a. has immunity to future infection.
    b. has persistent active infection.
    c. is a chronic carrier of HBV.
    d. is in the early stage of reinfection.

19. A false-negative TB PPD test may be the result of:
    a. dormant infection.
    b. immunosuppression.
    c. intradermal injection.
    d. prior BCG vaccination.

20. A patient with cholecystitis would most likely have a(n):
    a. decreased alkaline phosphatase.
    b. decreased indirect bilirubin.
    c. increased albumin level.
    d. increased direct bilirubin.

21. Measuring waist circumference is most appropriate when a patient's BMI places them in which of the following categories?
    a. Underweight
    b. Normal weight
    c. Overweight
    d. Extreme obesity

22. Which of the following lab values is not normally affected by pregnancy?
    a. Cholesterol
    b. MCV
    c. T_4
    d. Triglycerides

23. A 65-year-old female has a bone densitometry test, with the results of the T-score being −2.0. This indicates she has:
    a. bone density that is greater than that of most females her age.
    b. bone density that is equal to that of a young normal adult.
    c. bone loss that is at the level for a diagnosis of osteopenia.
    d. bone loss that is at the level for a diagnosis of osteoporosis.

24. Appropriate management for a 45-year-old patient who has no diabetes risk factors and no symptoms of diabetes with a fasting glucose of 130 mg/dL would include which of the following?
    a. Inform the patient she has impaired glucose tolerance.
    b. Order HbA_{1c} level.
    c. Repeat glucose testing on another day.
    d. Repeat glucose screening in 3 years.

25. A patient who either has acute active HBV infection or who is a carrier (chronic active state) would have a positive test for:
    a. HBsAg.
    b. HBsAb.
    c. HBeAg.
    d. HBeAb.

26. Tests for cerebellar function include:
    a. deep tendon reflex evaluation.
    b. short-term memory evaluation.

c. discriminatory sensation tests.
d. Romberg test for balance.

27. Which of the following statements is correct regarding autosomal recessive inheritance of a genetic disorder?
    a. Both parents are unaffected but are carriers of the mutated gene.
    b. Disorder tends to occur in every generation of the affected family.
    c. Male offspring are more likely to be affected than females.
    d. One parent has the genetic disorder with the mutated gene.

28. Obtaining a Z-score on a bone mineral density test might be appropriate for evaluating:
    a. a 40-year-old female with a nontraumatic hip fracture.
    b. a 46-year-old female with a strong family history of osteoporosis.
    c. a 60-year-old female who smokes cigarettes and has low body weight.
    d. a 70-year-old female with osteoporosis being treated with a bisphosphonate.

29. A patient who was treated for primary syphilis 1 year ago now has the following test results: VDRL nonreactive and FTA-ABS positive. These findings indicate that the patient most likely:
    a. was not adequately treated for primary syphilis 1 year ago.
    b. has become reinfected since the completion of the treatment 1 year ago.
    c. has some other condition that is causing a false-positive FTA-ABS.
    d. was treated adequately for syphilis and has not become reinfected.

30. Which of the following heart sounds may be a normal finding in the third trimester of pregnancy?
    a. Diastolic murmur
    b. Fixed split S_2
    c. S_3
    d. S_4

31. Pelvic findings on examination of a 22-year-old nulliparous patient are uterus 7 cm in length and ovaries 3 cm × 2 cm × 1 cm. These findings are consistent with:
    a. an enlarged uterus and enlarged ovaries.
    b. a normal-size uterus and enlarged ovaries.
    c. an enlarged uterus and normal-size ovaries.
    d. a normal-size uterus and normal-size ovaries.

32. A laboratory test finding of increased immature neutrophils (shift to the left) is consistent with a(n):
    a. acute bacterial infection.
    b. acute viral infection.
    c. allergic reaction.
    d. chronic bacterial infection.

33. An elderly patient has had gastroenteritis with vomiting and diarrhea for the past 3 days. The patient's mucous membranes appear dry and has not urinated yet today. Expected laboratory test findings related directly to these signs and symptoms might include:
    a. decreased urine specific gravity.
    b. decreased hematocrit.

c. increased blood glucose.

d. increased blood urea nitrogen.

34. The blood type in which an individual has no antigens on their RBCs is:
    a. AB+.
    b. AB–.
    c. O+.
    d. O–.

35. The heart sound heard best at the base of the heart is:
    a. S_1.
    b. S_2.
    c. S_3.
    d. S_4.

36. A patient who was sexually assaulted 3 weeks ago by an individual known to be HIV positive has a nonreactive HIV antibody test result. The most appropriate next step would be to:
    a. advise the patient to return for repeat testing in 3 months.
    b. order an HIV-1 p24 antigen test.
    c. order a Western blot test to confirm the nonreactive EIA test result.
    d. reassure the patient that she does not have HIV infection.

37. An abnormal finding on ophthalmoscopic examination would be:
    a. arterioles smaller than veins.
    b. a yellow optic disc.
    c. presence of a red reflex.
    d. tapering of the veins.

38. When examining the cervix of a 20-year-old patient, you note that most of the cervix is pink, but there is a small ring of dark-red tissue surrounding the os. This is most likely:
    a. an endocervical polyp.
    b. due to cervical dysplasia.
    c. due to cervical infection.
    d. the squamocolumnar junction.

39. The laboratory test that is done for definitive diagnosis of sickle cell disease is:
    a. Hgb electrophoresis.
    b. peripheral blood smear.
    c. RBC indices.
    d. sickle cell preparation.

40. An individual who is currently 18 weeks, pregnant and has had two full-term deliveries and one first-trimester abortion would be considered:
    a. gravida 2 para 2.
    b. gravida 3 para 2.
    c. gravida 3 para 3.
    d. gravida 4 para 2.

41. The best position for palpating the axilla is with the patient:
    a. lying down with the arm above the head on the side you are examining.
    b. lying down with the arm down at the side on the side you are examining.

c. sitting up with the arm raised above the head on the side you are examining.

d. sitting up with the arm down on the side you are examining.

42. Which of the following would be considered a positive PPD result?
    a. General population: 5 mm induration
    b. General population: 10 mm induration
    c. Moderate-risk population: 5 mm induration
    d. High-risk population: 5 mm induration

43. Abnormal findings on a urinalysis would include:
    a. pH 5.0.
    b. specific gravity 1.5.
    c. WBCs 3 per HPF.
    d. protein 4 mg/dL.

44. Adding KOH to a wet mount slide before viewing it under the microscope is useful in the detection of:
    a. clue cells.
    b. pseudohyphae.
    c. trichomonads.
    d. WBCs.

45. A 42-year-old patient is concerned about the possibility of a pregnancy because of being 12 days late for a period. The best initial pregnancy test to obtain is a:
    a. qualitative sensitive urine hCG test.
    b. qualitative serum hCG test.
    c. quantitative sensitive urine hCG test.
    d. quantitative serum hCG test.

46. A patient presents with no symptoms but is concerned because she had sexual intercourse 3 weeks ago with a new partner who has recently disclosed having a history of genital herpes. The patient wants to know if a test can be performed at this visit to see if she has been infected. Which of the following would be the best response?
    a. A Pap test can be done at this visit to show if she has been infected.
    b. A blood test can be done at this visit to see if she has recently been infected.
    c. If she does not develop lesions in the next 4–8 weeks, she is not infected.
    d. She can have a blood test in 1–2 months to determine whether she has herpes antibodies.

47. The glands located posteriorly on each side of the vaginal orifice are the:
    a. Bartholin's glands.
    b. Bulbar glands.
    c. Nabothian glands.
    d. Skene's glands.

48. Which of the following statements regarding gene mutations is correct?
    a. All gene mutations occur at the time of conception.
    b. Germ cell mutations occur after conception.
    c. Germ cell mutations may occur as a result of exposure to radiation.
    d. Somatic mutations may occur at any time in a person's life.

49. The CDC-recommended diagnostic test for *Trichomonas* is:
    a. culture.
    b. NAAT.
    c. vaginal fluid sialidase test.
    d. wet mount evaluation for motile trichomonads.

50. Which of the following statements concerning testing for strep throat in an adult patient with sore throat, fever, and tonsillar exudate is correct?
    a. A positive rapid streptococcal antigen test indicates the need for antibiotic treatment.
    b. No testing is indicated, as these findings indicate a viral infection.
    c. Throat culture is recommended rather than a rapid streptococcal antigen test.
    d. Throat culture is indicated if a rapid streptococcal antigen test is negative.

51. A premenopausal individual with which of the following conditions would be most likely to have a low FSH and low estradiol level?
    a. Adrenal tumor
    b. Anorexia nervosa
    c. Premature ovarian failure
    d. Turner's syndrome

52. Minimizing risks of retraumatization may include:
    a. adjusting lighting in the exam room.
    b. gather a patient's history during the physical exam.
    c. not addressing the history of trauma.
    d. developing the plan of care for the patient.

53. Which question is **not** an example of a strength-focused questioning to foster resilience?
    a. What creative ways have you learned to deal with painful feelings?
    b. What specific behaviors do you believe helped you survive during and after your traumatic experience?
    c. What specific problems have you had since your traumatic experience?
    d. What coping tools have you learned from your spiritual practices?

54. Using a trauma-informed model of care, who is responsible for screening and/or identifying patients with trauma?
    a. Clinician
    b. Student
    c. Receptionist
    d. All of the above

55. What should always be obtained prior to any physical exam?
    a. Consent
    b. Insurance information
    c. Last menstrual period
    d. Pregnancy test

56. Instructions for a patient who is going to be doing a fecal immunochemical test at home should include:
    a. avoid consumption of red meat for 3 days prior to testing.
    b. eat only cooked vegetables with no raw vegetables for 3 days prior to testing.
    c. only one stool sample is required for the test.
    d. a positive test requires a follow-up with a guaiac-based fecal occult blood test.

57. The most likely diagnosis for a patient who presents with an acutely painful, tender, swollen testicle retracted upward in the scrotum is:
    a. acute epididymitis.
    b. Peyronie's disease.
    c. torsion of spermatic cord.
    d. varicocele.

58. The test used to screen for the presence of any circulating antibodies against RBCs during pregnancy is a(n):
    a. antinuclear antibodies test.
    b. direct Coombs test.
    c. hemoglobin electrophoresis.
    d. indirect Coombs test.

59. Genetic testing for *BRCA 1 or 2* gene mutations is considered:
    a. carrier testing.
    b. karyotype testing.
    c. predictive testing.
    d. susceptibility testing.

60. Which of the following is recommended as a component of cultural assessment?
    a. Avoid silence so as not to make the patient uncomfortable.
    b. Do not make generalized assumptions based on what you know about the culture.
    c. Explain there is no evidence for supernatural forces causing illness.
    d. Use touch and sitting close to the patient to promote trust.

Answers with Rationales

1. **c.** "I feel sick to my stomach and have diarrhea."
   In the health history, the reason for a patient's visit/chief concern should be documented as a brief statement in the patient's own words.

2. **d.** Vaginal itching
   Subjective information is obtained as part of the health history and is what the patient or caregiver tells you.

3. **b.** 25-year-old patient with abdominal pain; no nausea, vomiting, or diarrhea

The description of presenting symptoms should include pertinent negatives. When a symptom suggests that an abnormality may exist or may develop in that area, include documentation of the absence of symptoms that may help eliminate some of the possibilities.

4. **c.** occasional loss of urine with coughing
   The review of systems is used to assess common symptoms for each major body system to avoid missing any potential or existing problems.

5. **d.** Mucopurulent cervicitis
   The A section of the SOAP charting format includes your diagnosis or prioritized list of problems determined from your assessment of subjective and objective data.

6. **b.** carotid bruits
   The bell of the stethoscope is best for listening to low-pitched sounds, such as those heard over large blood vessels.

7. **c.** the six cardinal fields of gaze
   EOM function is evaluated by assessing symmetry, lid lag, and nystagmus as the patient holds their head still and follows your finger through the six cardinal fields of gaze.

8. **d.** wheezes
   Wheezes are high-pitched (sound like a squeak), continuous adventitious lung sounds that may be heard when air flows through constricted passageways in conditions such as asthma.

9. **d.** vesicular
   The lung sound over most of the lung fields is vesicular, with inspiratory sounds lasting longer than expiratory sounds.

10. **c.** lobar pneumonia
    Tactile fremitus refers to the palpable transmission of vibrations through the bronchus to the chest wall when the patient speaks. There is increased transmission through consolidated tissue, as is found with lobar pneumonia.

11. **c.** friction rub
    A pericardial friction rub may be heard over the cardiac area as a grating sound throughout the cardiac cycle when inflammation of the pericardium is present.

12. **d.** Splenic dullness at the left anterior axillary line
    Splenic dullness may be percussed at the sixth to tenth ICS just posterior to the midaxillary line on the left side, with the patient in the supine position. Splenic dullness at the anterior axillary line is indicative of an enlarged spleen.

13. **b.** CN V—trigeminal nerve
    The cranial nerves with both motor and sensory functions are CN V (trigeminal nerve), CN VII (facial nerve), CN IX (glossopharyngeal nerve), and CN X (vagus nerve). Routinely, CN V is the only cranial nerve in which you test both motor and sensory function.

14. **b.** iron deficiency
    RBC indices provide information about the size, weight, and Hgb concentration of RBCs and are useful in classifying anemia when the individual has a low Hgb level. Iron-deficiency anemia is characterized by abnormally small (microcytic) and pale (hypochromic) RBCs.

15. **c.** lymphocytes
    The WBC count with differential provides information useful in evaluating an individual with infection, neoplasm, allergy, or immunosuppression. Lymphocytes and monocytes are increased with acute viral infections and chronic bacterial infections.

16. **c.** increased TSH and decreased FT_4
    An increased TSH level is seen with primary hypothyroidism and thyroiditis. A decreased FT_4 level is seen with hypothyroidism.

17. **a.** HAI titer of 1:10 at their initial visit 1 month earlier
    The HAI test is used to detect immunity to rubella and to diagnose rubella infection. Titers of 1:10 or greater indicate immunity to rubella. High titers (1:64 or greater) may indicate current rubella infection.

18. **c.** is a chronic carrier of HBV
    HBsAg rises before the onset of clinical symptoms, peaks during the first week of symptoms, and returns to normal by the time jaundice subsides. An individual is considered a carrier (remains infectious) if HBsAg persists.

19. **b.** immunosuppression
    False-negative TB PPD tests may result from incorrect administration (must be intradermal) or immunosuppression.

20. **d.** increased direct bilirubin
    An elevated direct (conjugated) bilirubin level occurs with gallstones and obstruction of the extrahepatic duct.

21. **c.** Overweight
    Waist circumference provides measurement of abdominal fat as an independent prediction of risk for type 2 diabetes, dyslipidemia, hypertension, and cardiovascular disease in individuals with a BMI between 25 and 39.9 (overweight and obesity). Waist circumference has little added value in disease risk prediction in individuals with a BMI of 40 or greater (extreme obesity).

22. **b.** MCV
    Cholesterol and triglyceride levels may be elevated during pregnancy. T_4 levels are affected by the amount of TBG, which is increased during pregnancy. The MCV is the average volume or size of a single RBC. Although the Hgb/Hct levels may be lower during pregnancy, the size of the RBCs should not change unless the patient has iron-deficiency anemia, thalassemia, vitamin B_{12} deficiency, or folic acid deficiency.

23. **c.** bone loss that is at the level for a diagnosis of osteopenia
    Osteopenia is defined as BMD between 1 and 2 SD below that of a young average adult. This is a T-score of between -1 and -2.5.

24. **c.** Repeat glucose testing on another day.
    A fasting glucose of 126 mg/dL or greater is diagnostic for diabetes. Repeat testing should be done on a subsequent day to confirm the diagnosis.

25. **a.** HBsAg
    HBsAg is present with both acute active infection and a chronic active (carrier) state.

26. **d.** Romberg test for balance
    The cerebellum coordinates motor activity, maintains equilibrium, and helps to control posture.

27. **a.** Both parents are unaffected but are carriers of the mutated gene.
    In autosomal recessive inheritance of a genetic disorder, the affected individual has two mutated copies of the responsible gene in each cell. The affected individual usually has unaffected parents (carriers), each carrying a single copy of the mutated gene.

28. **a.** a 40-year-old female with a nontraumatic hip fracture
    A Z-score may be used to compare bone density in a premenopausal female to an age-, sex,-, and ethnicity-matched

reference population to evaluate for secondary causes of osteoporosis.

29. **d.** was treated adequately for syphilis and has not become reinfected
Nontreponemal tests (VDRL, RPR) usually become nonreactive with time after treatment. Treponemal tests (FAT-ABS, TPI) usually remain positive indefinitely after treatment.

30. **c.** S_3
An increased S_3 may be audible in late pregnancy. This heart sound is heard early in diastole during rapid ventricular filling.

31. **d.** a normal-size uterus and normal-size ovaries
The uterus is 5.5–8 cm long and pear shaped in the nulliparous patient. During the reproductive years, the ovaries are approximately 3 cm × 2 cm × 1 cm.

32. **a.** acute bacterial infection
Neutrophils are increased with acute bacterial infections and trauma. Increased immature neutrophil forms (band or stab cells), referred to as a "shift to the left," are seen with ongoing acute bacterial infection.

33. **d.** increased blood urea nitrogen
BUN is an indirect measure of renal and liver function. Increased levels may be seen with hypovolemia, dehydration, reduced cardiac function, GI bleeding, starvation, sepsis, and renal disease.

34. **d.** O–
Blood types are grouped according to the presence or absence of antigens A, B, and Rh on RBCs. Blood type O negative has no antigens on RBCs.

35. **b.** S_2
The S_2 heart sound is heard best at the base of the heart using the diaphragm of the stethoscope.

36. **b.** order an HIV-1 p24 antigen test
The HIV-1 p24 antigen test detects HIV-1 antigen at 15 days, peaks at 25–30 days, then declines with antibody development. HIV antibodies are detectable as early as 21–28 days and in 95% of individuals within 6 months of infection. A combined HIV antibody and p24 antigen test is available.

37. **d.** tapering of the veins
The average retinal artery wall is transparent except for the column of blood going down the middle, so a vein crossing beneath the artery can be seen up to the column of blood on either side (arteriovenous crossing). When narrowing of the retinal artery occurs (as with hypertension), the arterial wall thickens and becomes less transparent. The vein crossing under the narrowed artery appears to taper down on either side of the artery.

38. **d.** the squamocolumnar junction
The squamocolumnar junction is where the squamous epithelium (pink) and columnar epithelium (dark red) of the cervix meet. The junction may be inside the cervical os, so that only squamous epithelium is visible, or a ring of columnar tissue may be visible to a varying extent around the os.

39. **a.** Hgb electrophoresis
The sickle cell preparation is used to screen for sickle cell disease and trait. A positive test indicates the presence of Hgb S, indicating either sickle cell disease or trait. Hgb electrophoresis is the definitive test performed if the screening test is positive, as it identifies Hgb type and quantity.

40. **d.** gravida 4 para 2
Gravida denotes the total number of pregnancies, including a current pregnancy. *Para* denotes the total number of pregnancies reaching 20 weeks or longer gestation.

41. **d.** sitting up with her arm down on the side you are examining
The examiner palpates the axillary lymph nodes and the breast tissue that extends into the axillary area (tail of Spence) with the patient sitting with arms relaxed at their side. The examiner supports the lower arm and uses the palmar surface of the fingers to palpate the entire area.

42. **d.** High-risk population: 5 mm induration
In the individual considered at high risk for tuberculosis, a PPD skin test resulting in a 5-mm or greater area of induration is a positive reaction.

43. **b.** specific gravity 1.5
Normal values are as follows: specific gravity 1.005–1.030, pH 4.6–8.0, WBCs 0–4 per HPF, and protein 0–8 mg/dL.

44. **b.** pseudohyphae
The addition of KOH to the vaginal wet mount slide facilitates visualization of *Candida* pseudohyphae and buds.

45. **a.** qualitative sensitive urine hCG test
Sensitive urine hCG tests may detect pregnancy as early as 28 days from the last menstrual period. Cross-reactions with other hormones are not a problem. A qualitative (positive/negative) test is the appropriate pregnancy test choice.

46. **d.** She can have a blood test in 1–2 months to determine whether she has herpes antibodies.
Type-specific serologic tests detect HSV-1 and HSV-2 antibodies. Seroconversion may take 4–12 weeks to occur.

47. **a.** Bartholin's glands
The glands located posteriorly on each side of the vaginal orifice are the Bartholin's glands.

48. **d.** Somatic mutations may occur at any time in a person's life.
Somatic mutations are acquired and occur after conception. A DNA copying mistake may occur during cell division or from exposure to ionizing radiation, chemicals, or viruses during gestation or later in life.

49. **b.** NAAT
The CDC-recommended test for *Trichomonas* is the NAAT. It is more sensitive than a wet mount or culture.

50. **a.** A positive rapid streptococcal antigen test indicates the need for antibiotic treatment.
A positive rapid streptococcal antigen test indicates the presence of GABHS requiring antibiotic treatment. A negative test indicates that the infection is more

likely viral. A culture is not needed to confirm a negative test.

51. **b.** Anorexia nervosa

The premenopausal patient with anorexia nervosa may have both a low FSH and low estradiol level.

52. **a.** adjusting lighting in the exam room

After addressing the history of trauma, the clinician may find that dim or harsh lighting may be a triggering event during a sensitive physical exam, and lighting adjustments may be required to minimize retraumatization.

53. **c.** What specific problems have you had since your traumatic experience?

Promoting resilience and fostering trauma-resistant skills focuses on developing those self-care skills, coping strategies, identifying supportive networks, focusing on their strengths, and a sense of competence with oneself.

54. **d.** All of the above

Universal screening should be performed on all patients, and all members of the healthcare team and staff should utilize a trauma-informed approach.

55. **a.** Consent

Consent should always be obtained prior to any physical exam.

56. **c.** only one stool sample is required for the test

Fecal immunochemical testing only requires one stool sample. There are no dietary or medication restrictions prior to testing.

57. **c.** torsion of spermatic cord

Twisting of a testicle on its spermatic cord causes acute pain, tenderness, swelling, and retraction of the testicle upward in the scrotum.

58. **d.** indirect Coombs test

An indirect Coombs test is used to screen for any circulating antibodies against RBCs during pregnancy.

59. **d.** susceptibility testing

Genetic testing for *BRCA 1 or 2* gene mutations is considered susceptibility testing. Susceptibility testing determines whether an individual carries a genetic variation that increases the potential risk of developing a condition. Only some people with the variant will develop the conditions.

60. **b.** Do not make any generalized assumptions based on what you know about the culture.

Generalized assumptions can lead to unintentional biases and culturally insensitive care.

Bibliography

American College of Obstetricians and Gynecologists. (2017). Committee Opinion No. 691. Carrier screening for genetic conditions. *Obstetrics and Gynecology, 129*(3), e41–e55.

American College of Obstetricians and Gynecologists. (2018). Committee Opinion No. 729: Importance of social determinants of health and cultural awareness in the delivery of reproductive health care. *Obstetrics and Gynecology, 131*(1), e43–e48.

American Diabetes Association. (2021). Standards of medical care in diabetes. *Diabetes Care, 44*(suppl 1), S1–S232.

Ball, J., Dains, J., Flynn, J., Solomon, B., & Stewart, R. (2019). *Seidel's guide to physical examination* (9th ed.). Mosby.

Beloff, M. S., Greenspan, S. L., Insogna, K. L., Lewiecki, E. M., Saag, K. G., Singer, A. J., & Siris, E. S. (2022). The clinician's guide to prevention and treatment of osteoporosis. *Osteoporosis International, 33*, 2049–2102.

H. Carcio, & M. Secor (2018). *Advanced health assessment of women: Clinical skills and procedures* (4th ed.). Springer.

Centers for Disease Control and Prevention. (2020). *Testing recommendations for hepatitis C virus infection.* https://cdc.gov/hepatitis/hcv/guidelinesc.html

Centers for Disease Control and Prevention. (2021). *Diagnostic tests: Newer, improved HIV tests allow for earlier HIV detection.* https://www.cdc.gov/hiv/clinicians/screening/diagnostic-tests.html

Institute of Medicine. (2015). *Cognitive aging: Progress in understanding and opportunities for action.* National Academies Press.

Iverson, K. M., King, M. W., Resick, P. A., Gerber, M. R., Kimerling, R., & Vogt, D. (2013). Clinical utility of an intimate partner violence screening tool for female VHA patients. *Journal of General Internal Medicine, 28*(10), 1288–1293. https://doi.org/10.1007/s11606-013-2534-x

Jarvis, C. (2020). *Physical examination and health assessment* (8th ed.). Elsevier.

Lab Tests Online. (n.d.). *Home page.* https://labtestsonline.org/

Lewinsohn, D., Leonard, M., LeBue, P., Cohn, D., Daley, C., Desmond, E., & Woods, G. (2017). Official American Thoracic Society/Infectious Diseases Society of America/Centers for Disease Control and Prevention clinical practice guidelines: Diagnosis of tuberculosis in adults and children. *Clinical Infectious Diseases, 64*(2), e1–e33.

National Human Trafficking Resource Center. (2016, February). *Framework for a human trafficking protocol in healthcare settings.* https://humantraffickinghotline.org/resources/framework-human-trafficking-protocol-healthcare-settings

National Institute of Child Health and Human Development. (2016). *How are obesity and overweight diagnosed.* https://www.nichd.nih.gov/health/topics/obesity/conditioninfo/diagnosed

National Library of Medicine. *Genetics.* https://medlineplus.gov/genetics

Pagana, K. D., Pagana, T. J., & Pagana, T. N. (2021). *Mosby's manual of diagnostic and laboratory tests* (7th ed.). Mosby.

Phillippi, J. & Kantrowitz-Gordon, I. (Eds.). (2025). *Varney's midwifery* (7th ed.). Jones & Bartlett Learning.

Rhoads, J. & Petersen, S. (2021). *Advanced health assessment and diagnostic reasoning* (4th ed.). Jones & Bartlett Learning.

Schuiling, K., & Likis, F. (2022). *Women's gynecologic health* (4th ed.). Jones & Bartlett Learning.

Substance Abuse and Mental Health Services Administration. (2014). Trauma-informed care in behavioral health services. *Treatment Improvement Protocol. TIP 57.* HHS Publication No. (SMA) 14-4816. Substance Abuse and Mental Health Services Administration. Retrieved October 2022, from https://store.samhsa.gov/sites/default/files/d7/priv/sma14-4816.pdf

Touhy, T., & Jett, K. (2020). *Ebersole and Hess' toward healthy aging: Human needs and nursing response* (10th ed.). Mosby Elsevier.

University of Washington STD Prevention Training Center. (2019). *National STD curriculum.* https://www.std.uw.edu/

U.S. Department of Veterans Affairs. (n.d.). *PTSD: National Center for PTSD: Trauma and Stressors Exposure Measures.* https://www.ptsd.va.gov/professional/assessment/te-measures/index.asp

Workowski, K. A., Bachmann, L. H., Chan, P. A., Johnston, C. M., Muzny, C. A, Park, I., Reno, H., Zenilman, J. M., & Bolan, G. A. (2021). Sexually transmitted infections treatment guidelines. *MMWR Recommendations and Reports, 70*(4), 1–187.

CHAPTER 3

Primary Care

Heather C. Quaile

Komkwuan P. Paruchabutr

Beth M. Kelsey

Health Screening, Education, and Counseling: Risk Assessment, Disease Prevention, Counseling, and National Screening Guidelines

- Key concepts and terms
  1. Health—a human condition with physical, social, and psychological dimensions, each characterized on a continuum with positive and negative poles (Centers for Disease Control and Prevention [CDC])
  2. Primary prevention—delivery of healthcare services focused on preventing disease from occurring (e.g., immunizations, health promotion counseling/education)
  3. Secondary prevention—delivery of healthcare services focused on early detection of disease states, as well as interventions that limit severity and morbidity (e.g., identification of risk factors, screening tests, counseling/education)
  4. Tertiary prevention—delivery of healthcare services focused on restoring optimal function, improving health status, and limiting long-term disability following the diagnosis of disease (e.g., treatment of the disease, counseling/education)
  5. Health screening—laboratory or other tests conducted on asymptomatic individuals for early detection of health problems (secondary prevention)
  6. Behavioral counseling interventions—education and counseling focused on assisting individuals maintain

healthy behaviors, change existing behaviors, or adopt new behaviors with the goal of improving health status and health outcomes

  7. Resources for health screening, education, and counseling recommendations—U.S. Preventive Services Task Force (USPSTF), American Cancer Society (ACS), American College of Obstetricians and Gynecologists (ACOG), American Diabetes Association (ADA), American Heart Association (AHA), CDC

- Cancer screening recommendations
  1. Breast cancer screening
     a. **Table 3-1**—breast cancer screening recommendations
     b. Breast cancer screening recommendations for transgender males are the same as for cisgender females.
     c. Breast cancer screening recommendations for transgender people assigned male at birth but who have received estrogen-containing, gender-affirming hormones are as follows:
        (1) Initiate routine mammograms every 1–2 years starting at age 50. Discontinue per guidelines outlined for cisgender women.
        (2) For those at higher risk due to genetic and family history, consider initiating screening 10 years prior to the youngest age of family member diagnosis, or per guidelines for cisgender women.
     d. See the Breast Carcinoma section in Chapter 5, *Gynecologic, Reproductive, and Sexual Disorders*, for information on breast cancer risk assessment and follow-up.
  2. Cervical cancer screening
     a. **Table 3-2**—cervical cancer screening recommendations
     b. Screening recommendations are for individuals at average risk; individualized screening decisions

Table 3-1 Breast Cancer Screening Recommendations

Screening Method	American Cancer Society (ACS)	American College of Obstetricians and Gynecologists (ACOG)	U.S. Preventive Services Task Force (USPSTF)
Clinical breast examination (CBE)	Does not recommend among average-risk people assigned female at birth at any age; average risk is no personal history of breast cancer, no suspected or confirmed genetic mutation known to increase risk of breast cancer, no previous radiotherapy to the chest at a young age	May be offered every 1–3 years for people assigned female at birth aged 25–39 and annually for those aged 40 and older. Offer in the context of a shared, informed decision-making approach that recognizes the uncertainty of additional benefits and harms of CBE beyond screening mammography	Insufficient evidence to assess the balance of benefits and harms of CBE if a person is being screened with mammograms (Grade I)
Mammogram	Yearly beginning at age 45 years for people assigned female at birth at average risk; those age 55 and older can transition to biennial screening or continue annual screening if they prefer; individuals in this risk group should have the opportunity to begin mammograms between age 40 and 44 years. No definitive age to discontinue screening; based on the individual's health and whether the individual would be a candidate for treatment of breast cancer	Offer starting at age 40 years; initiate at ages 40–49 years after counseling, if individual desires; recommend no later than age 50 years if screening has not already initiated; annual or biennial interval. Decision between options to be made through shared decision making after appropriate counseling. No definitive age to discontinue screening; based on the individual's health and whether the individual would be a candidate for treatment of breast cancer	Biennial screening from age 50 to 74 years (Grade B)* *As of December 2023, the draft of new recommendations to start biennial screening starting at age 40 is currently being finalized. Insufficient evidence to assess the balance of benefits and harms of screening in people assigned female at birth aged 75 years or older (Grade I)
Breast self-awareness (BSA)	Educate people assigned female at birth age 20 and older about BSA and when to seek further evaluation; encourage individuals to know normal appearance and feel of their breasts so they can be alert to any changes; no systematic or regular technique of self-examination	Same as ACS	

Data from American College of Obstetricians and Gynecologists. (2017, reaffirmed 2019). Practice Bulletin 179: Breast cancer risk assessment and screening in average-risk women. *Obstetrics and Gynecology, 130,* e1–e16; Smith, R., Andrews, K. Brooks, D., Fedewa, S., Manassaram-Baptiste, D., et al. (2019). Cancer screening in the United States, 2019: A review of current American Cancer Society guidelines and current issues in cancer screening. *CA Cancer Journal for Clinicians, 69* (3), 184–210; U.S. Preventive Services Task Force. (2016 2019). *Breast cancer: Screening.* Retrieved from https://www.uspreventiveservicestaskforce.org/Page/Document/RecommendationStatementFinal/breast-cancer-screening1.

may be different if higher risk (e.g., exposure in utero to diethylstilbestrol, previous history of high-grade precancerous lesion, positive for human immunodeficiency virus [HIV], otherwise immunocompromised)

c. Screening recommendations are the same for all individuals with a cervix, regardless of gender identity or hormone milieu.

3. Colorectal cancer screening—ACS
   a. Adults aged 45 years and older should undergo regular screening with either a high-sensitivity stool-based test or a structural (visual) exam
   b. More frequent testing and starting at a younger age is recommended for those with risk factors including inflammatory bowel disease, personal or family history of colonic polyps or colon cancer, known or suspected presence of Lynch syndrome (hereditary nonpolyposis colon cancer)
   c. All positive results on noncolonoscopy screening tests should be followed up with timely colonoscopy

d. Adults in good health with a life expectancy greater than 10 years should continue screening through the age of 75 years
   e. Stool-based tests
      (1) Guaiac fecal occult blood test—multiple-stool sample, at-home test detects hidden blood in stool; yearly screening
      (2) Stool DNA test—single-sample, at-home test detects DNA from cancer or polyp cells as well as blood; screening every 3 years
      (3) Fecal immunochemical test (FIT), yearly screening
   f. Structural (visual) examination
      (1) Colonoscopy every 10 years
      (2) Flexible sigmoidoscopy every 5 years
      (3) Computed tomography (CT) colonography (virtual colonoscopy) every 5 years

4. Lung cancer screening—USPSTF and ACS
   a. Screen individuals age 55–74 years of age (USPSTF—upper age 80 years) in fairly good health who have risk factors for lung cancer

Table 3-2 Cervical Cancer Screening Recommendations

Age Range (Years)	American Cancer Society (ACS)	American College of Obstetricians and Gynecologists (ACOG)	U.S. Preventive Services Task Force (USPSTF)
<21	Screening is not recommended	Same as ACS Exception: If human immunodeficiency virus (HIV) infected, begin screening within 1 year after beginning sexual activity or if already sexually active within 1 year of HIV diagnosis and no later than age 21	Same as ACS
21–29	Start screening at age 25; primary HPV test every 5 years preferred; cytology and HPV co-testing every 5 years or cytology alone every 3 years acceptable	Cytology alone every 3 years	Cytology alone every 3 years
30–65	Primary HPV test every 5 years preferred; cytology and HPV co-testing every 5 years or cytology alone every 3 years acceptable	Primary HPV test every 5 years or cytology and HPV co-testing every 5 years or cytology alone every 3 years	Primary HPV test every 5 years or cytology and HPV co-testing every 5 years or cytology alone every 3 years
>65	Stop screening if individual has adequate prior negative screening results—defined as 3 consecutive negative cytology results or 2 consecutive co-testing results within previous 10 years and most recent test within past 5 years Once screening has stopped, it should not resume in those older than 65 years, even if they report having a new sexual partner. If history of cervical intraepithelial neoplasia 2 (CIN2) or higher, continue screening for 20 years after spontaneous regression or appropriate management	Same as ACS	Same as ACS
Any age with total hysterectomy (cervix removed)	No further screening necessary unless has history of CIN2, cervical intraepithelial neoplasia 3 (CIN3), adenocarcinoma in situ, or cervical cancer in past 20 years	Same as ACS	Same as ACS

Data from American College of Obstetricians and Gynecologists. (2016, 2021). *Updated cervical cancer screening guidelines.* www.acog.org/clinical/clinical-guidance/practice-advisory/articles/2021/04/updated-cervical-cancer-screening-guidelines. Fontham, E., Wolf, A., & Church, T. (2020). Cervical cancer screening for individuals at average risk: 2020 guideline update from the American Cancer Society. *CA Cancer Journal for Clinicians, 70*(5), 321–346. U.S. Preventive Services Task Force. (2018a). *Cervical cancer: Screening.* Retrieved from https://www.uspreventiveservicestaskforce.org/Page/Document/RecommendationStatementFinal/cervical-cancer-screening2.

   b. Risk factors—30+ pack-year smoking history and still smoking or quit within last 15 years
   c. Low-dose CT scan every year
5. Testicular cancer—USPSTF and ACS do not recommend clinical or self-testicular examination for testicular cancer screening
   Prostate cancer
   a. USPSTF—for all individuals with a prostate aged 55–69 years, the decision to undergo periodic prostate-specific antigen (PSA)–based screening should be based on client–clinician discussion of benefits and harms based on family history, race/ethnicity, other medical conditions, and client values (Grade C); USPSTF recommends against PSA-based screening for those 70 years and older (Grade D)
   b. ACS—recommends client–clinician discussions about screening uncertainties, risks, and potential benefits beginning at age 50 years and earlier for Black individuals and those with a family history of prostate cancer before age 65 years
   c. Transgender individuals assigned male at birth should follow the same recommendations and still maintain a prostate even after gender-affirming genital surgeries.

- Diabetes screening recommendations—ADA
  1. Every 3 years starting at age 45
  2. More frequent testing and starting at a younger age with body mass index (BMI) >25 and one or more other risk factors
  3. Risk factors—obesity; hypertension; dyslipidemia; cardiovascular disease; physical inactivity; polycystic ovarian syndrome; diabetes in first-degree relative; Black, Asian, Hispanic, Native American, Pacific Islander; history of gestational diabetes or baby weighing more than 9 lb at birth
  4. Individuals diagnosed with gestational diabetes should have lifelong screening at least every 3 years
  5. Use HbA$_{1c}$, fasting glucose, or a 2-hour 75-g glucose tolerance test—see Chapter 2, *Health Assessment and Diagnostic Tests*, for more information on the use of these tests
  6. See the Diabetes section in this chapter for information on the assessment, diagnosis, and management of diabetes
- Cardiovascular disease (CVD)—USPSTF
  1. CVD risk factors for women—55 years of age or older, family history of premature coronary heart disease (CHD; male relative <55 years, female relative <65 years), cigarette smoking, hypertension, high-density lipoprotein cholesterol (HDL-C) <40 mg/dL, diabetes mellitus, history of hypertensive disorder of pregnancy
  2. Prevention focuses on behavioral counseling to decrease modifiable risk factors and treatment for conditions placing the individual at high risk
  3. Blood pressure (BP) screening
     a. Screen adults 18 years or older with office blood pressure measurement (Grade A)
     b. Obtain blood pressure measurements outside the clinical setting for diagnostic confirmation before starting treatment (Grade A)
     c. Evidence on optimal screening intervals is limited, reasonable options include
        (1) Screen every year in adults 40 years or older and in younger adults at increased risk for hypertension (e.g., Black persons, persons with high-normal blood pressure, persons who are overweight or obese)
        (2) Screen every 3–5 years as appropriate for adults aged 18–39 years not at increased risk for hypertension and with a prior normal blood pressure reading
     d. See the Hypertension section in this chapter for information on the assessment, diagnosis, and management of hypertension
- Hyperlipidemia/dyslipidemia screening recommendations— American College of Cardiologists (ACA)/AHA
  1. Age 20 and older check cholesterol and other risk factors every 4–6 years as long as risks remain low
  2. After age 40, add ASCVD Risk Calculator to calculate the 10-year risk of having a heart attack or stroke
  3. USPSTF—Insufficient evidence that screening for dyslipidemia before age 40 years has an effect on either short- or longer-term cardiovascular outcomes

  4. See Chapter 2, *Health Assessment and Diagnostic Tests*, for more information on lipid profile testing
  5. See the Dyslipidemia section in this chapter for information on the assessment, diagnosis, and management of this condition
- Obesity/weight management
  1. Obesity is associated with an increased risk of coronary heart disease, type 2 diabetes, various types of cancer, gallstones, and disability
  2. See Chapter 2, *Health Assessment and Diagnostic Tests*, for information on BMI measurement and classifications.
  3. Provide individual-centered counseling with concrete strategies and goals to improve overall health
  4. Offer or refer adults aged 18 and older with a BMI of 30 or higher (obesity) to intensive, multicomponent behavioral interventions
  5. Most successful intensive behavioral weight-loss interventions have multiple sessions over 1–2 years, including a support or maintenance phase; interventions should be tailored with attention to social, environmental, and individual factors
  6. Individuals with a BMI of 40 or greater are considered Class 3 Obesity and meet the criteria for weight-loss surgery if desired by the individual; individuals with a BMI of 35 or greater (Class 2) accompanied by a high-risk comorbid disease (e.g., hypertension, diabetes) may also meet criteria

     Offer management strategies and support for all health concerns of individuals in bigger bodies regardless of their ability or desire for weight loss.
- Osteoporosis screening recommendations—National Osteoporosis Foundation
  1. Screen all women 65 years of age or older for osteoporosis/ osteopenia with bone mineral density (BMD) test
  2. Screen postmenopausal people younger than 65 years of age with risk factors associated with increased fracture risk
  3. Risk factors—low BMI, history of low-trauma fracture, smoking, alcohol intake ≥3 drinks/day, family history of hip fracture or osteoporosis
  4. There is a lack of evidence about whether repeated screening is of value or necessary if the initial screen was normal
  5. If considering repeated screening, a minimum of 2 years may be needed to reliably measure any change in BMD.
  6. There is no recommended age after which screening should stop. See Chapter 2, *Health Assessment and Diagnostic Tests*, for more information on BMD testing and interpretation of results
  7. See the Osteoporosis section in this chapter for information on the assessment, diagnosis, and treatment for osteopenia/osteoporosis
- Hepatitis C screening
  1. Screen all adults aged >18 years at least once in a lifetime
  2. Screen all pregnant individuals during each pregnancy
  3. Provide routine periodic testing for people with ongoing risk factors

a. Risk factors—current injection or intranasal drug use, blood transfusion prior to 1992, long-term hemodialysis, born to parent with hepatitis C virus (HCV) infection, receipt of an unregulated tattoo, other percutaneous exposures, HIV infection, men who have sex with men (MSM)

b. Screening test—Hepatitis C Virus Antibody (anti-HCV) test

- Healthy lifestyles
  1. Nutrition
     a. Evaluation of nutritional status
        (1) Anthropometric measurements—height, weight, BMI, waist circumference
        (2) General appearance—skin, hair, muscle mass
        (3) Biochemical measurements—hemoglobin (Hgb)/hematocrit (Hct), lipid analysis, serum albumin, serum glucose, serum folate
        (4) 24-hour diet recall or 3- to 4-day food diary
        (5) Use of vitamin, mineral, and herbal supplements
     b. *Dietary Guidelines for Americans 2020–2025* (U.S. Department of Health and Human Services) key recommendations
        (1) Choose a healthy dietary pattern at an appropriate caloric level to help achieve and maintain a healthy body weight, support nutrient adequacy, and reduce the risk of chronic disease
        (2) Choose nutrient-dense foods and beverages—nutrients and other beneficial substances not diluted by the addition of calories from added solid fats, sugars, or refined starches, or by solid fats naturally present in the food
        (3) A healthy eating dietary pattern includes:
            (a) Variety of vegetables from all subgroups—dark green, red and orange, legumes, starchy, and others
            (b) Fruits, especially whole fruits
            (c) Fat-free or low-fat dairy products—milk, yogurt, cheese, and/or fortified soy products
            (d) Variety of protein foods—seafood, lean meats and poultry, eggs, legumes, nuts, seeds, and soy products
            (e) Oils
            (f) Minimize processed meats, refined carbohydrates, and sweetened beverages
            (g) Limit total fat intake to no more than 20%–35% of daily calories
            (h) Less than 10% of calories each day from saturated fats; trans fats as low as possible
            (i) Limit cholesterol to 300 mg or less daily
            (j) No more than 2,300 mg (about 1 teaspoon) each day of sodium
            (k) Alcohol only in moderation—up to one drink per day for women and two drinks for men; one drink = 12 ounces of beer, 5 ounces of wine, 1.5 ounces of hard liquor
     c. Calcium and vitamin D recommendations for people assigned female at birth or with estrogen-dominant sex hormone
        (1) Institute of Medicine
            (a) 14 to 18 years of age—1,300 mg/day of calcium; same amount if pregnant or lactating
            (b) 19 to 50 years of age—1,000 mg/day of calcium; same amount if pregnant or lactating
            (c) 51 years of age and older—1,200 mg/day of calcium
            (d) 14 to 70 years of age—600 IU/day of vitamin D
            (e) 71 years of age and older—800 IU/day of vitamin D
        (2) National Osteoporosis Foundation
            (a) Adults age 50 and younger—1,000 mg/day of calcium; 400–800 IU/day of vitamin D
            (b) Adults age 51 and older—1,200 mg/day of calcium; 800–1,000 IU of vitamin D
        (3) Sources of calcium—milk, yogurt, soybeans, tofu, canned sardines and salmon with edible bones, cheese, fortified cereals and orange juice, supplements
        (4) Sources of vitamin D—fortified milk, egg yolks, saltwater fish, liver, supplements, regular exposure to direct sunlight
     d. Folate requirements for people of childbearing potential
        (1) 0.4 mg folic acid/day
        (2) Those of childbearing age who are taking anticonvulsant medication, have insulin-dependent diabetes, or have had an infant with neural tube defect may benefit from a higher dose of up to 4 mg folic acid/day starting at least 1 month before trying to become pregnant and continuing through first 2–3 months of pregnancy
        (3) Sources—dried beans, leafy green vegetables, citrus fruits and juices, fortified cereals; most multivitamins contain 0.4 mg folic acid
     e. Iron requirements for nonpregnant individuals
        (1) 14 to 18 years of age—15 mg/dL each day
        (2) 19 to 50 years of age—18 mg/dL each day
        (3) 51 years of age or older—8 mg/dL each day
        (4) Sources—meat, fish, poultry, fortified cereals, dried fruits, dark green vegetables, supplements
     f. Special concerns
        (1) Eating disorders—see the Eating Disorders section in this chapter
        (2) Vegetarians—plan diet to avoid deficiencies in protein, calcium, iron, vitamin B12, and vitamin D
        (3) Older adults—consider effects of chronic illness, medications, isolation, decrease in ability to taste and smell, limited income
        (4) Need for more limited sodium intake (no more than 1,500 mg/day)—sodium intake may have a greater effect on blood pressure for some individuals (e.g., age older than 50 years; Black

individuals; individuals with hypertension, diabetes, chronic kidney disease)

(5) Increased risk for vitamin D deficiency—age older than 59 years, darker pigmented skin, residing in northern areas, overweight/obese, milk allergy/lactose intolerance, digestive diseases, such as Crohn's disease or celiac disease

(6) Postbariatric surgery—requires consultation with a nutritionist or bariatric specialist; see the Obesity/Weight Management section in this chapter

2. Physical activity

a. Strong evidence that regular physical activity lowers risk for heart disease, stroke, high BP, adverse lipid profile, type 2 diabetes, metabolic syndrome, colon and breast cancers; prevents weight gain and promotes weight loss; improves cardiovascular and muscular fitness; reduces depression; improves cognitive function in older adults

b. *Physical Activity Guidelines for Americans*

(1) Engage in at least 150–300 minutes of moderate-intensity aerobic physical activity, or 75–150 minutes of vigorous-intensity aerobic physical activity, each week, or equivalent combination of moderate and vigorous aerobic activity; spread throughout the week

(2) Moderate-intensity exercise achieves 50%–69% of maximum heart rate—maximum average heart rate equals 220 minus age

(3) Examples of aerobic physical activity—brisk walking, running, bicycling, jumping rope, swimming

(4) Engage in muscle-strengthening activities of moderate or high intensity involving all major muscle groups 2 or more days each week

(5) Examples of muscle-strengthening activities—weight-lifting, exercises with elastic bands, or the use of body weight (push-ups, tree climbing) for resistance

(6) Include bone-strengthening activity in the exercise regimen—running, brisk walking, weight training, tennis, dancing

3. Stress management—see the Psychosocial Problems section in this chapter for information on stress and stress management

- Substance use disorders (SUDs)

1. Substance use transitions from use to a disorder when there is continued use of a substance despite the existence of use-related health problems

2. The severity of an SUD is based on the number of criteria met—loss of control over use, impact on social function, risky use, development of tolerance or dependence

3. Tobacco and nicotine

a. Tobacco use is the leading preventable cause of disease, disability, and death in the United States contributing to approximately 1 in every 5 deaths. Smoking during pregnancy increases risks for congenital anomalies, preterm birth, fetal growth restriction, placental abruption, spontaneous abortion, stillbirth, and impaired lung function

b. Ask all adolescents and adults about tobacco use of all forms as well as e-cigarettes and provide FDA-approved pharmacotherapy or behavioral interventions alone or in combination for cessation of use

c. Ask all pregnant individuals about tobacco use of all forms as well as e-cigarettes and provide behavior interventions for cessation.

d. Smoking-cessation interventions should be individualized in relation to the smoker's physical and psychological dependence and the stage of readiness for change

e. Behavior-modification strategies—provide self-help materials and/or refer to a smoking-cessation class or hotline

f. Five As of smoking cessation—**A**sk about tobacco use, **A**dvise to quit, **A**ssess willingness to attempt to quit, **A**ssist in quit attempt, **A**rrange follow-up

g. Pregnant individuals who smoke should be encouraged to attempt cessation using behavioral interventions before pharmacological approaches are used

h. Pharmacologic aids

(1) Nicotine replacement therapy (gum, patches, inhalers, nasal spray, lozenges)—helps to reduce the physical withdrawal symptoms and cravings that occur with smoking cessation

(a) Major side effects—local skin reactions with patch; mouth and throat irritation with gum, lozenges, or inhaler; hiccups with gum or lozenges; nasal irritation; headache; dizziness; nausea

(b) Contraindications—serious cardiac arrhythmias, severe angina, recent myocardial infarction, concurrent smoking, pregnancy

(c) Avoid using for at least 1 hour before providing human milk.

(d) Client education

i. Individual must stop smoking before initiating nicotine replacement therapy

ii. Provide specific instructions for the chosen route of delivery

(2) Bupropion hydrochloride sustained-release tablets (Zyban)—reduces cravings that smokers experience; the exact manner of action unknown; probably acts on brain pathways involved in nicotine addiction and withdrawal

(a) Major side effects—insomnia, anxiety, dry mouth, nausea, skin rash

(b) Contraindications—seizure disorder, eating disorder, use of a monoamine oxidase (MAO) inhibitor, concomitant use of other forms of bupropion

(c) Data from animal reproductive studies and epidemiologic studies of pregnant individuals exposed to bupropion in the first trimester show no increased risk of congenital malformation overall; bupropion should be used during pregnancy only if the potential benefit justifies the potential risk to the fetus; bupropion is transmitted in human milk with insufficient evidence available to evaluate safety, advise to discuss risks/benefits with infant care provider

(d) Client education
   i. Individual should initiate medication 1–2 weeks before smoking cessation
   ii. Recommended duration of therapy is up to 6 months

(3) Varenicline tablets—reduces withdrawal symptoms; blocks effect of nicotine if individual resumes smoking; nicotinic acetylcholine receptor partial agonist

(a) Major side effects—nausea, changes in dreaming, constipation, gas, vomiting, neuropsychiatric symptoms

(b) Contraindications—precautions with major psychiatric disorders and renal impairment

(c) Data from animal reproductive studies and epidemiologic studies of pregnant people exposed to varenicline in the first trimester show no increased risk of congenital malformation overall; varenicline should be used during pregnancy only if the potential benefit justifies the potential risk to the fetus; varenicline is transmitted in human milk; insufficient evidence available to evaluate safety

(d) Client education
   i. Individual should initiate medication 1 week before smoking cessation
   ii. Concomitant use of nicotine replacement may increase side effects
   iii. Discontinue medication and report any agitation, depression, and suicidal ideation

4. Alcohol
   a. Unhealthy alcohol use reflects a spectrum of behaviors from risky drinking to alcohol use disorder (e.g., harmful alcohol use, abuse, dependence)
   b. Risky or hazardous alcohol use means drinking more than the recommended daily, weekly, or per-occasion amounts, resulting in increased risk for health consequences not meeting the criteria for alcohol use disorder
      (1) Three or more drinks per day or seven or more drinks per week for all individuals aged 65 years and older
      (2) Four or more drinks per day or 14 or more drinks per week for men younger than age 65 years
      (3) Binge drinking is generally defined as when a male consumes five or more drinks or a female consumes four or more drinks on one occasion and within a couple of hours
   c. Screen for unhealthy alcohol use in adults aged 18 and older, including pregnant individuals

   d. Screening instruments with demonstrated accuracy in assessing unhealthy alcohol use in adults include AUDIT-C and the Single Alcohol Screening Question
   e. Provide individuals engaged in risky or hazardous drinking with brief behavioral counseling interventions to reduce unhealthy alcohol use make referrals to specialty care as needed
   f. Any alcohol use is considered unhealthy/risky in pregnant individuals and adolescents
   g. There is no safe amount, type, or time to drink alcohol during pregnancy; alcohol is a known teratogen; use during pregnancy is one of the major preventable causes of congenital disabilities and developmental disabilities
   h. To avoid fetal alcohol exposure before a person might be aware of being pregnant, encourage individuals who are trying to conceive to not drink; encourage individuals who are sexually active, drink alcohol, and could become pregnant to consider using effective contraception

5. Other drugs
   a. Marijuana is the most frequently used illicit drug in the United States; it is legal in some states for medical and/or recreational use
   b. E-cigarette delivery devices are being used for inhalation (vaping) of marijuana and/or its psychoactive component tetrahydrocannabinol (THC); many samples tested by the Food and Drug Administration (FDA) as part of the investigation of vaping-related respiratory illnesses and deaths contain THC, and most of these also contain vitamin E acetate with limited data on its effects after inhalation
   c. Opioid use—in 2018, 1.7 million U.S. individuals age 12 and older were diagnosed with an opioid use disorder (prescription opioid pain relievers and/or heroin); 1.9 million individuals age 12 and older misused opioid pain relievers
   d. Screen all individuals annually—at wellness visits, initial prenatal visits, and other visits when indicated for substance use/SUD; use a validated screening tool
   e. Screening, brief intervention, and referral to treatment (SBIRT) for SUDs
      (1) Effective means for identifying individuals who engage in substance misuse including alcohol and determining the severity of the misuse/use disorder
      (2) Incorporates motivational interviewing to provide a brief intervention, with referral to treatment as needed ˙

6. See the Substance Use Disorders section in this chapter for assessment, diagnosis, and management of substance use disorders

7. See Chapter 7, *Complex Pregnancy*, for relevant information on screening and interventions for substance misuse/use disorders

- Reproductive life planning
1. Offer to discuss reproductive goals (life planning) with reproductive-age individuals

2. One Key Question® is designed for clinicians to screen individuals for pregnancy intention—Would you like to become pregnant in the next year?
   a. If the answer is yes, proceed to prepregnancy care/counseling—see the Prepregnancy Care section in this chapter
   b. If the answer is no, ask about current contraception method use, satisfaction with the method, and/or discuss contraception options
   c. If the answer is unsure or okay either way, offer a combination of contraception and prepregnancy care; discuss relevant issues
3. PATH questions were developed to use with individuals of any gender identity or sexual orientation
   a. Pregnancy/Parenthood Attitudes—Do you think you might like to have (more) children at some point?
   b. Timing—When do you think that might be?
   c. How important—How important is it to you to prevent pregnancy (until then)?
   d. As with One Key Question®—provide prepregnancy care/counseling and/or contraception dependent on answers to PATH questions
4. Recognize some individuals hold beliefs/values or live in circumstances that make planning impossible or irrelevant; clinicians should be nonjudgmental and respectful
- Prepregnancy care (also referred to as preconception care)
  1. Goals of prepregnancy care
     a. Reproductive life planning and provision of contraception as desired
     b. Health promotion/disease prevention to optimize parental and fetal health in future pregnancy
     c. Identification and management of existing chronic medical conditions to optimize disease control and parental health
     d. Identification of any complications during previous pregnancies and implementation of interventions to reduce risk for future pregnancies
     e. Identification of social, cultural, and structural barriers to health care and implementation of interventions to increase access to needed resources
  2. Timing of prepregnancy care—integrate into routine wellness and postpartum visits
  3. Components of prepregnancy care
     a. Health assessment—family history; medical/surgical history; infectious disease history; obstetric history; environmental history; cultural health beliefs/practices; psychosocial history including violence, substance use disorders, and depression; nutrition assessment; health history of other genetic contributors to a potential pregnancy
     b. Assessment of social determinants of health—factors associated with marginalization, discrimination, and healthcare disparities; financial resources; housing; safety in home and community; English proficiency; health literacy
     c. Carrier screening for genetic conditions
        (1) Carrier screening—determines whether an asymptomatic individual has a variant within a gene associated with a particular disorder (e.g., sickle cell disease, cystic fibrosis disease)
        (2) May be part of prepregnancy or prenatal screening
        (3) Expanded carrier screening evaluates an individual's carrier state for multiple conditions at one time
        (4) Expanded carrier screening more commonly used now rather than ethnic or targeted screening
        (5) All individuals considering pregnancy should be offered carrier screening
        (6) After counseling, an individual may decline any or all carrier screening
        (7) If an individual is found to be a carrier for a specific condition, the reproductive partner should be offered screening to determine risk of having an affected child
            (i) All pre- and posttest counseling should be provided by trained personnel
     d. Education/counseling and interventions
        (1) Reproductive life planning/contraception
        (2) Health promotion, disease prevention, risk reduction
            (a) Rubella, varicella, hepatitis B, human papillomavirus (HPV), Td (tetanus/diphtheria)/Tdap (tetanus/diphtheria/pertussis), MMR, influenza, COVID vaccinations, if needed
            (b) Nutrition counseling and folic acid supplementation
            (c) Smoking cessation
            (d) Discontinuation of alcohol use prior to pregnancy
            (e) Treatment for substance use disorders
            (f) Safe sex practices, sexually transmitted infection (STI)/HIV/HCV screening, if indicated, including for any current sex partners
            (g) Management of chronic health conditions to optimize disease control and parental health—optimal glucose control for diabetes, reduction of weight if obese, treatment for mental health conditions including depression
            (h) Medication changes as needed to avoid teratogenic/fetotoxic exposures (e.g., some antiseizure medications, some antihypertensives, some acne treatment medications)
            (i) Avoidance of environmental/occupational exposures that may be teratogenic
        (3) Resources/referrals
            (a) Local and community resources for financial, housing, transportation, legal, and social support concerns
            (b) Genetic testing and counseling as indicated
            (c) Dietary counseling—obesity, eating disorders, restricted diets
            (d) Mental health resources—substance use disorders, psychiatric disorders
            (e) Intimate-partner violence resources

- Abuse and violence
  1. Intimate-partner violence (IPV)—physical or sexual violence, psychological aggression (e.g., coercive, demeaning or threatening tactics), or stalking by a romantic or sexual partner
     a. IPV is more common in younger individuals; those of reproductive age have a higher prevalence of IPV than older individuals
     b. Screen all reproductive-age patients (aged 14 to 46 years) for IPV and provide or refer those who screen positive to support services; insufficient evidence to recommend for or against screening younger or older individuals
     c. Several reliable screening tools are available (e.g., HITS—Hurt, Insult, Threaten, Scream; HARK—Humiliation, Afraid, Rape, Kick; WAST—Woman Abuse Screen Tool)
     d. No valid, reliable screening tools in primary care setting to identify IPV in men without recognized signs or symptoms
     e. See the Psychosocial Problems section of this chapter for more detailed information on IPV and sexual violence
     f. Also see Chapter 7, *Complex Pregnancy*, for relevant information on IPV
  2. Elder abuse—acts by a trusted person (e.g., caregiver, family member) that cause or create risk of or actual harm to an older adult who because of age and/or disability is not able to protect themself; may include, but is not limited to, physical abuse, sexual abuse, emotional or psychological abuse, neglect, abandonment, and financial or material exploitation
     a. Risk factors for elder abuse—isolation, lack of social support, functional impairment, poor physical health
     b. Signs and symptoms of elder abuse—depression; agitation; becoming withdrawn; weight loss for no apparent reason; unexplained bruises, burns, scars; unkempt appearance, such as unwashed hair or dirty clothes
     c. No valid, reliable screening tools in primary care setting to identify abuse of older adults without recognized signs or symptoms
     d. Elder abuse reporting requirements vary from state to state
- Parenting
  1. Infant–parent attachment—process by which parent and infant develop an affectionate, reciprocal relationship that endures over time
  2. Conditions promoting attachment
     a. Parental emotional well-being and ability to trust
     b. Social support system
     c. Competent level of communication and caregiving skills
     d. Proximity with the infant
  3. Risk factors for abuse or neglect
     a. Immaturity of parent(s)—adolescent parents at high risk
     b. Isolation/lack of support system
     c. Parent rejected or abused as a child

d. Emotional instability
e. Lack of knowledge about the development and care of children
f. Low self-esteem
g. Stressful situations—intimate-partner abuse, poverty, unemployment
  4. Anticipatory guidance (birth to 1 year)
     a. Growth and development
        (1) Physical growth—height and weight
        (2) Motor development—early reflexive responses, gross and fine motor skills
        (3) Cognitive development—sensorimotor and language
        (4) Psychosocial development—temperament, emotional development, attachment
     b. Immunization schedule and health maintenance visits
     c. Nutritional needs—nutritional requirements, introduction of solid foods, weaning
     d. Safety promotion/injury prevention—shaken baby syndrome, sudden infant death syndrome, use of infant car seats, accident prevention, prevention of abduction, prevention of secondhand smoke exposure
- Sexual health
  1. Sexuality encompasses a wide range of values, beliefs, attitudes, thoughts, and behaviors experienced and/or expressed throughout life
  2. Biological, psychological, physical, social, religious, and cultural factors interact to influence one's sexuality and sexual health
  3. Gender and sex terminology
     a. Assigned sex—designation based on chromosomes and genitalia at birth
     b. Natal sex—sex designation assigned at birth based on the appearance of genitalia
     c. Gender—social construct assigning roles and attributes to an individual based on natal sex
     d. Gender identity—internal understanding of oneself regarding gender
     e. Cisgender—individuals whose gender identity is the same as the sex assigned at birth
     f. Transgender—individuals whose gender identity is different than the sex assigned at birth
     g. Transgender woman—individual assigned as male sex at birth who has a female gender identity
     h. Transgender man—individual assigned as female sex at birth who has a male gender identity
     i. Gender nonconforming—Describes a person whose gender presentation differs from the societal expectations and assumptions of either the person's assigned sex or current gender identity. This may apply to cisgender or transgender individuals.
     j. Nonbinary—an identity used by people who are not male or female and may live as both, either, or neither. They may identify as nonbinary, genderqueer, gender nonconforming (GNC), agender, genderfluid, two-spirit (if from native/aboriginal cultural background) and/or other terms.

k. Gender-affirming therapy—medical, surgical, or other intervention used to better align gender expression, social perception, and/or physical appearance with gender identity

l. Sexual orientation—individual's pattern of emotional, romantic, and sexual attraction; common labels include heterosexual (straight), gay or lesbian, bisexual, pansexual, asexual

m. Queer—umbrella term to describe all individuals with noncisgender and nonheterosexual identities; historically derogatory term now reclaimed by some members in the LGBTQ+ community

4. Sexual drive—biological component of desire, based on neuroendocrine mechanisms

5. Sexual motivation—intrapsychic and interpersonal component, influenced by quality of relationship, emotional/psychological health, past sexual history, cultural and religious values

6. Sexual response
   a. Linear model (Masters & Johnson, 1966)—applied to both men and women; excitement (sensory stimulation leads to vasocongestion), plateau (increased vasocongestion and pelvic floor muscle tension), orgasm (widespread genitopelvic muscle contraction), resolution (return to nonstimulated state)
   b. Nonlinear model (Basson, 2000)—focuses on women; emotional intimacy and physical satisfaction, not necessarily orgasm, may be the goal; recognizes female sexual motivation as complex and not an innate physiologic phenomenon
   c. Neither of these models explicitly studied the sexual responses of LGBTQ+ individuals.

7. PLISSIT model—used by clinicians who are not sex therapists to address sexual concerns and make appropriate referrals; *P*ermission giving, *L*imited Information giving, *S*pecific *S*uggestions, *I*ntensive *T*herapy

8. STI and HIV screening and counseling recommendations—CDC and USPSTF
   a. Chlamydia and gonorrhea—routine annual screening for women age <25 years and in those >25 years with risk factors (e.g., new sex partner, more than one sex partner, sex partner with concurrent partners, transactional sex); routine annual screening for MSM age <25 years; more frequent than annual screening based on individual risk; chlamydia screening for all pregnant individuals at first prenatal visit and in third trimester if at risk; adapt screening recommendation based on anatomy and risk for transgender and nonbinary individuals
   b. Trichomoniasis
      (1) Consider screening for persons receiving care in high-prevalence settings (e.g., STD clinics and correctional facilities)
      (2) Consider screening for asymptomatic people assigned female at birth at high risk for infection (e.g., multiple sex partners, transactional sex, drug misuse, a history of STIs, or history of incarceration)

(3) Screen asymptomatic individuals living with HIV annually
(4) Adapt screening recommendations based on anatomy for transgender and gender-diverse individuals

c. HIV
   (1) Screen all adolescents and adults in all health care settings unless the patient declines (opt-out screening)
   (2) Screen persons at high risk for HIV infection at least annually
   (3) Include in the routine panel of prenatal screening tests for all pregnant people unless the patient declines (opt-out screening)
   (4) Repeat screening in the third trimester in areas with elevated rates of HIV infection

d. See Chapter 2, *Health Assessment and Diagnostic Tests*, for information on STI and HIV tests; see Chapter 5, *Gynecologic, Reproductive, and Sexual Disorders*, for information on the assessment, diagnosis, and treatment of STIs; see the Immunologic Disorders section of this chapter for information on the assessment, diagnosis, and treatment of HIV infection

e. Safer sex practices for the prevention of STIs and HIV infection
   (1) Counseling regarding safer sex practices for the prevention of STIs and HIV infection should be based on behaviors and risk factors, not on sexual orientation or gender identity
   (2) Safe = all unprotected sexual activities when both partners are monogamous and known by testing to be free of HIV and other STIs
   (3) Low, but potential risk = all sexual activities when both partners are monogamous but have not been tested for HIV or other STIs; intact skin (no lesions in areas of contact); use of latex or plastic condom/barrier for oral, vaginal, and anal intercourse
   (4) Unsafe in the absence of mutual monogamy and STI/HIV testing of both partners = blood contact of any kind; oral, vaginal, or anal intercourse without latex or plastic condom/barrier; shared sex toys; digital penetration of vagina or anus

- Immunizations—CDC
  1. Hepatitis B
     a. Effective in 95% of cases in preventing hepatitis B virus (HBV) infection
     b. High-risk groups for whom HBV vaccination is recommended include, but are not limited to, individuals who have multiple sex partners, men who have sex with men, household contacts or sex partners of those with HBV infection, people who inject drugs, healthcare workers or workers otherwise at occupational risk, individuals in long-term correctional institutions
     c. Individuals not at risk but who want protection from hepatitis B may receive a vaccine—identification of a risk factor is not required

d. Either a three-dose series of conventional hep b vaccine, with the second and third doses at 1 and 6 months after the first dose

e. If three-dose series is interrupted, the series does not need to be restarted; give the second dose as soon as possible and third dose at least 8 weeks later

f. Or a two-dose series of the HepB-CpG vaccine, with the second dose at 1 month after the first dose. Not recommended for pregnant people.

2. Influenza

a. Recommended seasonally each year for all individuals age 6 months and older, including pregnant and lactating individuals

b. Healthy nonpregnant adults under age 50—live attenuated influenza vaccine (LAIV) intranasally or inactivated influenza vaccine (IIV) IM or intradermal

c. Pregnant individuals and adults age 50+—IIV only

d. Lactating individuals—IIV preferred over LAIV

e. High dose/adjuvanted IIV recommended for adults age 65+

3. Pneumococcus—pneumococcal conjugate 20-valent vaccine (PCV20) and pneumococcal polysaccharide vaccine (PPSV23)

a. The ACIP recommends the 20-valent PCV (PCV20) alone or the 15-valent PCV (PCV15) followed by the 23-valent PPSV (PPSV23) for all adults with indications for vaccination. For most adults, including healthy older adults, those with predisposing medical conditions, and those with a history of IPD, we prefer to administer PCV20, when available, due to the simplicity and lower cost of a single-dose vaccine.

b. PCV20 recommended for all individuals age 65 and older, repeat every 5–10 years

c. PCV20—recommended for adults younger than 65 years of age with immunocompromising conditions, functional or anatomic asplenia, cerebrospinal fluid leaks, or cochlear implants

d. PPSV23—consider for adults younger than 65 years of age with chronic illness, functional or anatomic asplenia, immunocompromising conditions, organ or bone marrow transplant recipients; residents of nursing homes or long-term care facilities; or people who smoke cigarettes. Administer 1 year after PCV20.

4. Rubella

a. Recommended for all nonpregnant individuals of childbearing age who lack documented laboratory evidence of immunity or prior immunization after 12 months of age; documentation of provider-diagnosed rubella is not considered acceptable evidence of immunity

b. Contraindications—pregnancy (advise not to become pregnant for 4 weeks after vaccination), known severe immunodeficiency, individuals with HIV infection who are severely immunocompromised

c. May be given during lactation

5. Tetanus, diphtheria, and acellular pertussis (Td/Tdap)

a. Recommended three-dose vaccination series including a Tdap dose for adults with unknown or incomplete history of primary Td vaccination

b. Recommended one dose of Tdap for all adults who have not previously received Tdap

c. Recommended one dose of Tdap vaccine for pregnant individual during each pregnancy regardless of number of years since prior Td or Tdap vaccination; preferred timing between 27 and 36 weeks' gestation to offer optimal protection to infant in first few months of life when high risk exists for severe illness or death from pertussis

d. Booster Td vaccination every 10 years for adults

6. Varicella

a. Recommended for all nonpregnant adolescents and adults without evidence of immunity; given in two doses 4–8 weeks apart

b. Evidence of immunity—documentation of two-dose vaccination; history of varicella based on diagnosis by healthcare provider, history of herpes zoster based on diagnosis of healthcare provider; laboratory evidence of immunity or confirmation of disease, U.S. born before 1980 except for pregnant individuals and healthcare personnel

c. Pregnant individual should be assessed for evidence of immunity and, if not immune, give the first dose of vaccine upon completion or termination of pregnancy and the second dose 4–8 weeks later

d. May be given during lactation

e. Contraindications—pregnancy (advise not to become pregnant for 4 weeks after vaccination), known severe immunodeficiency, individuals with HIV infection who are severely immunocompromised

7. Zoster (shingles)

a. Recommended two-dose series recombinant zoster vaccine (RZV) 2–6 months apart for individuals 50 years and older regardless of previous history of herpes zoster (shingles) or previously received zoster vaccine live (ZVL)

b. Recommended two-dose series 2–6 months apart for individuals >18 years old living with HIV or other immune compromise.

c. Contraindications—pregnancy, known severe immunodeficiency, individuals with HIV infection who are severely immunocompromised

8. Hepatitis A

a. Recommended for individuals who live in or are traveling to countries with high levels of hepatitis A infection, men who have sex with men, people who use illicit drugs (injection or noninjection), those with occupational exposure risks, food handlers, and individuals with chronic liver disease or clotting factor disorders

b. Individuals not at risk but who want protection from hepatitis A may receive the vaccine—identification of a risk factor is not required

c. Two doses at least 6 months apart

  d. Combination hepatitis A and hepatitis B vaccine given in three doses, with the second dose 1 month after the first dose and the third dose 6 months after the first dose
 9. Human papillomavirus (HPV)—CDC and American Society for Coloposcopy and Cervical Pathology (ASCCP)
  a. Nine-valent HPV vaccine (9vHPV) targets HPV types 16 and 18 (responsible for 66% of cervical cancer), types 6 and 11 (cause most anogenital warts), and an additional five types protecting against 90% of HPV-associated cancers
  b. 9vHPV recommended as routine vaccination for individuals 11–12 years of age; may be given as young as 9 years of age
  c. Recommended as a catch-up vaccination for individuals 13–26 years of age who did not receive it when younger
  d. For individuals younger than 15 years of age, administer two doses, with the second dose 6–12 months after the first dose
  e. For individuals 15 years of age and older, administer three doses, with second dose 2 months after the first dose and the third dose 6 months after the first dose
  f. Individuals already infected with one or more HPV types will still get protection from types not yet acquired
  g. Individuals living with HIV should be offered HPV vaccination up to age 45.
  h. Routine pregnancy testing prior to initiation of the HPV vaccination series is not recommended; if found to be pregnant after initiation, delay the remainder of the three-dose series until completion of pregnancy
  i. 9vHPV vaccine was FDA approved in 2018 for adults up to age 45; recommendations have not changed; public health benefit of HPV vaccination in immune-competent adults aged 27 through 45 is minimal; shared decision-making is recommended because some individuals not previously vaccinated might benefit
 10. Meningococcal
  a. Recommended initial vaccination at age 11–12 as a one-time dose
  b. Recommended booster vaccination at age 16; booster not needed if initial vaccination done at age 16 or older
  c. Recommended for all first-year college students living in dormitories if not previously vaccinated at age 16 years or older, military recruits, individuals with anatomic or functional asplenia, those living with HIV, individuals traveling to regions where meningococcal disease is common
 11. COVID-19—recommended for everyone aged 6 months and older including pregnant and lactating individuals; may be administered on the same day as other routinely recommended vaccines, including influenza vaccine; refer to CDC for updates on booster vaccinations

 12. Immunizations during pregnancy and lactation
  a. Live attenuated-virus vaccines (LAIV) should not be given during pregnancy: varicella, zoster, measles/mumps/rubella (MMR)
  b. Varicella, zoster, and MMR may be given during lactation; IIV preferred over LAIV
  c. Inactivated virus vaccines, bacterial vaccines, toxoids, and tetanus immunoglobulin may be given, if indicated
- Vision—American Academy of Ophthalmology (AAO) recommendations for screening for visual acuity and glaucoma by an ophthalmologist
 1. Every 3–5 years for Black individuals aged 20–39 years
 2. Every 2–4 years for individuals aged 40–64 years and every 1–2 years beginning at age 65 regardless of race
 3. Yearly for diabetic individuals regardless of age
- Dental—American Dental Association (ADA) recommends that adults should have routine dental care and preventive services, including oral cancer screening, at least once every year
- Safety—address the use of seat belts, safety helmets, smoke alarms, occupational safety, and other injury prevention

Cardiovascular Disorders

Hypertension
- Definition
 1. Hypertension (HTN) constitutes the level of blood pressure in the vessels that can cause target organ damage (TOD), morbidity, and mortality
 2. In 2020, AHA issued updated clinical practice guidelines and lowered the standard definition of HTN; rationale is that earlier treatment with lifestyle changes and, in some individuals, medication can reduce complications
  a. Normal BP = SBP less than 120 mm Hg and DBP less than 80 mm Hg
  b. Elevated BP (EBP) = SBP of 120–129 mm Hg and DBP of less than 80 mm Hg
  c. Stage I HTN = SBP 130–139 mm Hg and DBP 80–89 mm Hg
  d. Stage II HTN = SBP ≥140 mm Hg and DBP ≥ 90 mm Hg
 3. Evaluation of patients with documented HTN has three objectives
  a. To identify secondary causes
  b. To assess for TOD—eye, brain, blood vessels, heart, and kidney
  c. To identify other cardiovascular risk factors or concomitant disorders that may define prognosis and guide therapy
   (1) Smoking
   (2) Obesity (BMI ≥ 30)
   (3) Physical inactivity
   (4) Dyslipidemia
   (5) Diabetes mellitus

(6) Microalbuminuria or estimated glomerular filtration rate (GFR) of less than 60 mL/min

(7) Age older than 55 years in men and older than 65 years in women

(8) Family history of premature cardiovascular disease (men age <55 and women age <65)

- Etiology/incidence
  1. Etiology
     a. Primary or essential
        (1) No discernible cause; a complex polygenic and multifactorial disorder
        (2) Accounts for 90%–95% of diagnosed cases
     b. Secondary
        (1) Underlying disease or condition identified; requires separate treatment
        (2) Accounts for 5%–10% of adult cases
  2. Incidence/prevalence
     a. Statistics are based on 2017 AHA/ACC definitions for HTN, which did not explicitly study transgender individuals
     b. Prevalence of HTN among U.S. adults—45.6%
     c. Approximately 6% of adults have undiagnosed HTN
     d. Men and women have similar prevalence of HTN during ages 45–64 years
        (1) Women are more likely to develop HTN in the fifth decade of life and have higher rates than men in later life
        (2) Menopause is associated with a two-fold increase in the risk of HTN, with the prevalence of 75% in postmenopausal people in the United States
     e. The prevalence of HTN overall in women is highest in non-Hispanic Blacks (56%) compared with non-Hispanic whites (41%) and Hispanic individuals (42%)
- Symptoms
  1. Symptoms usually not present
  2. In cases of secondary hypertension, may be symptoms associated with a secondary condition
     a. Weakness in primary aldosteronism
     b. Truncal obesity and purple striae in Cushing's syndrome
     c. Palpitations, tremors, and sweating in pheochromocytoma
  3. In chronic HTN, may be symptoms associated with TOD
     a. Symptoms associated with peripheral vascular disease, coronary artery disease, and heart failure
     b. Symptoms associated with stroke or transient ischemic attack
- Physical findings
  1. Elevated blood pressure as noted in the definition
  2. Findings associated with secondary causes or TOD
     a. Retinopathy
     b. S_4 gallop, S_3 gallop, precordial heave, and displaced point of maximal impulse
     c. Renal artery bruit in renal artery stenosis
     d. Delayed or absent femoral pulses and decreased blood pressure in lower extremities in coarctation of the aorta

e. Diminished or absent peripheral pulses, edema
f. Neurologic findings

- Differential diagnosis/secondary causes
  1. Sleep apnea
  2. Chronic kidney disease (CKD)
  3. Primary aldosteronism
  4. Renovascular disease
  5. Chronic steroid therapy and Cushing's syndrome
  6. Pheochromocytoma
  7. Coarctation of the aorta
  8. Thyroid or parathyroid disease
  9. Drug-induced or drug-related
     a. Drug use—cocaine, amphetamines, alcohol
     b. Combination hormonal contraceptives
     c. Sympathomimetics—over-the-counter cold remedies
- Diagnostic tests/findings
  1. Recommended before initiating therapy to rule out secondary causes, determine the presence of risk factors, and assess for TOD
  2. Recommended initial laboratory tests
     a. Urinalysis
     b. Complete blood count (CBC)
     c. Blood glucose, serum potassium, creatinine or estimated GFR, calcium, lipid profile
        (1) Hypokalemia in primary aldosteronism
        (2) Elevated creatinine in renal disease
     d. Electrocardiogram (ECG) to assess evidence of ischemic heart disease or left ventricular hypertrophy (LVH)
  3. Optional studies
     a. Measurement of urinary albumin excretion or albumin/creatinine ratio
     b. Thyroid-stimulating hormone (TSH)
     c. Intravenous pyelogram (IVP) to rule out renovascular disease
     d. Twenty-four-hour urine for metanephrines and catecholamines to rule out pheochromocytoma
     e. Chest radiograph to rule out cardiomegaly and coarctation of the aorta
     f. Echocardiogram is a more sensitive study to detect LVH
- Management/treatment
  1. Goal of therapy—prevent/minimize TOD
  2. Nonpharmacologic—lifestyle modifications recommended for all patients with HTN
     a. Lifestyle modifications are recommended first-line therapy for
        (1) EBP (SBP 120–129 mm Hg and DBP less than 80 mm Hg)
        (2) Stage I HTN (SBP 130–139 mm Hg and/or DBP 80–89 mm Hg) and calculated 10-year risk of atherosclerotic CVD (ASCVD) less than 10%
        (3) Recheck BP in 3–6 months
     b. Weight reduction—maintain ideal body weight
     c. Adopt Dietary Approaches to Stop Hypertension (DASH) eating plan—diet rich in fruits, vegetables, and low-fat dairy products with a reduced content of saturated and total fat; other acceptable diets

include Mediterranean diet and plant-based eating patterns

  d. Dietary sodium reduction—no more than 1,500 mg/day but also aim to reduce by at least 1,000 mg/day

  e. Physical activity—engage in aerobic physical activity at least 40 minutes per day most days of the week

  f. Moderation of alcohol consumption—no more than one drink/day for women

  g. Smoking cessation

3. Pharmacologic

  a. Stage I HTN (SBP 130–139 mm Hg and/or DBP 80–89 mm Hg) and calculated 10-year risk of atherosclerotic CVD (ASCVD) ≥10% or with CVD, diabetes, or chronic kidney disease

    (1) Start with one antihypertensive medication—thiazide diuretic, calcium channel blocker (CCB), angiotensin-converting enzyme (ACE) inhibitor, angiotensin II receptor blocker (ARB)

    (2) ACC/AHA guidelines provide more detailed information on factors influencing the initial choice of medication

    (3) Advise also on lifestyle modifications

    (4) Follow up in 1 month to assess adherence and response to treatment

    (5) If a BP goal of <130/80 mm Hg is not achieved, consider titration of dose and/or sequential addition of other agents

    (6) Follow up monthly until control is achieved, then every 6 months

  b. Stage II HTN (SBP ≥ 140 mm Hg and/or DBP ≥ 90 mm Hg)

    (1) Start with two antihypertensive medications from two different classes

    (2) ACC/AHA guidelines provide more detailed information on factors influencing the choice of medications

    (3) Advise on lifestyle modifications

    (4) Follow up in 1 month to assess adherence and response to treatment

    (5) If a BP goal of <130/80 mm Hg is not achieved, consider titration of doses and/or sequential addition of other agents

    (6) Follow up monthly until control is achieved, then every 3–6 months

4. Special considerations for reproductive-age individuals

  a. Uncontrolled chronic HTN can lead to increased risks for parental, fetal, and neonatal morbidity and mortality

  b. Counsel reproductive-age patients with HTN who could become pregnant regarding risks of uncontrolled HTN in pregnancy

  c. Review antihypertensive medications—ACE inhibitors and ARBs are contraindicated during pregnancy; patients taking these medications should be counseled regarding the use of highly effective contraception

  d. Estrogen-containing contraceptive methods are contraindicated if the individual has uncontrolled HTN or vascular disease; not recommended even if adequately controlled unless no other method is available or acceptable

  e. Long-acting reversible contraceptive methods (i.e., intrauterine device [IUD], progestin implant) and progestin-only pills are options

5. Classification of drugs for hypertension by drug action (**Table 3-3**)

6. Patient education

  a. Asymptomatic nature of hypertension

  b. Adherence to treatment regimens important even if the individual is asymptomatic to avoid/reduce damage to eyes, brain, blood vessels, heart, and kidneys

  c. Lifestyle modification recommendations

  d. Instructions on use and common side effects of medications

  e. Follow-up plan to monitor treatment effectiveness and any need for medication modifications

- Referral

1. Evaluation and management of secondary causes

2. Hypertensive crisis (BP > 180/120 mm Hg)

3. Resistance to drug therapy

Heart Murmurs

- Definition

1. Prolonged extra heart sounds produced by the turbulent flow of blood heard during either systole or diastole; commonly associated with dynamics of regurgitation or stenosis

2. Classification

  a. Innocent or functional murmurs

    (1) Transient; pose no direct threat to health

    (2) Most frequently heard during systole

    (3) No structural or functional cardiac abnormality

    (4) Often noted in pregnancy because of increased cardiac output

  b. Pathologic murmurs (systolic and diastolic) are indicative of heart or valvular disease (e.g., aortic or pulmonary stenosis, atrial septal defect, rheumatic heart disease)

- Etiology/incidence

1. Etiology

  a. Turbulent blood flow into, through, or out of the heart can result in an audible murmur

  b. Characteristics of sound depend on the following factors:

    (1) Size of valve opening

    (2) Integrity of valve

    (3) Vigor of contraction

    (4) Rate of flow

    (5) Thickness of chest wall

2. Incidence

  a. Innocent systolic murmurs occur in 50%–70% of children and as many as 50% of adults at some time

Table 3-3 Hypertension Pharmacology (Representative List)

Drug Name	Action	Side Effects	Interactions	Contraindications/ Precautions
Thiazide Diuretics				
Hydrochlorothiazide (Esidrex, HydroDIURIL) Indapamide (Lozol) Chlorthalidone (Hygroton)	Inhibits sodium reabsorption from distal renal tubules; reduced sodium results in decreased vascular tone	Hypokalemia and other electrolyte disorders, hyperglycemia, hyperuricemia, orthostatic hypotension, volume depletion, worsening kidney function, transient hyperlipidemia	Enhances other classes of antihypertensives; may decrease oral sulfonylurea and insulin drug efficacy; digitalis and lithium toxicity; nonsteroidal anti-inflammatory drugs (NSAIDs) may reduce effect of thiazide and increase risk of acute renal failure	Sulfonamide allergy; use caution in patients with impaired renal function, diabetes, history of gout, and elderly who may be at more risk for orthostatic hypotension Second line as treatment choice during pregnancy; theoretical potential for intravascular volume depletion; other risks to fetus include decreased glucose, platelets, sodium, potassium levels, and possible death resulting from complications with the parent.
Beta-Adrenoreceptor Antagonists: Beta Blockers				
Propranolol (Inderal) Atenolol (Tenormin) Labetalol (Trandate)	Inhibits sympathetic stimulation of the heart; reduces sympathetic outflow to peripheral vasculature; blocks renin release from kidney	Bronchospasm, bradycardia, hypotension, heart failure; may mask insulin-induced hypoglycemia; insomnia, fatigue, decreased exercise tolerance Rebound hypertension	Additive effect with other antihypertensive agents and alcohol; altered effectiveness of hypoglycemic drugs	Asthma, atrioventricular (AV) block, heart failure; use caution with diabetes, older adults Labetalol may be considered if needed for initial treatment of pregnant people with chronic hypertension; low concentrations of labetalol and propranolol in breast milk, high concentrations of atenolol. May cause hypoglycemia in the newborn.
Calcium Channel Antagonists: Calcium Channel Blockers (CCBs)				
Nifedipine (Procardia XL) Amlodipine (Norvasc) Diltiazem (Cardizem, Triazac) Verapamil (Calan, Veralan)	Blocks influx of calcium through transmembrane calcium channels that trigger smooth muscle contraction; results in prolonged vascular smooth muscle relaxation	Dizziness, hypotension, headache, gastrointestinal (GI) symptoms, peripheral edema, heart failure	Side effects less common with sustained-release forms Additive effect with other antihypertensive agents and alcohol; risk of digoxin and lithium toxicity Drugs that inhibit CYP3A4 and grapefruit juice may increase free drug levels	Heart failure, AV block; significant peripheral edema Avoid in individuals with gastroesophageal reflux disease (GERD), as may make worse Nifedipine or amlodipine may be considered if needed for initial treatment of pregnant people with chronic hypertension

Drug Name	Action	Side Effects	Interactions	Contraindications/ Precautions
Angiotensin-Converting Enzyme (ACE) Inhibitors				
Captopril (Capoten) Enalapril (Vasotec)	Inhibits angiotensin-converting enzyme; prevents conversion of angiotensin I to angiotensin II, thereby enhancing vasodilation	Cough, hypotension, rash, angioedema	Additive effect with other antihypertensive agents and alcohol; increased risk for renal toxicity with NSAIDs; increased risk for hyperkalemia with potassium-sparing diuretics	Associated with other angioedema, bilateral renal artery stenosis, hyperkalemia Associated with fetal anomalies; not recommended for pregnant people
Angiotensin II Receptor Blockers (ARBs)				
Losartan (Cozaar, Hyzaar) Valsartan (Diovan) Olmesartan	Block binding of angiotensin II to receptor, thereby enhancing vasodilation	Similar to ACE inhibitors but not likely to cause cough and less likely to cause angioedema	Same as with ACE inhibitors	Same as with ACE inhibitors, with exception of angioedema Associated with fetal anomalies; not recommended for pregnant people

Data from American College of Obstetricians and Gynecologists. (2013). *Hypertension in pregnancy.* Washington, DC: Author; Brucker, M., & King, T. (Eds.). (2017). *Pharmacology for women's health* (2nd ed.). Burlington, MA: Jones & Bartlett Learning; Sachs, H. C., & American Academy of Pediatrics. (2013). The transfer of drugs and therapeutics into human breast milk: An update on selected topics. *Pediatrics,132*(3), e796–e809; Woo, T., & Robinson, M. (2020). *Pharmacotherapeutics for advance practice nurse prescribers* (5th ed.). Philadelphia, PA: F. A. Davis.

b. Pathologic murmurs are less common, but incidence increases with age
   (1) Congenital—Marfan's syndrome, valve malformation
   (2) Acquired—rheumatic heart disease, mitral valve prolapse (MVP)

- Symptoms
  1. Innocent murmurs—not symptomatic
  2. Pathologic
     a. Possible chest pain
     b. Shortness of breath on exertion
     c. Orthopnea
     d. Cough or wheeze
     e. Paroxysmal nocturnal dyspnea

- Physical findings
  1. Innocent
     a. Usually none except audible murmur
     b. Soft (grade 1 or 2 intensity), medium pitch, systolic murmur
     c. Heard best when the patient is supine
     d. Disappears with standing or straining
     e. Increases with increased cardiac output (e.g., fever, exercise)
  2. Pathologic
     a. Diastolic or pansystolic murmur or any murmur above grade 3
     b. Intensifies with exercise or Valsalva maneuver
     c. Mid- or late systolic click, associated with MVP
     d. Cyanosis
     e. Jugular vein distention
     f. Hepatomegaly
     g. Pedal edema
     h. Diminished femoral pulses or unequal blood pressure in left and right arms

- Differential diagnosis—focused on differentiating innocent versus pathologic murmur

- Diagnostic tests/findings—indicated only if a pathologic murmur suspected
  1. Echocardiography—confirms severity, location of clinically detected lesions
  2. Chest radiograph—suspected cardiac enlargement
  3. CBC—rule out anemia
  4. Thyroid function tests—rule out hyperthyroidism or hypothyroidism
  5. Other, if indicated (e.g., stress electrocardiogram, cardiac catheterization)

- Management/treatment
  1. Low-grade, asymptomatic systolic murmur with low-risk history can be assumed innocent and followed up at the next visit
  2. Pharmacologic—bacterial endocarditis prophylaxis for susceptible patients
     a. Patients with valvular heart disease, prosthetic heart valves, or other structural cardiac abnormalities
     b. Indicated with dental, upper respiratory, gastrointestinal, and genitourinary procedures
     c. Give oral amoxicillin 2 g 1 hour before the procedure
  3. Patient education
     a. Self-knowledge and self-disclosure in future encounters
     b. Follow-up schedule if indicated

- Referral
  1. Diastolic murmurs
  2. Suspected pathologic systolic murmurs

Thromboembolic Disease

- Definitions
  1. Thrombosis—blood clot that forms abnormally within blood vessels
  2. Embolus—blood clot that breaks free from its site of formation
  3. Deep vein thrombosis (DVT)—formation of blood clots in deep veins of legs; may break off and lead to pulmonary embolism
  4. Thromboembolism—DVT plus systemic embolism
  5. Thrombophilia—tendency to develop thrombosis from either acquired or inherited causes, or both
  6. Superficial phlebitis—inflammation of superficial veins as a result of local trauma, venous stasis, or infection
- Etiology/incidence/risk factors
  1. Etiology
     a. Origin of most venous thrombi is Virchow's triad—endothelial damage, stasis, hypercoagulability
        (1) Endothelial damage secondary to trauma
        (2) Stasis secondary to immobility
        (3) Hypercoagulability secondary to protein deficiency states, such as protein C or S, antithrombin III, nephrotic syndrome, chronic liver disease, and certain malignancies
     b. DVT occurs as blood clots form within the deep venous plexus of the calf or within the popliteal, femoral, and iliac veins
     c. Approximately 40% of DVTs embolize to pulmonary circulation when thigh veins are involved; risk is minimal when only calf veins are involved
     d. Prevention of pulmonary embolus (PE) necessitates prompt diagnosis and treatment of DVT
     e. Superficial thromboses usually occur in varicose veins
  2. Incidence of DVT/PE—900,000 cases annually
  3. Risk factors (acquired)
     a. Recent surgery—gynecologic or orthopedic procedures of the hip or knee
     b. Immobilization or venous stasis
     c. Trauma or fractures
     d. Malignancies
     e. Pregnancy and early postpartum
     f. Combination hormonal contraceptives
     g. Congestive heart failure or recent myocardial infarction (MI)
     h. Prior history of thromboembolic disease
     i. Obesity
     j. Inflammatory diseases
     k. Antiphospholipid syndrome
     l. Smoking
  4. Risk factors (inherited)
     a. Factor V Leiden
     b. Homocysteine abnormalities
     c. Prothrombin gene mutation
     d. Protein C or S deficiency

- Symptoms
  1. Superficial phlebitis—localized area of edema, erythema, and tenderness over superficial vein
  2. DVT
     a. Acute onset of unilateral leg pain (calf)
     b. Leg edema
     c. As many as 50% of affected individuals have no symptoms
  3. PE
     a. Unilateral chest pain
     b. Anxiety, restlessness
     c. Dyspnea
- Physical findings
  1. Superficial phlebitis
     a. Localized area of edema, erythema, and tenderness over a superficial vein
     b. Increased temperature in surrounding skin
  2. DVT—often no findings
     a. Calf tenderness to compression; pain elicited with dorsiflexion of foot (Homan's sign); nonspecific finding
     b. Palpable venous cord
     c. Unilateral leg edema; skin may be warm and erythematous
  3. PE
     a. Cyanosis
     b. Diminished breath sounds over the involved area
     c. Tachypnea
     d. Cough with hemoptysis
     e. Tachycardia
     f. Fever
- Differential diagnosis
  1. DVT
     a. Muscle strain or contusion
     b. Cellulitis—more diffuse redness
     c. Popliteal (Baker's) cyst
     d. Superficial phlebitis
  2. PE
     a. Myocardial infarction
     b. Pneumothorax
     c. Pneumonia
- Diagnostic tests/findings
  1. Superficial phlebitis—usually none indicated
  2. DVT
     a. Duplex ultrasound—used as initial test when the probability of DVT is intermediate to high; good sensitivity and specificity in symptomatic patients; negative test in individuals with intermediate to high probability of DVT requires further testing
     b. Plasma d-dimer enzyme-linked immunosorbent assay (ELISA)
        (1) Measures active breakdown of thrombi
        (2) Elevated in 95%–98% of DVT; useful in ruling out DVT if negative
        (3) Positive results are not diagnostic because several other conditions cause positive results (e.g., atrial fibrillation, impaired renal function, pregnancy, ongoing blood loss)
        (4) Best used as an initial test if the probability of DVT is low

c. Contrast venography—best used for suspected calf vein thrombus or when clinical findings conflict with ultrasound

d. Other lab tests for inherited or acquired anticoagulation deficiencies

    (1) Protein C, Protein S

    (2) Antithrombin III

    (3) Antiphospholipid antibodies

    (4) Factor V Leiden

3. PE

    a. Ventilation–perfusion (V/Q) lung scan

    b. Arterial blood gases

    c. ECG and chest radiograph

    d. Plasma d-dimer ELISA

    e. Pulmonary angiogram

- Management/treatment
  1. Refer suspected DVT or PE for immediate medical management
  2. Superficial phlebitis
     a. Nonpharmacologic—elevation of leg and compression with an ace wrap
     b. Pharmacologic—nonsteroidal anti-inflammatory drugs (NSAIDs)
  3. Patient education—for high-risk patients
     a. During prolonged, confined travel—support hose, adequate fluids, passive intermittent contraction of calf muscles; rest breaks to ambulate, stretch, and exercise the legs
     b. May consider low-dose aspirin (81–365 mg) for individuals with a risk for DVT who travel long distances
     c. Do not smoke
     d. Do not use estrogen-containing contraceptives

Dyslipidemia

- Definition
  1. Increased levels of total blood cholesterol and LDLs or triglycerides (TGs); suppressed HDLs, or any combination; risk factor for the development of CHD in adults
  2. Classifications using National Cholesterol Education Program (NCEP) Adult Treatment Panel III (ATP III) Guidelines
     a. Elevated LDL-C: greater than 100 mg/dL
     b. Hypertriglyceridemia: greater than 150 mg/dL
     c. Low HDL-C: less than 40 mg/dL
     d. Metabolic syndrome: any three risk factors
        (1) Abdominal obesity/waist circumference
           (a) Cisgender men, greater than 40 inches
           (b) Cisgender women, greater than 35 inches
           (c) Waist circumference risk factors for transgender individuals is not known.
        (2) Triglycerides: 150 mg/dL or greater
        (3) HDL-C
           (a) Cisgender men, less than 40 mg/dL
           (b) Cisgender women, less than 50 mg/dL
           (c) Cutoff for transgender individuals should be based on hormone milieu (estrogen vs. testosterone dominance).
        (4) Blood pressure: 130/85 mm Hg or greater
        (5) Fasting glucose: 110 mg/dL or greater

- Etiology/incidence/prevalence
  1. Etiology
     a. Genetic predisposition
     b. Secondary causes
        (1) Obesity
        (2) Disease processes (e.g., endocrine and metabolic disorders, obstructive liver disease, renal disorders)
        (3) Drugs (e.g., corticosteroids, thiazide diuretics, beta blockers, antipsychotics)
  2. Incidence/prevalence—dyslipidemia affects more than 50% of all adult women in the United States
- Symptoms—none except those associated with CHD
- Physical findings
  1. Xanthomas—slightly raised, yellowish, well-circumscribed plaques along nasal portion of eyelids
  2. Corneal arcus—thin grayish white arc or circle near edge of cornea
  3. Central obesity
- Differential diagnosis—focused on ruling out secondary causes
- Diagnostic tests/findings
  1. Cholesterol and triglycerides classification
     a. Total cholesterol
        (1) Less than 200 mg/dL—desirable
        (2) 200–239 mg/dL—borderline high
        (3) 240 mg/dL or greater—high
     b. LDL cholesterol
        (1) Less than 100 mg/dL—optimal
        (2) 100–129 mg/dL—near or above optimal
        (3) 130–159 mg/dL—borderline high
        (4) 160–189 mg/dL—high
        (5) 190 mg/dL or greater—very high
     c. HDL cholesterol
        (1) Less than 40 md/dL—low
        (2) 60 or greater mg/dL—high (protective against CHD)
     d. Triglycerides
        (1) Less than 150 mg/dL—normal
        (2) 150–199 mg/dL—borderline high
        (3) 200–499 mg/dL—high
        (4) 500 mg/dL or greater—very high
- Management/treatment
  1. Heart-healthy lifestyle habits are the foundation for prevention of CHD
  2. Treatment of dyslipidemia is based on the risk of CHD events
     a. Determine if the patient has clinically manifested CHD or CHD risk equivalents—peripheral vascular disease, abdominal aortic aneurysm, symptomatic carotid artery disease, diabetes
     b. Determine the presence of major risk factors (other than high LDL)
        (1) Cigarette smoking
        (2) Hypertension (BP > 140/90 mm Hg or on antihypertensive medication)
        (3) Low HDL cholesterol (<40 mg/dL); HDL >60 mg/dL counts as a negative risk factor—remove one risk factor from the total count

(4) Family history of premature CHD (CHD in male first-degree relative <55 years; CHD in female first-degree relative <65 years)

(5) Age (men ≥45 years; women ≥55 years)

c. If the patient has two or more risk factors, without CHD or CHD risk equivalent, determine the 10-year risk of a CHD event with the ASCVD Risk Calculator

(1) CHD or CHD risk equivalents = 10-year risk >20%

(2) 2+ risk factors without CHD or CHD risk equivalents = 10-year risk ≤20%

(3) 0–1 risk factors = 10-year risk <10%

d. Assign a treatment goal for LDL-C based on risk category (American College of Cardiology 2018 Guidelines)

(1) In very high-risk ASCVD, use an LDL-C threshold of 70 mg/dL to consider the addition of nonstatins to statin therapy

(2) In patients with severe primary hypercholesterolemia (LDL-C level ≥190 mg/dL, without calculating 10-year ASCVD risk, begin high-intensity statin therapy

(3) In adults 40–75 years of age without diabetes mellitus and with LDL-C levels ≥70 mg/dL, at a 10-year ASCVD risk of ≥7.5%, start a moderate-intensity statin if a discussion of treatment options favors statin therapy

3. Nonpharmacologic/therapeutic lifestyle changes

a. In patients without clinical CHD, no diabetes, age 40–75 years of age, LDL-C <190 mg/dL, and estimated CHD risk <7.5%, emphasize nonpharmacologic therapeutic lifestyle changes

b. Patients who meet the criteria for treatment with statins should also follow therapeutic lifestyle changes

c. Dietary modification to lower LDL cholesterol—AHA

(1) Reduce saturated fat to no more than 5%–6% of total calories

(2) Reduce trans fat to less than 1% of calories

(3) Emphasize fruits, vegetables, whole grains, low-fat dairy products, poultry, fish, and nuts

(4) Limit red meat and sugary foods and beverages

d. Encourage moderate-intensity exercise for 30 minutes/day for most days of the week—this can be walking

e. Aggressive smoking cessation program

f. Weight loss for patients who are overweight or obese (goal BMI < 25); initial weight loss goal of 5%–10% of current weight

4. Pharmacologic

a. Drug initiation and choice directed by risk factors

(1) Lipid laboratory values

(2) Presence (or not) of CHD or diabetes

(3) Estimated 10-year CHD risk

(4) Individual preference after discussion of benefits and risks, adverse effects, drug–drug interactions

b. Statin (HMG-CoA reductase inhibitor) therapy

(1) First-line treatment for reducing LDL levels in adults

(2) Drug action—inhibits HMG-CoA reductase, the enzyme that controls cholesterol biosynthesis in cells; effective in decreasing LDL-C, moderately effective in increasing HDL, moderately effective in decreasing triglycerides

(3) Contraindications/precautions

(a) Severe liver disease is a contraindication—monitor liver function for elevated liver enzymes

(b) Myopathy is a potential side effect, with increased risk if combined statin with fibrate or niacin

(c) Use is contraindicated during pregnancy and lactation

(4) **Table 3-4**—choice of initial statin based on LDL-C level, presence or not of CHD or diabetes, estimated 10-year CHD risk, ability to tolerate statin

(5) **Table 3-5**—levels of statin intensity, examples with daily doses

---

Table 3-4 **Choice of Initial Statin Based on LDL-C Level**

Low-density lipoprotein cholesterol (LDL-C) ≥190 mg/dL, regardless of coronary heart disease (CHD) or diabetes or estimated 10-year CHD risk, 21–75 years of age	High-intensity statin
LDL-C ≤190 mg/dL, no CHD or diabetes, estimated CHD risk ≥7.5%, 40–75 years of age	Moderate- to high-intensity statin
Individuals with diabetes and 40–75 years of age	May need either moderate- or high-intensity statin depending on LDL-C level and estimated CHD risk
Individuals with CHD and ≤75 years of age	High-intensity statin
≥75 years of age or if not a candidate for high-intensity statin	Moderate-intensity statin

Data from Stone, N., Robinson, J., Lichtenstein, A., Bairey Merz, C., Blum, C., Eckel, R., . . . Wilson, P. (2014). 2013 ACC/AHA guideline on the treatment of blood cholesterol to reduce atherosclerotic cardiovascular risk in adults: A report of the American College of Cardiology/American Heart Association Task Force on Practice Guidelines. *Journal of the American College of Cardiology, 63*(25), 2889–2934.

Table 3-5 Levels of Statin Intensity

High Intensity	Moderate Intensity	Low Intensity
Lowers low-density lipoprotein cholesterol (LDL-C) on average ≥50%	Lowers LDL-C on average 30%–50%	Lowers LDL-C on average <30%
Atorvastatin (Lipitor) 40–80 mg Rosuvastatin (Crestor) 20–40 mg	Atorvastatin 10–20 mg Rosuvastatin 5–10 mg Simvastatin (Zocor) 20–40 mg Pravastatin (Pravachol) 40–80 mg Lovastatin (Mevacor) 40 mg	Simvastatin 10 mg Pravastatin 10–20 mg Lovastatin 20 mg

Data from Stone, N., Robinson, J., Lichtenstein, A., Bairey Merz, C., Blum, C., Eckel, R., . . . Wilson, P. (2014). 2013 ACC/AHA guideline on the treatment of blood cholesterol to reduce atherosclerotic cardiovascular risk in adults: A report of the American College of Cardiology/American Heart Association Task Force on Practice Guidelines. *Journal of the American College of Cardiology, 63*(25), 2889–2934.

c. Ezetimibe (Zetia)—cholesterol absorption inhibitor considered in combination with moderate-intensity statin for selected individuals with risk factors who cannot tolerate high-intensity statins or for whom high-intensity statins do not sufficiently lower LDL.

d. No high-quality evidence supports the use of other pharmacologic options in the management of dyslipidemia—specifically fibrates, nicotinic acid, bile acid sequestrants, omega-3 fatty acids

5. Patient education
   a. Therapeutic lifestyle changes
   b. Medication regimens, side effects, adverse reactions
   c. Monitoring schedule
   d. Use of highly effective contraception if on statin and could become pregnant

- Referral
  1. Nutritional consultation
  2. Lipid specialist with severe, refractory, or complex disorders

Coronary Heart Disease (CHD)

- Definition—atherosclerotic changes to coronary vasculature; decreased blood flow through coronary arteries due to partial obstruction or vasospasm
- Etiology, incidence, and risk factors
  1. Etiology
     a. Atherosclerosis develops with the formation of fatty streaks, fibrous plaques, and complicated lesions that narrow the lumen of the coronary arteries
     b. Angina pectoris—myocardial ischemia secondary to inability of the coronary arteries to supply oxygenated blood to meet myocardial oxygen demands
     c. Acute coronary syndromes—a plaque may rupture with thrombus formation that impedes or completely occludes the coronary lumen
        (1) Unstable angina
        (2) Acute myocardial infarction
  2. Incidence—CHD is the leading killer of women; CHD is the cause of one out of every three deaths in this population each year; known as the silent killer because symptoms may not manifest until the disease is well advanced

3. Risk factors
   a. Cigarette smoking
   b. Hypertension
   c. Dyslipidemia
   d. Diabetes mellitus
   e. Genetic predisposition
   f. Obesity
   g. Sedentary lifestyle
   h. Sleep apnea

- Symptoms
  1. May be asymptomatic
  2. Chronic stable angina pectoris
     a. Clinical syndrome characterized by discomfort in the chest, jaw, shoulder, back, or arm precipitated by exertion and relieved by rest or nitroglycerin
     b. Predictable frequency, severity, duration, and provocation
     c. Pattern remains the same unless there is an acceleration of disease process
  3. Acute coronary syndromes—unstable angina and myocardial infarction
     a. May have a constellation of symptoms including nonspecific fatigue and nausea
     b. Chest pain—pressure, heaviness, squeezing, crushing, aching
     c. Pain generally involves sternum and/or epigastrium
     d. Pain may radiate to shoulder, arm, jaw, neck, back
     e. Associated nausea, vomiting, diaphoresis, dyspnea

- Physical findings
  1. May be no specific findings
  2. Elevated blood pressure
  3. Dyspnea, tachycardia, pallor, diaphoresis
  4. Heart—changes in point of maximum impulse(s) and heart sounds may occur depending on the extent of heart damage or dysfunction

- Differential diagnosis
  1. Chronic stable angina
  2. Unstable angina
  3. Myocardial infarction
  4. Pulmonary disease—pulmonary embolism, pneumothorax, pneumonia
  5. Gastrointestinal (GI) disorders—gastroesophageal reflux disease (GERD), cholecystitis, peptic ulcer

6. Musculoskeletal conditions—costochondritis, muscle strain
7. Anxiety disorders
8. Acute aortic dissection
9. Herpes zoster
- Diagnostic tests/findings
  1. ECG
     a. Acute episode of chronic stable angina—ST-segment depression, symmetric T-wave inversion in affected leads; reverts to normal during pain-free intervals
     b. Unstable angina, myocardial infarction—changes depend on the location of involved vessel, amount of myocardium involved, duration of ischemia
  2. Exercise or pharmacologic stress testing—ischemic changes or angina during test is clinically diagnostic
  3. Myocardial perfusion imaging—used to confirm and assess the extent and location of coronary artery disease
  4. Coronary angiography—definitive test for coronary artery disease
  5. Laboratory tests—myocardial markers
     a. Troponin I and T—high sensitivity and specificity; become elevated within 3–4 hours of an event and continue to be released for as long as 7–14 days after a cardiac event
     b. Myoglobin—released within 1–3 hours of myocardial cell injury; not as cardiac specific as troponins; normalizes in 24 hours
- Management/treatment
  1. Nonpharmacologic
     a. Primary prevention—smoking cessation; dietary management of hypertension, dyslipidemia, diabetes, obesity; regular aerobic exercise
     b. Secondary prevention—surgical revascularization
        (1) Percutaneous transluminal coronary angioplasty (PTCA)
        (2) Coronary artery bypass graft (CABG)
  2. Pharmacologic—the treatment of chronic stable angina has two major purposes: to prevent myocardial infarction and to reduce the symptoms of angina
     a. Primary prevention
        (1) Medications for treatment of hypertension, diabetes, dyslipidemia, obesity, and smoking cessation
        (2) Aspirin 81–325 mg/day—inhibits platelet aggregation
     b. Secondary management of angina—may use a combination of medications for increased effectiveness—for example, sublingual nitroglycerine, beta-adrenergic blockers, CCBs
        (1) Sublingual nitroglycerine 0.4 mg as needed for symptomatic relief of anginal episodes
        (2) Beta-adrenergic blockers—metoprolol, propranolol, atenolol; preferred initial therapy in the absence of contraindications; decrease myocardial demand by decreasing heart rate, systolic BP, and contractility
        (3) CCBs—verapamil, amlodipine/long-acting formulations only; promote peripheral arterial vasodilation, thereby decreasing oxygen demand

by decreasing afterload; also decrease coronary vasospasm
        (4) Long-acting nitrates—nitropaste, nitro-patches, isosorbide dinitrate; cause venous dilation, which decreases venous return to heart and leads to modest arterial vasodilation; results in decreased myocardial oxygen demand
  3. Patient education—education and support for lifestyle changes
- Referral
  1. Patients with new-onset angina
  2. Patients with unstable angina

Eye, Ear, Nose, and Throat Disorders

Allergic Rhinitis

- Definition—inflammation of mucous membranes of nose in response to contact with specific allergens, triggering production of immunoglobulin E (IgE) antibodies, causing histamine release and subsequent edema, itching, discharge, and sneezing; the eyes, ears, sinuses, and throat can also be involved
- Etiology/incidence
  1. Affects approximately 10%–20% of adults; onset typically between ages 10 and 20 years

Classification	
Seasonal	Occurs specific times of the year when pollen/allergens are present (hay fever) a. Trees—April to July b. Grasses—May to July c. Ragweed—August to October
Perennial	year-round symptoms usually related to dust mites, mold, cockroaches, and animal dander
Episodic	exposures not usually encountered in a clients' environment (i.e. visiting house with animals)
Frequency	
Intermittent	<4 days/week *or* <4 weeks/year
Persistent	>4 days/week *and* >4 weeks/year
Severity	
Mild	symptoms are present and quality of life not affected
More severe	Symptoms affect quality of life Examples: exacerbation of coexisting asthma; sleep disturbance; impairment in performance at school or work

- Symptoms
  1. Nasal congestion, clear rhinorrhea, sneezing
  2. Pruritus of nose, throat, eyes
  3. Sore throat and cough from postnasal drip

- Physical findings
  1. Pale, boggy nasal mucosa
  2. Clear, thin rhinorrhea
  3. Nasal crease—horizontal crease across lower bridge of nose caused by repeated upper rubbing of tip of nose with palm of hand
  4. Injected conjunctiva, tearing
  5. "Allergic shiners" or dark discoloration beneath both eyes
- Differential diagnosis
  1. Vasomotor rhinitis—triggered by nasal irritants; smoke, perfume, certain medications, alcohol, spicy foods
  2. Rhinitis medicamentosa (rebound rhinitis)—caused by excessive topical use of intranasal vasoconstrictors (e.g., decongestants, cocaine)
  3. Septal obstruction—nasal polyps, deviated septum, nasal neoplasms
- Diagnostic tests/findings
  1. Usually none indicated for diagnosis
  2. Skin tests to determine specific allergens; gold standard test
  3. Serum allergy tests—radioallergosorbent test (RAST); measures amount of specific IgE to individual allergens, which correlates with the allergic sensitivity to that substance; can determine specific IgE to a number of different allergens at one time; expensive and not as sensitive as specific skin testing
- Management/treatment
  1. Nonpharmacologic—allergen avoidance
     a. Bedroom must be the most allergen free
     b. Environmental control—vacuum; dust; remove carpeting, feather pillows, stuffed animals
     c. Eliminate or restrict exposure to pets; pets should not be in bedroom
     d. Air conditioning/air filters
  2. Pharmacologic (see **Table 3-6**)
     a. Antihistamines
        (1) Generally considered first-line therapy
        (2) Highly effective in reducing itching, sneezing, rhinorrhea; minimal effect on nasal congestion
        (3) More effective if given before the onset of symptoms

Table 3-6 Antihistamines, Decongestants, and Anti-inflammatory Medications for Respiratory Disorders (Representative List)

Drug	Action	Adverse/Side Effects	Interactions	Contraindications/Precautions
Antihistamines				
First generation (short acting, 4–6 hours) Chlorpheniramine (Chlor-Trimeton) Diphenhydramine (Benadryl)	Block action of histamine; anticholinergic effects	Drowsiness, dry mucous membranes, blurred vision	Additive effects with alcohol, sedatives, antianxiety agents, monoamine oxidase (MAO) inhibitors, tricyclic antidepressants	Avoid use in elderly—sedative effect may cause adverse effects on cognition and balance. No fetal malformations associated with use; diphenhydramine is the antihistamine drug of choice in pregnancy. Not recommended during lactation, as can cause neonatal sedation
Second generation (long acting, about 24 hours) Loratidine (Claritin) Fexofenadine (Allegra) Cetirizine (Zyrtec)	Selective peripheral histamine receptor antagonist; no anticholinergic effects	Fewer sedating effects (with exception of cetirizine)	Additive central nervous system (CNS) depressant effects with alcohol, barbiturates, tricyclic antidepressants, and loratadine and cetirizine	Caution in patients with renal or hepatic dysfunction. Limited data; no known teratogenic associations
Azelastine HCl (Astelin) Intranasal	Inhibits histamine release from mast cells	Bitter taste, somnolence, headache	Potentiates other CNS depressants	No controlled human data on use in pregnancy. Only use in pregnancy if benefit outweighs risk to the fetus
Decongestants				
Pseudoephedrine (Sudafed) Phenylephrine (Neo-Synephrine, Sudafed PE)	Alpha-adrenergic agonists; vasoconstriction reduces engorgement of mucosa	Increases heart rate and BP, CNS stimulation	Hypertensive crisis with MAO inhibitors	Contraindicated with severe hypertension, cardiovascular disease, MAO inhibitor use. Some evidence of association between first-trimester use of pseudoephedrine and risk of infrequent specific congenital disabilities. No controlled human data on use of phenylephrine during pregnancy

(continues)

Table 3-6 Antihistamines, Decongestants, and Anti-inflammatory Medications for Respiratory Disorders (Representative List)   *(continued)*

Drug	Action	Adverse/Side Effects	Interactions	Contraindications/Precautions
Corticosteroids				
Intranasal				
Budesonide (Rhinocort) Fluticasone propionate (Flonase Allergy Relief), Triamcinolone acetonide (Nasacort Allergy 24 hr)	Anti-inflammatory effects; therapeutic benefit not immediate	Local irritation, epistaxis, headache, sore throat, Candida infections, Headache, pharyngitis, cough, nasal burning/irritation, asthma symptoms	Cytochrome P-450 effect; Use not recommended with CYP3A4 inhibitors (i.e. ketoconazole)	increases intraocular pressure (caution with glaucoma and cataracts) avoid with Cushing's syndrome Very little of nasal corticosteroid is absorbed systemically
Mast Cell Stabilizers				
Cromolyn (NasalCrom)	Prevents degranulation of mast cells and release of histamine; prophylactic drug	Local reactions: burning, stinging, sneezing	None known	Available data suggest no association with fetal toxicity or teratogenicity

Data from Brucker, M., & King, T. (Eds.). (2017). *Pharmacology for women's health* (2nd ed.). Burlington, MA: Jones & Bartlett Learning; Sachs, H. C., & Drugs.com (2022). *Azelastine nasal Pregnancy and Breastfeeding Warnings.* Retrieved from https://www.drugs.com/pregnancy/azelastine-nasal.html; Seidman, M. D., Gurgel, R. K., Lin, S. Y., Schwartz, S. R., Baroody, F. M., Bonner, J. R., ... & Nnacheta, L. C. (2015). Clinical practice guideline: Allergic rhinitis. *Otolaryngology–Head and Neck Surgery, 152*(1_suppl), S1–S43; Woo, T., & Robinson, M. (2020). *Pharmacotherapeutics for advance practice nurse prescribers* (5th ed.). Philadelphia, PA: F. A. Davis.

b. Decongestants—use alone or in combination with antihistamines to treat nasal congestion
c. Topical (nasal) corticosteroids
   (1) Given their effectiveness, increased use as first-line treatment
   (2) Not helpful with ocular symptoms
   (3) Slow onset of effect; may use as needed; maximal effectiveness with daily use as maintenance therapy
d. Mast cell stabilizers/intranasal cromolyns—no direct anti-inflammatory or antihistamine effects; effective for prophylaxis
e. Montelukast (**Table 3-7**)
3. Patient education
   a. Identify and eliminate or avoid allergens (e.g., remove carpeting, pets; install air filters)
   b. Appropriate use of medications; combinations, side effects, and overuse syndromes
- Referral—refer for skin tests to determine specific allergens

Conjunctivitis

- Definition—encompasses a broad group of conditions presenting as inflammation of the conjunctiva
- Etiology/incidence
  1. Viral conjunctivitis—adenovirus most common; herpes simplex and herpes zoster
  2. Bacterial conjunctivitis—staphylococci, streptococci, *Chlamydia trachomatis*, *Neisseria gonorrhea*
  3. Allergic conjunctivitis—type I, IgE-mediated hypersensitivity reaction precipitated by small airborne allergens (e.g., pollen, animal dander, dust)

  4. Most common eye complaint in primary care
- Symptoms
  1. Sensation of grit in eye, "scratchy"; mild discomfort
  2. Pain, photophobia, blurred vision that fails to clear with a blink are not typical features of the primary conjunctival process—may indicate corneal involvement
  3. Viral conjunctivitis
     a. Acute onset; may be unilateral or bilateral with a watery discharge
     b. Preauricular adenitis
     c. May be associated with upper respiratory infection (URI)
  4. Bacterial conjunctivitis
     a. Acute onset; symptoms begin in one eye and spread to the other eye
     b. Mucopurulent discharge; patient reports eyelids are matted together on awakening
     c. Marked conjunctival injection of abrupt onset with copious purulent discharge associated with gonococcal infection; sight-threatening ocular infection
  5. Allergic conjunctivitis
     a. Major cause of chronic conjunctivitis
     b. Complaints of bilateral itching, tearing, redness, and mild eyelid swelling
     c. Discharge is clear and watery, or stringy and mucoid
     d. Personal or family history of atopic disease
- Physical findings
  1. Dilation of superficial conjunctival blood vessels resulting in hyperemia; hyperemia greatest at the periphery
  2. Discharge (see Symptoms section)
  3. Cornea clear; pupils equal, round, reactive to light (PERRL)

Table 3-7 Asthma Quick-Relief and Long-Term Control Medications (Representative List)

Drug	Action	Adverse/Side Effects	Interactions	Contraindications/Precautions
Short-Acting Inhaled β_2 Agonists				
Albuterol—metered-dose inhaler (MDI), nebulizer solution	Relaxes bronchial smooth muscle by selective action on β_2 receptors Duration 2–6 hours	Tachycardia, nervousness, skeletal muscle tremor	May have increased cardiovascular effects with MAO inhibitors, tricyclic antidepressants, sympathomimetic agents; antagonized by beta blockers	Caution with cardiovascular disease, diabetes, hyperthyroidism, seizure disorders No evidence of fetal harm with use; albuterol is short-acting beta agonist of choice, if needed, during pregnancy
Inhaled Corticosteroids				
Fluticasone (Flovent) MDI/dry powder inhaler (DPI) Budesonide (Pulmicort) DPI	Inhibits inflammatory response	Minimal systemic effects; oropharyngeal candidiasis, hoarseness	Cytochrome P-450 effect; caution with CYP3A4 inhibitors (e.g., ketoconazole)	Not for treatment of acute attack Very little of nasal corticosteroid is absorbed systemically; budesonide is inhaled corticosteroid of choice, if needed, during pregnancy
Oral Corticosteroids				
Prednisone	Inhibits inflammatory response	Adrenal suppression; masks infection	Effects may be decreased by barbiturates, rifampin, other hepatic enzyme inducers; may be potentiated by ketoconazole, oral contraceptives, nonsteroidal anti-inflammatory drugs (NSAIDs)	Contraindicated with systemic mycoses; live vaccination Several studies show possible association between fetal orofacial clefts and use of prednisolone in the first trimester of pregnancy
Long-Acting Inhaled β_2 Agonists				
Salmeterol (Serevent) DPI	Relaxes bronchial smooth muscle by selective action on β_2 receptors; duration 12 hours	Headache, pharyngitis, upper respiratory infection (URI), tachycardia, tremor	May have increased cardiovascular effects with MAO inhibitors, tricyclic antidepressants, sympathomimetic agents; antagonized by beta blockers	Allergy to milk proteins; should not be used for symptom relief or acute exacerbation; caution with cardiovascular disease, diabetes, hyperthyroidism, seizure disorder Preliminary data from human studies do not support an association with fetal harm
Combination Corticosteroid and Long Acting Beta$_2$ Agonist				
Budesonide and formoterol fumerate dihydrate (Symbicort)	Long-term control of asthma, inhibits inflammatory response and long-acting selective beta$_2$-adrenergic agonist (LABA)	Headache, backpain, throat pain/irritation, candida infections, stomach discomfort, vomiting, nausea, and upper respiratory infections	May have increased cardiovascular effects with MAO inhibitors, tricyclic antidepressants, sympathomimetic agents; antagonized by beta blockers; Cytochrome P-450 effect; Use not recommended with CYP3A4 inhibitors (i.e. ketoconazole)	May cause pneumonia and lower respiratory infections with those with COPD Use cautions with glaucoma and cataract clients Not indicated for primary treatment of status asthmaticus or acute episodes of asthma or COPD
Leukotriene Modifiers				
Montelukast (Singulair)	Suppresses leukotriene Biosynthesis; leukotrienes cause the inflammation component of asthma	Headache, fatigue, fever, gastrointestinal (GI) upset, depression	Effects may be decreased with phenobarbital, erythromycin, theophylline; effects may be increased by aspirin, rifampin	Not for treatment of acute attack No evidence of teratogenicity in animal studies; no human data from controlled trials in pregnancy

(continues)

Table 3-7 Asthma Quick-Relief and Long-Term Control Medications (Representative List)   *(continued)*

Drug	Action	Adverse/Side Effects	Interactions	Contraindications/Precautions
Mast Cell Stabilizers				
Cromolyn (Intal) Nedocromil (Tilade)	Prevents mast cells' release of histamine, leukotrienes; inhibits antigen-induced bronchospasm	Throat irritation, bad taste, cough	None identified	Not for treatment of acute attacks No evidence of teratogenicity in animal studies; no human data from controlled trials in pregnancy; use only if benefits outweigh risks in pregnancy
Methylxanthines				
Theophylline	Relaxes bronchial smooth muscle	GI upset, headache, central nervous system (CNS) stimulation, diuresis, arrhythmias, seizures	Cytochrome P-450 effect; numerous drugs may affect serum concentration via induction or inhibition of P-450 enzymes	Peptic ulcer disease, arrhythmias, seizure disorders Some teratogenicity in animal studies; no human data from controlled trials during pregnancy

Data from Drugs.com (2022). *Nedocromil Pregnancy and Breastfeeding Warnings.* Retrieved from https://www.drugs.com/pregnancy/nedocromil.html Brucker, M., & King, T. (Eds.). (2017). *Pharmacology for women's health* (2nd ed.). Burlington, MA: Jones & Bartlett Learning; Woo, T., & Robinson, M. (2020). *Pharmacotherapeutics for advanced practice nurse prescribers* (5th ed.). Philadelphia, PA: F. A. Davis.

4. Visual acuity with no acute change
5. Preauricular adenopathy—most common with viral etiology
- Differential diagnosis
  1. Foreign body
  2. Subconjunctival hemorrhage
  3. Blepharitis
  4. Episcleritis/scleritis
  5. Keratitis
  6. Uveitis
  7. Acute angle closure glaucoma
- Diagnostic tests/findings
  1. Typically, none indicated
  2. Fluorescein stain—stain uptake suggests corneal involvement
  3. Cultures, if suspected, gonococcal or chlamydial infection; chronic or recurrent infection; failure to respond to treatment
- Management/treatment
  1. Viral
     a. Self-limited
     b. Cold compresses and lubricants (liquid tears) for comfort
  2. Bacterial
     a. Broad-spectrum topical antibiotic—erythromycin; sodium sulfacetamide; polymixin B/trimethoprim
     b. Systemic antibiotics for gonococcal and chlamydial infections—ceftriaxone, azithromycin; doxycycline, erythromycin base
  3. Allergic
     a. Removal of offending allergen, if possible
     b. Short-term treatments for acute episodes—dual treatment with topical antihistamines (Neo-Synephrine) and vasoconstrictors (Clear Eyes)
     c. Extended therapy for seasonal/perennial allergic conjunctivitis—combination of topical antihistamine and a mast cell stabilizer, or combination oral antihistamine and a mast cell stabilizer (olopatadine HCl/Olopatadine, bepotastine/Bepreve)
     d. Topical NSAIDs—ketorolac (Acular)
  4. Prevention of transmission of viral or bacterial conjunctivitis
     a. Frequent, thorough handwashing for patients and close contacts
     b. Avoid close contact and sharing linens during the acute phase when drainage occurs
     c. Discard opened eye makeup; replace contact lenses, cases, and opened solutions
- Referral
  1. Patients with pain, photophobia, blurred vision; circumcorneal erythema/ciliary flush
  2. Conjunctivitis caused by herpes simplex or herpes zoster
  3. No improvement after 48 hours of treatment

Acute Otitis Media

- Definition—infection of the middle ear that is often preceded by URI or allergies
- Etiology/incidence/risk factors
  1. Etiology
     a. Eustachian tube dysfunction secondary to URI (often viral) or allergies causes edema and congestion that impede the flow of middle ear secretions; accumulation of secretions promotes the growth of pathogens
     b. Common pathogens—*Streptococcus pneumoniae, Haemophilus influenzae, Moraxella catarrhalis,* rhinovirus, respiratory syncytial virus
  2. Highest incidence in childhood, younger than age 10 years; seen infrequently in adults

3. Risk factors
   a. Recent/current URI
   b. Exposure to cigarette smoke, active or passive
- Symptoms
   1. Rapid onset, short duration, if uncomplicated
   2. Ear pain, decreased hearing, fever (adults less likely to have fever)
   3. Aural pressure
   4. Vertigo, nausea, and vomiting
- Physical findings
   1. Full or bulging tympanic membrane (TM) with absent or obscured landmarks
   2. Distorted light reflex
   3. Decreased/absent mobility of TM on pneumatic otoscopy
   4. Erythema of TM is an inconsistent finding
   5. Bullae on TM; often associated with *Mycoplasma pneumoniae*
   6. Postauricular or cervical lymphadenopathy
- Differential diagnosis
   1. Otitis externa
   2. Otitis media with effusion
   3. Temporomandibular joint (TMJ) syndrome
   4. Dental abscess
   5. Mastoiditis
- Diagnostic tests/findings
   1. Usually none indicated
   2. Tympanometry for recurrent infections; indicator fluid posterior to TM
- Management/treatment
   1. Most uncomplicated cases of acute otitis media resolve spontaneously without antibiotic treatment
   2. Weigh factors of symptoms lasting slightly longer if antibiotics are not used versus increase in antibiotic resistance
   3. Pharmacologic
      a. Analgesics—acetaminophen, NSAIDs
      b. Antibiotics
         (1) Amoxicillin (Amoxil) is the first-line choice; if inadequate response, change to amoxicillin–clavulanate (Augmentin); azithromycin (Zithromax), or trimethoprim–sulfamethoxazole (TMP/SMX/Bactrim DS/Septra) if penicillin-allergic
         (2) Contraindications/precautions
            (a) TMP/SMX may potentiate anticoagulants and hypoglycemic agents
            (b) Avoid use of TMP/SMX during the first and third trimesters of pregnancy
      c. No demonstrated benefit with the use of decongestants
   4. Patient education
      a. Appropriate ear canal hygiene
      b. Antibiotic use and side effects
      c. Need for additional care if no improvement in 2–3 days
      d. Cessation of smoking and avoidance of second-hand smoke exposure
- Referral
   1. For suspected extension of infection, mastoiditis, or perforation of TM

   2. Persistent hearing loss after adequate treatment
   3. Adults with recurrent otitis media need ears, nose, and throat (ENT) referral to rule out underlying process (e.g., malignancy)

Sinusitis

- Definition—inflammation of the mucosal surface of the paranasal sinuses
- Etiology/incidence
   1. Etiology
      a. Acute sinusitis—caused by viral or bacterial infections and allergies; bacterial causes include *Streptococcus pneumoniae, Haemophilus influenzae, Moraxella catarrhalis*
      b. Infection usually involves maxillary and ethmoid sinuses
      c. Chronic sinusitis occurs with episodes of prolonged infection that resist treatment and/or repeated or inadequately treated acute infection; treatment failure secondary to failure of sinuses to drain, which may be associated with anatomic defect
   2. Incidence—accounts for 6% of primary care office visits
- Symptoms
   1. Acute sinusitis
      a. Nasal congestion, facial pain, toothache, headache, fever, yellow/green nasal drainage
      b. Increased pain with bending over or sudden head movement
      c. Common cold and allergic/vasomotor rhinitis may precede infection
      d. "Double sickening"—URI symptoms with initial improvement, followed by increasing nasal symptoms
   2. Chronic sinusitis
      a. Nasal congestion, discharge, and cough that last longer than 30 days
      b. Dull ache or pressure across forehead and/or midface
      c. Constant postnasal drip and chronic cough
- Physical findings
   1. Afebrile or low-grade fever
   2. Mucopurulent nasal discharge; postnasal discharge
   3. Nasal mucosa swollen, pale, dull red to gray
   4. Pain on firm palpation over sinus areas
- Differential diagnosis
   1. Uncomplicated URI
   2. Migraine headaches
   3. Allergic/vasomotor rhinitis
   4. Nasal polyps
   5. Dental abscess
   6. Trigeminal neuralgia
- Diagnostic tests/findings
   1. None for typical presentation
   2. Maxillofacial CT scan—reserved for complicated disease and search for ethmoidal disease in patients with refractory symptoms
- Management/treatment
   1. Nonpharmacologic
      a. Saline nasal spray

b. Steam inhalation

c. Warm compresses

d. Hydration

2. Pharmacologic

a. Antibiotics

(1) If symptoms are present 10 or more days without any clinical improvement

(2) If symptoms worsen after 5–6 days when patient was initially improving

(3) If high fever (>102°F) and facial pain or purulent nasal discharge for 3 or more days

(4) First-line therapy—amoxicillin–clavulanate (Augmentin) for 5–7 days; if penicillin allergic—doxycycline; levofloxacin

(5) If no improvement on antibiotics within 72 hours, reevaluate and consider a change in antibiotic

b. Oral/topical decongestants

(1) Oral decongestants (see Table 3-6)

(2) Topical decongestant/oxymetazoline spray 0.05%

(a) Provides rapid relief

(b) Should not be used for longer than 3–5 days to prevent rebound congestion

c. Nasal steroids—to reduce mucosal inflammation (see Table 3-6)

d. Antihistamines not recommended unless patient has allergies

e. Pain management as needed with acetaminophen, NSAIDs

3. Patient education

a. Avoidance of allergens, environmental irritants (e.g., cigarette smoke)

b. Importance of maintaining adequate hydration

- Referral

1. Severe facial pain, periorbital swelling

2. Failure to respond to two courses of antibiotic

3. Suspected anatomic abnormality

4. Chronic sinusitis or more than three episodes of acute sinusitis per year

Upper Respiratory Infection/Common Cold

- Definition—an acute, mild, self-limited viral infection of the upper respiratory tract (nasal cavity, pharynx, and larynx) mucosa,

  **Important to note that acute otitis media and sinusitis also included in URI; however, included in Eye, Ear, Nose, and Throat Disorders*

- Etiology/incidence/risk factors

1. Etiology

a. Inflammation of the mucosal membranes: nasal cavity, pharynx, and larynx

b. Rhinovirus, adenovirus, influenza, parainfluenza, coronavirus, Streptococcus pyrogenes (group A streptococcus), Epstein Barr Virus

c. Spread by airborne droplets and contact with infectious secretions on hands and environmental surfaces

d. Incubation period of 1–5 days

2. Incidence

a. Peaks in winter months

b. Children—six to eight infections per season

c. Adults—two to four infections per season

3. Risks

a. Repeated exposure to groups of children

b. Close quarters, contact

- Symptoms

1. General malaise

2. Nasal congestion and clear rhinorrhea

3. Sneezing, coughing, sore throat, hoarseness

4. Tearing, burning sensation of eyes

- Physical findings

1. Low-grade fever

2. Nasal mucosa swollen and erythematous

3. Conjunctiva slightly red

4. Throat erythematous with cervical lymphadenopathy

- Differential diagnosis

1. Allergic rhinitis

2. Streptococcal pharyngitis

3. Influenza

4. COVID-19

5. Otitis media

- Diagnostic tests/findings

1. Generally, none recommended

2. Rapid strep screen/throat culture if streptococcal pharyngitis suspected

3. If >65, consider Respiratory Synctial Virus (RSV) Nucleic Acid Amplification Test (NAAT)

4. COVID-19 Rapid Antigen Test or NAAT

- Management/treatment

1. Nonpharmacologic

a. Inhalation of warm vapors

b. Saline nasal drops or sprays

c. Saline gargles/throat lozenges

d. Increase fluids

2. Pharmacologic

a. Acetaminophen or NSAIDs

b. Topical/oral decongestants (see Table 3-6)

c. Cough suppressants—e.g., dextromethorphan (Robitussin)

(1) Drug action—depresses cough reflex by direct inhibition of cough center in the medulla

(2) Contraindications/precautions

(a) Potential for hyperpyretic crisis if used with MAO inhibitors

(b) Do not use for persistent or chronic cough

(c) Animal reproduction studies have shown an adverse effect on the fetus, but there are no adequate and well-controlled studies in humans; use during pregnancy only if the benefits outweigh potential risk to the fetus

d. Expectorants—e.g., guaifenesin (Mucinex)

(1) Drug action—may increase output of respiratory tract secretions, facilitating removal of mucus

(2) Contraindications/precautions

(a) May increase toxicity/effect of disulfiram, MAO inhibitors, metronidazole

(b) Animal reproduction studies have not shown any adverse effect on the fetus, but there are no adequate and well-controlled studies in humans; use during pregnancy only if benefits outweigh potential risk to fetus
3. Patient education
   a. Infection control
   b. Self-limited nature of infection
   c. Symptoms of complications; secondary bacterial infection

Pharyngitis

- Definition—inflammation of the pharynx and tonsils
- Etiology/incidence
  1. Etiology
     a. Viral—most common cause is rhinovirus and adenovirus
     b. Bacterial
        (1) Group A beta-hemolytic streptococci (GABHS)
        (2) *Neisseria gonorrhoeae*
     c. Noninfectious causes—allergic rhinitis or postnasal drip
  2. Incidence
     a. One of the most frequent reasons for outpatient care in the United States
     b. Accounts for 16 million office visits per year; 2.5% of visits to primary care providers
- Risks—crowded work or living conditions, exposure to children
- Symptoms
  1. Viral pharyngitis
     a. Sore throat, fever, malaise, cough, headache, myalgia, fatigue
     b. May also complain of rhinitis, congestion, conjunctivitis
  2. GABHS
     a. Sudden onset of sore throat, fever, chills, headache, nausea/vomiting (occasionally)
     b. Rhinitis, cough, conjunctivitis typically absent
- Physical findings
  1. Viral pharyngitis—mild erythema of the pharynx with little or no exudates
  2. Bacterial pharyngitis
     a. Marked erythema of the throat, exudates, tender anterior cervical lymphadenopathy
     b. Erythematous "sandpaper" rash/accentuation in groin and axillae with scarlet fever
- Differential diagnosis
  1. Peritonsillar abscess
  2. Infectious mononucleosis
  3. Pharyngeal candidiasis
  4. Diphtheria
  5. Epiglottitis
- Diagnostic tests/findings
  1. GABHS testing is not indicated in all adults with pharyngitis—5% to 15% of adult pharyngitis cases are caused by GABHS

2. Rapid streptococcal antigen test is recommended for adult with pharyngitis that meets two or more of the following criteria
   a. Fever
   b. Lack of cough
   c. Tonsillar exudates
   d. Tender anterior cervical adenopathy
3. Cultures are not recommended for routine evaluation of adult pharyngitis or for confirmation of negative rapid antigen tests
4. Culture is useful if other pathogens (e.g., gonococcus) are being considered
- Management/treatment
  1. Nonpharmacologic
     a. Adequate hydration
     b. Saline gargles
     c. Topical anesthetics (e.g., lozenges, sprays)
  2. Pharmacologic
     a. GABHS
        (1) Penicillin V PO/benzathine penicillin IM
           (a) Drug action—bactericidal
           (b) Side effects—hypersensitivity reactions
           (c) Contraindications/precautions—penicillin allergy
        (2) Erythromycin if penicillin allergy
     b. Gonococcal pharyngitis—ceftriaxone IM
        (1) Drug action—bactericidal
        (2) Contraindications/precautions
           (a) Known anaphylactic penicillin allergy is generally a contraindication
           (b) Alternative agent is IM gentamycin;
           (c) obtain pharyngeal NAAT test for GC 2 weeks after either treatment.
- Referral
  1. Suspected peritonsillar abscess
  2. Epiglottitis

Coronavirus Disease 2019 (COVID-19)

As this remains a fluid situation, please stay up to date with any changes to recommendations at the CDC, NIH, ACOG, and Society for Maternal Fetal Medicine (SMFM).

- Definition—a mild to severe respiratory illness caused by a coronavirus called severe acute respiratory syndrome coronavirus 2 (SARS CoV-2). It is in the same family of coronaviruses that are the causes of common viruses responsible for head and chest colds to more severe diseases like severe acute respiratory syndrome (SARS) and Middle East respiratory syndrome (MERS). Discovered in December 2019, and The World Health Organization declared a pandemic in March 2020.
  1. Severe COVID-19 is primarily a lower respiratory tract infection in earlier phases of the pandemic
  2. Early and mild cases MAY have features of upper respiratory tract viral infection. This can be seen in omicron cases and those with breakthrough infections in the immunized populations.
- Etiology/incidence
  1. Etiology
     a. Causal pathogens

    (1) SARS-CoV-2
      (a) Variants
- Alpha
- Delta
- Omicron—50%–70% more transmissible than earlier variants
- Sub-variants of Omicron-BA.5 and BA.4.6

  b. Transmission
    (1) droplet transmission and/or aerosolization—inhalation of infectious particles (especially indoors/prolonged exposure, areas with poor ventilation)
      (a) recommendation of mask wearing and 6-foot social distancing to minimize the risk of transmission
    (2) Fomite transmission- risk is considered low
    (3) Viral shedding of asymptomatic people may occur
    (4) Viral shedding appears to occur approximately 48 hours prior to symptom onset
    (5) Viral titers are the highest 1–2 days prior to symptom onset and within the first 4–6 days of illness in patients without immunosuppression

  c. Incubation
    (1) Omicron—4.3 days, median 3–4 days, range 2–14 days

  d. Isolation and Quarantine recommendations—*As this remains a fluid situation, please stay up to date with any changes to recommendations at CDC.gov*
    (1) Quarantine—if partially exposed
      (a) No longer recommended as of August 2022 if up to date with immunization
      (b) If exposed (close contact <6 feet from infected person × 15 minutes cumulatively >24 hours) and not up to date on immunization (to include booster recommendations) or unimmunized
- Stay home × 5 days or wear a well-fitted mask if client cannot stay at home; no travel and get tested 5 days after close contact
- Monitor for symptoms × 10 days and avoid travel
- If symptoms develop, isolate and get tested
- Wear a mask for a full 10 days
- Avoid high-risk people
    (2) No travel, regardless of immunized status, for 10 days
      (a) Monitor for symptoms × 10 days

2. Incidence
  a. Approximately affecting more than 70% of the U.S. population with approximately 500 million confirmed cases and attributing to 6 million deaths
  b. >65 years old and people with comorbidities are more likely to develop an infection and severe symptoms and are at higher risk for death
  c. >85 years highest risk

  d. 81% of the U.S deaths are people aged >65 years with 80× greater mortality risk than 18–29 year olds
  e. CDC reports that 95% of COVID-19-related deaths have at least one comorbidity.
  f. Children <1 years of age are at higher risk for severe illness
  g. Approximately 80% of infections are not considered severe and recover without special treatment.
  h. Approximately 20% develop severe infection (elderly and comorbidities)
    (1) Approximately 15% require hospitalization
    (2) Approximately 5% require admission to the ICU
  i. Pregnant people
    (1) 41% higher risk for ICU admission during the Delta period (June 27, 2021–December 25, 2021) than compared to pregnant persons during the pre-Delta period (January 1, 2020–June 26, 2021)
    (2) 83% higher for invasive intubation or ECMO (extracorporeal membrane oxygenation) in the Delta period
    (3) 3.3 times higher risk of death in the pre-Delta period
      (a) Compared to non-pregnant people between the ages 15–44 years old—5 times the risk of admission to an ICU and a 76% increased risk for invasive intubation or ECMO
      (b) Death rate was 1.3 times higher than those who were not pregnant in the Delta period
  j. Health equity
    (1) Communities of color have been disproportionately affected by the COVID-19 pandemic
    (2) Individuals in communities of color are more likely to have severe illness and die from COVID-19
    (3) Largely related to social and structural factors
      (a) Including disparities in socioeconomic status, access to care, rates of chronic conditions, occupational exposures, systemic racism, and historic and continued inequities in healthcare systems
    (4) Black and Hispanic populations have lower vaccination rates compared to other populations

- Symptoms—may be milder with omicron infection and immunized
1. Cough, fever, myalgias, chills, sweats, fatigue, sore throat, GI symptoms, conjunctivitis, loss of taste or smell, rash
2. Serious/warning symptoms
  a. Shortness of breath
  b. Chest pain/pressure
  c. Confusion
  d. Lethargy
  e. Cyanosis
- Physical findings
1. Fever, tachypnea, tachycardia, rhinorrhea, nasal congestion, pharyngeal erythema and inflammation, dry

cough, rales, focal wheezing, high or low jugular venous pressure, decreased breath sounds, fluid retention, hypoxia
- Differential diagnosis
  1. Respiratory syncytial virus infection
  2. Influenza
  3. Community-acquired pneumonia
- Diagnostic tests/considerations/findings
  1. Viral Tests
     a. NAATs—highly sensitive and specific.
        (1) Detects one or more viral ribonucleic acid (RNA) genes and indicates a current infection
        (2) Viral RNA may remain in one's body for 90 days. DO NOT use this test if the patient was positive within the last 90 days.
        (3) Can be performed in a lab or point-of-care test
     b. Antigen tests
        (1) Immunoassays that detect the presence of specific viral antigen
        (2) Have similar specificity but less sensitive than most NAATs
        (3) Less expensive than NAATs and results in minutes
        (4) Negative results do not rule out SARS-CoV-2 infection
     c. Antibody (serologic) tests
        (1) Used to detect previous infection
        (2) Used for public health surveillance and epidemiologic purposes
        (3) Detects specific antibodies that target different parts (nucleocapsid or spike protein) of the virus
        (4) Consideration for discerning if antibodies present from COVID-19 vaccines versus a past infection
  2. Chest X-ray
     a. With severe COVID-19 demonstrate bilateral airspace consolidation
  3. Chest computed tomography (CT)
     a. Bilateral, peripheral ground glass opacities and consolidation
     b. Less common findings
        (1) intra-interlobular septal thickening with ground glass opacities (crazy paving pattern)
        (2) focal and rounded areas of ground glass opacity surrounded by a ring or arc of denser consolidation (reverse halo sign)
- Management/treatment
  1. Nonpharmacologic—lozenges, gargles for relief of pharyngitis; treatment largely supportive and monitor symptoms
  2. Pharmacologic
     a. It is important to note that as of September 26, 2022, guidance from the Centers for Disease Control and Prevention and the American College of Obstetricians and Gynecologists, and the Society for Maternal–Fetal Medicine recommend against withholding COVID-19 treatments or vaccination from pregnant or lactating individuals.
     b. They also recommend therapeutic management of pregnant people with COVID-19 should be the same as for nonpregnant patients with the exception including:
        (1) Non-recommendation of molnupiravir in pregnant persons unless there are no other options available and therapy is clearly indicated
        (2) Pregnancy and recent pregnancy are comorbidities the CDC classifies as risk factors for severe COVID-19 and is an indication for pharmacotherapy treatment.
        (3) Insufficient evidence to recommend therapeutic anticoagulation in pregnant persons with COVID-19 who do not have evidence of venous thromboembolism
     c. Although therapeutic recommendations for pregnant people should be the same as nonpregnant people, it is important to note that there is limited evidence and shared decision-making will need to take place with the client and multidisciplinary team.
     d. Acetaminophen, NSAIDs to reduce fever, aches
     e. Corticosteroids—prescribed for significant pharyngeal edema
     f. Antiviral drug
        (1) Nirmatrelvir/ritonavir (Paxlovid)—received Emergency Use Authorization (EUA) in December 2021
           (a) Outpatient treatment for mild/moderate symptoms and eligible
           (b) Begin ideally within 72 hours of onset of symptoms and no more than 5 days after symptom onset
        (2) Remdesivir—FDA approved October 2020 for COVID-19 hospitalized patients, age > 12 years or 40 hg
           (a) EUA issued for children <12 years
           (b) 3-day infusion and face barriers due to lack of staffing, room for patients while infusing, and patient demands
           (c) Similar efficacy to nirmatrelvir/ritonavir in limiting hospitalizations and deaths in the unvaccinated populations
        (3) Molnupiravir—received FDA EUA December 2021
           (a) 30% less effective than all other therapies in avoiding hospitalizations and death in unvaccinated patients
           (b) Good alternative option for those with significant renal impairment or drug–drug-interactions with other therapy options.
           (c) Need a pregnancy screen for genotoxicity concerns
           (d) No drug interactions noted
  3. Patient education
     a. Recommendation of vaccination and boosters to include pregnant persons
     b. Recommendation of booster in third trimester of pregnancy to provide antibody protection to newborn after birth
     c. Use supportive measures and stay home

- Referral
  1. Refer to hospital/ER if atypical presentation and/or symptoms are suggestive of complications of COVID-19 (i.e., ARDS, pneumonia, etc.)

Influenza

- Definition—acute respiratory viral infection that is responsible for significant global morbidity and mortality
- Etiology/incidence
  1. Etiology
     a. Causal pathogens
        (1) Influenza A—infects multiple species (humans, swine, equines, and birds). Most responsible for major pandemics. Many subtypes (i.e., H3N2, H5N1, H1N1)
        (2) Influenza B
        (3) Influenza C
     b. Mode of transmission
        (1) Large droplet transmission—inhalation of infectious particles
        (2) Airborne—small particle transmission by speaking or exhalation
        (3) Fomite transmission
  2. Incidence
     a. Affects approximately 8% of the U.S. population, ranging from 3% to 11% depending on the year
     b. Children (0–17 years old) and those 65 and older more likely to get sick from influenza
     c. Children (<18 years old) are more than twice as likely to develop symptomatic influenza
- Symptoms
  1. Cough, fever, myalgias, chills, sweats, fatigue, rhinitis, sore throat
  2. Vomiting/diarrhea—more likely to occur in children than adults
- Physical findings
  1. Fever, tachypnea, tachycardia, rhinorrhea, nasal congestion, pharyngeal erythema and inflammation, dry cough, rales, focal wheezing
- Differential diagnosis
  1. Respiratory syncytial virus infection
  2. COVID-19
  3. Rhinovirus
  4. Parainfluenza
  5. Adenovirus
  6. Dengue
  7. Legionnaires' disease
- Diagnostic tests/findings
  1. Rapid Influenza Diagnostic Tests (antigen detection)
     a. Tests influenzas A and B
     b. Nasopharyngeal swab, nasal swab, aspirate, or wash, throat swab
     c. <15 minutes for results
  2. Rapid molecular assay (influenza viral RNA or nucleic acid detection)
     a. Tests Influenza A and B
     b. Nasopharyngeal swab, nasal swab
     c. 15–30 minutes for results

3. Immunofluorescence, Direct (DFA) or Indirect (IFA) Fluorescent Antibody Staining (antigen detection)
   a. Tests Influenza A and B
   b. Nasopharyngeal swab or wash, bronchial wash, nasal or endotracheal aspirate
   c. 1–4 hours for results
4. RT-PCR (singleplex and multiplex; real-time and other RNA based) and other molecular assays (influenza viral RNA or nucleic acid detection)
   a. Tests Influenza A and B
   b. Nasopharyngeal swab, throat swab, nasopharyngeal or bronchial wash, nasal or endotracheal aspirate, sputum
   c. 1–8 hours return of results (depending on the assay)
5. Rapid cell structure
   a. Tests Influenza A and B
   b. Nasopharyngeal swab, throat swab, nasopharyngeal or bronchial wash, nasal or endotracheal aspirate, sputum
   c. 1–3 days for results
6. Viral tissue cell culture
   a. Tests Influenza A and B
   b. Nasopharyngeal swab, throat swab, nasopharyngeal or bronchial wash, nasal or endotracheal aspirate, sputum
   c. 3–10 days for results
- Management/treatment
  1. Nonpharmacologic—lozenges, gargles for relief of pharyngitis; treatment largely supportive
  2. Pharmacologic
     a. Acetaminophen, NSAIDs to reduce fever, aches
     b. Corticosteroids—prescribed for significant pharyngeal edema
     c. Antiviral drug
        (1) Treatment is recommended as soon as possible for patients suspected or confirmed who:
           (a) Are hospitalized
           (b) Have severe, complicated, or progressive illness
           (c) Are at higher risk for influenza complications
        (2) Oral oseltamivir initial recommendation for outpatient suspected or confirmed influenza with complications or progressive disease (i.e. pneumonia, exacerbation of chronic medical conditions)
        (3) Outpatient treatment for those who meet approved age groups with suspected or confirmed influenza
           (a) Oral oseltamivir
           (b) Inhaled zanamivir
           (c) IV peramivir
           (d) Oral baloxavir
        (4) Obstetric clients
           (a) Pregnant people and postpartum people up to 2 weeks are at increased risk for hospitalization with influenza compared to nonpregnant people
           (b) Initiate antiviral treatment as soon as possible after illness onset (i.e., within 48 hours of illness likely to be more beneficial)

(c) Do not wait for confirmation with laboratory testing if suspected

(d) Oral oseltamivir is the antiviral of choice for pregnant people and postpartum for up to 2 weeks since it has the most studies and the data suggest that it is safe and beneficial.

(e) Treat for 5 days

3. Co-circulation of Influenza and SARS-CoV-2
   a. Empiric antiviral treatment of influenza is recommended as soon as possible for priority groups:
      (1) Hospitalized patients with respiratory illness
      (2) Outpatients with severe, complicated, or progressive respiratory illness
      (3) Outpatients at higher risk for influenza complications who present with any acute respiratory illness symptoms (with or without fever)
   b. Co-infection with influenza and SAR-CoV-2 can occur and should be considered particularly with severe respiratory disease—see up-to-date CDC recommendations for further treatment recommendations

4. Patient education
   a. Recommendation of vaccination
   b. Use supportive measures and stay home until not symptomatic and feeling better typically around 5 days of symptom onset

- Referral
  1. Refer to hospital/ER if atypical presentation and/or symptoms are suggestive of complications of influenzas (i.e., pneumonia)

Infectious Mononucleosis (IM)

- Definition—an acute, self-limiting viral syndrome characterized by fever, malaise, pharyngitis, and lymphadenopathy
- Etiology/incidence
  1. Etiology
     a. Causal agent is most often Epstein-Barr virus (EBV)
     b. Mode of transmission is oropharyngeal route via saliva
  2. Incidence—rarely symptomatic in children younger than 5 years; most clinically apparent infections occur in individuals 10–30 years old; peak rate ages of 15–19 years
- Symptoms
  1. Prodrome of headache, malaise, fatigue, anorexia
  2. Fever, sore throat, swollen lymph nodes (classic triad)
- Physical findings
  1. Tonsillar enlargement with exudate
  2. Palatal petechiae at the junction of hard and soft palates (25% of cases)
  3. Lymphadenopathy; particularly posterior cervical chain
  4. Fever compatible with the severity of infection
  5. Hepatomegaly (25% of cases)
  6. Splenomegaly (50% of cases)
- Differential diagnosis
  1. Streptococcal pharyngitis

2. Other viral causes of pharyngitis
3. Acute cytomegalovirus (CMV) infection
4. Acute HIV infection

- Diagnostic tests/findings
  1. Monospot/heterophile antibody test
     a. Sensitivity 63%–84%; specificity 84%–100%
     b. Initially negative, usually positive by 1–2 weeks after onset of symptoms
  2. CBC—lymphocytic leukocytosis; atypical lymphocytes common
  3. Liver function tests (LFTs)—may have elevated aminotransferases (alanine aminotransferase [ALT], aspartate aminotransferase [AST]), bilirubin
  4. Throat culture—secondary infection with GABHS in about 30% of cases
  5. CT scan—may reveal splenomegaly and/or hepatomegaly; not required for diagnosis

- Management/treatment
  1. Nonpharmacologic—lozenges, gargles for relief of pharyngitis; treatment largely supportive
  2. Pharmacologic
     a. Acetaminophen, NSAIDs to reduce fever, aches
     b. Corticosteroids—prescribed for significant pharyngeal edema and obstructive tonsillar enlargement
  3. Patient education
     a. Rest during acute phase of illness; activity as tolerated
     b. Contact sports, heavy lifting, and strenuous activity should be avoided for at least 1 month if the patient has splenomegaly
     c. Avoid alcohol for at least 1 month
     d. Seek immediate care with sudden onset of severe abdominal pain

- Referral
  1. Onset of abdominal pain—possible ruptured spleen
  2. Airway obstruction from pharyngeal edema
     See **Table 3-8** for an overview of upper respiratory tract infections.

Lower Respiratory Disorders

Community-Acquired Pneumonia

- Definition—acute infection of the lower respiratory tract (trachea, primary bronchi, and lungs) that is associated with at least two symptoms of active pneumonia infection in an individual who has not been hospitalized or resided in a long-term care facility for 14 days before the onset of symptoms
- Etiology/incidence/risk factors
  1. Etiology
     a. Bacterial—*Streptococcus pneumoniae, Haemophilus influenzae, Legionella pneumophila*
     b. Atypical, nonbacterial—*Mycoplasma pneumoniae, Chlamydia pneumoniae*
     c. Viral—influenza, adenovirus
  2. Incidence—sixth leading cause of death; leading cause of death from infectious disease

Table 3-8 Overview of Upper Respiratory Tract Infections

Conditions	Pathogens	Symptoms/Physical findings	Treatment
Pharyngitis	Viral (most common): adenovirus, Epstein-Barr virus, influenza A/B, parainfluenza, rhinovirus Bacterial: *Streptococcus pyrogenes* (group A *Streptococcus*), SARS CoV-2	Viral: Sore throat, fever, malaise, cough, myalgia, fatigue, rhinitis, conjunctivitis Bacterial (GABS): sudden onset sore throat, fever, enlarged lymph node, erythema of tonsils, tender anterior cervical lymphadenopathy	Viral: Supportive measures, antiviral medication Bacterial: Penicillin or Amoxicillin if group A *Streptococcus* confirmed
Laryngitis	Viral (most common): Parainfluenza virus, influenza, rhinovirus, adenovirus, coronavirus	Viral: Sore throat, dry throat, dry cough	Supportive measures
Common Cold	Adenovirus, rhinovirus, parainfluenza, RSV, SARS CoV-2	Rhinorrhea, headache, sore throat, loss of smell, malaise, congestion	Supportive measures

3. Risk factors
   a. Preceding viral URI
   b. Cigarette smoking
   c. Age older than 65 years
   d. Chronic lung disease
   e. Corticosteroid use
   f. Immunosuppression
- Symptoms
  1. May be masked or absent in very young, elderly, immunosuppressed, coexisting chronic disease
  2. Fever, chills, sweats
  3. Cough with/without sputum production
  4. Dyspnea, pleuritic chest pain
  5. Associated symptoms—lethargy, headache, anorexia, nausea, vomiting
- Physical findings
  1. Tachycardia
  2. Tachypnea, dyspnea, hypoxia
  3. Percussion
     a. Often normal in early disease
     b. Dullness over area of consolidation
  4. Auscultation
     a. Coarse rhonchi may clear or shift with cough
     b. Nonclearing rales
     c. Diminished breath sounds over consolidation
  5. Fever with chills, high spikes ($\geq$ 102.2°F) especially if bacterial etiology
  6. Small areas of pneumonia cannot always be detected by physical examination
- Differential diagnosis
  1. Bronchitis
  2. Atelectasis
  3. Chronic obstructive pulmonary disease (COPD)
  4. Congestive heart failure
  5. Malignancy
  6. Tuberculosis
  7. Pulmonary embolism
  8. COVID-19
- Diagnostic tests/findings
  1. Chest radiograph
     a. Establishes diagnosis by revealing an infiltrate; helps distinguish pneumonia from acute bronchitis

   b. Demonstrates the presence of complications, such as pleural effusion and multilobar disease
2. Value of sputum collection for Gram stain and culture is controversial—not recommended as routine for outpatients diagnosed with community-acquired pneumonia
3. CBC with differential—white blood cell (WBC) elevation (10,000/mm^3 to 25,000/mm^3) with a shift to the left (e.g., bandemia, neutrophilia, especially if bacterial etiology)
4. Tuberculosis (TB) test
- Management/treatment
  1. Nonpharmacologic
     a. Oral hydration and humidification
     b. Improve oxygenation (e.g., smoking cessation)
  2. Pharmacologic
     a. Empiric antimicrobial therapy—American Thoracic Society (Mandell et al., 2007)
        (1) Patients who are otherwise healthy with no risk factors for drug-resistant streptococcal pneumonia (DRSP)—advanced-generation macrolide (azithromycin or clarithromycin)
           (a) Drug action—inhibits bacterial protein synthesis
           (b) Contraindications/precautions—contraindicated if allergy to macrolide antibiotics; alternative antibiotic is doxycycline, which is contraindicated during pregnancy
        (2) Patients with comorbidity, risk factors for DRSP, including age older than 65 years or nursing home residence, or use of antimicrobials within previous 3 months (use alternative from different class)—fluoroquinolone (levofloxacin, moxifloxacin, emifloxacinacin)
     b. Antipyretics—acetaminophen, NSAIDs
  3. Patient education
     a. Infection containment principles
     b. Need for hydration
     c. Rest
     d. Avoid cough medicines if a productive cough can clear thick secretions
     e. Medication schedules and side effects

f. Prevention—annual influenza vaccination; pneumonia vaccination for individuals age 65 years or older or at high risk for pneumonia; smoking cessation
- Referral/physician consult
  1. Fever >102°F, pallor or cyanosis, nasal flaring
  2. No improvement in 24 to 36 hours
  3. CURB-65 criteria—hospitalize for treatment if patient has two or more of the following five criteria
     a. *Confusion*
     b. *Uremia* (blood urea nitrogen [BUN] >19 mg/dL)
     c. *Respiratory rate* >30 bpm
     d. *Blood pressure* <90 mm Hg systolic or 60 mm Hg diastolic
     e. *65 years old*

Asthma

- Definition
  1. A lower respiratory chronic inflammatory disorder of the airways in which many cells and cellular elements play a role—characterized by recurring symptoms, airflow obstruction, bronchial hyperresponsiveness; airflow obstruction is widespread, variable, and usually reversible with an improvement of forced expiratory volume in 1 second (FEV_1) >12% with short-acting bronchodilator. Characterized by episodes of shortness of breath, cough, wheezing, and chest tightness that are recurrent and reversible.
  2. Classifications—intermittent (stage 1), mild persistent (stage 2), moderate persistent (stage 3), severe persistent (stage 4) used as basis for treatment decisions
     a. Frequency and timing of symptoms
     b. Degree of variation in pulmonary function throughout the day
     c. Degree of impairment that patient experiences from having asthma
     d. Intermittent—stage 1
        (1) Daytime symptoms two times/week or less; nocturnal symptoms two times/month or less
        (2) Use of short-acting beta-agonist inhaler 2 days/week or less
        (3) Either no or one exacerbation requiring oral corticosteroids over the last year
        (4) No interference with normal activity
        (5) FEV_1 greater than 80% predicted; normal FEV_1/FVC (forced vital capacity) ratio for age between exacerbations
     e. Mild persistent—stage 2
        (1) Daytime symptoms greater than two times/week but not daily; nocturnal symptoms three to four times/month
        (2) Use of a short-acting beta-agonist inhaler to manage symptoms greater 2 days/week, no more than one time a day and not daily
        (3) Two or more exacerbations requiring oral corticosteroids over last year
        (4) Mild interference with normal activity
        (5) FEV_1 greater than 80% predicted; normal FEV_1/FVC ratio for age between exacerbations
     f. Moderate persistent—stage 3
        (1) Daily symptoms; nocturnal symptoms more than once per week but not nightly
        (2) Daily use of a short-acting beta-agonist inhaler to manage symptoms
        (3) Two or more exacerbations requiring oral corticosteroids over last year
        (4) Some limitation in performing normal activities
        (5) FEV_1 60%–80% predicted; normal FEV_1/FVC ratio for age reduced by >5%
     g. Severe persistent—stage 4
        (1) Continual daily symptoms; frequent nocturnal symptoms
        (2) Use of short-acting beta-agonist throughout the day for symptom control
        (3) Two or more exacerbations requiring oral corticosteroids over the previous year
        (4) Major limitations in performing normal activities
        (5) FEV_1 less than 60% predicted; normal FEV_1/FVC ratio for age reduced by >5%
- Etiology/incidence
  1. Etiology
     a. Caused by single or multiple triggers
        (1) Allergic triggers
           (a) Airborne pollens, molds, dust mites, cockroaches, animal dander
           (b) Food additives or preservatives
           (c) Feather pillows
        (2) Nonallergic triggers
           (a) Smoke and other pollutants
           (b) Viral respiratory infections
           (c) Medications—acetylsalicylic acid (ASA, aspirin), NSAIDs, beta blockers
           (d) Exercise
           (e) Gastroesophageal reflux
           (f) Emotional factors
           (g) Menses, pregnancy
           (h) Obesity
     b. In children, generally a strong history of atopy; adult-onset asthma may be related to allergens, but nonallergic triggers likely to be a factor
  2. Incidence
     a. Affects approximately 10% of children and 5% of adults
     b. Can occur at any age; increasing in prevalence in the United States
- Symptoms
  1. Episodic wheeze, chest tightness, shortness of breath or cough; cough may be the sole symptom
  2. Symptoms worsen in the presence of aeroallergens, irritants, and exercise
  3. Symptoms occur or worsen at night; cause nighttime awakening
- Physical findings
  1. Hyperexpansion of thorax; hyperresonance with percussion
  2. Wheezing; prolonged respiratory phase
  3. Diminished breath sounds

4. Tachypnea, dyspnea
5. Atopic dermatitis/eczema or other skin manifestations of allergic skin disorders
6. Increased nasal secretions, mucosal swelling, nasal polyps
- Differential diagnosis
  1. Acute infection—bronchitis, pneumonia
  2. COPD; may overlap with asthma
  3. Heart disease—heart failure
  4. Foreign body aspiration
  5. Pulmonary emboli
  6. Cough secondary to drugs such as ACE inhibitors
  7. Cough secondary to GERD
- iagnostic tests/findings
  1. Pulmonary function tests/spirometry—useful to differentiate between restrictive lung disease and obstructive lung disease and to determine the severity of airway obstruction
     a. FVC—normal is >80% of predicted value; useful for diagnosing restrictive lung disease
     b. FEV_1 used to determine the severity of airway obstruction—normal is >80% of the predicted norm for age, sex, height; measured with spirometry
     c. FEV_1/FCV ratio used to detect airway obstruction—normal is >70% for middle-aged adult; measured with spirometry
  2. Peak expiratory flow (PEF) with peak flow meter—obstruction suggested by <80% of personal best; measured at home or office
  3. Chest radiograph, if infection, large airway lesions, heart disease, or foreign body obstruction suspected
- Management/treatment
  1. Goals
     a. Minimize symptoms, normalize daily activity
     b. Maintain near-normal pulmonary function
     c. Minimal use of short-acting β_2-agonist
  2. Nonpharmacologic
     a. Peak flow monitoring
        (1) Establish the patient's personal best and develop Asthma Action Plan
        (2) A drop in peak flow below 80% indicates an acute exacerbation and the need to contact the clinician for medication adjustment
        (3) A drop in peak flow below 50% indicates the need for emergency treatment
     b. Avoidance of known allergens, triggers
     c. Adequate hydration and humidity
     d. Annual influenza vaccine; pneumococcal vaccine
  3. Pharmacologic—see Table 3-7
     a. Staged approach for treatment (see **Box 3-1**)
     b. Severe exacerbation (peak flow <60%) can occur with any category of asthma; consider a short course of oral corticosteroids of 40–60 mg/day for 5–10 days
     c. Treatment of asthma in pregnancy
  4. Uncontrolled asthma increases the risk of perinatal mortality, preeclampsia, preterm birth, and low-birth-weight infants
  5. It is safer for pregnant people to be treated for asthma than to have asthma symptoms and exacerbations

---

Box 3-1 Staged Approach for Treatment

Intermittent: Stage 1
- No daily medications
- Short-acting inhaled β_2-agonist as needed for symptoms
- Course of systemic corticosteroids recommended for severe exacerbations

Mild Persistent: Stage 2
- Low-dose inhaled corticosteroids
- Alternative treatments—mast-cell stabilizer, leukotriene modifier, theophylline
- Short-acting inhaled β_2-agonist as needed for symptoms

Moderate Persistent: Stage 3
- Low- to medium-dose inhaled corticosteroids and long-acting inhaled β_2-agonist
- Alternative treatments: add leukotriene or theophylline; increase inhaled corticosteroid within medium dose range
- Short-acting inhaled β_2-agonist as needed for symptoms

Severe Persistent: Stage 4
- High-dose inhaled corticosteroids and long-acting inhaled β_2-agonist; oral corticosteroid if needed
- Short-acting inhaled β_2-agonist as needed for symptoms

Data from National Heart, Lung, and Blood Institute. (2007). *Expert panel report 3: Guidelines for the diagnosis and management of asthma.* (NIH Publication No. 07-4051). Bethesda, MD: Author

---

6. Albuterol is the preferred short-acting inhaled β_2-agonist; inhaled corticosteroids may be used; use the lowest dose needed to maintain normal respiratory function and have good control of symptoms
7. Patient education
   a. How to recognize signs of worsening asthma
   b. Use of peak flow meter
   c. Clear instructions on the use of a written Asthma Action Plan
   d. Proper use of inhaler for effective dosing
   e. Prophylactic medication (e.g., preexercise dosing)
   f. Control of environmental factors (e.g., allergens and irritants)
- Referral
  1. Arrange for immediate emergency treatment if signs of severe obstruction present—peak flow reduced by 50%, pulsus paradoxus, inaudible breath sounds, inability to lie flat, cyanosis
  2. Difficulty controlling asthma

Tuberculosis (TB)

- Definition—necrotizing bacterial infection caused by *Mycobacterium tuberculosis*; most commonly infects the lungs, but any organ can be affected
  1. Active TB disease (ATBD)—signs, symptoms, and radiographic findings secondary to *M. tuberculosis*; disease may be pulmonary or extrapulmonary

2. TB infection/latent TB infection (LTBI)
   a. Positive tuberculin skin or blood test with no signs or symptoms of disease
   b. Chest radiograph negative or only granulomas/calcifications in lungs and/or regional lymph nodes
   c. Not infectious to others
- Etiology/incidence/risk factors
  1. Etiology—*M. tuberculosis;* spread by small airborne particles
  2. Incidence
     a. In the United States, 10–15 million infected
     b. Most primary TB infections remain in a latent or dormant stage—90% to 95%
  3. Risk factors
     a. Individuals with weakened immune systems—presence of HIV, severe kidney disease, organ transplant, long-term corticosteroid therapy
     b. Individuals who are incarcerated, in long-term institutional living, or in crowded conditions
     c. Individuals with active substance use disorder
     d. Individuals who have emigrated from countries with high TB rates
     e. Individuals who work in institutions or facilities that serve high-risk individuals—hospitals, long-term care, correctional facilities, homeless shelters
     f. Household contacts of diagnosed cases
- Symptoms
  1. TB infection/LTBI
     a. Asymptomatic state may last months to years
     b. Approximately 10% go on to develop active TB
  2. Active TB/ATBD
     a. Generalized symptoms
        (1) Night sweats, fever
        (2) Malaise, weakness
        (3) Anorexia
        (4) Weight loss
     b. Pulmonary symptoms
        (1) Productive cough, possible hemoptysis
        (2) Chest pain
        (3) Dyspnea
     c. Systemic symptoms (extrapulmonary sites)
        (1) Pelvic pain
        (2) Flank pain
- Physical findings
  1. Generally normal appearance in early disease, progressing to cachectic
  2. Unexplained fever
  3. Lung findings—increased tactile fremitus and dullness to percussion over consolidated areas; apical rales
  4. Advanced disease—purulent green or yellow sputum
  5. Hemoptysis
- Differential diagnosis
  1. Pneumonia
  2. Malignancy
  3. COPD
  4. Silicosis
  5. Sarcoidosis
- Diagnostic tests/findings
  1. Purified protein derivative (PPD) skin test (antigen response)

a. Positive test indicates exposure, not active disease
b. Individual must return to the office in 48 to 72 hours to interpret test results
c. PPD interpretation—measure area of induration, not erythema
   (1) A reaction of 5-mm induration or greater is considered positive in patients who meet one of these criteria:
      (a) HIV infection or in immunocompromised/immunosuppressed individuals
      (b) Those with abnormal chest radiographs consistent with healed TB lesions
      (c) Recent close contact with an infected person
   (2) A reaction of 10-mm induration or greater is considered positive in patients who meet one of these criteria:
      (a) Recent arrivals (<5 years) from high-prevalence areas
      (b) Low socioeconomic status, homeless
      (c) Aged, nursing home residents, incarcerated individuals
      (d) Individuals with chronic disease or predisposing conditions (e.g., gastrectomy, diabetes mellitus, or corticosteroid therapy)
   (3) A reaction of 15-mm induration or greater is considered positive among individuals without risk factors
d. False negative
   (1) PPD administered after recent live virus vaccination
   (2) Immunosuppressed
   (3) Elderly
   (4) Incorrect administration—needs to be intradermal
e. False positive
   (1) Previous Bacillus Calmette–Guérin (BCG) vaccination
   (2) Nontuberculosis mycobacterium
f. Positive converter—previous negative PPD
2. Interferon-gamma release assay (IRGA) blood test—measures immune reaction to bacteria causing TB
   a. Requires only one visit; test results within 24 hours
   b. Not affected by prior BCG vaccination
   c. Reported as positive or negative
   d. More expensive
3. Chest radiography, both anteroposterior and lateral views; indicated by a positive skin or blood TB test result
   a. Identifies active pulmonary disease; negative chest radiograph rules out active TB
   b. Radiologic findings include apical scarring, hilar adenopathy with peripheral infiltrate and upper lobe cavitation
4. Three sputum samples required for both smear and culture in patients suspected of pulmonary TB
   a. A presumptive diagnosis of TB can be made with detection of acid-fast bacilli in sputum smear
   b. A positive culture for *M. tuberculosis* is essential to confirm diagnosis

- Management/treatment
  1. LTBI
     a. Nonpharmacologic—not applicable
     b. Pharmacologic
        (1) It is recommended to test individuals only if they would be candidates for treatment of LTBI
        (2) Treatment goal—stop progression to active disease state
        (3) Recommended for individuals at high risk of exposure and those at high risk of progression from LTBI to active disease—same as risk factors for acquiring infection
        (4) Treatment with isoniazid for 9 months
            (a) Drug action—inhibition of mycolic acid synthesis resulting in disruption of bacterial cell wall
            (b) Contraindications/precautions/ considerations
                i. Contraindicated with severe hepatic disease; monitor transaminase levels at baseline and at 3, 6, and 9 months
                ii. Risk for peripheral neuropathy; supplement with vitamin B_6 (pyridoxine) 50 mg each day
                iii. Considered safe during pregnancy and lactation; may consider delaying treatment of LTBI in low-risk pregnant people until postpartum
  2. Active disease treatment—consult/referral to specialist
     a. Nonpharmacologic
        (1) Well-balanced diet; additional caloric intake may be needed to maintain or gain weight
        (2) Outdoor exercise
     b. Pharmacologic
        (1) Typical regimen includes isoniazid, rifampin, pyrazinamide for 2 months; isoniazid and rifampin for 4 months; given resistance concerns, include ethambutol in initial regimen until drug susceptibility tests are known
        (2) Directly observed therapy (DOT) is one method to ensure compliance; the healthcare provider/designee observes the patient ingest medications
  3. Patient education
     a. Importance of continuous treatment
        (1) Possibility of microbial resistance
        (2) Signs of developing side effects, drug interactions
     b. Infection control principles
        (1) Reducing respiratory droplet broadcast
        (2) Care with disposal of infected wastes, tissues
        (3) Avoiding crowded conditions, contact with susceptible individuals while infectious
     c. Follow-up requirements, liver function monitoring
     d. Necessity for contact evaluation and treatment, including involvement of the Health Department.
     e. Importance of general health maintenance
- Referral
  1. Patients with ATBD
  2. Report all cases to state and local health departments

Gastrointestinal Disorders

Constipation

- Definition—infrequent or difficult evacuation of stool
  1. Constipation is a symptom rather than a disease
  2. May include incomplete evacuation of stool, straining during bowel movement, hard stools, fewer than three bowel movements in a week
- Etiology/incidence
  1. Etiology
     a. Functional causes—Most common cause
        (1) low-fiber diet, motility disorders (irritable bowel syndrome), sedentary lifestyle, dehydration
     b. Structural abnormalities—anal disorders (anal fissure), colon polyps or tumors, diverticulosis
     c. Hypothyroidism
     d. Neurologic, neuromuscular disorder—multiple sclerosis, spinal cord disorders
     e. Celiac disease
     f. Medications—laxative overuse, anticholinergics, opioids, iron supplements
     g. Pregnancy
  2. Prevalence—unknown because of frequent self-treatment; commonly reported by patients, especially elderly adults
  3. Risks—see Etiology/Incidence section; more common in elderly
- Symptoms
  1. Typically, fewer than three bowel movements per week
  2. Hard feces, difficult to pass
  3. Abdominal bloating or pain
  4. Hemorrhoids
  5. Sense of incomplete evacuation
  6. Having to use fingers to help stool passage
- Physical findings
  1. Firm-to-hard stool in rectum
  2. Fecal impaction
  3. Abdomen
     a. Normal bowel sounds
     b. Nontender with simple constipation
- Differential diagnosis—see Etiology/Incidence section; constipation is a symptom, not a disease
- Diagnostic tests/findings—indicated when "red flags" identified, constipation is persistent or fails to respond to treatment, or a particular disorder suspected
  1. Red flags
     a. Abdominal pain, nausea/vomiting
     b. Weight loss
     c. Melena, rectal bleeding
     d. Rectal pain
     e. Fever
     f. New onset older than age 50 years
  2. Diagnostic tests
     a. Typically none needed
     b. CBC, TSH
     c. Stools for occult blood test
     d. Flexible sigmoidoscopy/colonoscopy

- Management/treatment
  1. Nonpharmacologic
     a. Increased fluid intake
     b. Increased physical activity
     c. High-fiber diet—bran, fruits, vegetables, whole-grain cereals and bread
     d. Plan time for elimination, consistent time each day
  2. Pharmacologic
     a. Bulk-forming agents—psyllium husk, methylcellulose, calcium polycarbophil
        (1) Drug action
            (a) Increased stool bulk, retention of stool water, reduced transit time
            (b) Used to prevent constipation; not useful treatment of acute constipation
        (2) Contraindications/precautions
            (a) May result in decreased absorption of some medications
            (b) Do not use if the patient has signs of fecal impaction or GI obstruction
            (c) May use during pregnancy
     b. Stool softeners—docusate sodium (Colace)
        (1) Drug action
            (a) Act as surfactants; lower surface tension, which facilitates penetration of water into stool
            (b) Useful for patients complaining of hard stools and those for whom straining at stool should be avoided
        (2) Contraindications/precautions
            (a) Do not use if the patient has acute abdominal pain, signs of GI obstruction
            (b) May use during pregnancy
     c. Osmotic laxatives—sorbitol, lactulose, polyethylene glycol
        (1) Drug action
            (a) Nonabsorbable disaccharide that acts as an osmotic diuretic
            (b) Drug of choice after bulk-forming laxatives for chronic constipation
        (2) Contraindications/precautions
            (a) Do not use if the patient has acute abdominal pain or signs of GI obstruction
            (b) Do not use if the patient is on a galactose-restricted diet
            (c) May use short term during pregnancy if unresponsive to bulk-forming laxatives or stool softeners
     d. Saline laxatives—magnesium hydroxide/milk of magnesia
        (1) Drug action
            (a) Variety of poorly absorbed salts that draw water into intestinal lumen, causing fecal mass to soften and swell; swelling stretches intestinal lumen and stimulates peristalsis
            (b) Treatment of acute constipation
        (2) Contraindications/precautions
            (a) Decreased absorption of some medications
            (b) Do not use if the patient has acute abdominal pain or signs of GI obstruction

            (c) May use short term during pregnancy if unresponsive to bulk-forming laxatives or stool softeners
     e. Chloride channel activator—lubiprostone (Amitiza)
        (1) Drug action
            (a) GI motility enhancer; increases fluid in the intestines
            (b) Treatment of chronic idiopathic constipation
        (2) Contraindications/precautions
            (a) Avoid use if the patient has renal or hepatic impairment
            (b) Confirm absence of GI obstruction before use
            (c) Take with food and water
            (d) Reevaluate periodically for need to continue—established as safe for up to 12 months
            (e) Animal reproduction studies have shown an adverse effect on the fetus; there are no adequate and well-controlled studies in humans; use during pregnancy only if benefits outweigh potential risk to the fetus
  3. Patient education
     a. Plan time for defecation; do not ignore the urge to defecate
     b. Avoid overuse of laxatives
     c. Drink adequate amounts of fluid to avoid dehydration
     d. Increase fiber in diet
- Referral—any suspected obstructive or serious systemic pathology

Diarrhea

- Definition—defecation of loose, watery stools three or more times a day
  1. Diarrhea is a symptom rather than a disease
  2. Acute—less than 1–2 weeks' duration
  3. Chronic—more than 3 weeks' duration, continuous or intermittent
- Etiology/incidence/risk factors
  1. Etiology
     a. Acute
        (1) Viral—Norwalk
        (2) Bacterial—*Salmonella, Shigella, Escherichia coli* (traveler's diarrhea)
        (3) Protozoa—*Giardia lamblia, Entamoeba histolytica*
        (4) Bacterial toxins—*Staphylococcus, Clostridium*
        (5) Medications—antibiotics, laxatives, antacids
     b. Chronic or recurrent
        (1) Protozoa—*Giardia lamblia, E. histolytica*
        (2) Inflammatory—ulcerative colitis, Crohn's disease, ischemic colitis
        (3) Medications—antibiotics, laxatives, antacids
        (4) Functional—irritable bowel syndrome
        (5) Malabsorption—sprue, pancreatic insufficiency, lactase deficiency
        (6) Postsurgical—gastric bypass, dumping syndrome

(7) Hyperthyroidism
2. Incidence—estimated that the average adult in the United States experiences one to two acute diarrheal episodes per year
3. Risk factors
   a. Travel to some countries in Africa, Asia, Latin America, Caribbean
   b. Close contact with infected persons (e.g., day care, institutionalization)
   c. Decreased immunity—more susceptible to organisms that generally do not cause symptoms in immunocompetent hosts
- Symptoms
   1. Increased frequency and volume of stools
   2. Crampy abdominal pain
   3. May be associated with nausea and vomiting
   4. Dehydration if severe
- Physical findings
   1. Acute
      a. Occasionally—low-grade fever; postural changes in pulse, blood pressure
      b. Abdominal examination—hyperactive bowel sounds; diffuse tenderness to palpation
   2. Chronic—signs associated with specific causes (e.g., thyromegaly, lymphadenopathy, rectal mass, impaction)
- Differential diagnosis—see Etiology section; diarrhea is a symptom, not a disease
- Diagnostic tests/findings
   1. Usually none indicated for symptoms lasting less than 72 hours unless associated with bloody diarrhea or the patient appears ill
   2. If persistent or chronic
      a. Stool evaluation
         (1) For fecal leukocytes
         (2) For occult blood
         (3) For culture for bacterial pathogens
         (4) For ova and parasites
         (5) *Giardia* antigen assay
         (6) *Clostridium difficile* toxin assay
         (7) Qualitative fat (Sudan stain)—fat content increased in presence of small bowel disease or pancreatic insufficiency
      b. HIV testing
      c. CBC, electrolytes, and sedimentation rate for indications of infection, dehydration
      d. TSH low in hyperthyroidism
- Management/treatment
   1. Nonpharmacologic
      a. Observation—acute diarrhea is usually self-limited
      b. Hydration/electrolyte replacement
      c. Normal diet as soon as the patient able to tolerate
      d. For lactase deficiency, limit milk products and consider exogenous lactase
   2. Pharmacologic
      a. Antimotility agents—loperamide (Imodium), diphenoxylate (Lomotil)
         (1) Drug action—slows intestinal transit, allowing more time for absorption
         (2) Contraindications/precautions
            (a) May have anticholinergic effects
            (b) Use contraindicated if the patient has bloody diarrhea, acute dysentery, ulcerative colitis
            (c) Safe during pregnancy and lactation
      b. Antisecretory agents—bismuth subsalicylate (Kaopectate, Pepto-Bismol)
         (1) Drug action—may involve adsorption of bacterial toxins and/or local anti-inflammatory effect
         (2) Contraindications/precautions
            (a) May potentiate oral anticoagulants and hypoglycemic agents
            (b) Avoid use if hypersensitivity to salicylates
            (c) Not recommended during pregnancy because of salicylate component
      c. Antibiotics
         (1) Indicated only when a pathogen is identifiable
         (2) May exacerbate simple episode
         (3) Traveler's diarrhea—ciprofloxacin or trimethoprim–sulfamethoxazole for 3 days
   3. Patient education
      a. Maintain adequate fluid intake
      b. Normal diet when tolerated
      c. Limit use of antidiarrheal agents
      d. Prevention of traveler's diarrhea
         (1) Don't drink tap water or use tap water for brushing teeth or as ice in drinks
         (2) Don't eat raw fruits and vegetables unless you have to peel them
         (3) Don't drink unpasteurized milk or milk products
         (4) Don't eat raw or rare cooked meats or fish
- Indications for referral
   1. Blood in stools
   2. Diarrhea accompanied by severe abdominal pain
   3. Worsening symptoms
   4. Definitive diagnosis and management of underlying disease

Hemorrhoids

- Definition—varicosities of the hemorrhoidal plexus in lower rectum or anus
   1. Internal
      a. Originate above the anorectal line
      b. Covered by nonsensitive rectal mucosa
   2. External
      a. Originate below the anorectal line
      b. Covered by well-innervated epithelium
- Etiology, incidence, and risk factors
   1. Etiology
      a. Thin-walled, dilated vessels; engorge with increased intra-abdominal pressure
      b. Prolapse may occur secondary to passage of a large, hard stool; increase in venous pressure from pregnancy or heart failure; straining due to lifting or defecation
   2. One of the most commonly encountered anorectal conditions in general practice

3. Risk factors
   a. Constipation, straining at stool
   b. Pregnancy or childbirth with a prolonged second stage
   c. Low-fiber diet
   d. Pelvic congestion
   e. Poor pelvic musculature
   f. Loss of muscle tone with advanced age
- Symptoms
  1. Internal—painless, bright red bleeding with defecation
  2. External—itching, pain, and bleeding with defecation
- Physical findings
  1. Internal
     a. Usually not palpable unless thrombosed
     b. Usually not visible unless prolapsed
  2. External
     a. Protrude with straining or standing
     b. Blue, shiny masses at the anus if thrombosed
     c. Painless, flaccid skin tags (resolved thrombotic hemorrhoids)
- Differential diagnosis
  1. Condyloma accuminata
  2. Rectal prolapse
  3. Rule out other causes for bleeding
     a. Colorectal cancer
     b. Polyps
     c. Anal fissures
     d. Inflammatory bowel disease
     e. Colonic diverticulitis
- Diagnostic tests/findings
  1. Anoscopic examination—with internal hemorrhoids, bright red to purplish bulges
  2. Additional testing if underlying pathology suspected
- Management/treatment—no treatment necessary if asymptomatic
  1. Nonpharmacologic
     a. Increase bulk/fiber/fluids in diet
     b. Sitz baths
     c. Witch hazel pads or gel—may provide transient relief and help reduce inflammation
  2. Pharmacologic
     a. Topical anesthetic/steroid suppositories and ointments
        (1) Drug action—anesthetic and anti-inflammatory action
        (2) Contraindications/precautions—may be used during pregnancy
     b. Bulk-forming agents (see Constipation section in this chapter)
     c. Stool softeners (see Constipation section in this chapter)
  3. Patient education
     a. Regulation of bowel habits
     b. Dietary changes to maintain hydration, bulk
     c. Appropriate use of bulk laxatives, stool softeners, hemorrhoidal preparations
- Referral
  1. Acute thrombosis of an external hemorrhoid
  2. Failure to respond to conservative management

Irritable Bowel Syndrome (IBS)

- Definition
  1. A chronic functional disorder characterized by altered bowel habits and abdominal pain
  2. Rome IV (replaced Rome III criteria in 2016) Criteria for diagnosis of irritable bowel syndrome
     a. Diagnostic criteria
        (1) Recurrent abdominal pain on average at least 1 day/week in the last 3 months, associated with two or more of the following criteria
           (a) Related to defecation
           (b) Associated with a change in the frequency of the stool
           (c) Associated with a change in the form (appearance) of the stool
        (2) The criteria described above should be fulfilled for the last 3 months with symptom onset at least 6 months prior to diagnosis
     b. Predominant (no longer an average) bowel habits >25% of occasions for subgroup identification
        (1) IBS-C-IBS with predominant constipation
        (2) IBS-D-IBS with predominant diarrhea
        (3) IBS-M-IBS with mixed bowel habits
        (4) IBS, untyped
     c. Stool classification utilizing the Bristol Stool Form Scale
        (1) Type 1: Separate hard lumps, like nuts (hard to pass)
        (2) Type 2: Sausage-shaped, but lumpy
        (3) Type 3: Like a sausage but with cracks on its surface (considered normal stools)
        (4) Type 4: Like a sausage or snake, smooth and soft (considered normal stools)
        (5) Type 5: Soft blobs with clear-cut edges (passed easily)
        (6) Type 6: Fluffy pieces with ragged edges, a mushy stool
        (7) Type 7: Watery, no solid pieces, entirely liquid
- Etiology/prevalence/risk factors
  1. Etiology—proposed
     a. Altered bowel motility
     b. Visceral hypersensitivity
     c. Imbalance of neurotransmitters
  2. Prevalence—as high as 15% in the general population; female-to-male ratio, 2:1; onset usually late teens, early adulthood
- Symptoms
  1. Refer to the Rome criteria
  2. Presence of the following symptoms suggests organic disease (alarm symptoms)
     a. Pain/diarrhea that interferes with sleep
     b. Recurrent nausea and vomiting
     c. Evidence of GI bleeding
     d. Unintentional weight loss (>10% of body weight)
     e. Persistent diarrhea or severe constipation
- Physical findings—mild left lower quadrant (LLQ) tenderness on abdominal examination
- Differential diagnosis
  1. Food intolerance—lactose, fructose, sorbitol

2. Colon cancer
3. Infectious disease/parasitic infestation (*Giardia*)
4. Inflammatory disease (ulcerative colitis, Crohn's disease)
5. Laxative abuse
- Diagnostic tests/findings
   1. Not indicated for patients younger than 50 years or who meet Rome criteria, have normal physical examination, or lack alarm symptoms
   2. Consider the following, dependent on other history or physical examination findings
      a. CBC, chemistry panel, sedimentation rate, celiac panel
      b. Stool studies including fecal leukocytes, occult blood, ova, and parasites
      c. Flexible sigmoidoscopy
   3. Colonoscopy, if the patient is older than 50 years, has weight loss, anemia, evidence of GI bleeding, or risk factors for colon cancer or inflammatory bowel disease
- Management/treatment
   1. Nonpharmacologic
      a. Reassurance of benign nature of disease
      b. Diet
         (1) Decrease caffeine, alcohol, fatty foods, gas-forming foods, or products containing sorbitol; limit dairy products if lactose intolerance suspected
         (2) Increase fiber in diet or in the form of supplements if the patient has constipation-IBS
      c. Mindfulness-based cognitive therapy, psychotherapy, stress management, relaxation techniques, identification of triggers
      d. Regular physical activity
      e. Probiotics—theorized that they may ameliorate IBS symptoms by stimulating immune response, reducing inflammation, altering the composition of gut flora
   2. Pharmacologic—use patient's symptoms as a guide
      a. Pain predominant
         (1) Antispasmodic/anticholinergic—dicyclomine hydrochloride (Bentyl), *L*-hyoscyamine sulfate (Hyosine, Anaspaz)
            (a) Drug action—selectively inhibits GI smooth muscle and may reduce pain and bloating
            (b) Contraindications/precautions/considerations
               i. May cause drowsiness, anticholinergic effects
               ii. Do not use if the patient has glaucoma, unstable cardiovascular disease, GI or urinary tract obstruction
               iii. Animal reproduction studies have not shown any adverse effect on the fetus, but there are no adequate and well-controlled studies in humans; use during pregnancy only if the benefits outweigh potential risk to the fetus
         (2) Tricyclic antidepressants—amitriptyline, nortriptyline, desipramine (not FDA approved for this indication)

            (a) Drug action—analgesic and mood-enhancing properties; anticholinergic effects
            (b) Contraindications/precautions/considerations
               i. May have anticholinergic effects
               ii. Do not use during or within 14 days of MAO inhibitors
               iii. Do not use postacute MI
               iv. Animal reproduction studies have shown an adverse effect on the fetus, and there are no adequate and well-controlled studies in humans; use during pregnancy only if the benefits outweigh the potential risk to the fetus
      b. Diarrhea predominant
         (1) Loperamide (Imodium), diphenoxylate (Lomotil)
         (2) Alosetron (Lotronex)
            (a) Drug action—a 5-HT$_3$ receptor antagonist, decreases intestinal secretion, motility, and afferent pain signals
            (b) Limited use for those with severe chronic diarrhea and predominant IBS; unresponsive to conventional therapy and not caused by anatomic or metabolic abnormality
            (c) Contraindications/precautions/considerations
               i. May have severe adverse GI effects, including ischemic colitis and serious complications of constipation that could result in hospitalization and rarely blood transfusion, surgery, and death
               ii. Only healthcare providers enrolled in Lotronex (alosetron) prescribing program should prescribe
               iii. Discontinue immediately in patients who develop constipation or symptoms of ischemic colitis
               iv. Animal reproduction studies have not shown any adverse effect on the fetus, but there are no adequate and well-controlled studies in humans; use during pregnancy only if the benefits outweigh the potential risk to the fetus
      c. Constipation predominant
         (1) Fiber supplements—psyllium, polycarbophil, methylcellulose
         (2) Osmotic laxative—lactulose, sorbitol, polyethylene glycol, magnesium hydroxide
         (3) Lubiprostone (Amitiza)
   3. Patient education
      a. Appropriate implementation of the nonpharmacologic measures
      b. Education on the gut/brain access
      c. Reassurance of the relative benign nature of disorder
      d. Need for reevaluation if symptoms progress or change
- Referral—onset in those older than 50 years; presence of symptoms suggestive of organic disease/alarm symptoms

Appendicitis

- Definition—inflammation of the wall of the vermiform appendix that may result in perforation with subsequent peritonitis
- Etiology/incidence
  1. Etiology
     a. Based on operative findings, classified as simple, gangrenous, or perforated
     b. Acute appendicitis secondary to obstruction due to fecal material, lymphoid hyperplasia, foreign bodies, or parasites with secondary bacterial infection
     c. Gangrene and perforation develop within 24–36 hours; perforation results in the release of luminal contents into the peritoneal cavity
  2. Incidence—occurs in all age groups; highest incidence in males 10–30 years of age
- Symptoms—classic sequence of symptoms
  1. Pain is the initial symptom; begins in the epigastrium or periumbilical area
  2. Anorexia, nausea, or vomiting
  3. Pain localizes to the right lower quadrant (RLQ) after several hours
  4. Sense of constipation; infrequently diarrhea
- Physical findings
  1. Temperature of 99°F–100°F (>100°F may indicate peritonitis)
  2. Tenderness localized to McBurney's point; pain worsened and localized with cough
  3. Signs of peritoneal irritation—guarding, rigidity, and rebound tenderness in RLQ
  4. Absent bowel sounds
  5. Positive psoas sign—pain with flexion at the hip against resistance or hyperextension
  6. Positive Rovsing's sign—RLQ pain elicited when LLQ is deeply palpated and pressure is released
  7. Positive obturator sign—pain with passive internal rotation of flexed right hip/knee
  8. Rectal examination may reveal tenderness/mass
- Differential diagnosis
  1. Ovarian (e.g., mittelschmerz, cyst)
  2. Ectopic pregnancy
  3. Pelvic inflammatory disease
  4. Pyelonephritis, calculi
  5. Gallbladder or pancreatic inflammation
  6. Gastroenteritis
- Diagnostic tests/findings
  1. WBC count—moderate leukocytosis 10,000–18,000 cells/mm^3
  2. Validated diagnostic tools
     a. The Alvarado Score
        (1) Eight item, 10-point tool and the best-studied clinical decision tool in adults and children
        (2) Stratifies risk into low, moderate, high risk
     b. Appendicitis Inflammatory Response Score
        (1) Includes fewer symptoms than the Alvarado score but adds an inflammatory biomarker (C-reactive Protein)
  3. Pregnancy test—rule out ectopic pregnancy
  4. Ultrasound is diagnostic in 85% of patients

5. CT is the most commonly used (~75% of cases); however, ultrasonography recommended by multiple professional organizations as the initial modality, especially for pediatrics and pregnancy
  6. CT is specific and sensitive but time consuming and costly. Must consider its usefulness in routine diagnosis
- Management/treatment
  1. Nonpharmacologic—none
  2. Pharmacologic—Acetaminophen and NSAIDs should be considered for pain management, especially for those who have contraindications to opioids while awaiting referral/transfer
  3. Patient education
     a. Need for emergency care if pain or other symptoms change during observation, evaluation period
     b. Postoperative care instructions
- Referral—immediate surgery; consult for acute abdomen

Peptic Ulcer Disease (PUD)

- Definition—chronic mucosal ulcerative disorder involving the upper GI tract (stomach or duodenum); imbalance both in the amount of acid–pepsin production and in the ability of gastric and duodenal mucosa to protect itself
- Etiology/incidence/risk factors
  1. Etiology
     a. Acid and pepsin activity overpower mucosal defenses to produce ulcers when mucosal defense is impaired by exogenous factors/*Helicobacter pylori* and NSAIDs
     b. *H. pylori*—established causative factor
        (1) 90%–95% of duodenal ulcer patients and 70%–80% of gastric ulcer patients are infected with *H. pylori*
        (2) gram-negative bacterium; produces urease, which breaks down urea, forming ammonia and CO_2, and allowing an organism to control the pH of its environment
     c. NSAIDs—damage mucosa through direct action and systemically by inhibiting endogenous prostaglandin synthesis; NSAID-related ulcers more likely to be gastric
  2. Incidence
     a. Estimated 5%–10% of the general population
     b. Male/female ratio nearly equal
     c. Duodenal ulcers more common, with peak incidence at 25–55 years of age; peak incidence of gastric ulcers at 55–65 years of age
  3. Risk factors
     a. Family history
     b. Cigarette smoking—delays healing and increases the risk of recurrence
     c. Medications—corticosteroids, NSAIDs
     d. Alcohol use—delays healing and increases the risk of recurrence
- Symptoms
  1. Burning or deep epigastric pain that occurs 1–3 hours after meals; relieved by ingestion of food or antacids
  2. Pain commonly causes early morning awakening

3. Other dyspeptic symptoms—nausea, vomiting, belching, bloating
4. Symptomatic periods occur in clusters lasting a few weeks, followed by symptom-free periods for weeks/months
5. Gastric ulcer presentation more variable; food may make symptoms worse
6. Complications—hemorrhage, perforation, obstruction
7. Alarm symptoms for gastric cancer or complicated PUD
   a. Bloody or black stools
   b. Unintended weight loss
   c. Dysphagia
   d. Persistent, severe epigastric or stomach pain
   e. Bloody or coffee-ground-type vomit
- Physical findings
  1. Usually none in uncomplicated PUD
  2. Occasionally, well-localized epigastric tenderness
- Differential diagnosis
  1. Gastroesophageal reflux disease
  2. Nonulcer dyspepsia
  3. Gastric carcinoma
  4. Angina
- Diagnostic tests/findings
  1. Stool for occult blood—positive if bleeding present
  2. *H. pylori* testing
     a. Unless indications for endoscopy, use stool antigen test or urea breath test to determine presence, as well as cure, if indicated
        (1) Serologic test—ELISA detects immunoglobulin G (IgG) antibodies, indicating current or past infection; may or may not revert to negative after treatment; nonpreferred test
        (2) Stool antigen test—reverts to negative within 5 days or a few months after eradication of organism
        (3) Urea breath test—detects presence or absence of active infection
  3. CBC with differential
  4. Mucosal biopsy during endoscopy indicated if age older than 50 years, alarm symptoms, family history of gastric cancer, no improvement with treatment
- Management/treatment
  1. Nonpharmacologic
     a. Avoid aspirin and NSAIDs
     b. Smoking cessation
     c. Decrease alcohol intake
     d. Decrease intake of any identified irritants that make symptoms worse—coffee, caffeine, spicy foods
     e. Use stress management, relaxation techniques
  2. Pharmacologic
     a. Disease not due to *H. pylori*
        (1) Histamine-2 receptor antagonists (H₂RA)—cimetidine (Tagamet), ranitidine (Zantac), nizatidine (Axid), famotidine (Pepcid)
            (a) Drug action—inhibits acid secretion by blocking H₂ receptors in parietal cell
            (b) Contraindications/precautions
                i. May alter absorption of some drugs secondary to changes in gastric pH

ii. Contraindicated in patients with renal insufficiency or hepatic impairment
iii. Animal reproduction studies have not shown any adverse effect on the fetus, but there are no adequate and well-controlled studies in humans; use during pregnancy only if the benefits outweigh the potential risk to the fetus
(2) Proton pump inhibitors (PPIs)—omeprazole (Prilosec), lansoprazole (Prevacid), rabeprazole (AcipHex), pantoprazole (Protonix), esomeprazole (Nexium)
   (a) Drug action—inhibits gastric acid secretion by altering the activity of the proton pump; virtual cessation of acid production
   (b) Contraindications/precautions
      i. May alter the absorption of some drugs secondary to changes in gastric pH
      ii. Long-term use of PPIs
         - can lead to increased gastric pH, hypochlorhydria (decreased gastric secretions/hydrochloric acid) and in some cases achlorhydria (absence of gastric secretions/hydrochloric acid)
         - Increases risk for gastric carcinoma
            - Decreased bone density
            - Iron deficiency anemia
            - Community-acquired pneumonia
            - Clostridium difficile
            - Magnesium or vitamin B₁₂ deficiency
      iii. Animal reproduction studies have not shown any adverse effects on the fetus, but there are no adequate and well-controlled studies in humans; use during pregnancy only if the benefits outweigh the potential risk to the fetus
      iv. Long-term use of PPIs in pregnant persons may impose a potential risk of congenital malformations
   b. Ulcers caused by *H. pylori*—eradication of *H. pylori* to reduce the risk of recurrent duodenal ulcer
      (1) PPI triple therapy—PPI, amoxicillin, clarithromycin
      (2) Bismuth quadruple therapy—bismuth subsalicylate, metronidazole, tetracycline, PPI
      (3) Persistent *H. pylori* infection—retreat with alternative combination
3. Patient education
   a. Importance of positive lifestyle changes (e.g., smoking cessation, decreased alcohol consumption)
   b. Purpose, dosage, side effects of medications
   c. Importance of compliance with medication regimen
- Referral
  1. Patients with unintended weight loss, dysphagia, anorexia, vomiting, hematemesis/melena; new-onset pain in patients older than 45 years

2. If treatment for *H. pylori* fails a second time, referral indicated
3. Obtain surgical consultation for patients with evidence of bleeding, gastric outlet obstruction, or perforation

Viral Hepatitis

- Definition—a group of systemic infections involving the liver with common clinical manifestations caused by different viruses with distinctive epidemiologic patterns
- Etiology/incidence/risk factors
  1. Hepatitis A virus (HAV)
     a. Spread via fecal–oral route by person-to-person contact or eating and/or drinking contaminated food and/or water; spreads readily in households, childcare centers, and through anal–oral sexual contact.
     b. Mean incubation time, 25 days; range, 15–60 days; maximum infectivity, 2 weeks before jaundice; acute onset
     c. Infections in infancy and childhood are generally mild without jaundice; adult infections can be severe
     d. Self-limited; no carrier state or chronic liver disease results
     e. Accounts for as many as one-third of acute viral hepatitis cases
  2. Hepatitis B virus (HBV)
     a. Transmitted via percutaneous or mucosal contact with infectious blood or body fluids (saliva, vaginal secretions, semen) by parenteral, sexual, perinatal exposure
     b. Mean incubation time, 75 days; range, 28 to 160 days
     c. Spectrum of illness ranges from asymptomatic seroconversion to acute illness; fulminant hepatitis occurs in fewer than 1% of cases
     d. As many as 10% of people infected as adults and 90% infected as neonates become chronic carriers; increased risk of cirrhosis, hepatocellular carcinoma
  3. Hepatitis C virus (HCV)
     a. Transmitted most efficiently via large or repeated percutaneous exposure to infected blood through transfusion prior to 1992 or IV drug use; transmitted much less frequently through occupational, sexual, or perinatal exposures; most common chronic bloodborne infection in the United States
     b. Mean incubation time, 50 days; range, 2–22 weeks; onset insidious
     c. Acute disease often mild in adults; asymptomatic in children
     d. As many as 80% of infected individuals develop chronic hepatitis; 20%–30% with untreated chronic infection will eventually develop cirrhosis or hepatocellular carcinoma
  4. Hepatitis D virus (HDV)
     a. An incomplete virus that requires the helper function of HBV to replicate
     b. Transmitted via percutaneous or mucosal exposure to infectious blood as a coinfection with HBV or superinfection in person with HBV
     c. Incubation period for superinfection is 2–8 weeks
     d. Contributes to the severity of HBV infection
     e. Suspect superinfection with HDV in a patient who presents with fulminant hepatitis and chronic HBV
  5. Hepatitis E virus (HEV)
     a. Spread via fecal–oral route
     b. Endemic in developing countries
     c. Mean incubation time, 27 days; range, 2–9 weeks
     d. More common in children and young adults; infection during pregnancy can lead to liver failure
     e. No risk of chronicity or carcinoma
  6. Miscellaneous viral causes
     a. Herpes simplex virus
     b. EBV
     c. CMV
- Symptoms—all viral types produce very similar syndromes; the severity of illness can vary widely
  1. Phase 1—incubation
     a. Asymptomatic
     b. Weeks to months
  2. Phase 2—pre-icteric (prodromal)
     a. Three to 10 days in length
     b. Malaise, fatigue
     c. Anorexia, nausea, vomiting
     d. Flulike aches, headache
     e. Skin rash
     f. Change in sense of smell or taste; aversion to cigarettes
  3. Phase 3—icteric
     a. One to 4 weeks in length
     b. Right upper quadrant (RUQ) pain
     c. Dark-colored urine
     d. Clay-colored stools
     e. Jaundice of skin, sclera, nail beds
  4. Phase 4—convalescence
     a. May last weeks to months
     b. Chronic disease develops in certain types
     c. Hepatitis B, C, D may be fatal; HEV has 10%–20% mortality rate in pregnant individuals
- Physical findings
  1. Rash—maculopapular and urticarial lesions
  2. Low-grade fever
  3. Slight jaundice, yellow sclera
  4. Hepatomegaly
  5. Splenomegaly
- Differential diagnosis—noninfectious causes of hepatitis (e.g., hepatotoxic drugs, alcohol)
- Diagnostic tests/findings
  1. Viral serologies (**Table 3-9**)
  2. Urinalysis—positive for protein, bilirubin
  3. LFTs
     a. Marked elevation—ALT, AST
     b. Mild increase or normal lactate dehydrogenase (LDH), serum bilirubin, alkaline phosphatase (ALP), prothrombin time
- Management/treatment
  1. Nonpharmacologic
     a. Activity as tolerated; avoid strenuous activities or contact sports

Table 3-9 Serologic Diagnosis and Markers of Hepatitis

Test Name	Hepatitis A Virus (HAV)	Hepatitis B Virus (HBV)	Hepatitis C Virus (HCV)	Hepatitis D Virus (HDV)
HAV IgM antibody (IgM anti-HAV)	Positive: current or recent infection, resolves in 6 months	N/A	N/A	N/A
HAV IgG antibody (IgG anti-HAV)	Positive: indicates immunity due to prior infection or vaccination	N/A	N/A	N/A
HBV surface antigen (HBsAg)	N/A	Positive: acute and chronic infection; indicates person is infectious	N/A	Positive with HBV/HDV coinfection or superinfection
HBV surface antibody (anti-HBs)	N/A	Positive: immune due to prior infection or vaccination	N/A	N/A
HBV core antibody (anti-HBc)	N/A	Positive: acute and chronic infection, persists for life		
HBV core IgM antibody (IgM anti-HBV)	N/A	Positive: acute infection, resolves in 4–6 months	N/A	Positive with HBV/HDV coinfection or superinfection
HBV e antigen	N/A	Positive: acute infection, highly infectious	N/A	N/A
HBV DNA	N/A	Positive: acute and chronic infection	N/A	Positive with HBV/HDV coinfection or superinfection
HCV antibody (anti-HCV)	N/A	N/A	Positive: current or resolved infection, persists for life	N/A
HCV RNA	N/A	N/A	Positive: confirms current infection, persists with chronic infection	N/A
HDV antibody	N/A	N/A	N/A	Positive with positive HBV surface antigen, current or past HBV/HDV coinfection or superinfection
HDV IgM antibody	N/A	N/A	N/A	Positive: positive HBV surface antigen, current or past HBV/HDV coinfection or superinfection Negative: resolved HDV infection

IgM, immunoglobulin M; IgG, immunoglobulin G; N/A, not applicable.
Data from Centers for Disease Control and Prevention. (2015b). *Viral hepatitis serology training*. Retrieved from https://www.cdc.gov/hepatitis/resources/professionals/training/serology/training.htm

b. Hydration
c. Maintain adequate caloric intake and a balanced diet; small feedings may be better tolerated
d. Discontinue all but essential medications
e. Avoid alcohol
2. Pharmacologic
a. Antiemetics if indicated for nausea
b. Chronic hepatitis B—recombinant interferon alfa-2b; direct inhibitor of HBV replication;

tenofovir-based antiviral regimens; treatment rarely produces permanent remission of disease
c. Chronic hepatitis C—8 to 12 week course of antiviral medication; initiate at onset of chronic infection (detectable viral load for 6 months), rather than waiting for cirrhosis or other adverse health outcomes. Medication has a 90% cure rate. Patients should be counseled on the risk of reinfection.
d. Prevention

(1) HAV

    (a) Immune globulin—recommended for travelers going to countries for longer than 6 months where HAV is endemic; give as prophylaxis within 2 weeks of known exposure

    (b) HAV vaccine

(2) HBV

    (a) Hepatitis B immune globulin (HBIG)—given as a prophylaxis to infants born to HBsAg (surface antigen of HBV)–positive people; given within 14 days of sexual exposure

    (b) HBV vaccine

(3) HCV—prophylaxis with immune globulin is not effective in preventing infection after exposure; no vaccine is available

3. Patient education

  a. Careful disposal of infected wastes and needles

  b. Scrupulous handwashing, food-handling techniques

  c. Need for prophylactic immunization of contacts, household members

  d. Safer sexual practices

  e. Safer substance use practices

  f. Avoidance of blood contamination—no sharing toothbrushes, razors, needles

  g. Laboratory follow-up

    (1) Monitor aminotransferase at 1- to 4-week intervals during acute illness

    (2) Monitor HBsAg and anti-HBsAg until anti-HBs (hepatitis B surface antibody) present with HBV infection

- Referral

1. Fulminant disease—patients presenting with altered mental state

2. Patients with chronic HBV who require treatment

3. HCV—early identification/referral important because evidence suggests that early treatment reduces risks associated with chronic infection

Cholecystitis

- Definition—acute or chronic distention and inflammation of the gallbladder, most commonly related to obstruction of cystic or bile ducts by gallstones

- Etiology/incidence/risk factors

1. Etiology

  a. Gallstones may be the result of an imbalance in bile components; about 90% composed of cholesterol; the majority of patients are asymptomatic

  b. Gallstone may become impacted in cystic or common bile duct, causing obstruction; may be transient (acute) or chronic

  c. Continued blockage of the cystic or common bile duct results in inflammation; usually bacterial infection also contributes to the inflammation

  d. Gangrene of the gallbladder and possible perforation can occur

2. Risk factors for gallstone formation

  a. Female sex and/or estrogen-dominant hormone milieu

  b. Advanced age

  c. Obesity

  d. Pregnancy

  e. Rapid weight loss

  f. History of gastric bypass surgery

  g. Family history

  h. Medications/oral contraceptives

- Symptoms

1. Biliary colic—presenting symptom in more than 90% of patients

  a. Severe, steady pain localized to the epigastrium or RUQ; may radiate to the back or scapula

  b. Pain is precipitated by a spasm of a dilated cystic duct obstructed by gallstone(s)

  c. Attacks of biliary colic are more common at night

  d. Pain typically has a sudden onset and may last 3 hours; may be accompanied by nausea/vomiting

2. Acute cholecystitis

  a. Pain similar to biliary colic but lasts longer; associated with nausea/vomiting and fever

  b. Symptoms of local inflammation and systemic toxicity

  c. Most patients have had previous attacks of biliary colic

- Physical findings—acute cholecystitis

1. Fever

2. Murphy's sign—inspiratory arrest secondary to pain during deep palpation of right subcostal region; relatively specific finding

3. Gallbladder distended and palpable in 20%–30% of cases

4. Jaundice—mild, 20% of cases

5. Localized tenderness may be only finding in elderly patients; pain and fever may be absent

- Differential diagnosis

1. Appendicitis

2. Pancreatitis

3. Ruptured ectopic pregnancy or ovarian cyst

4. Peptic ulcer disease

- Diagnostic tests/findings

1. Ultrasound

  a. Has a 95% sensitivity for detecting stones in the gallbladder; detects bile duct stones in only 50% of cases

  b. Best noninvasive imaging technique to diagnose acute cholecystitis

2. CT, magnetic resonance imaging (MRI), cholescintigraphy, endoscopic retrograde cholangiopancreatography (ECRP), possible follow-up tests based on ultrasound and lab test findings

3. ECG if cardiac risk factors or cardiac involvement suspected; chest radiograph to rule out pneumonia

4. Pregnancy test if indicated to rule out ectopic and prior to any teratogenic imaging studies

5. CBC with differential—mild leukocytosis with a "left shift" observed in acute cholecystitis

6. LFTs—elevation of serum bilirubin and ALP with bile duct stones

7. Pancreatic enzymes—increased amylase and lipase associated with concomitant pancreatitis

- Management/treatment
    1. Expectant management for patients with asymptomatic gallstones
    2. Initial management of symptomatic gallstones may include IV rehydration and correction of electrolyte imbalance, antispasmodic and antiemetic medications, injected nonsteroidal anti-inflammatory prostaglandin inhibitor for pain
    3. Elective cholecystectomy for most patients with symptomatic gallstones
    4. Acute cholecystitis managed with hospital admission; cholecystectomy once the patient is stable
    5. Bile duct stones should be removed whether the patient is symptomatic or asymptomatic because of the high rate of complications

Gastroesophageal Reflux Disease (GERD)

- Definition
    1. *Gastroesophageal reflux*—movement of gastric contents from the stomach into the esophagus
    2. *GERD*—symptomatic clinical condition or histologic alteration that results from episodes of reflux
    3. When the esophagus is repeatedly exposed to refluxed material for prolonged periods of time, inflammation of esophagus can occur
    4. Complications—esophagitis; strictures; Barrett's esophagus, which carries a 10% risk of progression to adenocarcinoma
- Etiology/incidence/risk factors
    1. Etiology
        a. Contributing factors include reflux of caustic gastric contents, a breakdown in the defense mechanism of the esophagus, and a functional abnormality that results in reflux
        b. Most common etiology—prolonged esophageal acid exposure due to transient lower esophageal relaxation
        c. Less common mechanisms—pathologically weak lower esophageal sphincter (LES) tone, hiatal hernia, esophageal motility disorder, Zollinger–Ellison syndrome, and delayed gastric emptying
    2. Incidence
        a. Approximately 20% of adults report reflux symptoms that occur at least weekly
        b. Approximately 1% of adults with GERD have Barrett's esophagus
    3. Risk factors
        a. Foods that lower LES pressure—high fat, chocolate, peppermints
        b. Foods that irritate esophageal mucosa—citrus fruits, spicy tomato drinks
        c. Drugs that lower LES pressure—calcium channel blockers, progesterone
        d. Cigarette smoking, alcohol
        e. Pregnancy
        f. BMI >30
- Symptoms
    1. "Heartburn"—retrosternal burning sensation radiating upward

2. Acid regurgitation—effortless return of gastric contents into pharynx; bad taste in mouth
3. Symptoms usually occur 30–60 minutes after eating
4. Symptoms aggravated by reclining, straining, bending, or stooping
5. Nocturnal aspiration—causes coughing
6. Atypical symptoms
    a. Odynophagia—burning, squeezing pain with swallowing
    b. Dysphagia—sensation of food lodged in the chest secondary to stricture
    c. Globus sensation—sensation of lump in the throat
7. Extraesophageal symptoms
    a. Hoarseness
    b. Chronic cough
    c. Bronchospasm

- Physical findings
    1. Usually normal examination
    2. Occasionally epigastric tenderness with palpation
- Differential diagnosis
    1. Cardiac chest pain
    2. Peptic ulcer disease
    3. Infectious esophagitis—viral, fungal
    4. Medication-induced esophagitis—antibiotics
    5. Esophageal/gastric malignancy
    6. Hepatobiliary disease
- Diagnostic tests/findings
    1. Diagnosis of GERD based on clinical findings and confirmed by response to therapy
    2. Diagnostic evaluation if symptoms are chronic or refractory to therapy or if esophageal complications are suspected
        a. Endoscopy
    3. Useful for diagnosis of complications—esophagitis, strictures, Barrett's esophagus
    4. Indications
        a. Dysphagia or odynophagia
        b. Unplanned weight loss
        c. Evidence of GI bleeding or iron-deficiency anemia
        d. Screen for Barrett's if 10 years or more of GERD symptoms
        e. Upper GI may demonstrate structural problems; evaluation of dysphagia
        f. Ambulatory esophageal pH monitoring—best test to establish abnormal acid reflux
- Management/treatment
    1. Nonpharmacologic—target to specific patient circumstances
        a. Weight loss if BMI >30
        b. Smoking cessation
        c. Elevate head of bed (HOB); sleep on wedge-shaped bolster if have nocturnal symptoms
        d. Avoid recumbency for 3 hours after eating if symptoms worse when supine
        e. Reduce fat to no more than 30% of calories
        f. Reduce consumption of alcohol, chocolate, colas, coffee, peppermint, citrus juices, tomato products
    2. Pharmacologic
        a. Commercially available antacids are useful for mild, infrequent symptoms

b. H_2-receptor antagonists (acid reducers)—effective treatment for less severe GERD; see the section about PUD earlier in this chapter

c. PPIs (acid suppressant agents)—most effective agents for healing esophagitis and preventing complications; see the section about PUD earlier in this chapter

3. Patient education—lifestyle modifications

- Referral
  1. Symptoms of dysphagia, weight loss, blood loss, obstructive symptoms including nausea/vomiting, early satiety, anorexia
  2. Long-standing or refractory cases
  3. Candidates for surgical intervention

Urinary Tract Disorders

Lower Urinary Tract Infections (UTIs)

- Definition—a term that encompasses infections affecting the bladder and urethra
  1. Cystitis—infection of the bladder
  2. Urethritis—infection and/or inflammation of the distal urethra
- Etiology/incidence
  1. *Escherichia coli* is the most common organism (80%–90%) in cystitis; less common causative organisms include *Staphylococcus saprophyticus*, *Proteus mirabilis*, *Klebsiella*, *Pseudomonas*, *Enterobacter* species
  2. Most cases of cystitis are caused by ascending infection from the urethra into the bladder
  3. More than half of women will develop cystitis in their lifetime
  4. Urethritis is associated with chlamydia, gonorrhea, trichomoniasis, genital herpes
- Risk factors—cystitis
  1. Frequent or recent penetrative sexual activity with new partner
  2. Vaginal atrophy
  3. Diabetes
  4. Congenital anatomic abnormalities
  5. Rectocele, cystocele, uterine prolapse
  6. Urinary tract calculi
  7. Instrumentation/catheterization
  8. Infrequent voiding or incomplete bladder emptying
  9. Diaphragm, tampon, and spermicide use
  10. Immunosuppression
  11. Sickle cell disease or trait
  12. First UTI prior to age 15
  13. Mother with a history of recurrent UTI
- Symptoms
  1. Range from mild to severe
  2. Acute cystitis
     a. Abrupt onset
     b. Dysuria
     c. Frequency of urination
     d. Urgency of urination
     e. Suprapubic pain
     f. Painful bladder spasms
     g. Cloudy, malodorous urine

h. Hematuria (gross)
i. New or worsening incontinence

3. Urethritis
   a. Dysuria
   b. Frequency of urination
   c. Urethral pruritus
   d. Mucopurulent penile or vaginal discharge

- Physical findings
  1. Cystitis—may have suprapubic tenderness
  2. Urethritis—erythema, mucopurulent penile or vaginal discharge
- Differential diagnosis
  1. Vaginitis
  2. STI
  3. Pelvic inflammatory disease
  4. Interstitial cystitis
  5. Urinary tract obstruction
  6. Urinary tract malignancy
- Diagnostic tests/findings
  1. Urine culture and sensitivity
     a. Clean catch-midstream urine sample or catheterization
     b. Traditional criterion for infection—a colony count of 10^5 single-isolate bacteria per milliliter
     c. Using a colony count of 10^3–10^4 bacteria per milliliter in symptomatic patients improves sensitivity (fewer false negatives) without significantly compromising specificity
     d. Provides information on sensitivity or resistance to specific medications
  2. Microscopic urinalysis
     a. Clean catch-midstream urine sample or catheterization
     b. More than five WBCs per high-powered field and the presence of bacteria
     c. Presence of epithelial cells suggests contamination of the sample
  3. Enzymatic (dipstick) testing—less reliable (75% sensitivity)
     a. Indicates hematuria; nitrites indicate the presence of bacteria; leukocyte esterase indicates the presence of WBCs
     b. Send urine for urinalysis and culture and sensitivity if dipstick is negative in symptomatic patient and other cause of symptoms is not apparent
  4. Test for vaginitis and STIs in all sites used for sex (oral, vaginal/penile, and anal) if indicated; in people with penises under age 50, acute simple cystitis is an unlikely diagnosis
- Management/treatment
  1. Uncomplicated cystitis
     a. Initial treatment of uncomplicated cystitis can be based on the presence of typical symptoms and urinalysis or dipstick testing without urine culture
     b. If culture is done, may start treatment before results are available
     c. Suggested first-line medical regimens for nonpregnant individuals
  2. Trimethoprim–sulfamethoxazole (TMP/SMX) orally—3-day regimen

3. Nitrofurantoin orally—5-day regimen
4. Fosfomycin orally—single dose, may have lower efficacy than the first two options
   a. Second-line or alternative therapies, including β-lactam agents and fluoroquinolones, should be used only in case of resistance to first-line therapies or allergies
5. Recurrent UTI—at least two culture-proven symptomatic uncomplicated acute cystitis episodes in 6 months or three episodes within 1 year in which symptom resolution occurred between culture-proven events
   a. Retest and retreat—culture confirmation of infection is important to avoid unnecessary overuse of antibiotics and to confirm the correct diagnosis
   b. Use the same medications as for uncomplicated cystitis for up to 7 days
   c. Review potential lifestyle risk factors that can be reduced or eliminated
   d. Review antibiotic-sparing prophylactic regimens of either cranberry tablets 500–1,000 mg PO daily or methenamine 1 g orally twice daily
   e. Consider a 6–12 months' prophylaxis regimen if two infections in past 6 months or three infections in the prior 12 months and insufficient response to antibiotic-sparing regimens—recommended antibiotics include TMP/SMX, trimethoprim, nitrofurantoin, cephalexin, fosfomycin; dosing may be daily, 3 times per week, or weekly depending on dosage and specific medication
   f. If related to coitus, consider a single-dose antibiotic regimen after sex—recommended antibiotics include TMP/SMX, nitrofurantoin, cephalexin, norfloxacin
   g. Consider vaginal estrogen for postmenopausal individual with vaginal atrophy/genitourinary syndrome of menopause
6. Urethritis—treat for identified infection (e.g., chlamydia, gonorrhea, genital herpes)
7. Prevention/prophylaxis—cystitis
   a. Liberal fluid intake of 2–3 L per day
   b. Void after intercourse
   c. Discontinue use of spermicides and diaphragm
   d. Intravaginal estrogen in individuals with atrophy of genitalia
   e. Avoid delay in emptying bladder
8. Referral
   a. Patients with possible pyelonephritis or a history of pyelonephritis with UTI symptoms
   b. Patients with acute or recurrent cystitis associated with urine cultures resistant to oral antibiotics
   c. Suspected renal calculus, urinary tract obstruction, urinary tract malignancy

Acute Pyelonephritis

- Definition—infection of the renal pelvis and kidney
- Etiology/incidence
  1. Usually results from the ascent of bacterial pathogen up the ureters from the bladder to the kidneys

2. Incidence is highest in otherwise healthy people with natal vulvas 15–29 years of age, followed by infants and older persons
3. *Escherichia coli* most common responsible pathogen (80%); less common causative organisms include *Klebsiella pneumoniae*, *Staphylococcus saprophyticus*
4. Risk factors
   a. Frequent sexual intercourse, new partner in the previous year
   b. Cystitis in the previous 12 months
   c. Stress incontinence
   d. Complicated urinary tract infection
   e. Antibiotic-resistant urinary tract infections
   f. Pregnancy
   g. Diabetes
- Symptoms
  1. Chills, fever
  2. Dysuria
  3. Frequency of urination
  4. Urgency of urination
  5. Nausea, vomiting
  6. Flank and/or abdominal pain
  7. Hematuria (gross)—less common than with acute cystitis
- Physical findings
  1. Unilateral or bilateral costovertebral angle tenderness
  2. Fever
- Differential diagnosis
  1. Abdominal abscess
  2. Appendicitis
  3. Pancreatitis
  4. Pelvic inflammatory disease
- Diagnostic tests/findings
  1. Urine culture and sensitivity—more than 95% of patients will have a colony count of 10^5 single-isolate bacteria per milliliter
  2. Microscopic urinalysis—positive hematuria, pyuria
  3. Enzymatic (dipstick) testing—positive blood, leukocyte esterase, nitrites
  4. Blood cultures—if severely ill
- Management/treatment
  1. Oral fluoroquinolone—if the level of resistance to this antibiotic does not exceed 10% in the community, 7-day regimen
  2. Other option—TMP/SMX, 14-day regimen
  3. Test of cure with urine culture
  4. Hospitalize if severe illness, pregnancy, immunocompromised, unable to tolerate oral treatment, inability to return for follow-up, lack of notable improvement within 48–72 hours of antibiotic initiation

Urolithiasis

- Definition—renal or ureteral stones/calculi that can cause urinary tract obstruction
- Etiology/incidence
  1. May occur at any age
  2. Incidence is approximately 1% in the general population
  3. May be related to metabolic disorders, such as gout or inborn errors in calcium metabolism

4. May be related to chronic UTI and/or stasis of urine
5. Risk factors
   a. Genetic tendency
   b. Gout
   c. Pregnancy
   d. Certain medications
   e. Dehydration
- Symptoms
  1. Dull ache to severe paroxysms of pain on the side of the stone as it passes from the kidney to the ureter
  2. Flank pain, lower abdominal pain, groin pain
  3. Nausea and vomiting
- Physical findings—gross or microscopic hematuria
- Differential diagnosis
  1. Pyelonephritis
  2. Pelvic inflammatory disease
  3. Appendicitis
  4. Bladder or kidney carcinoma
- Diagnostic tests/findings
  1. Noncontrast CT scan—gold standard for diagnosis
  2. Ultrasound misses small stones but is recommended if pregnant
- Management/treatment
  1. Observation with pain medications and fluids while awaiting spontaneous passage for stones <5 mm
  2. Urgent intervention if the patient has fever, chills, nausea, vomiting, or pain uncontrolled by narcotics
  3. Endoscopic, surgical, laser, or shockwave lithotripsy for removal if the stones >10 mm
  4. Tamsulosin (0.4 mg PO once daily for up to 4 weeks) if stones >5 mm <10 mm

Urinary Incontinence (UI)

- Definition—involuntary loss of urine
  1. Stress incontinence (SUI)—leakage of urine during events that result in increased abdominal pressure, such as sneezing, coughing, physical exercise
  2. Urge incontinence (UUI)—involuntary leakage of urine accompanied by or immediately preceding an urgency
  3. Mixed incontinence—a combination of SUI and UUI symptoms
  4. Overactive bladder (OAB)—sense of urgency with or without incontinence; may be accompanied by frequency and nocturia
- Etiology/incidence
  1. SUI—inadequate pelvic floor support or weak tone of sphincter between bladder and urethra
  2. UUI and OAB—overactivity of detrusor muscle, causing inappropriate contraction during bladder filling
  3. Prevalence—approximately 25% of reproductive-age people assigned female at birth, 44%–57% in those middle-aged and postmenopausal, and 75% in older adults assigned female at birth
  4. Fifty percent of the nursing home population experience incontinence
  5. Fewer than 50% of individuals seek help; most suffer in silence

6. Risk factors
   a. Advancing age
   b. Childbearing (vaginal birth more than cesarean)
   c. Family history in a first-degree relative
   d. Hysterectomy
   e. Pelvic organ prolapse
   f. Obesity, pregnancy, chronic cough, straining from constipation—increased abdominal pressure
   g. Cognitive impairment, restricted mobility, neurologic disability, stroke, diabetes
   h. Medications (e.g., diuretics, anticholinergics, alpha adrenergic, alpha antagonists, sedatives)
   i. Genitourinary syndrome of menopause
- Symptoms
  1. SUI
     a. Loss of urine, usually in small amounts, with coughing, laughing, sneezing
     b. Vaginal dryness if atrophy is present
  2. UUI
     a. Involuntary loss of urine preceded by a sudden, strong urge to urinate
     b. Usually voids large amounts
     c. Difficulty in controlling once flow begins
     d. Occurs without warning—cold weather, physical activity, laughing, sexual intercourse, or placing a key in a door lock (as with latchkey incontinence subtype)
  3. OAB—frequency, urgency, nocturia
  4. Mixed urinary incontinence—presents with both symptoms of stress and urge incontinence
- Physical findings
  1. Urinary leakage with increased abdominal pressure—SUI, UUI
  2. Weak pelvic floor muscles—SUI
  3. Vaginal atrophy, perineal irritation—SUI, UUI
- Differential diagnosis
  1. UTI
  2. Prolapse of bladder
  3. Tumor-compressing bladder
  4. Inability to toilet because of cognitive or mobility impairments (functional incontinence)
  5. Stool impaction
- Diagnostic tests/findings
  1. Review prescription and nonprescription drugs for etiologic factors
  2. Voiding diary
  3. Urinary stress test to assess loss of urine when coughing and straining—immediate loss of urine (SUI), may have delayed loss of urine (UUI)
  4. Postvoid residual measurement using catheter or scan—rule out retention and overflow incontinence
  5. Urinalysis/culture to evaluate for infection
  6. Urodynamic testing if etiology of incontinence is unclear after a basic office evaluation
- Management/treatment
  1. Treat any identified transient causes for incontinence—DIAPPERS: delirium, infection (acute UTI or STI), atrophic vaginitis, pharmaceuticals (e.g., antihypertensives, diuretics), psychological disorder, excessive urine output (e.g., hyperglycemia), reduced mobility,

reversible (e.g., drug-induced) urinary retention, stool impaction

2. SUI
   a. Behavioral therapies—timed voiding, fluid management
   b. Pelvic floor physical therapy—Kegel exercises and biofeedback
   c. Weight loss if obese
   d. Pessaries
   e. No drugs approved specifically for the treatment of SUI in the United States
   f. Urethral bulking agents
   g. Surgical therapies

3. UUI/OAB
   a. Behavioral therapies—bladder retraining with timed voiding, fluid management, avoidance of bladder irritants
   b. Pelvic floor physical therapy—Kegel exercises, pelvic floor relaxation, and biofeedback
   c. Pharmacologic agents—anticholinergic antimuscarinic agents (e.g., oxybutynin chloride [Ditropan], tolterodine [Detrol]—see Chapter 11, *Principles of Pharmacology*, for detailed information on oxybutynin chloride; beta$_3$-adrenergic receptor agonists (e.g., mirabegron)
   d. Other therapies—Botox, percutaneous tibial nerve stimulation, sacral neuromodulation

4. Mixed incontinence—combine measures for urge and stress incontinence

5. Surgery decisions based on type and severity of symptoms, lack of response to conservative therapy, or preferring not to use conservative therapy

6. Referral to a urogynecologist

Interstitial Cystitis (IC)/Painful Bladder Syndrome

- Definition—unpleasant sensation (pain, pressure, discomfort) perceived to be related to the urinary bladder, associated with lower urinary tract symptoms, greater than 6 weeks' duration, absence of infection
- Etiology/incidence
  1. Etiology unknown—possible causes
     a. Defect in bladder epithelium that allows irritating substances in urine to penetrate into the bladder wall
     b. Autoimmune condition targeting bladder
     c. Allergic reaction—mast cells releasing histamine
     d. Neural hypersensitivity
     e. Associated with other chronic pain conditions—for example, IBS, fibromyalgia, vulvodynia
  2. Incidence—estimated 3 million U.S. women older than age 18 years; only about 10% diagnosed
- Symptoms
  1. Urinary frequency and urgency
  2. Suprapubic pain/pressure/discomfort related to bladder filling—may void to avoid or relieve pain
  3. Increased pain with ingestion of specific foods or beverages

4. Nocturia
5. Dyspareunia

- Physical findings
  1. Suprapubic tenderness
  2. Anterior vaginal wall/urethra tenderness
  3. Perineal tenderness
- Differential diagnoses
  1. UTI
  2. Endometriosis
  3. PID
  4. OAB
- Diagnostic test/findings
  1. Frequency/volume diary—often demonstrates frequent small voids of less the 150 mL each and as many as 20 voids per day
  2. Pelvic pain, urgency, frequency (PUF) patient symptom scale
  3. Urinalysis and urine culture—evaluate for infection or hematuria
  4. Postvoid residual urine measurement
  5. Cytology if hematuria or history of tobacco use
  6. Cystoscopy, urodynamic testing if diagnosis unclear
- Management/treatment
  1. Avoid foods that trigger symptoms—acidic, alcoholic, and carbonated beverages; spicy foods; coffee, tea, chocolate, tomatoes, vinegar, artificial sweeteners
  2. Physical therapy to release muscle contractures and trigger points
  3. Bladder retraining to increase the time interval between voiding
  4. Oral medications
     a. Pentosane polysulfate sodium (Elmiron)
        (1) FDA approved for treatment of IC/painful bladder syndrome
        (2) Decreases permeability of bladder lining
        (3) May take up to 6 months to show an effect
     b. Histamine blockers—cimetidine (Tagamet), hydroxyzine hydrochloride (Atarax, Vistaril)
     c. Tricyclic antidepressants—amitriptyline (Elavil), nortriptyline (Aventyl)
  5. Bladder instillation medications—dimethyl sulfoxide (DMSO), heparin, lidocaine
  6. Hydrodistention with cystoscopy under anesthesia
  7. Stress management, support groups

Hematologic Disorders
Anemias

- Definition
  1. Abnormally low hemoglobin concentration (<12 g/dL for estrogen-dominant hormone milieu, <13 g/dL for testosterone-dominant hormone milieu)
  2. Anemia occurs as a result of abnormal red blood cell (RBC) development, abnormal hemoglobin synthesis, or accelerated RBC destruction
  3. Usually classified according to RBC size—mean corpuscular volume (MCV)

a. Microcytic anemia (MCV < 80 fL) (e.g., iron-deficiency anemia, thalassemia trait)

b. Macrocytic anemia (MCV > 100 fL) (e.g., vitamin B_{12} deficiency, folate deficiency, liver disease, hypothyroidism)

c. Normocytic anemia (MCV 80–100 fL) (e.g., anemia of chronic disease, hemolysis, sickle cell disease, renal failure)

- Etiology/incidence—commonly encountered anemias
  1. Iron-deficiency anemia (IDA)—microcytic, hypochromic
     a. Etiology
        (1) Slow, persistent blood loss—GI overt/occult, heavy or prolonged menstrual bleeding
        (2) Inadequate dietary intake of iron-rich foods
        (3) Metabolic demands in excess of intake—pregnancy
     b. Incidence
        (1) Most common form of anemia; represents 25% of all anemia cases
        (2) Affects 10%–15% of premenopausal people who menstruate
  2. Anemia of chronic disease—normochromic, normocytic
     a. Etiology
        (1) A hypoproliferative anemia associated with underlying chronic disorders, such as infections, inflammatory disorders, malignancy
        (2) Reduced production and response to erythropoietin; decreased RBC lifespan
        (3) Defect in iron reutilization
     b. Incidence—most common anemia in the elderly population
  3. Vitamin B_{12}–deficiency anemia—megaloblastic, macrocytic, normochromic
     a. Etiology
        (1) Vitamin B_{12} deficiency alters DNA synthesis and maturation of RBCs
        (2) Vitamin B_{12} deficiency develops secondary to lack or relative deficiency of intrinsic factor that leads to impaired vitamin B_{12} absorption (pernicious anemia)
           (a) Autoimmune reaction involving gastric parietal cells
           (b) History of gastrectomy
        (3) Rarely secondary to nutritional deficiency of vitamin—risk with strict vegan diet, history of bariatric surgery, and other malabsorptive conditions.
     b. Incidence—usually presents around age 60; most common in whites of northern European descent; familial tendency
  4. Folate-deficiency anemia—megaloblastic, macrocytic, normochromic
     a. Etiology
        (1) Folate deficiency alters the synthesis of DNA and RBC maturation
        (2) Folate deficiency causes
           (a) Malabsorption syndromes
           (b) Increased demand—pregnancy
           (c) Inadequate intake—alcohol use disorder, elderly

(3) Certain drugs may inhibit folic acid absorption—antacids, histamine-2 antagonists, PPIs, metformin
     b. Incidence
        (1) Found in all races and age groups
        (2) Most common megaloblastic anemia in pregnancy
  5. Sickle cell anemia
     a. Etiology
        (1) A chronic hemolytic anemia characterized by sickle-shaped RBCs
        (2) Autosomal recessive genetic disorder
           (a) Hgb S develops instead of Hgb A
           (b) Individual is homozygous for Hgb S
     b. Incidence
        (1) Homozygous Hgb S—found in an estimated 0.5% of Black individuals
        (2) Heterozygous trait—found in an estimated 8% of Black individuals; asymptomatic carrier state
        (3) Prevalent in Black individuals, also to a lesser extent in persons of Mediterranean ancestry and among people from parts of the world where malaria is common.

- Symptoms
  1. Iron-deficiency anemia
     a. Asymptomatic unless severe, then nonspecific
     b. Fatigue, generalized weakness
     c. Dyspnea on exertion
     d. Headaches
     e. Pica
  2. Anemia of chronic disease
     a. Symptoms common to all anemias—fatigue, weakness, exertional dyspnea, lightheadedness, anorexia
     b. Other symptoms related to specific underlying disease
  3. Vitamin B_{12}–deficiency anemia
     a. None at first; insidious onset
     b. Fatigue, weakness, lightheadedness
     c. Dyspnea, palpitations
     d. GI disturbances—anorexia, bloating, diarrhea
     e. Sore tongue
     f. Neurologic—peripheral paresthesia, ataxia
     g. Loss of taste and smell
  4. Folate-deficiency anemia—symptoms similar to vitamin B_{12}–deficiency anemia except there is no neurologic involvement
  5. Sickle cell anemia
     a. Often none during remissions
     b. Vaso-occlusive crises—precipitating factors include infection, physical or emotional stress, blood loss, pregnancy, surgery, high altitudes
        (1) Malaise, chills
        (2) Pain, especially in bones, abdomen, chest, lower legs
        (3) Headaches, epistaxis, vomiting
        (4) Difficulty walking

- Physical findings
  1. Iron-deficiency anemia
     a. Often none with mild anemia

b. Skin or conjunctival pallor
c. Nail changes—spoon shaped (koilonychia); brittle
d. Brittle, fine hair
e. Tachycardia with or without systolic flow murmur
f. Tachypnea
2. Anemia of chronic disease
   a. Ill appearance
   b. Signs of precipitating illness
3. Vitamin B$_{12}$–deficiency anemia
   a. Skin pale, occasionally jaundiced
   b. Smooth, beefy-red tongue (glossitis)
   c. Tachycardia, arrhythmias, systolic flow murmur
   d. Hepatomegaly, splenomegaly
   e. Neurologic
      (1) Ataxia, positive Romberg test
      (2) Hyperactive reflexes
      (3) Peripheral loss of sensation, decreased vibratory sense, impaired proprioception
      (4) Changes in mental state with possible wide range of expression—mild confusion to acute psychosis
4. Folate-deficiency anemia
   a. Pallor and dryness of skin and mucous membranes
   b. Brittle nails; brittle fine hair
   c. Tachycardia, tachypnea
5. Sickle cell anemia
   a. In crises
      (1) Temperature, pulse, respiration elevated
      (2) Hypotension
      (3) Pallor, cyanosis secondary to poor oxygenation
      (4) Scleral jaundice
      (5) Decreased skin turgor
   b. Chronic findings due to anemia, vaso-occlusive events, end organ damage
      (1) Cardiomegaly
      (2) Skin ulcers, especially on lower extremities
      (3) Osteomyelitis
      (4) Retinopathy
      (5) Renal disease—hematuria
- Differential diagnosis
  1. Iron-deficiency anemia
     a. Anemia of chronic disease
     b. Thalassemia trait
     c. Sideroblastic anemia
  2. Anemia of chronic disease—diagnosis of exclusion
     a. Iron-deficiency anemia
     b. Anemia of renal disease

3. Vitamin B$_{12}$–deficiency anemia
   a. Nutritional deficiency
   b. Malabsorption
   c. Chronic alcohol use disorder
   d. Chronic gastritis (*H. pylori* infection)
   e. Folate deficiency
4. Folate-deficiency anemia
   a. Pernicious anemia
   b. Medication, toxins
5. Sickle crises
   a. Appendicitis
   b. Acute cholecystitis
   c. Pneumonia
- Diagnostic tests/findings
  1. World Health Organization (WHO) standard for anemia diagnosis
     a. Men—Hgb 13 g/dL or less (approximately 38% Hct)
     b. Women—Hgb 12 g/dL or less (approximately 35% Hct)
  2. Severe anemia (symptomatic) generally less than 25% Hct
  3. See **Table 3-10** for an overview of laboratory values in common anemias
  4. Iron-deficiency anemia—hypochromic microcytic RBCs
     a. RBC changes in early disease may be mild
     b. MCV less than 80 fL
     c. Increased red cell width (RDW)
     d. Serum ferritin less than 10 mg/L
        (1) Levels reflect iron stores; the single most useful test for diagnosing IDA
        (2) Ferritin is an acute-phase reactant; may be elevated in inflammatory disease
     e. Decreased reticulocyte count
  5. Anemia of chronic disease—normochromic–normocytic early in course; becomes microcytic
     a. Anemia is typically mild; Hct remains around 30%
     b. Normal or slightly reduced MCV
     c. Low serum iron levels; normal or low total iron-binding capacity (TIBC)
     d. Normal or increased serum ferritin
  6. Vitamin B$_{12}$–deficiency anemia—megaloblastic–macrocytic anemia
     a. MCV greater than 100 fL
     b. Serum B$_{12}$ decreased; less than 100 pg/mL
     c. Peripheral blood smear—RBCs of widely varying size (anisocytosis) and shape (poikilocytosis)

Table 3-10 Laboratory Values in Common Anemias

Anemia	MCV	MCH	Serum Iron	TIBC	Ferritin	Vitamin B$_{12}$	Folate
Iron-deficiency anemia	Low	Low	Normal/low	High	Low	Normal	Normal
Folate-deficiency anemia	High	Normal	High	Normal	High	Normal	Low
Vitamin B$_{12}$–deficiency anemia	High	Normal	High	Normal	High	Low	Normal

MCH, mean corpuscular hemoglobin; MCV, mean corpuscular volume; TIBC, total iron-binding capacity

d. Serum methylmalonic acid and homocysteine levels elevated

e. Assay for anti-intrinsic factor/parietal cell antibody—positive with autoimmune reaction; deficiency in intrinsic factor leading to malabsorption

7. Folate deficiency—megaloblastic–macrocytic anemia

  a. MCV greater than 100 fL

  b. Serum folate less than 3 ng/mL; normal serum vitamin B_{12}

  c. Elevated homocysteine level; normal methylmalonic acid level

8. Sickle cell anemia

  a. Hgb 7–9 g/dL; Hct 20%–30%

  b. Mild leukocytosis—12,000 to 15,000 cells/mm^3

  c. Reticulocytosis 10%–25%

  d. Irreversibly sickled cells on peripheral smear

  e. Platelets may be elevated

  f. Sickledex used for screening—sickle cells present in patients with disease and trait

  g. Hemoglobin electrophoresis—Hgb S, 85%–95% in sickle cell anemia; Hgb S, 40% in sickle cell trait

- Management/treatment

1. Iron-deficiency anemia—identify the cause of iron deficiency and correct it

  a. Nonpharmacologic

    (1) Diet with increased iron content

    (2) Hemoglobin-monitoring schedule

      (a) Check 3 weeks after initiation of treatment; recheck in 6–8 weeks

      (b) Ongoing monitoring every 3 months until stable

  b. Pharmacologic

    (1) Ferrous sulfate—may need to continue therapy 4–6 months to replenish iron stores; may discontinue when serum ferritin exceeds 50 mg/L

      (a) Drug action—replenishes depleted iron stores; incorporated into hemoglobin; allows the transportation of oxygen via hemoglobin

      (b) Contraindications/precautions

        i. Iron absorption may be inhibited with concurrent use of antacids or calcium supplements

        ii. Iron inhibits tetracycline absorption

        iii. Constipation and black stools are common side effects

2. Anemia of chronic disease

  a. Nonpharmacologic—treatment of underlying disorder; transfusion if severe anemia

  b. Pharmacologic—none; iron, folate, and vitamin B_{12} have not been shown to be effective

3. Vitamin B_{12}–deficiency anemia

  a. Nonpharmacologic—none

  b. Pharmacologic

    (1) Vitamin B_{12}/cyanocobalamin—dose intramuscular (IM) injection daily for 1 week, then weekly until Hct is normal, then monthly for life

    (2) Cyanocobalamin nasal gel—weekly dosing; alternative maintenance therapy

    (3) Drug action—required for hematopoiesis

    (4) Contraindication/precautions

      (a) Alcohol decreases vitamin B_{12} absorption

      (b) Avoid if hypersensitive to cobalt

4. Folate-deficiency anemia

  a. Nonpharmacologic—increased dietary sources of folic acid: legumes, leafy green vegetables, fruits, and liver

  b. Pharmacologic—folic acid

    (1) Drug action—cofactor in biosynthesis of nucleic acids needed for RBC synthesis

    (2) Contraindications/precautions

      (a) Long-term corticosteroid use increases folic acid requirements

      (b) Folic acid may inhibit the absorption of tetracyclines; decreases serum levels of some anticonvulsant drugs (e.g., phenobarbital, primidone)

5. Sickle cell anemia

  a. Nonpharmacologic

    (1) Treat all infections aggressively to decrease the risk of crises

    (2) Maintain hydration, oxygenation

  b. Pharmacologic—maintained continuously on folic acid supplement

  c. Therapy during crisis

    (1) Hydration and adequate oxygenation

    (2) Analgesics for pain control

    (3) Antibiotics for associated infections

6. Patient education

  a. Iron-deficiency anemia

    (1) Take iron with meals to alleviate GI distress; taking with orange juice or other vitamin C source enhances absorption

    (2) Dietary counseling to improve iron intake and overall nutrition

    (3) Need for follow-up blood monitoring

  b. Vitamin B_{12}–deficiency anemia—need for monthly supplementation

  c. Folate-deficiency anemia

    (1) Folate maintenance dosage

    (2) Avoid overcooking folate-rich foods

  d. Sickle cell anemia

    (1) Consider genetic counseling

    (2) Crises avoidance

      (a) Maintain good nutrition

      (b) Avoid temperature extremes

      (c) Immunizations for pneumococcus and influenza

    (3) Routine evaluation of body systems every 3–6 months

    (4) Report any infection symptoms

- Referral

1. Evaluation of suspected GI blood loss

2. Sickle cell crisis

3. Evaluation of resistant cases

Immunologic Disorders

Human Immunodeficiency Virus Infection

- Definition
  1. HIV infection produces a spectrum of diseases progressing from a clinically latent or asymptomatic state to a state of profound immunosuppression, with acquired immune deficiency syndrome (AIDS) as a late manifestation
  2. Stages of HIV infection
     a. Acute HIV infection/seroconversion—seroconversion, depending on the test type, somewhere between 5 and 50 days after exposure; may take up to 10 months to have initial acute symptoms; highly contagious
     b. Clinical latency—HIV remains active but reproduces at very low levels; without antiviral therapy may last up to a decade or more and remain contagious; with consistent antiviral therapy and follow-up, may remain in this stage for life with undetectable viral load and no risk for transmitting HIV
     c. AIDS, specific clinical conditions present or CD4$^+$ cell count less than 200 cells/mm^3
- Etiology/incidence
  1. Etiology
     a. HIV virus transmitted through direct contact with blood, blood products, and other body fluids
     b. Methods of transmission include sexual contact, sharing needles, blood transfusions, babies born to HIV-infected parents, occupational exposure
  2. Incidence (CDC, 2024)
     a. Prevalence of HIV infection in United States estimated to be 1.2 million, with one in eight undiagnosed
     b. Men who have sex with men, particularly young Black men, are most affected
     c. Women accounted for 19% (7,401) of diagnoses in 2017, with Black women disproportionally affected (59%)
     d. Diagnoses among women are primarily attributed to heterosexual contact (86%) or injection drug use (14%)
     e. Diagnoses among all women declined 21% from 2010 to 2016
  3. Risk factors
     a. Condomless or traumatic sexual activity (e.g., multiple partners or partners with other partners, anal intercourse, lack of condom use)
     b. Intravenous drug use, sharing needles
     c. Infant of HIV-positive parent (vertical transmission)—15%–25% if parent does not receive antiretroviral therapy during pregnancy
        (1) Risk of transmission may be reduced to less than 1% if the pregnant individual receives multi-agent antiretroviral therapy and has an undetectable viral load at delivery
        (2) Risk of transmission greater with parental CD4$^+$ counts of less than 200 cells/mm^3
     d. Transfusion of blood or blood products, artificial insemination, organ transplant recipient prior to 1985
     e. Healthcare worker or service worker exposed to blood or body fluids (e.g., needlestick injury, splash)
- Symptoms
  1. Acute HIV infection and seroconversion
     a. Moderate flulike syndrome 2–4 weeks after inoculation
     b. Fever, diarrhea, headache, oral lesions on palate, lethargy, muscle/joint pain, rash lasting 2–4 weeks, lymphadenopathy
     c. Self-limited; patients who seek care often misdiagnosed
  2. Clinical latency
     a. Asymptomatic
     b. At the end of latency stage, viral load starts to go up, and CD4 cell count begins to go down, the patient may begin to have constitutional symptoms—fatigue, headache, arthralgia, myalgia, weight loss, anorexia, diarrhea, fever, night sweats, chills, lymphadenopathy, oral/vulvovaginal candidiasis, folliculitis, seborrheic dermatitis, and more severe manifestations of HSV, HPV, and molluscum contagiousum
  3. AIDS
     a. CD4 cell count drops below 200 cells/mm^3
     b. Ongoing constitutional symptoms
     c. Opportunistic infections—caused by a spectrum of pathogens that rarely cause disease in healthy people, causative agents include bacterial, fungal, viral, and parasitic infections
        (1) Candidiasis—mouth, vagina, penis, esophagus, large intestine, skin
        (2) Toxoplasmosis
        (3) Malignancies
        (4) Kaposi's sarcoma
        (5) Lymphoma—late manifestation of HIV
        (6) Invasive squamous cell carcinoma—cervix, vulva, anus secondary to HPV
        (7) *Pneumocystis (carinii) jirovecii* pneumonia (PCP)—major AIDS-defining diagnosis
        (8) Tuberculosis
        (9) *Mycobacterium avium* complex (MAC)—occurs in late-stage HIV infection with CD4 count <50
- Physical findings
  1. Related to immunocompromised status
  2. Generalized lymphadenopathy
  3. Weight loss
  4. Skin lesions
  5. Oral hairy leukoplakia
  6. Genital and oral candidiasis
  7. Dementia
- Differential diagnosis
  1. Lymphomas
  2. Pneumonia

3. Tuberculosis
4. Chronic fatigue syndrome
5. Mononucleosis
- Diagnostic tests/findings
    1. Diagnosis—See Chapter 2, *Health Assessment and Diagnostic Tests*, for information on HIV screening/diagnostic tests
    2. Initial laboratory tests for individuals with established HIV infection—stage HIV infection, screen for comorbidities, screen for risk of opportunistic infections and need for prophylaxis, initiate antiretroviral (ARV) medications same day or as soon as patient is ready to begin
        a. Quantitative plasma HIV RNA
            (1) Useful for predicting progression of disease by indicating viral load
            (2) Used monitor response to medication
        b. CD4 cell count
            (1) Indicative of immune status; predictor of disease progression
            (2) Complements viral load assay; also used to monitor response to therapy
            (3) Normal is 800–1050 cells/mm^3
            (4) Patients with CD4 count of 200 cells/mm^3 or less are likely to have symptoms or an AIDS-defining condition
        c. Genotypic antiretroviral drug resistance tests even if not immediately initiating antiretroviral therapy
        d. CBC with differential and platelets
        e. Chemistry panel, transaminase levels, BUN, creatinine, urinalysis, lipid profile, fasting blood glucose
        f. Serology for hepatitis A, B (include core), and C
        g. Serology for syphilis, varicella
        h. TB testing and chest radiography if indicated
        i. Chlamydia and gonorrhea tests
        j. Cervical cancer screening
- Management/treatment
    1. Nonpharmacologic
        a. Symptom management
        b. Laboratory monitoring
        c. Nutrition counseling—identify and address symptoms that may affect appetite, chewing, swallowing; support overall health and immune system function
    2. Pharmacologic
        a. Antiretroviral therapy for HIV suppression
            (1) Highly active antiretroviral therapy (HAART)—combining two to three is the standard of care for the treatment of HIV infection to minimize development of drug resistance and maximize the therapeutic effect
            (2) Goal is to reduce HIV RNA to minimal levels for as long as possible (undetectable level <200 copies/mL)
            (3) Decisions regarding the need to change therapy based on:
                (a) Viral resistance to current medication
                (b) Immunological status (CD4 count)
                (c) Virologic status (HIV RNA levels)
                (d) Opportunistic infection identification
                (e) Symptoms indicating clinical deterioration or intolerance of adverse drug effects or difficulty with adherence
        b. Antiretroviral drug classes
            (1) Nucleoside reverse transcriptase inhibitors (NRTIs)—stall virus replication by providing a faulty version of the building blocks needed for HIV to make copies of itself
            (2) Nonnucleoside reverse transcriptase inhibitors (NNRTIs)—bind to and disable reverse transcriptase, a protein needed for HIV to make copies of itself
            (3) Protease inhibitors (PIs)—disable protease, a protein needed for HIV to make copies of itself
            (4) Integrase strand transfer inhibitors (ISTIs)—block integrase, an enzyme HIV uses to integrate its viral DNA into the DNA of the host CD4 cell and prevent replication
            (5) Chemokine receptor antagonists (CCR5)—antagonize the CCR5 receptor that is involved in the process by which HIV enters cells
            (6) Consideration: People with HIV, aged 40–75 years, receiving continuous antiretroviral medications, with low-to-intermediate risk of atherosclerotic cardiovascular disease (ASCVD), may benefit from statin therapy to reduce the risk of major adverse cardiovascular events over a median follow-up duration of 5 years
        c. HIV treatment in pregnancy is discussed in Chapter 7, *Complex Pregnancy*
    3. Patient education
        a. Natural history of HIV infection
        b. Explain modes of transmission
            (1) Discuss lifelong ability to transmit virus when off of medication, and that when medicated and receiving regular care and labs, and undetectable viral load means the patient cannot transmit the virus via sexual contact (Undetectable = Untransmissable)
            (2) Teach effective ways to reduce fluid exchange
                (a) People with HIV should receive evidence-based, patient-centered counseling to support shared decision-making about infant feeding. Discussion should include replacement feeding with formula or banked pasteurized donor human milk and the possibility of breastfeeding for individuals who are on ART with a sustained undetectable viral load.
                (b) Encourage safer sex practices—condom use, limiting the number of partners when desired, communication with partners about risk and PrEP
                (c) Eliminate needle sharing
        c. Emphasize behaviors that protect/enhance immune system
            (1) Maintain immunizations
                (a) Hepatitis B and A
                (b) Pneumococcal vaccine (repeat in 5 years)

(c) Influenza (annually)

(d) COVID-19

(e) Tetanus/diphtheria vaccine, Tdap vaccine if not done previously, booster every 10 years

(f) HPV vaccine

(g) Meningococcal vaccine

(h) Shingles vaccine

(i) Live vaccines contraindicated if severe immunosuppression (CD4 count < 200 cells/mm^3)

(2) Stop tobacco, alcohol, street drug use

(3) Follow nutritious diet, use clean food preparation techniques

(4) Reduce/manage stress

(5) Exercise as tolerated

(6) Avoid infectious individuals and high-risk environments depending on CD4 count and immune status (e.g., childcare settings, work settings such as hospitals)

(7) Control travel exposures

d. Drug regimens, interactions, and resistance—importance of adherence to medication schedule, CD4$^+$ monitoring

e. HIV and pregnancy implications—encourage antiviral medication to reduce vertical transmission

f. Contraception

(1) Barrier methods reduce transmission

(a) Condoms—external or internal for vaginal or anal penetrative sex

(b) Dental dams or plastic film for oral contact

(c) Stress need for consistent barrier use in addition to other contraception, especially when not on effective ARVs

(2) Hormonal contraceptives—not contraindicated; limited data indicate some antiretroviral drugs may have potential to decrease bioavailability of contraceptive hormones

(3) Spermicides—controversy regarding role in possible changes in vaginal mucosa with frequent use increasing risk for HIV transmission. May increase risk of transmission when used with anal intercourse.

(4) Intrauterine contraception (IUC)—not contraindicated if HIV positive or if has AIDS but is clinically well on antiretroviral therapy

- Referral

1. All cases initially for full evaluation

2. Monitoring and titration of medications

3. Evaluation of new symptomatology

- Preexposure prophylaxis (PrEP)

1. Combination of one or two antiretrovirals: tenofovir disoproxil fumarate and emtricitabine (Truvada) taken orally once daily or long-acting cabotegravir given IM once a month for 2 months, then every other month are approved for people of all genders for all types of sexual activity. Tenofovir alafenamide and emtricitabine (Descovy) daily oral medication is only approved in cisgender men and transgender people assigned female at birth.

2. Available to persons who are HIV negative but have an increased risk of exposure to HIV through sexual and/or injection drug use

3. Reduces transmission risk by as much as 96%

4. Laboratory tests for prospective PrEP recipients include HIV testing, HBV screening, and renal function tests

5. Oral PrEP medications also suppress replication of HBV; reactivation of HBV infection occurs if medications are discontinued or PrEP is taken inconsistently

6. Contraindications/precautions

a. May have loss of appetite; mild gastric upset; mild headaches initially for oral medications; may have pain at injection site

b. May cause increased serum concentrations of acyclovir, valacyclovir, aminoglycosides

c. Do not use if HIV positive

d. Injectables are contraindicated in individuals with silicone injections in the buttocks.

e. Contraindicated with severe renal function disorders. Descovy is a good option for those with reduced renal function.

f. Oral medications are FDA approved for use during pregnancy and lactation

7. Patient instructions

a. Must take consistently for effectiveness

b. Not immediately effective because it reaches maximum intracellular concentration in about 20 days

c. Important to use safer sex practices to reduce HIV infection risks and other STIs

d. Follow up every 3 months—repeat HIV testing, STI testing at all sexual sites used (oral, vaginal/penile, anal), and renal function tests every 6–12 months

Systemic Lupus Erythematosus (SLE)

- Definition—chronic, inflammatory, multisystem disorder of the immune system characterized by periods of remission and exacerbation, course of disease unpredictable and highly variable

- Etiology/incidence/risk factors

1. Etiology

a. An autoimmune disorder—abnormal immune response creates antibodies to normal tissue; familial connection

b. Associated with reaction to some medications—chlorpromazine, hydralazine, isoniazid, methyldopa

c. Criteria for diagnosis

(1) ANA (antinuclear antibodies) positive MUST be included as an obligatory entry criterion followed by:

(a) Scored system which includes 7 clinical domains

○ **Constitutional**—Fever

○ **Hematologic**—Leukopenia, Thrombocytopenia, autoimmune hemolysis

○ **Neuropsychiatric**—Delirium, psychosis, seizure

- **Mucocutaneous**—Nonscarring alopecia, oral ulcers, subacute cutaneous OR discoid lupus, acute cutaneous lupus
- **Serosal**—Pleural or pericardial effusion, acute pericarditis
- **Musculoskeletal**—Joint involvement
- **Renal**—Proteinuria, renal biopsy Class II or V lupus nephritis, renal biopsy class III or IV lupus nephritis
  (b) Score system which includes three Immunology domains and criteria
    - **Antiphospholipid antibodies**—Anti-cardiolipin antibodies OR Anti-βGP1 antibodies OR Lupus anticoagulant
    - **Complement proteins**—Low C3 OR low C4, Low C3 AND low C4
    - **SLE-Specific antibodies**—Anti-dsDNA antibody OR Anti-Smith antibody
  (2) Systemic Lupus Erythematous is classified with a score of 10 or more if the entry criterion of a positive ANA is fulfilled
2. Incidence/prevalence
   a. Approximately 5 per 100,000 individuals each year in the United States
   b. Primarily affects women of childbearing age
   c. Approximately 250,000 definitive cases of SLE in the United States
   d. Prevalence much higher in Black women (1 in 250) and Hispanic or Latina women (100 in 100,000) than in white women (12–39 in 100,000)
- Symptoms
  1. Early symptoms—vague, nonspecific, frequently misdiagnosed
  2. Constitutional—fever, fatigue, weight loss
  3. Arthralgia, arthritis
  4. Photosensitivity
  5. Headache, seizures
- Physical findings
  1. Malar rash—erythematous, flat or raised rash over malar eminences
  2. Discoid rash—erythematous raised patches with scaling
  3. Alopecia
  4. Mucosal ulcers
  5. Pleurisy
  6. Pericarditis
- Differential diagnosis
  1. Contact dermatitis, eczema
  2. Rheumatoid arthritis (RA)
  3. Infectious processes
  4. Chronic fatigue syndrome
- Diagnostic tests/findings
  1. ANA positive in 95% of cases
  2. Anti-dsDNA, anti-Sm, LE cell prep, biologic false-positive Venereal Disease Research Laboratory (VDRL) test
  3. CBC—anemia, leukopenia, lymphopenia, thrombocytopenia

4. Serum creatinine to assess kidney function
5. Urinalysis to determine the presence of hematuria, cellular casts, and proteinuria
6. Antiphospholipid antibodies (anticardiolipin IgG or IgM or lupus anticoagulant); 30%–50% of individuals with SLE have positive antiphospholipid antibodies
- Management/treatment
  1. Nonpharmacologic
     a. Moderate physical activity
     b. Adequate rest to avoid fatigue
     c. Protection from direct sunlight
     d. Proper diet and nutrition—low fat, low cholesterol, adequate vitamin D and calcium
     e. Avoiding medications that induce or aggravate symptoms
  2. Pharmacologic
     a. Treatment is generally symptomatic and variable, with many new medications available.
     b. NSAIDs—for fever, joint pain, serositis
     c. Topical corticosteroids—low-dose agents for skin lesions
     d. Oral or IV glucocorticoids—for major organ involvement
     e. Hydroxychloroquine (Plaquenil)
        (1) Drug action—antimalarial drug; may help treat lupus rashes and joint symptoms; evidence that it may decrease flares and organ damage with long-term use
        (2) Contraindications/precautions
           (a) Avoid use with hepatic dysfunction, alcoholism
           (b) Continue as needed at lowest therapeutic dose during pregnancy
     f. Anticoagulants may be indicated if patient has antiphospholipid syndrome
  3. Patient education
     a. Sunscreen, protective clothing to avoid ultraviolet (UV) light
     b. Relaxation, stress reduction
     c. Individualized exercise/rest program
     d. Prompt treatment of infections
     e. Effective contraception
        (1) Many individuals with SLE are good candidates for most contraceptive methods
        (2) Combination hormonal contraceptives are Category 4, progestin-only contraceptives are Category 3, and LNG-IUS is Category 3 if positive or unknown antiphospholipid antibodies; associated with higher risk for both arterial and venous thrombosis
        (3) Initiation but not continuation of DMPA or copper IUC is Category 3 if patient has severe thrombocytopenia
     f. Prepregnancy/intraconception care
        (1) Pregnancy outcomes best when parent has been in remission for at least 6 months prior to pregnancy and has normal renal function
        (2) Medication management and adjustments ideally done prior to pregnancy

(3) Risk of discontinuation of a medication may be more organ damage affecting both parent and fetus

g. Careful supervision of obstetric care

(1) Increased risk for premature birth, spontaneous abortion, intrauterine fetal death, fetal growth restriction, pregnancy-induced hypertension, venous thromboembolism, postpartum hemorrhage

(2) Exacerbation of symptoms may occur—usually mild to moderate in severity

h. Avoidance of surgery, dental procedures when SLE symptoms present

i. Immunizations

(1) Pneumococcal vaccine, meningococcal vaccine, annual influenza vaccine

(2) Live vaccines not advisable

j. Vitamin D supplementation

- Referral

1. Evaluation of new symptoms, exacerbations

2. When invasive procedures are indicated

3. Social services, family, or individual counseling regarding chronic disease coping strategies

Rheumatoid Arthritis (RA)

- Definition—chronic multisystem disease characterized by symmetrical joint inflammation, loss of normal synovial joint anatomy and mobility, pain

1. Classification criteria for RA—American College of Rheumatology (ACR)

a. Score-based algorithm with a total score of 6 out of 10 needed in four categories (A–D) for the classification of a patient as having definite RA

b. A (joint involvement)—score 0–5 dependent on number and size of joints with clinical synovitis (stiffness, swelling)

c. B (serology)—score 0–3 dependent on negative, positive, and level of rheumatoid factor (RF) and anti-citrullinated protein antibody (ACPA)

d. C (acute-phase reactants)—score 0–1 dependent on normal/abnormal C-reactive protein (CRP) and/or erythrocyte sedimentation rate (ESR)

e. D (duration of symptoms)—score 0–1, with 1 point if patient has had symptoms for 6 or more weeks

2. The ACR 2010 criteria do not include the presence of rheumatoid nodules, radiographic erosive changes, and symmetric arthritis because these may not be present in early RA

- Etiology/incidence

1. Etiology

a. Exact etiology unknown

b. May have an autoimmune component

c. Genetic predisposition

d. Environmental factors may trigger disease in susceptible individuals—viral or bacterial infections, exposure to asbestos and other pollutants

2. Incidence

a. Prevalence—approximately 1% of the adult population

b. Occurs twice as often in women as in men; typically presents between 30 and 50 years of age.

c. RA exists in both remitting–relapsing and progressive forms

d. Extra-articular manifestations—increased risk for cardiovascular disease, pulmonary disease, gastrointestinal bleeding, certain cancers, serious infection

- Symptoms

1. Morning stiffness in joints lasting more than 1 hour

2. Joint pain, constant or recurring; insidious development over weeks to months

3. Joint warmth and redness; functional impairment

4. Fatigue, weakness, anorexia, low-grade fever, malaise may precede arthritic symptoms

- Physical findings

1. Soft tissue swelling—most frequently in metacarpophalangeal (MCP) and proximal interphalangeal (PIP) joints; usually symmetric

2. Deformity of involved joints

3. Limited range of motion in affected joint

4. Subcutaneous nodules

5. Lymphadenopathy

6. Splenomegaly

7. Ocular disease—scleritis

8. Entrapment neuropathies

- Differential diagnosis

1. Polymyalgia rheumatica

2. Osteoarthritis

3. Systemic lupus erythematosus

4. Ankylosing spondylitis

5. Reiter's syndrome

- Diagnostic tests/findings

1. RF

a. Positive in 70%–80% of patients with RA; may not be positive in early disease

b. Not specific to RA

2. Anti-citrullinated protein antibody

a. Higher specificity for RA than RF

b. Similar or higher sensitivity; present in 40% of people with negative RF

3. Erythrocyte sedimentation rate—may be elevated; not useful in diagnosis or prognosis

4. Radiography—joint erosion, narrowing of joint space; may not be evident in early disease

- Management/treatment

1. Major goals

a. Reduce joint inflammation

b. Manage pain

c. Prevent joint destruction deformities

2. Nonpharmacologic

a. Physical therapy, occupational therapy, hydrotherapy

b. Rest

c. Exercise

d. Assistive devices

(1) Footwear—orthotics

(2) Canes, crutches

(3) Splints, braces

e. Surgery—replacement of destroyed joints

3. Pharmacologic
    a. Disease-modifying antirheumatic drugs (DMARDs)—nonbiologic
        (1) Drug action—interruption of inflammatory and immune-regulating pathways; slow disease progression; no analgesic effect
        (2) Methotrexate is most commonly used as a mainstay for individuals with moderate to severe RA
            (a) Avoid use with immunodeficiency, blood dyscrasias, alcoholism, chronic liver disease
            (b) Contraindicated during pregnancy
        (3) Other nonbiologic DMARDs—hydroxychloroquine (Plaquenil), leflunomide (Arava), sulfasalazine (Azulfidine)
    b. DMARDs—biologic (anti-tumor necrosis factor-alpha agents)
        (1) Drug action—block activity of pro-inflammatory cytokines; decrease pain, improve physical function, reduce bone erosion
            (a) Commonly used for individuals with toxicity, failure, or intolerance of nonbiologic DMARDs but may be used as initial therapy for individuals with severe RA
            (b) When used as monotherapy, has more rapid onset of action and is as effective as methotrexate
            (c) Combination with methotrexate or other nonbiologic DMARD may be considered
            (d) Infliximab (Remicade) recommended for combined therapy with methotrexate; adalimumab (Humira) and etanercept (Enbrel) may be used as monotherapy or with DMARDs
        (2) Contraindications/precautions
            (a) May have infusion reaction—fever, urticarial, dyspnea, hypotension
            (b) May cause exacerbation of congestive heart failure (CHF)
            (c) Do not use with CHF, active infections (e.g., HCV, HBV), live vaccines
            (d) Animal reproduction studies have not shown any adverse effect on the fetus, but there are no adequate and well-controlled studies in humans; use during pregnancy only if the benefits outweigh the potential risk to the fetus; however, do not combine with methotrexate
    c. NSAIDs—use for short-term pain management therapy until DMARDs take effect
    d. Corticosteroids—use for short-term therapy until DMARDs take effect
4. Patient education
    a. Safety issues—footwear, balance, transport, walking
    b. Discussion of long-term, chronic nature of disease with remission and exacerbations; support network helpful
    c. Pain control techniques—relaxation, drug therapy, rest, appropriate exercise
    d. Use of medications
        e. Monitoring for and reducing risks for extra-articular manifestations
- Referral
    1. Medications managed by a rheumatology specialist and/or specialists in care of people with autoimmune disorders
    2. Physical therapy, occupational therapy
    3. Surgical procedures

Endocrine Disorders

Diabetes

- Definition
    1. A heterozygous group of metabolic diseases characterized by hyperglycemia resulting from defects in insulin secretion, insulin action, or both
    2. Types
        a. Type 1—absolute insulin deficiency
        b. Type 2—combination of resistance to insulin action and inadequate compensatory insulin secretory response
        c. Gestational diabetes mellitus (GDM)—glucose intolerance diagnosed during pregnancy; excludes high-risk individuals found to have diabetes at initial prenatal visit using standard criteria
        d. Diabetes secondary to other causes
            (1) Genetic defects in beta-cell function/insulin action
            (2) Diseases of the pancreas or other endocrinopathies in which excess hormones antagonize insulin action (e.g., growth hormone, cortisol, glucagon, epinephrine)
            (3) Drug-, chemical-, or viral infection–induced
        e. Metabolic syndrome—group of metabolic components, synergistic in nature, that can lead to cardiovascular disease: abdominal adiposity, insulin resistance and hyperglycemia, elevated triglycerides and low HDL, hypertension, and pro-inflammatory state
    3. Complications
        a. Macrovascular
            (1) Coronary artery disease
            (2) Myocardial infarction; sudden cardiac death
            (3) Cerebrovascular disease
            (4) Peripheral vascular disease
            (5) Intestinal ischemia
            (6) Renal artery stenosis
        b. Microvascular
            (1) Retinopathy
            (2) Nephropathy
            (3) Peripheral neuropathy—paresthesia and glove-and-stocking neuropathy
            (4) Autonomic neuropathy—gastroparesis and sexual dysfunction (e.g., decreased vaginal lubrication, decreased frequency of orgasm, erectile dysfunction, retrograde ejaculation)
        c. Depression—three- to fourfold increase in prevalence of depression in patients with type 1 or type 2 diabetes

- Etiology/prevalence/risk factors
  1. Type 1
     a. Caused by autoimmune destruction of the pancreatic beta cells that produce insulin
        (1) Genetic predisposition, a hypothetical triggering event, and immunologically mediated beta-cell destruction
        (2) Typically begins in childhood or adolescence but can occur in adults of any age; obesity is rarely a factor when patients present with this type of diabetes
     b. Manifested by absolute insulin deficiency that results in elevation of blood glucose, breakdown of fats and proteins
     c. Predisposition to development of ketoacidosis—this may be the first manifestation of type 1 diabetes or first appear in the presence of infection or other stress
  2. Type 2
     a. Characterized by impaired insulin secretion, peripheral insulin resistance, and increased hepatic glucose production
     b. Typically occurs in those older than age 45 years, those who are overweight and sedentary, and those with a family history of diabetes; genetic predisposition plays a significant role in the risk of acquisition
     c. Racial/ethnic groups with increased prevalence likely due to systemic factors including racism—Native Americans, Hispanic, and Black individuals
  3. GDM
     a. Function of hormonal/metabolic demands of pregnancy; usually regresses after parturition
     b. Affected individuals have a 50% risk of developing type 2 diabetes within 5–10 years
  4. Prediabetes—impaired fasting glucose (IFG) and impaired glucose tolerance (IGT)
     a. Hyperglycemia not sufficient to meet the diagnostic criteria for diabetes
     b. Categorized as IFG if identified by fasting blood glucose or IGT if identified by oral glucose tolerance test in the 2-hour sample
     c. Both categories are risk factors for diabetes and cardiovascular disease
  5. Prevalence in the general population estimated at 6%–8% of individuals older than 40 years
     a. Type 1 accounts for approximately 10% of diagnosed cases
     b. Type 2 prevalence is estimated at more than 14 million cases; many undiagnosed
- Symptoms
  1. "Classic" symptoms—polyuria, polydipsia, polyphagia
  2. Weight loss
  3. Fatigue and/or weakness
  4. Persistent/recurrent vaginal candidiasis; candida balanitis
  5. Vision changes, blurred vision
  6. Type 2 often asymptomatic in early stages
- Physical findings
  1. Early

     a. Type 1: average or low BMI; type 2: BMI >25,
     b. Type 2: PCOS, acanthosis nigricans, hypertension, hyperglycemia, hyperlipidemia
     c. Skin infections—frequent or slow to heal
     d. More frequent UTIs or candidiasis
  2. With more advanced disease
     a. Skin—ulcerations of feet and legs; loss of hair on lower legs and toes
     b. Eyes—retinopathy/microaneurysms; exudates; neovascularization; cataracts; glaucoma
     c. Cardiovascular—diminished or absent peripheral pulses; orthostatic hypotension/ominous finding
     d. Neurologic—sensory loss; diminished/absent deep tendon reflexes
- Differential diagnosis
  1. Type 1 versus type 2
  2. Pancreatic disease
  3. Cushing's syndrome
  4. Hypothyroidism
  5. Secondary effects of drug therapy—corticosteroids, thiazide diuretics, COCs
- Diagnostic tests/findings
  1. Criteria for diagnosis of diabetes type 1 and type 2 (ADA, 2019a)
     a. Diabetes can be diagnosed in any one of four ways; must be confirmed on a subsequent day unless the patient also has classic symptoms of hyperglycemia or hyperglycemic crisis
        (1) Fasting plasma glucose—126 mg/dL or greater; fasting defined as no caloric intake for at least 8 hours
        (2) Oral glucose tolerance test (OGTT)—value of 200 mg/dL or greater in the 2-hour sample; using glucose load of the equivalent of 75 g glucose dissolved in water
        (3) Hemoglobin A_{1c} (HbA_{1c})—6.5% or greater
        (4) Random plasma glucose—200 mg/dL or greater with classic symptoms of hyperglycemia or hyperglycemic crisis
     b. Criteria for diagnosis of prediabetes/impaired glucose tolerance
        (1) IFG—fasting plasma glucose of 100–125 mg/dL
        (2) IGT—results of oral glucose tolerance test of 140–199 mg/dL in the 2-hour sample
        (3) HbA_{1c}—5.7% to 6.4%
     c. Criteria for diagnosis of GDM (American Diabetes Association [ADA])—test at 24–28 weeks in individuals not previously diagnosed with pregestational diabetes
        (1) One-step strategy—75 g OGTT at 24–28 weeks in those not previously diagnosed with pregestational diabetes with any of these values exceeded: fasting, 92 mg/dL; 1-hour, 180 mg/dL; 2-hour, 153 mg/dL
        (2) Two-step strategy
           (a) Step 1—1-hour 50 g glucose load test (nonfasting); if 130–140 mg/dL or greater, proceed to Step 2

(b) Step 2—100 g OGTT with at least two of the four plasma glucose levels (fasting, 1-hour, 2-hour, 3-hour) are met or exceeded: fasting, 95 mg/dL; 1-hour, 180 mg/dL; 2-hour, 155 mg/dL; 3-hour, 140 mg/dL

2. Criteria for screening asymptomatic adults (fasting plasma glucose, 2-hour 75-g OGTT, or HbA$_{1c}$) (ADA, 2019a)
   a. Anyone older than 45 years at 3-year intervals
   b. Consider testing younger than 45 years or more frequent screening in adults who are overweight or obese (BMI 25 or greater; for Asian Americans BMI 23 or greater) with one or more additional risk factors
      (1) Physical inactivity
      (2) First-degree relative with diabetes (parent, sibling)
      (3) Member of a race/ethnic population at high risk for systemic racism
      (4) Delivered infant of greater than 9 pounds or history of GDM
      (5) Hypertension
      (6) HDL cholesterol of 35 mg/dL or less and/or triglyceride level of 250 mg/dL or more
      (7) Cardiovascular disease
      (8) HbA$_{1c}$ 5.7%, IFG or IGT on previous testing
      (9) Polycystic ovarian syndrome
      (10) Other conditions associated with insulin resistance (e.g., class 2 or 3 obesity, acanthosis nigricans)
3. Criteria for screening pregnant and postpartum individuals
   a. Screen for undiagnosed type 2 diabetes at the initial prenatal visit in those with risk factors using standard diagnostic criteria
   b. Screen pregnant patients at 24–28 weeks if not previously diagnosed with overt diabetes
   c. Screen those with a history of GDM for persistent diabetes with a 75-g oral glucose tolerance test at 4–12 weeks postpartum using standard diagnostic criteria
   d. Screen patients with a history of GDM every 3 years for diabetes or prediabetes

- Management/treatment
1. Diabetes care is best managed by a multidisciplinary team that includes, but is not limited to, physicians, nurse practitioners, nurses, dieticians, exercise specialists, pharmacists, podiatrists, mental health professionals, the client, and family members.
2. Clinical trials have demonstrated that glycemic control is associated with decreased rates of microvascular complications; epidemiologic studies support reduction in cardiovascular disease
3. Recommended blood glucose, blood pressure, and lipid goals shown in **Table 3-11** for most adults with diabetes
4. Based on individual patient characteristics, glucose, blood pressure, and lipid goals may be lower
5. Nonpharmacologic—types 1 and 2
   a. Home glucose determinations to monitor glycemic control daily
   b. Diet
      (1) Evidence inconclusive on percentage of calories to come from carbohydrates, protein, and fat
      (2) Individualized diabetes nutrition therapy is needed to achieve treatment goals with registered dietician
      (3) Reduced caloric intake while maintaining healthful eating for weight loss as needed/desired by patient
   c. Regular aerobic exercise
      (1) Improves blood glucose control
      (2) Reduces cardiovascular risk factors
      (3) Contributes to weight loss
   d. Smoking cessation
   e. Refer those with type 2 diabetes at time of diagnosis and type 1 diabetes within 3–5 years for eye examination; annually thereafter
   f. Perform comprehensive foot examination annually; examination should include the use of a Semmes-Weinstein monofilament, tuning fork, and a visual examination
   g. Annual influenza vaccination; pneumococcal vaccination
   h. Diabetes self-management education (DSME) and diabetes self-management support (DSMS) according to national standards from ADA

Table 3-11 Recommended Blood Glucose, Blood Pressure, and Lipid Goals for Most Adults with Diabetes

Hgb A$_{1c}$	<7.0%
Preprandial capillary plasma glucose	80–130 mg/dL
Peak postprandial capillary plasma glucose (1–2 hours after beginning of meal)	<180 mg/dL
Blood pressure	<140/90 mm Hg (10-year risk for atherosclerotic cardiovascular disease [ASCVD] less than 15%) <130/80 mm Hg (10-year risk for ASCVD greater than 15%)
Lipids: LDL cholesterol	<100 mg/dL

Data from American Diabetes Association. (2019). Standards of medical care in diabetes—2019. *Diabetes Care, 39* (Suppl. 1), S1–S119.

6. Pharmacologic
    a. Insulin—type 1 diabetes, may be combined with oral medications for type 2 diabetes if needed; see **Table 3-12** for types and actions of insulin
        (1) Some patients may need more than three insulin injections per day and/or to use an insulin pump to maintain control
        (2) For patients with frequent nocturnal hypoglycemia and/or hypoglycemia unawareness, consider the use of sensor-augmented low glucose suspend threshold pump
    b. Oral agents—type 2 diabetes (**Table 3-13**)
        (1) May consider management with diet and exercise first; if glucose intolerance persists, begin noninsulin agent
        (2) Several classes of noninsulin agents with different mechanisms of action subdivided into two main categories
            (a) Hypoglycemic agents—for example, sulfonylureas, meglitinides
            (b) Antihyperglycemic agents—for example, biguanides, GLPs, dipeptidyl peptidase-4 inhibitors, alpha-glucoside inhibitors, thiazolidinediones, incretin mimetics
        (3) Choice of initial oral agent balances the mechanism of action with specific characteristics of the patient, such as BMI, HbA_{1c}, other lab values, risk factors for cardiovascular and renal disease, cost and insurance coverage
        (4) Initial treatment and subsequent treatment changes are assessed every 2–3 months with a review of self-monitoring glucose records and HbA_{1c}
        (5) If treatment goals not met, additional pharmacologic therapy, often combination therapy, is prescribed
    c. Consider aspirin therapy as a secondary prevention strategy in individuals with diabetes who have a history of cardiovascular disease
7. Patient education—DSME and support
    a. Family involvement in care, medication instruction
    b. Safety concerns, especially compensation for neuropathies
    c. Ensure compliance with the drug regimen
        (1) Appropriate injection technique for insulin
        (2) Importance of regular dosing, oral or parenteral

    d. Blood glucose monitoring
        (1) Routine schedule and glycemic target values
        (2) Aseptic technique for blood sampling
        (3) Medication dosage calculation based on blood glucose
    e. Risk factor management and screening
        (1) Smoking cessation, if appropriate
        (2) Annual comprehensive eye examination with an ophthalmologist
        (3) Foot care
        (4) Dental hygiene and annual examination
        (5) Nutritional counseling with a registered dietitian
    f. Preconception counseling emphasizing optimal glucose control, folic acid supplementation, early prenatal care, precautions in pregnancy concerning noninsulin diabetes medication
    g. Contraception counseling
        (1) Most contraceptive methods can be used by those who have diabetes with no complications
        (2) Combination hormonal contraceptives contraindicated (Category 4) if diabetes with nephropathy, retinopathy, neuropathy, other vascular disease or longer than 20 years' duration
        (3) DMPA not recommended unless other acceptable methods are not available or acceptable (Category 3) if diabetes with nephropathy, retinopathy, neuropathy, other vascular disease or longer than 20 years' duration
    h. Hypoglycemia—causes, symptoms, management
        (1) Cause—side effect of medications for diabetes, skipped or delayed meals or snacks, increased physical activity, alcohol intake, especially on an empty stomach
        (2) Symptoms
            (a) Caused by alteration in brain and central nervous system (CNS) function because of lowered glucose levels—mild, moderate, severe depending on blood glucose level
            (b) Mild—hunger, weakness, shakiness, sweating, difficulty concentrating, irritability, palpitations
            (c) Moderate—increased irritability, inability to complete tasks, some changes in mental status

Table 3-12 Types and Actions of Insulin

Type of Insulin	Onset	Peak	Duration
Rapid acting: aspart (NovoLog), glulisine (Aprida), lispro (Humalog)	10–30 minutes	½ hour–3 hours	3–5 hours
Short acting: regular (Humulin R, Novolin R)	30–60 minutes	1–5 hours	6–8 hours
Intermediate acting: NPH (Humulin N, Novolin N), combination NPH, and regular	1–2 hours	4–12 hours	14–24 hours

Data from Brucker, M., & King, T. (Eds.). (2017). *Pharmacology for women's health* (2nd ed.). Burlington, MA: Jones & Bartlett Learning; Woo, T., & Robinson, M. (2020). *Pharmacotherapeutics for advanced practice nurse prescribers* (5th ed.). Philadelphia, PA: F. A. Davis.

Table 3-13 Oral Medications Used to Treat Type 2 Diabetes Mellitus (Representative List)

Drug	Action	Side Effects	Interactions	Contraindications/Precautions
Biguanides (metformin [Glucophage]): Preferred initial agent for type 2 diabetes in nonpregnant individual if tolerated and not contraindicated	Decreases hepatic glucose production and intestinal absorption of glucose; increases peripheral glucose uptake and utilization; may be used as monotherapy or as combination therapy	Anorexia, nausea, diarrhea, abdominal bloating; lactic acidosis is serious, rare	Effects potentiated by cimetidine, ranitidine, nifedipine, digoxin, trimethoprim, alcohol	Renal disease or dysfunction, metabolic acidosis, high risk for lactic acidosis No evidence of harm to fetus
Sulfonylureas: Second generation—glipizide (Glucotrol), glyburide (DiaBeta), glimepiride (Amaryl)	Stimulates insulin secretion from pancreatic beta cells; may be used as monotherapy or as combination therapy	Hypoglycemia, weight gain, photosensitivity, gastrointestinal (GI) upset, cholestatic jaundice	Rare drug interactions with currently used second-generation sulfonylureas	Ketoacidosis, impaired renal, hepatic function Glyburide safe for use during pregnancy First-generation sulfonylureas not much used (chlorpropamide, tolbutamide); associated with multiple drug–drug interactions First-generation sulfonylureas associated with teratogenic risk in animal studies; no controlled human data in pregnancy
Dipeptidyl peptidase-4 inhibitors: sitagliptin (Januvia), linagliptin (Tradjenta)	Inhibits degradation of incretin GLP-1 with subsequent increase of insulin release from pancreas; action in response to elevated glucose; may be used as monotherapy or as combination therapy	Nasopharyngitis, headache, GI discomforts, arthralgia	Several drugs may reduce effects; beta blockers may prolong hypoglycemia	Contraindicated for type 1 diabetes; caution with renal function impairment No evidence of fetal harm in animal studies; no controlled human data in pregnancy
Glucagon-like peptide 1 (GLP-1) receptor agonists/incretin mimetic: exenatide (Bydureon), liraglutide (Victoza) (daily subcutaneous injection rather than oral medication) Semaglutide (Ozempic) (weekly subcutaneous injection)	Binds to GLP-1 receptor; stimulates production and secretion of insulin; may be used as monotherapy or as combination therapy	GI upset, hypoglycemia, jittery feeling, dizziness, headache	Increased risk for hypoglycemia in combination with meglitinides or sulfonylureas	Contraindicated for type 1 diabetes; caution with renal function impairment, GI disorders, history of pancreatitis, personal or family history No evidence of fetal harm in animal studies; no controlled human data in pregnancy
Alpha-glucosidase inhibitors: acarbose (Percose), miglitol (Glyset)	Delays absorption of carbohydrates; inhibits metabolism of sucrose to glucose and fructose; not used as monotherapy	Flatulence, diarrhea, abdominal discomfort (symptoms decrease over time); increases in aspartate aminotransferase (AST), alanine aminotransferase (ALT),	Digestive enzymes, intestinal absorbents decrease effect; may decrease effects of digoxin, propranolol	Inflammatory bowel disease, or any intestinal disease causing disordered digestion or absorption No evidence of fetal harm in animal studies; no controlled human data in pregnancy

(continues)

Table 3-13 Oral Medications Used to Treat Type 2 Diabetes Mellitus (Representative List) *(continued)*

Drug	Action	Side Effects	Interactions	Contraindications/Precautions
Meglitinides: repaglinide (Prandin)	Stimulates insulin release from pancreas; may be used as monotherapy or as combination therapy	Hypoglycemia, headache, dizziness	Several drugs may potentiate or reduce hypoglycemic effect	Caution in hepatic impairment No evidence of fetal harm in animal studies; no controlled human data in pregnancy
Thiazolidinediones: rosiglitazone (Avandia), pioglitazone (Actos)	Improves insulin sensitivity, glucose uptake in muscle and adipose tissue; inhibits gluconeogenes; may be used as monotherapy or as combination therapy	Edema, headache, myalgia, initial increase in low-density lipoprotein (LDL) and high-density lipoprotein (HDL)	Several drugs may potentiate or reduce hypoglycemic effect	Hepatotoxicity—monitor liver function tests (LFTs) at start of therapy, every 2 months, in first year; congestive heart failure No evidence of teratogenicity in animal studies; no controlled human data in pregnancy
Sodium-glucose co-transporter 2 (SGLT2) inhibitors: Brenzavvy (bexaglifloxin), Invokana (canagliflozin), Farxiga (dapagliflozin), Jardiance (empagliflozin), Steglatro (ertugliflozin)	SGLT2 is responsible for reabsorbing glucose and sodium in kidneys	Increased risk of serious urinary tract infection (UTI)—urosepsis and pyelonephritis; hypoglycemia; lower limb amputation and bone fractures	Rifampin, phenytoin, phenobarbital. ritonavir	Increased risk for amputations in those with diabetic foot infection

Data from Brucker, M., & King, T. (Eds.). (2017). *Pharmacology for women's health* (2nd ed.). Burlington, MA: Jones & Bartlett Learning; Woo, T., & Robinson, M. (2020). *Pharmacotherapeutics for advanced practice nurse prescribers* (5th ed.). Philadelphia, PA: F. A. Davis.

(d) Severe—confusion, drowsiness, progression to unconsciousness and coma

(3) Management

(a) Take simple carbohydrates—4 ounces of fruit juice or regular soft drink, five to six pieces of hard candy, a tablespoon of honey, three to four glucose tablets; test blood glucose in 10–15 minutes; if less than 60 mg/dL, take more simple carbohydrates

(b) Administration of subcutaneous glucagon by caregiver or family member if patient is not able to swallow or is unconscious

(c) Wear a medical identification bracelet or necklace

(d) Keep simple carbohydrates in the car if driving

    i. Hyperglycemia—causes, symptoms, management

(4) Cause—insulin deficiency precipitated by acute illness, injury, infection, lack of adherence to or errors in treatment, other medications

(5) Symptoms

(a) Early symptoms may include increased thirst, frequent urination, headache, blurred vision, fatigue, difficulty concentrating

(b) Progressive symptoms with diabetic ketoacidosis may include fruity breath, abdominal pain, nausea and vomiting, dehydration, changes in consciousness

(6) Management—medical emergency—insulin, hydration, electrolyte repletion

- Referral
1. All newly diagnosed cases for complete medical evaluation
2. Evaluation of suspected or developing complications

Hyperthyroidism

- Definition—a hypermetabolic syndrome affecting all body systems characterized by excess circulating thyroid hormone
- Etiology/incidence
1. Etiology
   a. Graves' disease
      (1) Accounts for 90% of cases
      (2) Autoimmune condition; excess synthesis and secretion of thyroid hormone caused by antibodies that stimulate TSH receptors
   b. Toxic multinodular goiter—accounts for most cases in middle-aged and elderly adults
   c. Toxic adenoma/solitary autonomous nodule—single hyperfunctioning nodule within thyroid tissue
   d. Thyroiditis—group of inflammatory diseases

Table 3-14 Thyroid Function Tests in Thyroid Disorders

Thyroid Disorder	Thyroid-Stimulating Hormone (TSH)	Free T$_4$	Antithyroid Peroxidase
Hyperthyroidism	Low	High	+ Graves' − Toxic multinodular goiter
Subclinical hypothyroidism	High	Normal	±
Primary hypothyroidism	High	Low	+ Hashimoto's/chronic autoimmune thyroiditis
Secondary hypothyroidism	Low or normal	Low	−

(1) Inflammation causes disruption of the follicles, resulting in the release of preformed thyroid hormone
(2) Usually self-limited
(3) Phases—thyrotoxicosis, transient euthyroid, hypothyroid, recovery
(4) Classification of thyroiditis
   (a) Subacute lymphocytic—autoimmune process
      ◦ Postpartum thyroiditis
      ◦ Painless/sporadic thyroiditis
   (b) Subacute granulomatous/de Quervain's thyroiditis—likely viral in origin and generally preceded by URI
2. Incidence
  a. Annual incidence 0.05%–1% in the general adult population
  b. Hyperthyroidism is 5–10 times more common in females than in males
  c. Postpartum thyroiditis occurs in 8%–10% of individuals within 1 year of delivery; increased incidence with diabetes or high microsomal antibody titers before pregnancy
- Symptoms—nonspecific, affecting all body systems; reflect increased stimulation from excess thyroid hormone
  1. Increased appetite, weight loss
  2. Irritability, nervousness, sleep disturbance
  3. Heat intolerance, sweating
  4. Fatigue, exertional shortness of breath
  5. Palpitations, chest pain
  6. Diarrhea
  7. Menstrual irregularities, amenorrhea, infertility
  8. Eye irritation, vision changes, double vision (Graves' disease)
  9. Proximal muscle weakness, tremor
- Physical findings
  1. Thyroid gland—enlarged/diffuse or asymmetric nodularity
  2. Neuromuscular system—hyperreflexia, tremor, muscle wasting
  3. Dermatologic system—skin moist, smooth
  4. Cardiovascular system—tachycardia, systolic flow murmur, atrial fibrillation in elderly adults
  5. Eyes—lid retraction, exophthalmos
  6. Gastrointestinal system—increased bowel sounds

7. Graves' disease
  a. Symmetrical and moderate thyroid enlargement/bruit
  b. Exophthalmos/proptosis and pretibial myxedema (nonpitting thickening of skin)
8. Toxic multinodular goiter—asymmetric nodularity
9. Toxic adenoma—single nodule
10. Thyroiditis—slight enlargement; tender with subacute granulomatous thyroiditis
- Differential diagnosis
  1. Neoplasm—because of associated weight loss and weakness
  2. Psychological disorders—panic disorder, generalized anxiety
- Diagnostic tests/findings—see **Table 3-14**
  1. Ultrasensitive serum TSH
    a. Best initial test for diagnosis
    b. Low or undetectable in response to excess circulation thyroid hormone
  2. Free T$_4$ usually elevated
  3. Serum T$_3$ elevated—useful when T$_4$ is normal, TSH is low, and the patient is symptomatic
  4. Antithyroid peroxidase (anti-TPO) may be detected in Graves' disease
  5. Radioactive iodine (RAI) scan with uptake if clinical presentation is not diagnostic of Graves' disease or in the presence of thyroid nodularity; contraindicated during pregnancy
    a. Uptake diffusely increased in Graves' disease
    b. Uptake decreased in thyroiditis
    c. Focal areas of increased and decreased uptake in multinodular goiter
    d. Hot nodule with little uptake in rest of gland in toxic adenoma
- Management/treatment
  1. Treatment depends on cause, severity, patient's age, goiter size, comorbid conditions, and treatment desires
  2. Goal is to correct the hypermetabolic state with the fewest side effects and the lowest incidence of hypothyroidism
  3. Total or partial thyroidectomy—option considered especially for older adults and pregnant individuals in second trimester. High percentage will progress to hypothyroidism.

4. Antithyroid drugs—thionamides (propylthiouracil [PTU], methimazole)
   a. Drug action
      (1) Blocks multiple steps in the synthesis of thyroid hormone
      (2) Permanent remission in half of patients and one-fourth of these hypothyroid in 15–20 years
      (3) Clinically euthyroid in 4–8 weeks
   b. Contraindications/precautions
      (1) May increase risk for leukopenia and agranulocytosis—monitor CBC; instruct patient to notify healthcare provider if fever or sore throat
      (2) May increase risk for hepatocellular damage—monitor LFTs; most risk is with PTU
      (3) May potentiate oral anticoagulants
      (4) Pregnant individuals with overt hyperthyroidism should be treated with a thionamide to reduce the risk of preterm delivery, low birth weight, fetal loss
      (5) PTU recommended in the first trimester—crosses placenta less readily than methimazole; no known teratogenic effects; does present higher risk for hepatotoxicity
      (6) Switch to methimazole in the second trimester—increased risk for major fetal anomalies when taken in the first trimester; less risk for hepatotoxicity than PTU
   c. RAI therapy
      (1) Drug action
         (a) Damages functioning thyroid tissue
         (b) Reduces symptoms in 6–12 weeks
      (2) Side effects
         (a) Long-term hypothyroidism; 70% of patients at 10 years
         (b) May exacerbate ophthalmopathy in the short term
      (3) Contraindications—pregnancy or lactation; use contraception for 6–12 months following RAI administration
   d. Beta blockers—propranolol, atenolol (see Table 3-3)
      (1) Decrease signs and symptoms by blocking the sympathetic nervous system
      (2) Indicated for symptomatic relief until more specific therapy initiated
   e. Management of thyroiditis—often no treatment required
      (1) Beta blockers for symptomatic treatment of thyrotoxicosis
      (2) Subacute granulomatous thyroiditis
         (a) NSAIDs for pain/inflammation
         (b) Prednisone for extreme cases (see Table 3-3)
5. Patient education
   a. Medication regimens, side effects
   b. Signs/symptoms of thyroid storm—an exaggeration of signs and symptoms of hyperthyroidism; acute, life-threatening exacerbation of hyperthyroidism that is a medical emergency

      c. Avoid pregnancy for 6–12 months after RAI administration to avoid fetal thyroid ablation and possible gonadal chromosomal damage secondary to radiation effect on ovaries
- Referral
  1. Evaluation of treatment options
  2. Ophthalmologist referral for ophthalmopathy
  3. Surgical referral for patients with obstructive symptoms

Hypothyroidism

- Definition—a metabolic syndrome affecting all organ systems characterized by deficient levels of circulating thyroid hormone
- Etiology/incidence/risk factors
  1. Etiology
     a. Primary thyroid failure
        (1) Hashimoto's thyroiditis—chronic autoimmune thyroiditis
        (2) Previous RAI treatment, surgery
     b. Secondary—pituitary or hypothalamic disease
     c. Transient
        (1) Subacute granulomatous thyroiditis/de Quervain's thyroiditis
        (2) Subacute lymphocytic thyroiditis occurs most often in the postpartum period, but may also occur sporadically
  2. Prevalence—estimated 1%–3% of the general population
     a. Increasing prevalence with age and in women
     b. Women older than 50 years have an estimated 5% prevalence
  3. Risk factors
     a. Age older than 50 years
     b. Female-to-male ratio is 8–10:1
     c. History of autoimmune disease
     d. Family or personal history of thyroid disease
- Symptoms—often subclinical; reflect slowed physiologic functioning of all organ systems
  1. Weakness, lethargy
  2. Skin changes—dry or coarse skin, skin pallor; coarse hair
  3. Slow speech, forgetfulness, depression
  4. Cold sensation, decreased sweating
  5. Eyelid, facial edema
  6. Constipation
  7. Irregular menses—menorrhagia, amenorrhea; infertility
  8. Weight gain
- Physical findings—depend on severity, duration of deficiency, and rapidity of development
  1. Thyroid gland may be atrophic, normal, or goitrous
  2. Neuromuscular system—diminished relaxation phase of reflexes, carpal tunnel syndrome, hearing loss
  3. Dermatologic system—skin cool, dry; hair dry, brittle; generalized hair loss, especially outer third of eyebrows
  4. Cardiovascular system—bradycardia; edema, especially periorbital; anemia
  5. Gastrointestinal system—diminished bowel sounds

6. Endocrine system—galactorrhea
7. Mentation may be slowed and may appear lethargic and expressionless
- Differential diagnosis
1. Primary versus secondary
2. Clinical depression
3. PCOS
4. Antithyroid drugs—lithium
- Diagnostic tests/findings—see Table 3-13
1. TSH—elevated in primary hypothyroidism
2. Free T_4—decreased
3. Decreased TSH and FT_4 in secondary hypothyroidism
4. Antithyroid peroxidase (anti-TPO), Hashimoto's thyroiditis
5. Those with positive TPO antibodies (even when euthyroid) have an increased risk for recurrent miscarriage with or without infertility
6. Other lab findings may include an elevated cholesterol level and mild normocytic, normochromic anemia
- Management/treatment
1. Most patients with primary hypothyroidism need lifelong thyroid hormone therapy
2. Levothyroxine
   a. Drug action—synthetic T_4
      (1) T_4 converted to T_3; administration of T_4 produces both hormones
      (2) Half-life is 6 days; slow rate of achieving steady state
      (3) Adjust the dose every 6 weeks until TSH normalizes
   b. Contraindications/precautions
      (1) Potentiates sympathomimetics
      (2) Contraindicated with thyrotoxicosis, acute MI, uncorrected adrenal insufficiency
3. Treatment of clinical hypothyroidism during pregnancy
   a. Untreated hypothyroidism is associated with low birth weight, preterm delivery, impaired neuropsychological development of the fetus, postpartum hemorrhage
   b. Levothyroxine is safe to use during pregnancy as well as during lactation
   c. Measure TSH at 4- to 6-week intervals; adjust levothyroxine dose as needed to maintain trimester-specific TSH levels
4. Treatment of subclinical hypothyroidism—defined as elevated TSH in the presence of normal thyroid hormone levels
   a. Majority progress to clinical hypothyroidism
   b. Treat if TSH greater than 10 μIU/mL
   c. Treat if TSH between 5 and 10 μIU/mL and elevated anti-TPO titers, symptoms of hypothyroidism, goiter, or depression
   d. Studies on adverse pregnancy outcomes associated with subclinical hypothyroidism are inconsistent, as are studies showing any improvement in outcomes when treated
5. Patient education
   a. Medication use and doses; need for long-term therapy
      b. Danger of increasing medication too rapidly or taking more than prescribed
      c. Preconception counseling—untreated hypothyroidism during pregnancy may adversely affect parental and fetal outcomes; early prenatal care and close monitoring of TSH levels for adjustments in medication are important
- Referral—all secondary cases for evaluation

Musculoskeletal Disorders

Low Back Pain (LBP)

- Definition—acute (<3 months), chronic, or recurrent pain occurring in the lumbosacral spine region; pain may be localized or radiate to the extremities
- Etiology/incidence/risk factors
1. Etiology
   a. Lumbosacral strain results from stretching, tearing of muscles, tendons, ligaments, and fascia due to trauma or repetitive mechanical stress
   b. Herniated intervertebral disc causes nerve root compression, resulting in pain below the knee and other neurologic signs and symptoms
   c. Other underlying medical conditions
2. Incidence
   a. One of the top 10 reasons for visit to primary care provider
   b. Estimated 60%–85% of individuals experience at least one episode
   c. All sexes equally affected
   d. Chronic LBP accounts for 2% of all cases
3. Risk factors—acute LBP
   a. Repetitive motion
   b. Poor body mechanics
   c. Poor strength of abdominal and back muscles
- Symptoms
1. Lumbosacral strain
   a. Pain located in the lower back, buttocks
   b. Pain characterized as spasms, aching
   c. Pain aggravated by standing/flexion; relieved with rest/reclining
2. Herniated intervertebral disc
   a. Pain felt in the buttock or radiating into the lower extremity (radicular) rather than localized to the lower back area
   b. Pain characterized as sharp, burning, shooting
   c. Pain increased with bending and maneuvers that increase intra-abdominal pressure—for example, straining for bowel movement
   d. Also associated with numbness and tingling over the distribution of the involved nerve root
   e. Most common disc ruptures involve the L5 or S1 nerve roots
      (1) L5 root/L4–5 disc—pain/numbness lateral calf
      (2) S1 root/L5–S1 disc—pain in buttocks, lateral leg, and malleolus; numbness in lateral foot and posterior calf

- Physical findings
  1. Lumbosacral strain
     a. Increased pain with back flexion
     b. Possible tenderness with palpation over paraspinal muscles
     c. Negative straight leg raise (SLR)
     d. Normal neurologic exam
  2. Herniated intervertebral disc
     a. Increased pain with back flexion
     b. Positive SLR—radicular pain when leg is passively raised 30°–60°
     c. L5 root—weakness of dorsiflexion of great toe; decreased sensation anterior/medial dorsal foot
     d. S1 root—weakness of plantar flexion/tiptoe walking; diminished/absent Achilles reflex; decreased sensation lateral foot
- Differential diagnosis
  3. Cauda equina syndrome
     a. Surgical emergency because of impingement on the cauda equina
     b. Characterized by saddle anesthesia, bladder or bowel incontinence, muscle weakness
     c. Immediate MRI and referral to neurosurgery
  4. Fracture
     a. Major trauma, such as motor vehicle accident or fall from high place
     b. Risks: ≥50 years of age, osteoporosis
  5. Osteoporosis/compression fracture—may be precipitated by minor trauma or lifting
  6. Neoplasm
     a. Constitutional symptoms, no relief with bed rest, chronic pain, urinary retention
     b. Risks: ≥ 50 years of age, male sex, history of cancer
  7. Infection—chills, fever, IV drug use, recent bacterial infection, immunosuppression, comorbidities
- Diagnostic tests/findings
  1. Indicated in the presence of "red flags"—fever, chills, weight loss, recent-onset bladder/bowel dysfunction, lower-extremity sensory or neurologic deficit
  2. ESR/CRP—if suspicion of malignancy
  3. Radiograph of lumbosacral spine
     a. Generally not necessary in acute phase—3 to 6 weeks duration
     b. Suspicion of fracture
     c. Suspicion of malignancy—patient older than 50 years; persistent bone pain unrelieved by bed rest; history of malignancy
  4. MRI or CT
     a. Severe persistent symptoms despite conservative treatment
     b. Suspected disc herniation
- Management/treatment
  1. Nonpharmacologic
     a. Encourage continuation of daily activities rather than bed rest
     b. Local application of heat, warm baths
     c. Prescribe physical therapy program to improve strength and conditioning
     d. Low-stress aerobic exercise—walking, biking, swimming
  2. Pharmacologic
     a. NSAIDs
     b. Muscle relaxant—cyclobenzaprine (Flexeril)
        (1) Drug action—reduces tonic somatic motor activity in the brain stem
        (2) Contraindications/precautions
            (a) May cause somnolence and not recommended when operating heavy machinery
            (b) Potentiates alcohol and other CNS depressants
            (c) Increased risk for hypertensive crisis with MAO inhibitors
            (d) Limit to 1–2 weeks at most
            (e) Avoid use in elderly adults
            (f) Use not recommended during pregnancy
     c. Opioid pain relievers—only use for acute pain and when other treatments do not relieve pain; limit use to no more than 72 hours
  3. Patient education
     a. Avoid bed rest
     b. Weight loss if indicated and desired to reduce lordosis—not a treatment for acute LBP but rather prevention and long-term potential treatment
     c. Good body mechanics; proper lifting
     d. Appropriate exercises
     e. Signs of deterioration
        (1) Loss of bladder control
        (2) Numbness or weakness in the groin or rectal area
        (3) Pain extending down leg past knee
     f. Reassurance
        (1) Excellent prognosis for complete resolution of acute LBP episodes
        (2) Recurrence likely at variable intervals
- Referral
  1. Urgently refer patients to neurosurgery with symptoms suggestive of cauda equina or cord compression
  2. Symptoms suggestive of spinal infection or malignancy
  3. Neurologic consultation if back pain remains severe after 4–6 weeks of conservative treatment or findings of neurologic deficits

Osteoarthritis

- Definition
  1. Noninflammatory joint disease characterized by degeneration of articular cartilage with new bone formation at the articular surface
  2. Most commonly involved joints are distal and proximal interphalangeal joints of hands, hips, knees, and cervical and lumbar spine
  3. Primary—no obvious cause
  4. Secondary—occurring in damaged or abnormal joints
- Etiology/incidence/risk factors
  1. Etiology
     a. Progressive degeneration and loss of articular cartilage and subchondral bone
     b. Bone ends thicken and osteophytes or spurs form where the ligaments and capsule attach to the bone
     c. Variable synovial inflammation results

2. Incidence
   a. Radiographic evidence in 80% of adults by age 60
   b. Clinical osteoarthritis affects approximately 25% of adults
3. Risk factors
   a. Increasing age
   b. Female assigned sex
   c. Obesity
   d. Major joint trauma
   e. Repetitive joint stress
   f. Congenital and developmental joint defects
   g. Metabolic and endocrine disorders
- Symptoms
  1. Gradual onset of joint pain, tenderness, and limited movement
  2. Pain aggravated by joint use and subsides with rest
  3. Morning joint stiffness or stiffness following a period of inactivity, lasting generally less than 30 minutes
  4. Symptoms often asymmetrical
- Physical findings
  1. Decreased range of motion
  2. Effusions of involved joint(s) with minimal local warmth and no erythema
  3. Enlargement of distal interphalangeal (DIP) joints (Heberden's nodes); enlargement of PIP joints (Bouchard's nodes)
  4. Crepitus with joint motion
- Differential diagnosis
  1. RA
  2. Infectious arthritis
  3. Tendonitis/bursitis syndromes
  4. Crystal-induced arthritis—gout, pseudogout
  5. Fracture
- Diagnostic tests/findings
  1. Radiography
     a. Does not demonstrate deterioration of cartilage
     b. Four cardinal radiologic features
        (1) Narrowed joint space
        (2) Sclerosis of subchondral bone
        (3) Bony cysts
        (4) Osteophytes
  2. Diagnostic joint fluid aspiration
     a. Indicated if joint effusion
     b. Synovial fluid analysis—WBC count with differential; culture; evaluation for crystals
     c. Findings in osteoarthritis—WBC count <2000 cells/mL; negative culture; negative for crystals
  3. Laboratory tests—normal in primary osteoarthritis
     a. RF/ANAs—if arthritis is inflammatory and symmetrical in distribution to exclude RA or SLE
     b. Erythrocyte sedimentation rate—elevated in many autoimmune, inflammatory, infectious diseases
     c. CBC—if an inflammatory or infectious arthritis suspected
- Management/treatment
  1. Nonpharmacologic
     a. Appliances (e.g., canes, crutches, orthotics)
     b. Exercise
        (1) Aerobic
        (2) Resistance training

(3) Muscle strengthening
   c. Yoga
   d. Supervised heat and cold therapy
   e. Weight loss if indicated
   f. Transcutaneous electrical nerve stimulation (TENS)
   g. Massage
   h. Acupuncture
   i. Rest during exacerbations
2. Pharmacologic
   a. Oral analgesics
      (1) Acetaminophen
      (2) Tramadol (not first line)
      (3) NSAIDs
   b. Topical analgesics
      (1) Capsaicin cream
      (2) Diclofenac (Voltaren, Cataflam)
   c. Intra-articular injection
      (1) Glucocorticoids—beneficial in patients with inflammation, effusion, or substantial pain
      (2) Hyaluronic acid—synovial fluid analogue
3. Patient education
   a. Symptomatic relief techniques (e.g., cold, heat, immobilization, rest)
   b. Medication regimens and precautions
- Referral
  1. Physical therapy, exercise
  2. Need for joint injection
  3. Surgery consultation—joint replacement

Osteoporosis

- Definition—disease characterized by low bone mass and structural deterioration of bone tissue, leading to bone fragility and an increased susceptibility to fractures of the hip, spine, and wrist
- Etiology/incidence
  1. Combination of factors—nutrition, genetics, level of physical activity, age, and estrogen status
  2. Approximately 10 million Americans have osteoporosis
  3. Approximately one out of every two women in the United States will experience a fracture related to osteoporosis
  4. Most common fracture sites are vertebrae, femur, and dorsal forearm; in older population, these fractures may lead to chronic pain, disability, and even death
  5. Conditions, diseases, and medications that cause or contribute to osteoporosis and fractures
     a. Advanced age
     b. Female assigned sex
     c. History of surgical or chemical gonadectomy without adequate sex hormone replacement and/or hypogonadism
     d. Lifestyle
        (1) Low calcium intake
        (2) Alcohol (intake of three or more drinks/day)
        (3) Current cigarette smoking (active or passive)
        (4) Vitamin D insufficiency
        (5) High salt intake
        (6) Inadequate physical activity, immobilization
        (7) Falling, prior history of osteoporotic fracture
        (8) Low BMI

e. Genetic disorders
   (1) Cystic fibrosis
   (2) Ehlers–Danlos syndrome
   (3) Gaucher's disease
   (4) Hemochromatosis
   (5) Marfan's syndrome
   (6) Osteogenesis imperfecta
   (7) Parental history of hip fracture
f. Hypogonadal states
   (1) Androgen insensitivity
   (2) Anorexia nervosa and bulimia
   (3) Athletic amenorrhea
   (4) Hyperprolactinemia
   (5) Panhypopituitarism
   (6) Premature ovarian failure
   (7) Turner's and Klinefelter's syndromes
   (8) Gonadectomy (chemical or surgical)
g. Endocrine disorders
   (1) Adrenal insufficiency
   (2) Cushing's syndrome
   (3) Diabetes mellitus
h. Medications
   (1) Glucocorticoids—long-term use
   (2) Aromatase inhibitors
   (3) Certain anticonvulsants
   (4) Excessive thyroxine doses
   (5) Cytotoxic agents
   (6) Gonadotropin-releasing agonists or analogues
   (7) Long-term use of certain progestin-only contraceptives

- Symptoms
  1. Often a silent disease
  2. Backache
  3. Spontaneous fracture or collapse of vertebrae
- Physical findings
  1. Loss of height > 1.5 inches
  2. Kyphosis
  3. Fractures—spine, hip, wrist
- Differential diagnosis
  1. Malignancy—bone neoplasms, metastatic carcinoma, multiple myeloma
  2. Osteomalacia
  3. Paget's disease
  4. Secondary causes of osteoporosis
     a. Hyperparathyroidism
     b. Hyperthyroidism
     c. Cushing's syndrome
- Diagnostic tests/findings
  1. BMD tests
     a. World Health Organization definitions based on bone mass measurement in women
        (1) Normal—BMD within 1 standard deviation (SD) of a young normal adult; T-score above –1.0
        (2) Osteopenia (low bone mass)—BMD between 1 and 2.5 SDs below that of a young normal adult; T-score between –1.0 and –2.5
        (3) Osteoporosis—BMD 2.5 SDs or more below that of a young normal adult; T-score at or below –2.5

b. Dual-energy X-ray absorptiometry (DXA)—most widely used; quick; radiation exposure one-tenth of standard chest radiograph; body sites measured include hip, spine, wrist; BMD testing at one or more of these body sites with DXA required for densitometric diagnosis of osteoporosis
c. Other bone densitometry technologies and measurements at peripheral body sites (e.g., finger, heel) may be used to predict fracture risk but are not diagnostic
2. Standard radiography—20% to 30% bone loss must occur for osteoporosis detection; used to detect osteoporotic fractures
3. Laboratory tests to consider to rule out secondary causes of osteoporosis and/or conditions that can exacerbate bone loss—CBC, metabolic panel, 25-hydroxyvitamin D, 24-hour urine for calcium and creatinine; other tests if clinically indicated may include parathyroid hormone (PTH) level, TSH, dexamethasone suppression test, and urine cortisol level for Cushing's syndrome
4. Biochemical markers for bone turnover (urine and serum) can aid in risk assessment and as an additional monitoring tool during treatment
5. Vertebral fracture assessment (VFA)—vertebral imaging is available on most modern DXA machines, can perform VFA at time of BMD assessment; vertebral fracture is consistent with diagnosis of osteoporosis independent of BMD results; consider VFA for women who are:
   a. Age 70 or older if BMD T-score is at or below –1.0
   b. Age 65–69 if BMD T-score is at or below –1.5
   c. Postmenopause with low-trauma fracture during adulthood, historical height loss of 4 cm or more, prospective height loss of 2 cm or more, recent or ongoing long-term glucocorticoid treatment
6. Fracture risk algorithm (FRAX)—developed to calculate the 10-year probability of hip fracture and the 10-year probability of a major osteoporotic fracture; takes into account femoral neck BMD and clinical risk factors; used to make decisions concerning preventive medications for postmenopausal women with osteopenia

- Management/treatment
  1. Nonpharmacologic—prevention and treatment
     a. Adequate intake of calcium and vitamin D—see Health Screening, Education, and Counseling section of this chapter for more information
     b. Regular weight-bearing exercise
        (1) Thirty minutes three to four times each week
        (2) Walking, stair climbing, dancing, tai-chi, jogging
     c. Regular muscle-strengthening exercise—lifting weights, swimming
     d. Avoidance of tobacco use and alcohol abuse
     e. Fall prevention strategies—correct impaired vision, assess medications for potential to cause orthostatic hypotension, supportive low-heeled shoes, assistive devices if needed (cane, walker), home safety measures

2. Pharmacologic
   a. Consider pharmacologic treatment for postmenopausal people presenting with any of the following (National Osteoporosis Foundation, 2014):
      (1) Hip or vertebral fracture
      (2) T-score of –2.5 or less at the femoral neck or spine after appropriate evaluation to exclude secondary causes
      (3) T-score between –1.0 and –2.5 at femoral neck or spine and 10-year probability of hip fracture of 3% or greater, or a 10-year probability of major osteoporotic-related fracture of 20% or greater based on FRAX algorithm
   b. Estrogen/hormone therapy (HT)—may be considered short term (5 years) for prevention if the patient needs treatment for vasomotor symptoms and/or vulvovaginal atrophy; not approved for treatment of existing osteoporosis
   c. Bisphonates—alendronate (Fosamax, Binosto)/risedronate (Actonel, Atelvia): indicated for prevention and treatment; ibandronate (Boniva): oral form approved for prevention and treatment, IV form approved for treatment; zoledronic acid (Reclast): IV form approved for treatment
      (1) Drug action—osteoclast-mediated bone resorption inhibitor; bone formation exceeds bone resorption, leading to progressive gains in bone mass
      (2) Contraindications/precautions
         (a) Rare occurrence of osteonecrosis of jaw; atypical femoral fracture
         (b) Antacids and calcium interfere with absorption
         (c) Do not use if patient has esophageal stricture or inability to stand/sit upright for at least 30 minutes after taking medication
         (d) Caution for use if patient has hypocalcemia or renal disease—measure serum calcium and creatinine prior to starting medication; check serum creatinine before each ibandronate injection
         (e) Animal reproduction studies have shown an adverse effect on the fetus, but there are no adequate and well-controlled studies in humans; use during pregnancy only if benefits outweigh potential risk to fetus
      (3) Client instructions
         (a) Take with 8 ounces of water in the morning at least 30 minutes before any beverage, food, or medication
         (b) Do not lie down for at least 30 minutes and until the first food of the day
         (c) May take acetaminophen prior to zoledronic acid injection to reduce risk of postinjection arthralgia, headache, myalgia, fever
   d. Estrogen agonist/antagonist (formerly known as selective estrogen receptor modulators [SERMs])—raloxifene (Evista): indicated for prevention and treatment
      (1) Drug action—estrogen-like effects on bones and lipid metabolism; lacks estrogen-like effect on uterus and breasts
      (2) Contraindications/precautions
         (a) May increase the risk for venous thromboembolic events (rare)
         (b) May cause hot flashes; leg cramps
         (c) Contraindicated in pregnancy; active or history of venous thromboembolic event; concurrent use of estrogen
   e. Denosumab (Prolia)—indicated for treatment of postmenopausal people with osteoporosis at high risk for fracture, if they have failed or are intolerant to other therapy, if they are receiving adjuvant aromatase inhibitor therapy for breast cancer; subcutaneous administration by healthcare professional every 6 months
      (1) Drug action—receptor activator of nuclear factor-B ligand (RANKL) inhibitor, inhibits osteoclasts
      (2) Contraindications/precautions
         (a) Rare occurrence of osteonecrosis of jaw; atypical femoral fracture
         (b) Increased risk of osteonecrosis of the jaw with concomitant use of corticosteroids or chemotherapy
         (c) Increased risk of infection with concomitant use of immunosuppressants
         (d) Contraindicated with hypocalcemia
         (e) Contraindicated in pregnancy
   f. Calcitonin—indicated for treatment only; increased risk of malignancy; European Medicines Agency (equivalent to FDA) removed indication of treatment for postmenopausal osteoporosis in 2012; March 2014—U.S. FDA required risk of malignancies be added to labeling, but FDA indication as a treatment remains; not to be used as a first-line drug, and not for more than 6 months
      (1) Drug action—directly inhibits bone resorption of calcium; administered as a nasal spray or injection
      (2) Contraindications/precautions
         (a) Contraindicated if hypersensitivity to salmon calcitonin
         (b) Animal reproduction studies have shown an adverse effect on the fetus, but there are no adequate and well-controlled studies in humans; use during pregnancy only if the benefits outweigh the potential risk to the fetus
   g. Parathyroid hormone—PTH (1–34), teriparatide (Forteo), abaloparatide (Tymlos): approved for treatment if patient is at high risk for fracture
      (1) Drug action—anabolic bone-building agent, PTH; administered as subcutaneous injection
      (2) Contraindications/precautions
         (a) Avoid if increased risk for osteosarcoma; prior radiation of skeleton; bone metastases
         (b) Contraindicated with hypercalcemia

(c) Animal reproduction studies have shown an adverse effect on the fetus, but there are no adequate and well-controlled studies in humans; use during pregnancy only if the benefits outweigh the potential risk to the fetus

h. Humanized monoclonal antibody (IgG2), romosozumab (Evenity): approved for treatment of postmenopausal people at high risk for fracture

(1) Drug action—inhibits sclerostin, a glycoprotein secreted by osteocytes that has anti-anabolic effects on bone; administered as a monthly subcutaneous injection

(2) Contraindications/precautions

(a) Anabolic effect wanes after 12 monthly doses of therapy; if osteoporosis therapy remains warranted after 12 doses consider therapy with an anti-resorptive agent

(b) May increase risk of myocardial infarction or stroke—contraindicated in patients who have had myocardial infarction or stroke within the preceding year, weigh benefits and risks in patients with other cardiovascular risk factors

i. Monitoring pharmacologic therapy effectiveness

(3) Baseline BMD before onset of therapy

(4) Repeat test every 2 years; more frequently if warranted by certain clinical situations

(5) Urine/serum biochemical markers of bone formation or resorption may be used as adjuncts to monitor response to therapy—variable results and precision error limit usefulness; changes must be large to be clinically meaningful

3. Patient education

a. Adequate calcium and vitamin D intake

b. Weight-bearing and muscle-strengthening exercises

c. Avoidance of tobacco and excessive alcohol

d. Fall prevention strategies

e. Medication use

Fibromyalgia

- Definition
  1. Syndrome characterized by chronic fatigue, and generalized, widespread musculoskeletal pain and stiffness associated with the finding of characteristic tender points of pain on physical examination
  2. Criteria for the classification of fibromyalgia— American College of Rheumatology (ACR)
     a. Widespread pain index (WPI) score of 7 or greater and symptom severity (SS) scale score of 5 or greater or WPI score of 3–6 and SS scale score of 9 or greater
     b. Symptoms present at a similar level for at least 3 months
     c. Exclusion of other disorders that would otherwise explain pain
     d. WPI—number of areas in which the patient has had pain over the last week (0–19)

e. SS scale score—presence and severity of fatigue, waking unrefreshed, cognitive symptoms over the past week (0–12)

- Etiology/incidence
  1. Etiology—unknown but classified as a rheumatic disease; several causal mechanisms postulated
     a. Physical or mental stress
     b. Sleep disturbances
     c. Decreased serotonin levels
     d. Metabolic factors
     e. Viral infection—EBV, CMV, herpes virus, enteroviruses
  2. Incidence—unknown in the general population because of misdiagnosis, self-treatment
     a. More common in women, with a 9:1 female-to-male ratio
     b. Most common in 30- to 50-year olds
- Symptoms
  1. Multiple, specific areas of muscle tenderness (trigger points)
  2. Fatigue, sleep disturbances
  3. Muscle weakness and generalized aching
  4. Pain typically worsens with cold
  5. Paresthesia
  6. Headaches
  7. Anxiety, stress
  8. Depression
- Physical findings
  1. Pain on digital palpation of characteristic tender points
  2. Normal muscle strength, range of motion
- Differential diagnosis
  1. Chronic fatigue syndrome
  2. RA
  3. SLE
  4. Somatization and depression
- Diagnostic tests/findings
  1. Unnecessary unless a coexisting condition is suspected
  2. Erythrocyte sedimentation rate normal; excludes inflammatory conditions
- Management/treatment
  1. Nonpharmacologic
     a. Low-impact exercise (e.g., walking, swimming, tai-chi, yoga)
     b. Supervised heat and cold therapy
     c. Massage, relaxation therapy
     d. Biofeedback
     e. Hypnotherapy
     f. Strength training
     g. Acupuncture
     h. Cognitive Behavioral Therapy
  2. Pharmacologic
     a. FDA-approved drugs to treat fibromyalgia
        (1) Gamma-aminobutyric (GABA) analogue— pregabalin (Lyrica)
        (a) Drug action—affects descending noradrenergic and serotonergic pain transmission pathways from the brain stem to the spinal cord
        (b) Contraindications/precautions
           ○ May potentiate CNS depressants

° Animal reproduction studies have shown an adverse effect on the fetus, but there are no adequate and well-controlled studies in humans; use during pregnancy only if benefits outweigh potential risk to fetus

(2) Selective serotonin–norepinephrine reuptake inhibitors (SNRIs)—duloxetine hydrochloride (Cymbalta), milnacipran HCl (Savella)

    (a) Drug action—mechanism by which these drugs reduce pain for people with fibromyalgia is unknown; data suggest that these drugs possibly affect the release of neurotransmitters

    (b) Contraindications/precautions

      ° May cause somnolence, dry mouth, dizziness

      ° Animal reproduction studies have shown an adverse effect on the fetus, but there are no adequate and well-controlled studies in humans; use during pregnancy only if benefits outweigh potential risk to fetus

b. Tramadol—not recommended as first-line treatment

  (1) Drug action—centrally acting analgesic; creates a weak bond to opioid receptors and inhibits reuptake of both norepinephrine and serotonin

  (2) Contraindications/precautions

    (a) Seizure risk if used with other agents that lower threshold

    (b) Abuse potential

    (c) Potentiated with alcohol and other CNS depressants

    (d) Animal reproduction studies have shown an adverse effect on the fetus, but there are no adequate and well-controlled studies in humans; use during pregnancy only if benefits outweigh potential risk to fetus

c. Over-the counter analgesics

  (1) Acetaminophen

  (2) NSAIDs

3. Patient education

  a. Reassurance regarding benign course of condition

  b. Supportive care for chronic pain

- Referral—physical therapy, rheumatologist

Strains/Sprains

- Definition—musculoskeletal injury of varying degrees
  1. *Strain*—injury to muscle or tendon
  2. *Sprain*—stretching or tearing of ligaments
- Etiology/incidence/risk factors
  1. Etiology
     a. Overuse of the muscle–tendon unit by stretching, tearing, hyperextension, forceful contraction
     b. Acute injury
     c. Chronic overuse as seen in sports injury, repetitive motion

2. Incidence—unknown because of frequent self-treatment, but common presenting complaint in primary care practice
3. Risk factors
   a. Increased physical activity
   b. New physical exercise program
   c. Overweight

- Symptoms
  1. Pain at site of injury
  2. Strain
     a. Temporary weakness
     b. Pain with stretch of muscle
     c. Pain and spasm with more severe strains
  3. Sprain
     a. Marked swelling
     b. Loss of function
- Physical findings
  1. Strain—temporarily reduced range of motion, muscle strength
  2. Sprain
     a. Contusion, hemorrhage
     b. Reduced range of motion, muscle strength
     c. Joint instability in severe sprain or ruptured ligament
- Differential diagnosis
  1. Other overuse syndromes—tendonitis, shin splints
  2. Fracture
- Diagnostic tests/findings
  1. Radiograph to rule out fractures—negative for bony abnormality in strains/sprains
  2. MRI
- Management/treatment
  1. Nonpharmacologic
     a. RICE—initial therapeutic strategy for first 48 hours
        (1) *Rest* or immobilization of injured part
        (2) *Ice* or application of cold
        (3) *Compression*, elastic wrap
        (4) *Elevation* of affected area
     b. Application of alternating heat and cold after first 2 days
     c. Topical heat-generating liniments for symptomatic relief
  2. Pharmacologic—NSAIDs as needed
  3. Patient education
     a. Physical training progression to avoid repeat injury
     b. Stretching and warm-up exercises
     c. Appropriate footwear, protective gear for exercise
- Referral
  1. Physical therapy for stretching and strengthening program
  2. Consult an orthopedic surgeon if no response to conservative management

Neurologic Disorders

Headaches

- Definition
  1. Headache/cephalgia is defined as diffuse pain in various parts of the head

2. Primary headaches—migraine, tension, cluster head-aches are not directly related to a specific underlying cause or secondary to another problem, and not showing any "red flag" signs and symptoms
3. Secondary headaches are the result of identifiable structural or physiologic pathology
- Etiology/incidence/risk factors
  1. Etiology
     a. Primary headaches—90% to 98% of headaches presenting in primary care
  1. Migraine headache
     a. Current understanding suggests genetic basis
     b. Those genetically predisposed inherit a nervous system that is more sensitive/easily aroused to a variety of internal/external factors—hormonal fluctuations, weather changes, diet, psychosocial disruptions
     c. Changes in serotonin activity result in release of vasoactive mediators; mediators produce an inflammatory response adjacent to cerebral blood vessels accompanied by vasodilation
     d. The dilated vessels and inflammatory response stimulate the trigeminal nerve to transmit impulses to the brain, resulting in migraine headache
  2. Tension headache
     a. Pathophysiology poorly understood; formerly attributed to contraction of the muscles of the scalp and neck
     b. Recent theories suggest tension headaches may involve changes in the intracranial neurotransmitter and vascular systems similar to migraine
     c. Symptom complex resulting from several simultaneous processes—muscle tension, psychological stress, neurovascular changes
  3. Cluster headache
     a. Secondary to serotonergic neurologic dysfunction
     b. Clustering of attacks suggests the involvement of circadian pacemakers of the anterior hypothalamus
     c. Tearing and nasal stuffiness suggests abnormality in the autonomic nervous system
     d. Secondary headaches
  4. Vascular disorders—subarachnoid, cerebral, cerebellar hemorrhage; acute ischemic cerebrovascular disorder; arteriovenous (AV) malformation; temporal arteritis; arterial HTN
  5. Nonvascular intracranial disorders—neoplasm; infection; low cerebrospinal fluid pressure/postlumbar puncture; benign intracranial HTN/pseudotumor cerebri
  6. Traumatic—concussion and postconcussion; hematoma/subdural and epidural
  7. Metabolic disorders—hypoxia, hypercapnia, hypoglycemia
  8. Substances that act as triggers—medications; foods: monosodium glutamate (MSG), alcohol; exposures: carbon monoxide; rebound: caffeine, analgesics
  9. Extracranial structures—eyes/glaucoma, refractive errors; sinusitis; TMJ dysfunction; neck/cervical disc disease; trigeminal neuralgia
  10. Systemic—infection; allergies/pollen; hormonal

11. Incidence
   a. Migraine
12. Reported in as many as 15%–17% of women; 5% of men
13. Estimated 10% of adults affected
   a. Tension—most common form of headache
   b. Cluster—relatively rare incidence compared to other types; six times more common in men
14. Risk factors—primary headache syndromes
   a. Migraine headaches—female assigned sex, family history
   b. Tension headaches—overuse of headache medications
   c. Cluster headaches—male sex, middle aged or older
- Symptoms
  1. Migraine
     a. Types
        (1) Migraine with aura/classic migraine
            (a) Aura consists of focal neurologic symptoms that may precede or accompany headache
            (b) Usually visual phenomenon; flashing lights, zigzag/jagged lines, difficulty focusing
            (c) May have a premonitory phase, occurring hours or days before the headache
        (2) Migraine without aura/common migraine—accounts for 75% of migraines
            (a) Attack lasting 4–72 hours untreated or unsuccessfully treated
        (3) Complicated migraine—basilar/hemiplegic migraine
     b. Phases
        (1) Prodrome—occurs 24 hours prior to onset of headache: fatigue, euphoria, difficulty concentrating, irritability
        (2) Aura
        (3) Early and late stages of migraine
        (4) Postdrome—individual feels "wiped out," fatigued, "hungover"
     c. Triggers
        (1) Stress
        (2) Hormonal changes
        (3) Certain foods, caffeine, alcohol, skipping meals
        (4) Fatigue, oversleeping
        (5) Medications
        (6) Changes in weather or barometric pressure
     d. Location—unilateral tendency
     e. Duration—four to 72 hours
     f. Character
        (1) Moderate to severe intensity; inhibits daily activities
        (2) Characterized as throbbing, pounding
     g. Associated symptoms—nausea, vomiting, photophobia, phonophobia, fatigue
     h. Frequency—recurrent, variable from two to three per year to two to three per week
  2. Tension headache
     a. Onset—gradual
     b. Location—diffuse, bilateral, generalized

    c. Duration—variable, hours to days

    d. Character

      (1) Mild to moderate severity; generally able to continue with daily activities

      (2) Dull, pressure, constant, viselike

    e. Associated symptoms—fatigue, irritability, difficulty concentrating, neck and shoulder spasm

    f. Frequency

      (1) Episodic—less than 15 days per month

      (2) Chronic—must be present 15 days or more a month for at least 6 months

3. Cluster headaches

    a. Onset

      (1) Abrupt

      (2) Often nocturnal, awakens patient; often recurs at same time of day

    b. Location

      (1) Unilateral

      (2) During a series, pain remains on same side

      (3) Retro-orbital, sometimes radiating

    c. Duration—usually 30–45 minutes

    d. Character—intense, severe

    e. Associated symptoms—facial pain, ptosis of the affected side, lacrimation, nasal congestion

    f. Frequency—occurs in clusters lasting a few weeks, with remission lasting weeks to months

- Physical findings

1. General appearance indicates discomfort
2. Neurologic assessment normal in primary headaches—temporary focal neurologic findings with migraine may be present, but not common
3. Blood pressure, vital signs normal
4. Cluster headache—unilaterally constricted pupil, nasal discharge

- Differential diagnosis—"red flags" suggesting secondary causes

1. Headache beginning after 50 years of age—temporal arteritis, infection, mass, lesion
2. Sudden onset, worst headache ever experienced—subarachnoid hemorrhage, bleeding into a mass or AV malformation
3. Headaches increasing in severity/frequency—mass, lesion, subdural hematoma, medication overuse
4. Headache initiated by exertion, such as coughing or straining or during sexual intercourse—mass, lesion, subarachnoid hemorrhage
5. Focal neurologic symptoms that do not resolve within 60 minutes of headache onset—intracranial mass or lesion
6. Headache subsequent to head trauma—intracranial hemorrhage, subdural/epidural hematoma, posttraumatic headache
7. Systemic illness/fever—meningitis, encephalitis, temporal arteritis

- Diagnostic tests/findings

1. None indicated when examination is consistent with primary headache syndromes
2. Erythrocyte sedimentation rate on all patients with new onset and older than 40 years to rule out temporal arteritis

3. CT/MRI

    a. Indicated if persistent focal neurologic findings or history of trauma

    b. CT—preferred to identify acute hemorrhage

    c. MRI—more sensitive in identifying pathologic intracranial changes

    d. Magnetic resonance angiography if aneurysm suspected, history of exertional headaches

- Management/treatment

1. Nonpharmacologic

    a. Regular sleep and meal schedules

    b. Daily exercise

    c. Avoiding known triggers

2. Pharmacologic

    a. Migraine—abortive therapy

      (1) First-line therapy—mild to moderate intensity

        (a) NSAIDs, acetaminophen

        (b) Combination analgesics—acetaminophen 250 mg/aspirin 250 mg/caffeine 65 mg—one tablet every 6 hours, not to take more than eight tablets/day

      (2) First-line therapy—moderate to severe intensity: triptans

        (a) Agents—sumatriptan (Imitrex), zolmitriptan (Zomig), rizatriptan (Maxalt); available in oral, nasal, and subcutaneous forms

        (b) Drug action—selective serotonin agonists

        (c) Contraindications/precautions

          ◦ May initially cause tightness of the throat/chest, flushing, numbness, tingling, dizziness

          ◦ Should not use within 24 hours of another triptan or any ergotamine-containing drug

          ◦ Contraindicated with coronary artery disease, hypertension

          ◦ Animal reproduction studies have shown an adverse effect on the fetus, but there are no adequate and well-controlled studies in humans; use during pregnancy only if benefits outweigh potential risk to fetus

          ◦ Some concerns about use in late pregnancy—association with preeclampsia, preterm birth, low birth weight, and postpartum hemorrhage

      (3) Second line—ergotamines

        (a) Agents—ergotamine, dihydroergotamine/parenteral and nasal spray

        (b) Drug action—nonspecific serotonin agonist and vasoconstrictor

        (c) Contraindications/precautions

          ◦ Do not give with triptan

          ◦ Contraindicated with coronary artery disease; hypertension

          ◦ Contraindicated during pregnancy

    b. Migraine headache—prophylactic therapy: consider in patients who experience more than two severe headaches per month, need acute treatment

medication more than two times per week, or are unable to tolerate abortive agents
  (1) Riboflavin (B2) 400 mg/day
  (2) Beta blocker—propranolol/timolol (see Table 3-3)
  (3) CCB—verapamil (see Table 3-3)
  (4) Antiepileptic agents—valproic acid (Valproate), divalproex (Depakote), topiramate (Topamax)
  (5) Antidepressants—amitriptyline, venlafaxine
  c. Tension—episodic
  (1) NSAIDs, acetaminophen
  d. Tension—chronic
  (1) Tricyclic antidepressants (TCAs)—amitriptyline, nortriptyline
    (a) Drug action—increases synaptic concentration of serotonin and norepinephrine in CNS
    (b) Contraindications/precautions
      ○ May cause sedation
      ○ Additive effect of anticholinergic drugs
      ○ Do not use with MAO inhibitors or if the patient has impaired liver function
      ○ Animal reproduction studies have shown an adverse effect on the fetus, but there are no adequate and well-controlled studies in humans; use during pregnancy only if the benefits outweigh the potential risk to the fetus
  (2) Selective serotonin reuptake inhibitors—less effective than TCAs; see the section about Major Depressive Disorder in this chapter
  3. Patient education
    a. Signs indicating need for emergency treatment
      (1) Acute fever with headache
      (2) Abnormal mental status or personality changes
      (3) Sudden onset; worst headache experienced
      (4) Neurologic symptoms (e.g., projectile emesis, visual disturbances)
    b. Self-medication for abortive therapy, injections
    c. Education regarding nonpharmacologic management—avoidance of precipitating factors
- Referral
  1. Abnormal neurologic findings on physical examination
  2. Secondary cause is suspected
  3. Chronic headaches develop new features
  4. New headaches in individuals older than 50 years

Dermatologic Disorders

Acne

- Definition—a common self-limited disease that presents with a variety of lesions, including open and closed comedones, papules and pustules, nodules, and cysts
- Etiology/incidence/risk factors
  1. Etiology
    a. Primary cause is obstruction of the pilosebaceous follicle
    b. Characterized by plugging of the hair follicle with abnormally cohesive desquamated cells, sebaceous gland hyperactivity, proliferation of bacteria (*Propionibacterium acnes*), and inflammation
    c. Obstruction of follicle leads to development of noninflammatory acne—closed comedones/white heads and open comedones/blackheads
    d. Proliferation of *P. acnes*/rupture of follicle wall results in inflammatory acne with papules, pustules, nodules, cysts
  2. Incidence
    a. Affects as many as 90% of teens; 15% have moderate to severe acne
    b. May persist to older than 40 years in some
  3. Contributing/aggravating factors—hormonal cycles, topical or oral corticosteroids, irritant oils or cosmetics
- Symptoms
  1. Erythematous lesions, sometimes tender
  2. May be episodic, cyclic in severity
  3. Distribution and severity tend to be similar in family members
- Physical findings
  1. Lesions occur primarily on the face, but the neck, shoulders, chest, and back may be involved
  2. Mild—open and closed comedones without inflammation
  3. Moderate—comedones with papules and pustules
  4. Severe—comedones, papules and pustules with nodules, cysts, and scarring
- Differential diagnosis
  1. Rosacea
  2. Pyoderma
  3. Drug eruptions
  4. Underlying endocrine disease—polycystic ovarian syndrome, Cushing's syndrome
  5. Folliculitis
  6. Perioral dermatitis
  7. Hidradenitis suppurativa
- Diagnostic tests/findings—none indicated
- Management/treatment
  1. Varies depending on the severity of the condition
  2. Nonpharmacologic—cleansing
  3. Pharmacologic
    a. Mild acne—topical medications alone or in combination
    (1) Benzoyl peroxide
      (a) Drug action—antibacterial and comedolytic properties
      (b) Contraindications/precautions
        ○ May cause skin irritation, allergic dermatitis
        ○ May bleach clothing/bed linens, hair
        ○ Use with para-aminobenzoic acid (PABA) sunscreens may temporarily discolor skin
        ○ Avoid eyes, mouth, mucous membranes
        ○ May use during pregnancy; minimal systemic absorption

(2) Retinoic acid derivatives—tretinoin/cream, gel, lotion, and microspheres; adapalene gel/solution; tazarotene gel

    (a) Drug action—comedolytic agent

    (b) Contraindications/precautions

       ∘ May cause local irritation, erythema, scaling

       ∘ Avoid UV light, sun, extreme weather

       ∘ Do not use with eczema

       ∘ Not recommended during pregnancy, although systemic absorption is likely minimal

  b. Moderate acne—topical antibiotics combined with benzoyl peroxide and retinoic acid derivative (clindamycin, erythromycin)

    (1) Drug action—bactericidal effects

    (2) Contraindications/precautions

      (a) Avoid eyes, mucous membranes

      (b) Do not use clindamycin if patient has history of regional enteritis, ulcerative or antibiotic-induced colitis

      (c) May use during pregnancy; minimal systemic absorption

  c. Moderate to severe acne—oral medications

    (1) Oral antibiotics—doxycycline, minocycline

      (a) Drug action (tetracycline and its derivatives)—antibacterial and anti-inflammatory effect

      (b) Contraindications/precautions

        ∘ May cause photosensitivity

        ∘ Reduced absorption with antacids

        ∘ Tetracycline and its derivatives are contraindicated during pregnancy

    (2) Oral combination hormonal contraceptives—some have FDA approval for treatment of moderate acne in women who also desire contraception; all with low androgenic or antiandrogenic progestin are likely effective

      (a) Drug action—antiandrogenic/decreases free testosterone available for metabolism in sebaceous glands

      (b) See Chapter 4, *Gynecologic, Reproductive, Sexual, and Menopause Health*, for side effects, drug interactions, contraindications

  d. Severe cystic acne—oral isotretinoin (Accutane)

    (1) Drug action—decreases size and secretion of sebaceous glands, normalizes follicular keratinization, inhibits *P. acnes*, and modulates the inflammatory response

    (2) Contraindications/precautions

      (a) May cause skin and mucosal dryness

      (b) Use with tetracyclines may increase the incidence of pseudotumor cerebri

      (c) Contraindicated during pregnancy and lactation

      (d) Must be on birth control if in reproductive years

4. Patient education

  a. Use of mild cleansers, noncomedogenic moisturizers, sunscreen

  b. Hands-off policy to avoid secondary infection, scarring

  c. Importance of avoiding pregnancy if using isotretinoin

- Referral—severe acne; may refer patients requiring treatment with isotretinoin

Contact Dermatitis

- Definition—skin inflammation due to irritants (irritant contact dermatitis) or allergens (allergic contact dermatitis)
- Etiology/incidence
  1. Irritant contact dermatitis
     a. Eczematous response that is nonallergic caused by irritants, including chemicals, dry and cold air, and friction
     b. May occur acutely; occurs more commonly after chronic exposure
  2. Allergic contact dermatitis
     a. A manifestation of cell-mediated hypersensitivity; causes delayed reaction on first exposure
     b. *Rhus* plant antigens (poison oak, poison ivy) result in clinical eruption in 12–72 hours and within minutes on reexposure
     c. Other common allergic sensitizers include nickel (jewelry), rubber compounds (gloves), cosmetics, topical medications
  3. Most (80%) of contact dermatitis cases are due to contact with local irritants
- Symptoms
  1. Report of recent exposure (within 24 hours) to known allergens; exposure to irritants
  2. Pruritus
- Physical findings
  1. Irritant contact dermatitis
     a. Mild irritants cause erythema, dryness, fissuring
     b. Chronic exposure may cause oozing, weeping lesions
  2. Allergic contact dermatitis
     a. Classic lesions—vesicles and blisters on erythematous base
     b. Linear eruption—hallmark of most plant dermatoses
  3. Distribution often provides clues to diagnosis
- Differential diagnosis
  1. Atopic dermatitis, eczema
  2. Tinea
  3. Scabies/pediculosis
  4. Herpes simplex/herpes zoster
- Diagnostic tests/findings
  1. Usually none indicated
  2. Negative potassium hydroxide (KOH) preparation of skin scraping
  3. Patch testing with suspected allergens in difficult cases
- Management/treatment
  1. Nonpharmacologic
     a. Compresses, soaks (e.g., Burow's solution, Epsom salt)
     b. Lubricants—lubricating ointments, petrolatum, no creams

2. Pharmacologic
   a. Topical corticosteroids—potency depends on severity and response
      (1) Drug action—anti-inflammatory effect
      (2) Contraindications/precautions
         (a) May cause local irritation; epidermal and dermal atrophy
         (b) Avoid prolonged use on large areas
         (c) May use during pregnancy; systemic absorption is minimal
   b. Systemic steroids for widespread or severe dermatitis (see Table 3-7)—avoid in first trimester of pregnancy
   c. Antihistamines—allergic pruritus (see Table 3-6)
3. Patient education
   a. Avoidance of allergens
   b. Protective garments, gloves

Eczema

- Definition—chronic or chronically relapsing pruritic inflammation of the skin; associated scratching is the cause of characteristic lichenification of the skin
- Etiology/incidence
  1. Etiology—exact cause unknown
  2. Incidence
     a. Affects 3.5% of the world's population
     b. Most prevalent in infants, reproductive-age people of childbearing potential
     c. Rates have risen particularly in lower-income countries
- Symptoms
  1. Extremely pruritic, erythematous, dry, scaly, excoriated, lichenified patches of skin
  2. Areas most commonly affected—arms, wrists, knees, face, hands, genitals
- Physical findings
  1. Lesions become more diffuse with an underlying background of erythema on the face, neck, upper trunk, and at bends of elbows and knees
  2. Face is commonly involved, becomes dry and scaly
  3. Lichenification may be present
- Differential diagnosis
  1. Seborrheic dermatitis
  2. Contact dermatitis
  3. Eczema herpeticum
  4. Scabies
  5. Superimposed bacterial infection
  6. Secondary causes
     a. Hay fever
     b. Asthma
     c. Limited exposure to allergens during childhood
     d. Having celiac disease or having a relative with celiac disease
- Diagnostic tests/findings—tests are not routinely ordered but may be indicated in some cases (significant bacterial infection)
  1. Culture for herpes
  2. CBC
- Management/treatment

1. Varies depending on the severity of the condition
2. Drying soaps and detergents should not be used on affected skin because they can remove oils, further exacerbating the itch
3. Avoid perfumes
4. Moisturize frequently, thick heavy moisturizer—oil-based products preferred over thinner products; use even when lesion free as prevention
5. Consider topical antibiotics (Bactroban) if at risk, or oral antibiotics (penicillin, erythromycin)—do not give for longer than 2 weeks
6. First-generation oral antihistamine (e.g., Benadryl) to control pruritus and aid in sleep
7. Daytime histamine (e.g., Claritin, Allegra, or Zyrtec)
8. Topical corticosteroid may be needed during exacerbations
9. Severity determines potency of steroid
10. Oral steroids—last option if numerous widespread lesions
11. When eczema is severe and does not respond to steroids or topical immunosuppressant, consider an oral immunosuppressant
12. May consider daily vitamin D 2000 IU to minimize symptoms
- Patient education
  1. Severe scratching may lead to skin infections due to breaks in skin integrity
  2. Severe scratching will injure skin cells, causing histamine to be released
  3. Warn patient about sedating effects of antihistamines
  4. Avoid irritants (wool and acrylic clothing)
  5. Trim nails to avoid excoriations
  6. Methods to reduce stress

Skin Cancer

- Definition—malignant neoplasms arising in skin cells
- Etiology/incidence
  1. Etiology
     a. Basal cell carcinoma (BCC)
        (1) Slow growing, rarely metastasizes, but may cause extensive local tissue damage
        (2) Tumor arises in the basal layer of the epidermis; causes include chronic sun exposure and genetic predisposition
     b. Squamous cell carcinoma (SCC)
        (1) Directly attributable to sun exposure or chronic irritation
        (2) Approximately 60% occur at the site of previous actinic keratoses
        (3) Low tendency for metastasis
     c. Malignant melanoma (MM)
        (1) Arises from cells of the melanocyte system; begins either de novo or develops from preexisting lesion; may have genetic predisposition
        (2) Initially grows superficially and laterally; enters vertical growth phase with potential to metastasize
  2. Incidence

a. BCC accounts for approximately 75% of all skin cancers, affects about 1 million people per year in the United States; increased risk in fair-skinned individuals with the tendency to sunburn easily

b. SCC second most common skin cancer in whites; most common skin cancer in Blacks, especially on the plantar surface of feet; increased risk of oral and lip SCC in people who smoke cigarettes and cigars

c. MM represents 1% of skin cancers; 77% of skin cancer deaths

- Symptoms
  1. BCC and SCC—painless, slow-growing lesion that will not heal on sun-exposed areas or skin damaged by burns or chronic inflammation
  2. MM
     a. Changing nevus; change in color, diameter increase, or border outline
     b. Pruritus is an early symptom
     c. Bleeding, ulceration, discomfort are late signs
     d. Location of melanoma commonly on the skin but also found in the eyes, ears, mucosal membranes of the mouth and genitals
- Physical findings
  1. BBC—several clinical variants; nodular basal cell most common
     a. Waxy, semitranslucent nodule with rolled borders
     b. Central ulcerations; telangiectasias
  2. SCC
     a. Red/reddish brown plaque/nodule
     b. Surface is scaly/crusted with erosions or ulcerations
  3. MM—tends to have *A*symmetry, *B*order irregularity, *C*olor variations, *D*iameter greater than 6 mm, and *E*levation (ABCDE)
     a. Superficial spreading type (70%)—prolonged horizontal growth phase; vertical growth occurs later
     b. Nodular—raised, pigmented (blue, black, dark brown, gray) nodules with normal surrounding skin
     c. Acral lentiginous—found on palms, soles, nail beds, mucous membranes
     d. Lentigo melanoma—occurs in preexisting lentigo maligna
- Differential diagnosis
  1. Common melanocytic nevus
  2. Seborrheic keratosis
  3. Dermatofibroma
- Diagnostic tests/findings—biopsy
- Management/treatment
  1. Nonpharmacologic/pharmacologic
     a. Excision and biopsy of lesions
     b. BCC/SCC—treatment options
        (1) Mohs' micrographic surgery—gradual lesion excision using serial frozen section analysis and mapping of excised tissue until tumor-free plane reached
        (2) Cryotherapy
        (3) Curettage with electrodesiccation/freezing
        (4) 5-FU (fluorouracil) or imiquimod
     c. MM
        (1) Excision of lesion

        (2) Lymph node dissection
        (3) Adjunctive therapy—chemotherapy, radiation, excision of metastasis
        (4) Long-term follow-up
  2. Patient education—focused on prevention
     a. Reduce exposure
        (1) Avoid UVB exposure—sun or tanning salon
        (2) Use of sunscreen with sun protective factor (SPF) of 15 or greater
        (3) Protective clothing
     b. Educate regarding the acronym ABCDE; useful reminder of the clinical features that should raise suspicion of melanoma in a pigmented lesion
     c. Total cutaneous examination (TCE)—recommended annually for populations with risk factors
        (1) Complete visual inspection of skin, scalp, hands, and feet for any suspicious lesions
        (2) Include questions regarding risk, exposures, family history
        (3) Best preventive practice to reduce mortality
     d. Self-examination for lesions, changing nevi
- Referral for ongoing care (chemotherapy, immunotherapy)

Tinea/Dermatophytosis

- Definition
  1. Superficial fungal infection caused by dermatophytes and yeasts
  2. Dermatophytes require keratin for growth; infection restricted to hair, superficial skin, and nails
  3. Classified according to the involved anatomic location
     a. Tinea capitis—scalp
     b. Tinea corporis—body
     c. Tinea cruris—upper inner thigh/spares scrotum
     d. Tinea pedis—toe webs; soles/heels
     e. Tinea unguium—toenails more frequently involved than fingernails
     f. Tinea versicolor—diffuse rash causing discolored patches of trunk (hypo or hyperpigmented)
- Etiology/incidence
  1. Etiology
     a. *Microsporum, Trichophyton, Epidermophyton* species
     b. Transmission via contact with infected persons, fomites (shoes, towels, shower stalls), animals, or soil
  2. Incidence
     a. Tinea capitis—more common in children
     b. Tinea cruris and tinea pedis—increased incidence in hot, humid conditions
     c. Tinea unguium—increased incidence in older adults, those with diabetes, use of poorly fitting shoes
- Symptoms
  1. Itching, burning—variable
  2. Inflamed, tender rash
  3. Dependent on area of involvement—hair loss on scalp, thickened nails
- Physical findings
  1. Classic presentation is a lesion with a central clearing surrounded by an advancing, red, scaly, elevated border

2. Scalp lesions characterized by hair loss/scaling
3. Maceration, especially intertriginous lesions
4. Involved nails are yellowish/thickened with subungual debris
- Diagnostic tests/findings
  1. KOH microscopy positive for hyphae
  2. Fungal culture for specific identification
  3. Wood's lamp of limited usefulness; most dermatophytes currently seen in the United States do not fluoresce
- Management/treatment
  1. Nonpharmacologic
     a. Careful nail and skin care
     b. Keep area dry; wear absorbent clothing
  2. Pharmacologic
     a. Topical antifungals—tinea corporis, tinea cruris, tinea pedis
        (1) Azoles—clotrimazole (Lotrimin), ketoconazole (Nizoral), miconazole (Monistat)
           (a) Drug action—fungicidal activity
           (b) Contraindications/precautions
              ○ May cause pruritus, irritation, stinging
              ○ May use during pregnancy; minimal systemic absorption
        (2) Allylamines—naftifine (Naftin), terbinafine (Lamisil), butenafine (Lotrimin Ultra)
           (a) Drug action—fungicidal activity
           (b) Contraindications/precautions
              ○ May cause burning, stinging, dryness
              ○ May use during pregnancy; minimal systemic absorption
     b. Oral antifungals—tinea capitis, tinea unguium
        (1) Griseofulvin (Gris-PEG)
           (a) Drug action—interferes with fungal microtube formation by disrupting mitosis and cell division
           (b) Contraindications/precautions
              ○ May cause photosensitivity
              ○ May reduce effectiveness of oral contraceptives
              ○ Contraindicated with porphyria; hepatic function impairment
              ○ Contraindicated during pregnancy
        (2) Itraconazole (Sporanox)
           (a) Drug action—decreases ergosterol synthesis, inhibiting cell membrane formation
           (b) Contraindications/precautions
              ○ Inhibits drug-metabolizing enzymes/CYP3A4; may increase levels of other drugs
              ○ Contraindicated with hepatic function impairment
              ○ Contraindicated during pregnancy
  3. Patient education
     a. Keep skin as dry as possible, especially intertrigal spaces
     b. Wear loose, clean, absorbent clothing
     c. Contagious nature of condition

Psoriasis

- Definition—chronic immune-mediated disorder with overgrowth of keratinocytes and accompanying inflammation; has recurrent exacerbations and remissions; associated with systemic manifestations, especially arthritis
- Etiology/incidence
  1. Genetic predisposition
  2. Environmental triggers for flares—stress, trauma, infection, medications, smoking
  3. Onset most common between ages 15 and 30 years
  4. Incidence in the United States is 2%–3% of the adult population
  5. Approximately 5% develop psoriatic arthritis; average of 12 years after the onset of skin lesions
  6. Prevalence of depression is as high as 60%; may improve with psoriasis treatment
- Symptoms
  1. Red papules and plaques, with elbows, knees, and scalp most commonly affected
  2. Severe pruritus when occurs in folds of skin—axillae, groin, antecubital, and popliteal fossae
  3. Constitutional symptoms—joint pain, fever, chills
- Physical findings
  1. Lesions have four prominent features
     a. Sharply demarcated with clear-cut borders
     b. Erythematous plaque base
     c. Overlapping silvery scales
     d. Removal of scales results in small blood droplets—Auspitz sign
  2. Fingernails—stippling or pitting; accumulation of yellow debris under nails; swelling and redness of paronychial margins
- Diagnostic tests/findings
  1. Generally not needed with classic presentation
  2. Biopsy for uncertain diagnosis
- Management/treatment
  1. Determined by type and severity
  2. Goals—improvement of skin, nail, and joint lesions and improvement of quality of life
  3. Nonpharmacologic—phototherapy with sun exposure or ultraviolet B radiation
  4. Pharmacologic
     a. Mild to moderate disease affecting <5% of the body, and sparing genitals, face, hands, and feet—generally treated with topical medications, either intermittent or continuous
        (1) Most commonly used are steroids, retinoid gel, vitamin D_3 analogues, and calcineurin inhibitors; less commonly used are nonmedicated moisturizers, salicylic acid, coal tar, and anthralin
        (2) Topical steroids—often combined with emollients to soften skin and prevent infection
        (3) Retinoid gel—tazarotene (Tazorac)
           (a) Drug action—blocks production of procollagen, decreases number of inflammatory mediators, unblocks clogged pores; exact mechanism of action unknown
           (b) Contraindications/precautions

i. May cause alopecia, skin dryness, peeling

ii. Contraindicated during pregnancy

(4) Topical vitamin D₃ analogues—calcipotriene ointment or solution

(a) Drug action—slows skin cell proliferation; exact mechanism of action not known; may be used in combination with phototherapy

(b) Contraindications/precautions

i. May cause itching, skin irritation, peeling

ii. Increased risk for kidney stones in susceptible individuals; avoid use for these individuals

iii. Animal reproduction studies have shown an adverse effect on the fetus, but there are no adequate and well-controlled studies in humans; use during pregnancy only if the benefits outweigh the potential risk to the fetus

(5) Calcineurin inhibitors (tacrolimus [Protopic], pimecrolimus [Elidel])—first-line therapy for facial psoriasis, with less skin atrophy than steroids

(a) Drug action—immunosuppressant agent selectively inhibiting inflammation through action on T-cell activation

(b) Contraindications/precautions

i. May cause skin irritation, erythema

ii. Conflicting data that long-term use may increase the risk of some cancers; only use for short term and if other topical therapies not effective

iii. Animal reproduction studies have shown an adverse effect on the fetus, but there are no adequate and well-controlled studies in humans; use during pregnancy only if the benefits outweigh the potential risk to the fetus

(c) Severe disease—generalized lesions covering >5% of body surface or involving hands, feet, face, or genitals; generally treated with systemic medications combined with phototherapy

(6) Most commonly used medications are biologic immune modulators, methotrexate, cyclosporine

(7) Biologic immune modulators—adalimumab (Humira), etanercept (Enbrel), infliximab (Remicade)

(a) Drug action—stimulate body's immune system to block the production of T cells or tumor necrosis factor alpha, affecting the progression of psoriatic plaques; administered by injection or infusion

(b) Contraindications/precautions

i. May cause flulike syndrome; injection-site inflammation

ii. Animal reproduction studies have not revealed any fetal damage or fertility impairment, but there are no adequate and well-controlled studies in humans; use during pregnancy only if the benefits outweigh the potential risk to the fetus

(8) Methotrexate—antimetabolite and antifolate agent that acts by decreasing the production of new skin cells, in turn interfering with cellular metabolism; contraindicated during pregnancy and lactation

(9) Cyclosporine—immunosuppressant that inhibits lymphocytes, decreasing T cells' infiltration of the dermis; contraindicated during pregnancy and lactation

5. Patient education

a. Chronic nature of the condition

b. Reduction of triggers

c. Emotional support

d. Medications

6. Referral

a. Dermatologist—for severe disease or mild to moderate disease not controlled with topical medications

b. Rheumatologist—if the patient has arthritis symptoms

Vitiligo

- Definition—a progressive condition in which melanocytes lose their ability to produce melanin, resulting in depigmentation of the skin
- Etiology/incidence
  1. Etiology
     a. Exact cause unknown, but possibly due to autoimmune disorder, genetics, or skin trigger—sun, virus, or stress
     b. If present in older women, other comorbidities, such as thyroid, RA, diabetes, and alopecia areata, should be considered.
  2. Incidence
     a. Affects less than 1% of the world's population
     b. Most prevalent before age 20
     c. All racial groups are affected, but is more noticeable in darker-skinned individuals
- Symptoms
  1. Discoloration patches on the skin that may occur anywhere on the body
  2. Sun-exposed areas show the discolorations first—face, lips, hands, feet, arms
  3. Can cause graying of the hair
  4. Loss of color in multiple areas—retina, axillae, genitals
- Physical findings
  1. Almost always diagnosed clinically upon physical examination
  2. Manifests as acquired depigmented patches surrounded by normal skin and may appear in many patterns
  3. Macules are chalk or milk-white in color, well demarcated

4. Lesions can be round, oval, or linear in shape
5. Borders may be convex
- Differential diagnosis
  1. Pityriasis alba
  2. Postinflammatory hypopigmentation
  3. Tinea versicolor
  4. Albinism
- Diagnostic tests/findings
  1. Diagnosis can usually be made with visual assessment
  2. Glowing skin under Wood's lamp
  3. May be an increased risk of hearing loss with this diagnosis; consider a hearing test
- Management and treatment
  1. Vitiligo is not curable; some treatments may help the appearance
  2. UVB light to repigment the affected skin
  3. Photochemotherapy with light therapy may help to repigment the skin affected by the condition
  4. Topical steroids may help with skin repigmentation if used in the early stages; best for small lesions and short-term use
- Patient education
  1. Protect skin from the sun; use sunscreen every day
  2. Wear clothing that protects skin from the sun
  3. Seek shade
  4. Do not use tanning beds or sun lamps
  5. Do not get a tattoo—can cause Koebner phenomenon, in which a new patch of vitiligo appears 10–14 days later

Psychosocial Problems

Stress

- Definition—Selye's theory of stress response and adaptation describes a continuum related to stress
  1. Eustress or good stress—degree of stress that is motivating and viewed as positive for the individual
  2. Distress—the point at which stress becomes psychologically or physically debilitating
- Etiology/incidence
  1. Major life events—marriage, divorce, job change, death of a family member
  2. Chronic situations—poverty, illness of self or family member, abuse
  3. Acute situations—acute pain, sudden threats to safety
  4. Environmental conditions—noise, pollution, overcrowding
  5. Daily hassles—minor events that occur on a regular basis
- Symptoms
  1. Irritability, anxiety, depression, chronic worrying
  2. Decreased productivity, sleep disturbances, appetite changes, loss of libido
  3. Vague or nonspecific physical complaints—headaches, nausea, diarrhea, chest pain, muscle tension
- Physical findings
  1. Muscle tension
  2. Increase in blood pressure

- Differential diagnosis
  1. Depression
  2. Anxiety disorders
  3. Other medical conditions that could account for signs and symptoms
- Diagnostic tests/findings—none
- Management/treatment
  1. Eliminate or modify stressors—assertiveness training, time management, positive thought strategies, communication skills
  2. Relaxation techniques—guided imagery, muscle relaxation exercises, biofeedback, massage, meditation, use of humor, physical exercise, mindfulness

Anxiety

- Definition—*Diagnostic and Statistical Manual of Mental Disorders*, fifth edition (*DSM-5*) lists several psychiatric syndromes of which anxiety is a primary component; interference with everyday function must be present to classify anxiety as a psychiatric syndrome
  1. Generalized anxiety disorder (GAD)
     a. Persistent, excessive, incapacitating worry over life events, occurring more days than not, for at least 6 months
     b. Anxiety and worry are associated with three or more of the following symptoms: restlessness, easy to fatigue, difficulty concentrating, irritability, muscle tension, sleep disturbance
  2. Panic attack
     a. Period of intense fear or discomfort, develops abruptly and peaks within 10 minutes
     b. At least four of the following symptoms must be present—palpitations, sweating, trembling, sensation of shortness of breath/smothering, choking sensation, chest pain, nausea/abdominal distress, dizziness/lightheadedness, derealization, fear of losing control, sense of impending doom, paresthesia, chills/hot flashes
  3. Panic disorder
     a. Recurrent, unexpected panic attacks—not due to substance use, medical condition, or other mental disorder
     b. At least one attack, followed by at least 1 month of one or more of the following:
        (1) Persistent concern about having other panic attacks
        (2) Worry about the implications of the attack and its consequences
        (3) Significant change in behavior related to attacks
     c. May occur with or without agoraphobia
  4. Agoraphobia—anxiety about, or avoidance of, places or situations in which the ability to leave suddenly may be difficult in the event of having a panic attack
  5. Specific phobia—anxiety elicited by a discrete stimulus, such as heights or specific animals; the individual recognizes that the fear is excessive or unreasonable
  6. Social phobia—fear of one or more social and performance situations that is excessive or incapacitating;

the individual recognizes the fear is excessive or unreasonable

7. Posttraumatic stress disorder (PTSD)—persistent anxiety lasting more than 1 month following an extremely traumatic event; symptoms may not start until several days or weeks after the event
   a. Exposure to a traumatic event in which the patient experienced, witnessed, or was confronted with an event that involved actual or threatened death, serious injury, or threat to the physical integrity of others
   b. Traumatic event persistently reexperienced through at least one of the following ways:
      (1) Intrusive distressing recollections of event
      (2) Distressing dreams
      (3) Feeling as if traumatic event was recurring
      (4) Psychological distress when exposed to cues symbolizing an event
      (5) Physiologic reaction on exposure to cues symbolizing event
   c. Avoidance of stimuli associated with trauma and numbing of general responsiveness
   d. Persistent symptoms of increased arousal
8. Acute stress disorder (ASD)—similar to PTSD, but more immediate and of shorter duration; lasts minimum of 2 days and maximum of 4 weeks, occurs within 4 weeks of traumatic event
9. Obsessive–compulsive disorder (OCD)—characterized by obsessions that cause marked anxiety or distress and/or by compulsions that serve to neutralize the anxiety

- Etiology/incidence/prevalence
  1. One of the most prevalent of all psychiatric disorders
  2. Prevalence varies—specific phobia most common (25%), social phobia (13%), PTSD (7.8%; 12% in women, 20% in victims of war trauma), GAD (5%), panic disorder (3.5%)
  3. Disrupted CNS modulation, with several neuroregulators implicated in the cause of anxiety (e.g., dopamine, serotonin, norepinephrine)
  4. May be a genetic predisposition
- Symptoms—vary with the particular anxiety disorder
- Physical findings
  1. Physical findings may be present with an acute anxiety attack
  2. Tachycardia, increased respirations, elevated BP
  3. Restlessness
  4. Diaphoresis
  5. Muscle tension
- Differential diagnosis
  1. Medical conditions that may account for symptoms of anxiety—cardiac arrhythmias, mitral valve prolapse, angina, pulmonary embolism, hypoglycemia, hyperthyroidism, asthma, COPD, Cushing's disease, pheochromocytoma
  2. Medication-induced symptoms of anxiety—steroids, anticholinergics, sympathomimetics, digoxin, thyroxine
  3. Substance use or withdrawal
  4. Other psychological disorders—depression, bipolar disorder

- Diagnostic tests/findings
  1. May be done to exclude other medical conditions suggested by history or physical examination findings
  2. TSH, urine toxicology, ECG, CBC, metabolic panel
- Management/treatment
  1. Nonpharmacologic—psychotherapy/cognitive-behavioral therapy
  2. Pharmacologic
     a. Benzodiazepines (lorazepam, diazepam, clonazepam, alprazolam) for short-term management if needed for severe impairment until acceptable reduction of symptoms is achieved with selective serotonin reuptake inhibitors (SSRIs) and/or cognitive-behavioral therapy
        (1) Drug action—produces an antianxiety effect by enhancing the action of the neurotransmitter GABA acid at the cortical and limbic areas of the brain
        (2) Contraindications/precautions
           (a) May cause sedation, impaired concentration, anterograde amnesia; dependence; misuse potential
           (b) Potentiates effects of other CNS depressants, including alcohol
           (c) May be potentiated by concomitant use of cimetidine
           (d) Risk for rebound anxiety with withdrawal of alprazolam because of short half-life
           (e) Not recommended for use during pregnancy; an increased risk of congenital malformations in humans has been suggested; withdrawal syndrome has been described in neonates whose parents took benzodiazepines during pregnancy
     b. SSRIs—escitalopram (Lexapro), sertraline (Zoloft); see the section about Major Depressive Disorder in this chapter; best tolerance and response rates for GAD, panic disorder, PTSD, OCD, social anxiety disorder
     c. SNRIs—duloxetine (Cymbalta), venlafaxine (Effexor); see the section about Major Depressive Disorder in this chapter
     d. Buspirone (BuSpar)—nonbenzodiazepine antianxiety agent
        (1) Drug effect—partial agonism or mixed agonism/antagonism at 5-HT_{1A} receptors
        (2) Contraindications/precautions
           (a) Increased risk for hypertensive crisis with concomitant use of MAO inhibitors
           (b) Animal reproduction studies have not revealed any fetal damage or fertility impairment; there are no controlled data on human pregnancy
           (c) Sexual side effects
  3. Client education
     a. Caution about the potential for physical/psychological dependence with the use of benzodiazepines
     b. Caution against the use of alcohol or other CNS depressants with benzodiazepines

c. Discuss the use of relaxation techniques and effective coping mechanisms
d. Reassurance that effective treatment is available, but patience required until the right combination of modalities is found

Major Depressive Disorder (MDD)

- Definition (*DSM-5*)—at least five of the symptoms listed must be present most of the day, nearly every day, for 2 weeks and number 1 or number 2 must be present for a diagnosis of major depression
  1. Sad or depressed mood most of the day, every day
  2. Loss of interest in usual activities
  3. Fatigue, weight gain/loss, sleep disturbance, difficulty concentrating, feelings of worthlessness/guilt, psychomotor retardation/agitation, suicidal ideation
- Etiology/incidence/prevalence/risk factors
  1. Lifetime prevalence of clinically significant MDD is 16%; cisgender women affected two to three times more than cisgender men. For transgender individuals, the prevalence may be closer to 33%, and up to 66% of transgender youth experience symptoms of depression
  2. First major depressive episode usually occurs in adolescence or early adulthood
  3. Bimodal curve of prevalence in cisgender individuals—one peak in late 20s and early 30s, and a second peak around 65–70 years of age
  4. Theories include biologic, sociologic, and neuroendocrine etiologies
  5. Risk factors for depression
     a. Prior incident of major depression
     b. Family history of depression
     c. Severe or chronic illness/chronic pain
     d. History of early trauma, abuse, neglect, deprivation
     e. Current high-stress burden (e.g., marital or family problems, abuse, experience of discrimination)
     f. Postpartum period—see Chapter 9, *Postpartum and Lactation*, on postpartum depression
  6. Approximately 15% of depressed individuals attempt suicide
  7. Risk factors for suicide
     a. Prior attempt/family history of suicide attempt
     b. Male sex
     c. Substance abuse/family history of substance abuse
     d. Living alone
     e. Medical illness
     f. Hopelessness
     g. Psychosis or panic disorder
     h. Advanced age
     i. Violence or impulsivity
- Symptoms
  1. As listed in the definition
  2. Vague pain, headaches, GI complaints, sexual complaints
  3. Substance use disorder or dependence
- Physical findings
  1. Poor eye contact, tearful, downcast
  2. Inattention to appearance/hygiene
  3. Slow, monotone speech
  4. Psychomotor retardation or agitation
  5. Impaired cognitive reasoning
- Differential diagnosis
  1. Adjustment disorder following a stressor event
  2. Bereavement or grief reaction
  3. Dysthymia
     a. Chronic low-grade depressive symptoms for 2 or more years
     b. Insufficient number and intensity of symptoms to qualify as MDD
     c. Often accompanies chronic, disabling medical disorders
  4. Other psychiatric syndromes
  5. Medical disorders—thyroid disorders, sleep apnea, Parkinson's disease, multiple sclerosis
  6. Medications—antihypertensives, benzodiazepines, chemotherapeutic drugs, and others
- Diagnostic tests/findings
  1. Laboratory/diagnostic tests may be done to exclude other diagnostic possibilities
     a. CBC
     b. TSH
     c. Glucose
  2. Screening tools—depression assessment scales
     a. Ask patients to rate the severity or frequency of various symptoms
     b. Beck Depression Inventory, Zung Self-Rating Depression Scale, Geriatric Depression Scale, Patient Health Questionnaire (PHQ) 9, Edinburgh Postnatal Depression Scale
- Management/treatment
  1. Nonpharmacologic—psychotherapy, regular exercise, light therapy for seasonal affective disorder (subtype of MDD), neuromodulation techniques (e.g., electroconvulsive therapy, vagus nerve stimulation); hospitalization may be required for severe depression or if the client has suicidal ideation
  2. Pharmacologic
     a. SSRIs—have replaced TCAs as the drugs of choice because of their improved tolerability and safety if taken in overdose
  3. Agents—fluoxetine (Prozac), sertraline (Zoloft), paroxetine (Paxil), escitalopram (Lexapro), citalopram (Celexa)
  4. Drug action—block reuptake of serotonin, enhancing serotonin neurotransmission
  5. Contraindications/precautions
     a. May cause sexual dysfunction
     b. Use with MAO inhibitors may cause hypertensive crisis
     c. Screen for symptoms of bipolar disorder before prescribing to avoid precipitating a manic episode
     d. Animal reproduction studies have shown an adverse effect on the fetus, but there are no adequate and well-controlled studies in humans; use during pregnancy only if benefits outweigh potential risk to fetus
     e. Discuss with pregnant individual the balance of benefits and risks of not treating depression versus use of SSRI during pregnancy
     f. SNRIs

6. Agents—venlafaxine (Effexor), duloxetine (Cymbalta)
7. Drug action—inhibits both serotonin and norepinephrine reuptake
8. Contraindications/precautions
   a. May cause sexual dysfunction
   b. Use with MAO inhibitors may cause hypertensive crisis
   c. Contraindicated with uncontrolled narrow-angle glaucoma
   d. Animal reproduction studies have shown an adverse effect on the fetus, but there are no adequate and well-controlled studies in humans; use during pregnancy only if the benefits outweigh the potential risk to the fetus
   e. Discuss with pregnant individuals the balance of benefits and risks of not treating depression versus the use of SSRI during pregnancy
   f. Other classes of antidepressants
      (1) Mirtazapine (Remeron)
          (a) Drug action—stimulates the release of norepinephrine and serotonin
          (b) Contraindications/precautions
              ° May cause dizziness, orthostatic hypotension, transient sedation
              ° Animal reproduction studies have shown an adverse effect on the fetus, but there are no adequate and well-controlled studies in humans; use during pregnancy only if the benefits outweigh the potential risk to the fetus
      (2) Bupropion (Wellbutrin)
          (a) Drug action—decreases reuptake of dopamine in the CNS
          (b) Contraindications/precautions
              ° May cause agitation, headache, nausea
              ° Contraindicated with seizure disorder, eating disorders
              ° Animal reproduction studies have shown an adverse effect on the fetus, but there are no adequate and well-controlled studies in humans; use during pregnancy only if the benefits outweigh the potential risk to the fetus
   g. Once full remission achieved, continue therapy for 6–12 months; for second episode, continue therapy for 1–2 years; a third episode requires indefinite maintenance
9. Client education
   a. SSRIs—usually taken in the morning to reduce the incidence of insomnia
   b. Antidepressants should be started slowly, and the dose increased to a therapeutic level that alleviates symptoms
   c. An adequate trial period and close follow-up are essential for successful treatment
   d. Caution concerning the use of medications with alcohol
   e. Encourage use of support systems, effective coping mechanisms

- Referral
  1. Patients requiring referral to a psychiatrist include those with suicidal ideation or severe depression; bipolar disorder; atypical depression, substance use disorder, treatment resistance
  2. Referral to a licensed counselor should be offered to most patients with depression

Domestic Violence/Intimate-Partner Violence (IPV)

- Definition—a pattern of coercive and controlling behavior that occurs in an intimate adult relationship; four main types: physical violence, sexual violence, threats of physical or sexual violence, psychological/emotional violence
- Etiology/incidence/prevalence
  1. Societal, community, relationship, and individual factors all contribute to the etiology of IPV and must be addressed as part of the ecological model of violence prevention
  2. One in three women has been the victim of severe physical violence by an intimate partner in her lifetime
  3. IPV is the single most common reason women go to emergency rooms
  4. Approximately 12% of teenagers and more than 20% of college students have experienced dating violence
  5. Evidence of whether IPV increases or decreases during pregnancy is conflicting
  6. Associated impacts on pregnancy include preterm delivery, low birth weight, delayed prenatal care, substance misuse
  7. Estimated 80% of women who have experienced IPV face significant short- or long-term psychological impacts, including PTSD, depression, fear of intimacy, inability to trust others, low self-esteem, sleep disturbances, suicidal behavior, substance abuse
  8. Gastrointestinal and gynecologic disorders, headaches, sexual dysfunction, and chronic pain syndromes are common in those who have experienced IPV
- Symptoms
  1. History of frequent visits to the emergency room
  2. Evidence of current or old injuries
  3. Delay in reporting an injury/explanation of cause inconsistent with injury
  4. Depression, anxiety, posttraumatic stress reactions, low self-esteem
  5. History of suicide attempts or ideation
  6. Alcohol or drug use disorders
  7. Vague or nonspecific physical complaints
  8. Late/sporadic prenatal care or other health care
  9. Controlling partner/increased anxiety in the presence of partner
  10. Behavioral problems in children who are witnessing the abuse
  11. Cycle of violence—tension building, serious battering incident, honeymoon phase
- Physical findings
  1. Facial lacerations
  2. Injuries to breasts, back, abdomen, and genitalia
  3. Bilateral injuries to arms/legs

4. Obvious patterns—bite marks, hand grip, cigarette burns
5. Injuries during pregnancy
6. Recurrent or chronic injuries
- Differential diagnosis
  1. Accidental injuries
  2. Self-inflicted injuries
- Diagnostic tests/findings—none
- Management/treatment
  1. Routine assessment for abuse in all patients
  2. Danger assessment—suicide or homicide
  3. Safety plan—where to go in an emergency or dangerous situation; what to do during violent incidents; what items/documents will be needed for a comfortable and safe escape
  4. ABCDEs of intervention
     a. *Alone*—assure the individual that the individual is not alone in being a person who has experienced domestic violence
     b. *Belief*—let the individual know that you believe no one deserves to be hurt or threatened in a relationship
     c. *Confidential*—assure the individual that the information the individual shares is confidential
     d. *Document*—record any findings that may be helpful to the individual at a later date; use accurate description of incident and/or threats in patient's own words; include all pertinent physical examination findings with body map and/or photographs, with individual's permission
     e. *Educate*—provide information about available resources, dangers of escalating violence, and safety plans
  5. Referrals
     a. Shelters
     b. Legal assistance
     c. Counseling
  6. Mandatory reporting—laws vary in each state

Sexual Violence

- Definition—any sexual act that is committed against someone without that person's freely given consent; may be physical, verbal, or psychological
  1. Types of sexual violence
     a. Completed or attempted forced penetration of a person
     b. Completed or attempted alcohol/drug-facilitated penetration of a person
     c. Completed or attempted forced acts in which a person is made to penetrate a perpetrator or someone else
     d. Completed or attempted alcohol/drug-facilitated acts in which a person is made to penetrate a perpetrator or someone else
     e. Nonphysically forced penetration that occurs after a person is pressured verbally or through intimidation or misuse of authority to consent or acquiesce
     f. Unwanted sexual contact—intentional touching, directly or through clothing, of genitalia, anus, groin, breast, inner thigh, or buttocks

g. Noncontact unwanted sexual experiences—voyeurism, exposure to exhibitionism, pornography, sexual harassment, threats of sexual violence
  2. Legal terminology—varies from state to state
     a. Sexual assault—force, threats, or coercion to engage in any unwanted sexual contact; includes contact or penetration of the intimate parts (sexual organs, anus, groin, buttocks, and breasts)
     b. Rape—sexual assault that involves penetration, however slight, of the labia by the penis; legal definitions of rape vary from state to state but typically include the use of force, threat, or coercion and lack of consent in relation to sexual intercourse
- Etiology/incidence
  1. Sexual violence occurs in all ages, races, ethnic and cultural groups
  2. Approximately 18% of women in the United States have experienced a completed or attempted act of sexual violence in their lifetime; the majority perpetrated by an acquaintance rather than a stranger
- Symptoms—sexual assault
  1. Genital injury may or may not be present and is often difficult to visualize
  2. Typical findings include lacerations, ecchymosis, abrasions, erythema, and edema in areas of assault
  3. Rape trauma syndrome describes the symptoms that occur in most survivors of sexual assault
  4. Sometimes the person may appear asymptomatic and show no signs of injury
     a. Acute phase—lasts a few days to a few weeks
        (1) Emotional responses may be expressed or controlled and may range from anger, fear, anxiety, and restlessness to a calm, composed, subdued affect
        (2) Physical responses include general soreness and soreness in the areas of assault, gastrointestinal and genitourinary symptoms, sleep disruption and nightmares, and sexual disruption
     b. Reorganization phase—wide range of emotions and physical responses with the purpose of reorganizing life after the assault
  5. PTSD occurs in 30%–65% of sexual assault survivors—see Anxiety section earlier in this chapter for diagnostic criteria
- Physical findings
  1. Physical findings may be minimal or not apparent until a day or more after the assault
  2. Lacerations, ecchymosis, abrasions, erythema, edema in areas of assault
  3. Colposcopic examination may be used to assist in the evaluation
- Differential diagnosis
  1. Accidental injuries
  2. Violence—nonsexual
- Diagnostic tests/findings
  1. Forensic evidence collection technique and requirements may vary from state to state—most states supply evidence collection kits that contain instructions and collection materials

2. STI and HIV testing is not required as part of routine care of sexual assault survivor and may be forgone to prevent risk for use against patient in future litigation. It is recommended in all children, those with symptoms, and those who choose to forego prophylactic STI treatment.

- Management/treatment
   1. Comprehensive care for sexual assault survivor is often provided by a multidisciplinary team that includes a sexual assault nurse examiner (SANE), survivor advocate, and law enforcement
   2. Triage and immediate treatment of any life-threatening injuries
   3. Attention to emotional needs of the survivor
   4. Collection of evidence per state and agency protocol
   5. Prophylactic treatment for STIs—chlamydia, gonorrhea, trichomoniasis
   6. Initiate hepatitis B and HPV vaccination series if patient has not had previously
   7. Prophylactic treatment for HIV—decision based on risk as a result of type of sexual contact, vaginal lacerations, multiple assailants, HIV prevalence in geographic area, and time from assault (<72 hours)
   8. Offer emergency contraception if pregnancy is a concern
   9. Discuss need for chlamydia and gonorrhea testing in 1–2 weeks if not treated prophylactically, along with testing for HIV and syphilis at 6 weeks, 3 months, and 6 months
   10. Referrals
       a. Legal and social services referrals
       b. Counseling for survivor and family
       c. Domestic abuse housing and/or safe house
   11. Screen all patients for history of sexual violence

Human Trafficking

- Definition—A crime involving compelling or coercing a person to provide labor or services, or to engage in commercial sex acts in a way that is subtle or overt, physical or psychological. It includes recruitment, transportation, transfer, harbor, or receipt of a person for exploitation. Any exploitation of a minor for commercial sex is human trafficking.
   1. Legal terminology—varies from state to state
   2. Must involve force, fraud, or coercion
   3. Labor trafficking—a form of modern-day slavery in which individuals perform labor or services through the use of force, fraud, or coercion
   4. Sex trafficking—the recruitment, harboring, transportation, provision, obtaining, patronizing, or soliciting of a person for the purposes of a commercial sex act, in which the commercial sex act is induced by force, fraud, or coercion, or in which the person induced to perform such an act has not attained 18 years of age
- Etiology/incidence
   1. Trafficking occurs in all ages, races, ethnic and cultural groups
   2. 600,000–800,000 people are trafficked annually, worldwide

3. Third largest illegal industry in the world, after drugs and weapons
4. Men are represented but often underreported; especially common for men in forced labor situations
5. 200,000 U.S. children are at risk every year
6. Runaways—one in three will be approached within 48 hours
7. Challenging to identify, often missed
   a. There are no evidence-based protocols on how to screen or identify
   b. Individual may present with risk factors but not disclose anything
   c. Individual may disclose details of trafficking but not identify as an individual who has been trafficked
- Risk factors
   1. Age (12–16 years)
   2. Runaway or homeless
   3. History of sexual or physical abuse or neglect
   4. Dysfunctional families
   5. Interactions with child protective services or the juvenile justice system
   6. Lesbian, gay, bisexual, transgender, queer, or questioning
   7. Substance use disorder, behavioral issues, mental health concerns
   8. Economically vulnerable
   9. Learning disabilities
   10. Living in high-crime areas, poverty, transient male population
   11. Living in a country with political or social unrest or corruption
   12. Living in a society with gender bias and discrimination or glorification of pimp culture
   13. No health care
   14. ACE (Adverse Childhood Experience) score greater than 4 poses an increased risk
   15. International adoptees
- Physical findings
   1. Branding/tattoo that the patient is unwilling to discuss
   2. Physical injuries in various stages of healing
   3. Physical exam findings that do not match the patient's history
   4. Multiple sexual partners, unintended pregnancies, STIs, or repeated visits for emergency contraception
   5. Signs of malnourishment or neglect
   6. Oral and dental injuries
   7. Central body pattern injuries
   8. Defensive posturing injuries
   9. Bilateral or multiple injuries
   10. Injuries during pregnancy
   11. Strangulation injuries
   12. Patterned injuries
   13. Pelvic/genital injuries
   14. Cigarette burns, chemical burns, or heated liquid burns
- Differential diagnosis
   1. Accidental injuries
   2. Violence—nonsexual
   3. Employment in voluntary sex work

- Diagnostic tests/findings
  1. Forensic evidence collection technique and requirements may vary from state to state—most states supply evidence collection kits that contain instructions and collection materials; sometimes individuals who have been trafficked may decline a forensic exam but still want treatment
  2. Individuals who have been trafficked may come to care to get STI and HIV testing only
- Management/treatment
  1. Provide trauma informed care that gives patient control of what is done or not done
  2. Offer STI/HIV testing and treatment; may decline STI testing due to potential marginalization within the patient's community
  3. Provide information on safer sex practices
  4. Bacterial and/or yeast infections are common—offer testing and treatment
  5. Comprehensive care for an individual who has been sexually assaulted is often provided by a multidisciplinary team that includes a SANE, an advocate for the individual, and law enforcement; offer this care if you suspect sex trafficking
  6. Triage and immediate treatment of any life-threatening injuries
  7. Attention to emotional needs of the individual, counseling resources
  8. Offer emergency contraception if pregnancy is a concern
  9. Referrals
     a. Legal and social services referrals
     b. Housing
     c. Counseling

Eating Disorders

- Definitions
  1. Anorexia nervosa—*DSM-5* criteria for diagnosis
     a. Restriction of intake relative to requirements, leading to significantly low body weight in context of age, sex, and physical health
     b. Intense fear of gaining weight and/or persistent behavior that interferes with weight gain, even though the patient is at a significantly low body weight
     c. Disturbed body image
  2. Bulimia nervosa—*DSM-5* criteria for diagnosis
     a. Recurrent episodes of binge eating
     b. Recurrent, inappropriate compensatory behavior to prevent weight gain (self-induced vomiting; misuse of laxatives, diuretics, or enemas; strict dieting or fasting; excessive exercise)
     c. Binge eating and inappropriate compensatory behaviors occur on the average at least twice a week for at least 3 months
     d. Persistent and exaggerated concern with body shape and weight
- Etiology/incidence/prevalence/risk factors
  1. Anorexia nervosa
     a. Etiology—biologic, psychological, social, and family factors

b. About 1% of female adolescents have anorexia
c. Age of onset—early to late adolescence
d. Has 10%–20% mortality due to cardiac arrest or suicide
e. Risk factors
   (1) Female sex
   (2) Parent or sibling with eating disorder
   (3) Career choice or aspiration that stresses thinness, perfection, or self-discipline
   (4) A difficult transition or loss (leaving home for college, breakup of an important relationship)
  2. Bulimia nervosa
     a. Etiology—biologic, psychological, social, and family factors
     b. Age of onset—late adolescence to early adulthood
     c. Occurs in 4% of college-age women
     d. Mortality rate lower than that for anorexia nervosa
     e. Approximately 30%–80% of patients with bulimia have a history of anorexia nervosa
- Symptoms
  1. Anorexia nervosa—fatigue, cold intolerance, muscle weakness and cramps, dizziness, fainting spells, bloating, amenorrhea, social isolation, excessive concerns about weight, compulsive exercising, odd food rituals, depression
  2. Bulimia nervosa—menstrual irregularities; depression; anxiety; impulsive behaviors (shoplifting, alcohol or drug use disorder, unsafe sexual behaviors); lack of meaningful relationships; excessive concerns about weight; requests for diet pills, diuretics, or laxatives
- Physical findings
  1. Anorexia nervosa—emaciation, dry skin, fine body hair (lanugo), muscle wasting, peripheral edema, bradycardia, arrhythmias, hypotension, delayed sexual maturation, stress fractures
  2. Bulimia—erosion of tooth enamel, calluses on dorsal surface of hands from inducing vomiting, swollen parotid glands, cardiac arrhythmias if syrup of ipecac used
- Differential diagnosis
  1. Gastrointestinal disorders
  2. Malignancies
  3. Depression
  4. Other psychiatric disorders
- Diagnostic tests/findings
  1. Anorexia—mild anemia; elevated BUN, cholesterol, and LFTs; electrolyte imbalance; low serum estrogen; abnormal ECG
  2. Bulimia—electrolyte imbalance, abnormal ECG
  3. Rating instruments—Eating Attitudes Test, Eating Disorders Inventory, Body Shape Questionnaire
- Management/treatment
  1. Outpatient treatment—individual/group/family therapy, nutritional counseling, treatment of any medical complications, treatment of any associated mood disorders
  2. Pharmacologic—SSRI fluoxetine (Prozac) approved for treatment of bulimia
  3. Hospitalization is indicated if any of the following apply:

a. Weight is less than 75% of ideal body weight
b. Client is experiencing suicidal thoughts or behavior
c. Rapid, persistent decline in oral intake or weight despite intensive outpatient interventions
d. Electrolyte or metabolic abnormalities, hematemesis, orthostatic hypotension, heart rate <40 beats per minute (bpm) or >110 bpm, inability to sustain core body temperature
4. Pregnancy considerations—individuals with anorexia nervosa may have fertility problems; pregnant individuals with eating disorders require special nutritional management to ensure adequate weight gain and nutrient intake

Substance Use Disorders (SUDs)

- Definition
  1. Substance use—use of any psychoactive substance that has a pharmacologic effect on the brain or CNS
  2. Psychoactive substance classifications and examples
     a. Stimulants—for example, cocaine, amphetamines, caffeine, nicotine
     b. Depressants or sedative hypnotics—for example, alcohol, barbiturates, benzodiazepines
     c. Narcotics—for example, heroin, opioid medications
     d. Hallucinogens—for example, LSD, PCP, ecstasy
     e. Cannabis—for example, marijuana, hashish
     f. Inhalants—for example, nitrous oxide, hydrocarbons
  3. Potential for harm—physical injury; body organ pathology; increased risk for cancer; transmission of communicable disease; negative social, legal, psychological consequences
  4. SUD occurs across a continuum, taking into account severity, evidence of physiologic dependence, and course of treatment
  5. Physiologic dependence—evidence of tolerance or withdrawal
  6. Severity of SUD is based on the presence of a number of the 11 *DSM-5* criteria
     a. Two to three criteria—mild disorder
     b. Four to five criteria—moderate disorder
     c. Six or more criteria—severe disorder
  7. SUD—*DSM-5* criteria
     a. Repeatedly unable to carry out major obligations at work, school, or home due to substance use
     b. Recurrent use of substance in physically hazardous situations
     c. Continued use despite persistent or recurrent social or interpersonal problems caused or made worse by substance use
     d. Tolerance—either a need for markedly increased amounts to achieve intoxication or desired effect or markedly diminished effect with continued use of the same amount
     e. Withdrawal—either characteristic syndrome or use of substance to avoid withdrawal
     f. Using greater amounts or over a longer time period than intended
     g. Persistent desire or unsuccessful attempts to cut down or control substance use
     h. Spending a lot of time obtaining, using, or recovering from using substances
     i. Stopping or reducing important social, occupational, or recreational activities due to substance use
     j. Consistent use of substances despite acknowledgment of persistent or recurrent physical or psychological difficulties from using substance
     k. Craving or strong desire to use substance
- Etiology/incidence
  1. Complex interplay of neurobiology, genetics, and psychosocial factors involved in SUD
  2. Approximately 8% of adults age 18 and older have alcohol use disorder meeting the criteria for SUD; the prevalence is greater among men than women with a 2:1 ratio
  3. Approximately 22% of adult women report binge drinking; 12% of whom report binge drinking 3 or more times a month; 1 in 5 adolescent females (under age 18) report binge drinking. Approximately 21.8% of sexual minority adults had an alcohol use disorder in the last year.
  4. Approximately 18% of individuals aged 12 years and older report use of illicit drugs or misuse of prescription drugs in the previous year.
  5. Opioid use disorder (OUD) is an epidemic in the United States; more than 4 million individuals misuse or are dependent on opioids, including prescription opioid pain relievers (OPRs), illicitly manufactured synthetic opioids, and heroin
  6. Approximately 67% of drug overdose deaths (intentional and unintentional) involve prescription and/or illicit opioids.
  7. Evidence suggests that women may progress to dependence on OPRs at a more accelerated rate than men.
- Symptoms
  1. Variable—depends on substance, amount, length of time used, and if going through withdrawal; refer to *DSM-5* criteria
  2. Screen all adolescents and adults at least annually for substance use; screen all pregnant individuals early in pregnancy and repeat as indicated
  3. Use of validated tools helps identify both those who are engaged in at-risk substance use and those with a probable SUD
  4. Examples of screening tools
     a. National Institute on Drug Abuse (NIDA) Quick Screen
        (1) In the past year, how many times have you used alcohol, tobacco products, prescription medication for nonmedical reasons, or illegal drugs? (Ask about each substance separately)
        (2) If answer indicates possible at risk with use of substance, proceed with further screening with another validated tool

b. NIDA Modified ASSIST (seven items)—not gender specific; covers alcohol, nonmedical use of prescription drugs, illicit drugs, tobacco; asks about frequency and pattern; asks questions specific to psychosocial and physical symptoms

c. CAGE-C (seven items)—not gender specific; focuses on alcohol use; asks about frequency, pattern, and quantity of use; asks questions specific to psychosocial and physical symptoms

d. AUDIT (10 items)—not gender specific; focuses on alcohol use; asks about frequency, pattern, and quantity of use; asks questions specific to psychosocial and physical symptoms

- Physical findings with SUD
  1. May not be any apparent physical findings; may be variable depending on substance, amount, length of time used, if going through withdrawal from the substance
  2. General—poor nutritional status, poor personal hygiene
  3. Mental status—memory loss, agitation, delirium tremors, hallucinations, lethargy
  4. Behavior—slurred speech, staggering gait, scratching, violent or bizarre behavior
  5. Mood—depression, anxiety, mood lability, euphoria
  6. Skin—signs of physical injury, needle marks, skin abscesses, cellulitis, jaundice, diaphoresis
  7. HEENT (head, eyes, ears, nose, throat)—conjunctival injection, pupil constriction or dilation, inflamed nasal mucosa, rhinorrhea, dental caries, gingivitis
  8. Cardiac—chest pain, increased blood pressure, tachycardia, arrhythmias
  9. Abdominal—enlarged liver, ascites
- Diagnostic test/findings
  1. Blood alcohol level—may be elevated
  2. Gamma glutamyl transferase (GGT)—elevated with heavy or chronic alcohol use
  3. Urine toxicology tests—may be positive for specific substance
  4. Consider other laboratory or diagnostic tests based on risk factors and clinical presentation
- Differential diagnosis
  1. Psychiatric disorders that could account for symptoms and physical exam findings—for example, depression, anxiety disorders, schizophrenia
  2. Medical conditions that could account for symptoms and physical exam findings—for example, endocrinopathies, seizure disorders, head trauma
- Management/treatment
  1. Follow federal and state laws regarding the protection of confidentiality for persons receiving alcohol and drug use disorder treatment services and treatment of minors for alcohol and drug use disorder without parental consent
  2. Nonpharmacologic
     a. Brief intervention (component of SBIRT— screening, brief intervention, referrals for treatment [CDC, 2014])—if screening reveals at-risk substance use, engage the patient in brief

motivation-enhancing intervention to reduce or stop the substance use

b. Further assessment and treatment if patient is not able to moderate the risky behavior independently

3. Pharmacologic
   a. Medications to assist in cessation of alcohol use
      (1) Naltrexone (ReVia)—long-acting opioid agonist injectable or oral daily pill; alcohol craving is reduced in about half of patients
      (2) Disulfiram (Antabuse)—alcohol antagonist; creates a toxic response when patient consumes alcohol
      (3) Acamprosate (Campral)—antagonizes glutamate receptors; restores chemical balance between excitatory and inhibitory neurotransmitters; prescribed to help in maintaining alcohol abstinence
   b. Medications for Opioid Use Disorder (MOUD): use of medications along with counseling and behavioral therapies to treat OUD and to prevent opioid overdose
      (1) Proven to be clinically effective, reduces the risk of overdose death by 50%
      (2) Often multidisciplinary, recovery-oriented treatment approach
      (3) Improves birth outcomes among pregnant people with OUD
      (4) Medications for MOUD
         (a) Buprenorphine (Buprenex, Subutex)— partial opioid receptor agonist; lower potential for misuse and less risk of overdose or respiratory depression than methadone; used for MOUD during pregnancy and lactation; neonate may need treatment for neonatal abstinence syndrome
         (b) Methadone (Dolophine)—long-acting, full opioid agonist; used for MOUD during pregnancy and lactation; neonate may need treatment for neonatal abstinence syndrome
         (c) Naltrexone (ReVia)—long-acting opioid agonist; not used for detoxification; may be used to help prevent relapse; should not be used in pregnancy
         (d) Naloxone—opioid antagonist used to reverse the physical effects of opioid overdose; reverses depression of CNS and respiratory system

- Referrals
  1. SUD inpatient or outpatient counseling and treatment, especially with polysubstance use
  2. Collaboration with maternal–fetal health specialists if the patient is pregnant and has SUD
  3. Support groups—Alcoholics Anonymous, Narcotics Anonymous, Smart Recovery
  4. Family involvement/support—counseling, Al-Anon, Ala-Teen, Nar-Anon

Questions

Select the best answer.

1. A systolic heart murmur present in an asymptomatic pregnant individual is likely:
   a. due to valvular disease
   b. associated with history of rheumatic fever
   c. a physiologic (innocent) murmur
   d. to intensify with a Valsalva maneuver

2. Which of the following, if left untreated, may progress to squamous cell carcinoma?
   a. Keratosis pilaris
   b. Seborrheic keratosis
   c. Actinic keratosis
   d. Lichen planus

3. Which one of the following is a finding in asthma?
   a. Shortened expiratory phase
   b. Vasoldilation
   c. Bradypnea
   d. Diminished lung sounds

4. Which one of the following is consistent with a diagnosis of mild persistent asthma?
   a. Symptoms fewer than twice a week
   b. Daily symptoms
   c. Symptoms cause mild interference with normal activities
   d. Nocturnal symptoms less than twice per month

5. Approximately what percentage of tuberculosis infections cause active disease?
   a. 75%
   b. 60%
   c. 30%
   d. 10%

6. Which one of the following is considered to have a positive PPD reaction?
   a. A 35-year-old healthy individual with a tuberculin reaction of 5 mm who has been in close contact with a TB-infected person
   b. A 45-year-old individual who was recently released from one year of incarceration with a tuberculin reaction of 5 mm
   c. A 28-year-old individual who has no risk factors with a tuberculin reaction of 10 mm
   d. A 40-year-old individual with a tuberculin reaction of 5 mm who has recently immigrated from a country with a high TB prevalence

7. Which one of the following is an anticipated symptom of active TB infection?
   a. Tachycardia
   b. Abdominal Pain
   c. Bulemia
   d. Night sweats

8. A 29-year-old female with migraine headaches receives subcutaneous sumatriptan for the first time. After the injection, she experiences tightness of the throat and chest, flushing, and dizziness. You recognize that these symptoms represent a(n):
   a. allergic reaction to the medication
   b. anxiety attack related to her headache
   c. contraindication to subcutaneous administration of the medication
   d. side effect that usually abates in a few minutes

9. Referral for neurologic evaluation of headaches is indicated when:
   a. new headaches occur in an individual older than 50.
   b. there is a family history of stroke.
   c. focal neurologic deficits precede headache episodes.
   d. migraine headache lasts more than 12 hours.

10. Important nonpharmacologic treatments for acute low back pain includes:
    a. high-intensity aerobic exercise
    b. ice application
    c. strength-building activity
    d. bed rest

11. Osteoarthritis may be distinguished from RA by:
    a. asymmetry of joint involvement
    b. erythema of affected joints
    c. constant pain not affected by rest
    d. presence of systemic symptoms

12. RICE therapy refers to a:
    a. nonpharmacologic therapy plan for muscle injuries
    b. bland diet therapy for nausea and vomiting
    c. weight-loss plan
    d. combination therapy for peptic ulcer disease

13. A 46-year-old individual presents with complaints of worsening low back pain after lifting a heavy object on the previous day. The individual has a history of intermittent low back pain in the last year but notes that the pain is now radiating down the right leg. The individual does not have any complaints of trouble with urination or bowel movements. On exam, you note a decreased range of motion of the spine in all planes. Straight leg raising at 35 degrees is positive on the right side. The Achilles tendon reflex on the right side is diminished compared to the left side, with decreased sensation over the right lateral foot. The most likely etiology of this patient's symptoms is:
    a. rupture of the Achilles tendon
    b. cauda equina syndrome
    c. herniated disc involving the L5 root
    d. herniated disc involving the S1 root

14. A 27-year-old patient presents with moderate sore throat, runny nose, cough, and general malaise for the past 2 days. Physical examination reveals temperature of 99.8°F, mild pharyngeal erythema, and no exudates. Appropriate management includes:
    a. CBC with differential
    b. rapid strep antigen test
    c. saline gargles
    d. antibiotic treatment

15. Risk of vertical transmission of the HIV virus has been reduced by:
    a. artificial rupture of membranes at 38 weeks' gestation
    b. antiretroviral treatment of infants
    c. stopping parental therapy in pregnancy so as to reduce CD4+ counts
    d. antiretroviral therapy during pregnancy

16. PrEP is contraindicated in individuals who:
    a. are not in a monogamous relationship
    b. are pregnant
    c. have hepatitis B
    d. have severe renal function disorders

17. An important principle of antiretroviral therapy is that:
    a. response to drug therapy is monitored with a p24 antigen/antibody test
    b. monotherapy is recommended as the initial treatment
    c. response to drug therapy is monitored by HIV RNA levels
    d. therapy should be started when symptoms first appear

18. A 34-year-old patient presents with a 2-month history of a nonproductive cough associated with shortness of breath. The patient reports fatigue and an intermittent fever for the past 6 weeks. Significant cervical, inguinal, and axillary lymphadenopathy is noted. The patient's HIV test is positive. Chest X-ray shows a bilateral infiltrate, and the patient is diagnosed with PCP. HIV infection produces a spectrum of the disease. This patient's symptoms place them in which stage of HIV infection?
    a. Acute HIV infection
    b. Asymptomatic infection
    c. Early symptomatic infection
    d. AIDS

19. For the client described in question 18, isoniazid prophylaxis would be recommended if the PPD was greater than or equal to:
    a. 5 mm
    b. 10 mm
    c. 15 mm
    d. 20 mm

20. Risk factors for SLE include:
    a. female assigned sex, reproductive age group, Hispanic descent
    b. reproductive age group, first-degree relative with SLE, white
    c. first-degree relative with SLE, female assigned sex, Asian race
    d. female assigned sex, small stature, white

21. Diagnosis of SLE is made by:
    a. abnormal ANA titer
    b. presence of at least four combined signs, symptoms, and laboratory findings
    c. presence of a specific hematologic disorder on a single occasion
    d. identification of an immunologic disorder such as abnormal anti-DNA

22. SLE is usually characterized by:
    a. periods of exacerbation and remission
    b. slow, steady disease progression
    c. initial symptoms of typical skin eruptions
    d. remission in pregnancy

23. Which one of the following is suspected in the etiology of RA?
    a. Congenital dysplasia
    b. Environmental factors
    c. Severe osteoarthritis
    d. Joint trauma

24. The World Health Organization standard for anemia diagnosis in nonpregnant women is hemoglobin less than:
    a. 10 g/dL
    b. 11 g/dL
    c. 12 g/dL
    d. 13 g/dL

25. Otitis media is suspected when deep ear pain develops concurrent with or following:
    a. airplane travel
    b. an asthma attack
    c. an upper respiratory infection
    d. persistent headache

26. A patient presents with moderate scratchy sensation in the right eye and a watery discharge that started about 24 hours ago. The patient reports to be just getting over a cold. Appropriate treatment would include:
    a. antibiotics
    b. comfort measures only
    c. mast cell stabilizer
    d. topical antihistamine

27. Antibiotic treatment should be initiated for the patient with sinusitis who has:
    a. increased pain when bending over or with sudden head movement
    b. symptoms present for 10 or more days without clinical improvement
    c. symptoms that started within the first week of onset of an upper respiratory infection
    d. yellow to green nasal discharge

28. A 21-year-old patient presents with symptoms suggestive of infectious mononucleosis. Which one of the following supports the diagnosis?
    a. Acute rhinitis
    b. Low hematocrit
    c. Lymphocytic leukocytosis
    d. Hoarse cough

29. Those individuals most often affected by infectious mononucleosis are:
    a. prepubertal children
    b. women of reproductive age
    c. adults at any age
    d. people in their teens to early twenties

30. The most common reason for painless rectal bleeding with defecation is:
    a. external hemorrhoids
    b. internal hemorrhoids
    c. rectal polyps
    d. colorectal cancer

31. A 21-year-old individual complains of intermittent abdominal pain, bloating, and loose stools three to four times per month for the past 3 months. Which of the following additional findings would lead you toward a diagnosis of irritable bowel syndrome?
    a. Abdominal pain is relieved with defecation.
    b. Antacids relieve the pain.
    c. The individual is awakened at night by the need to defecate.
    d. There is a small amount of bright red blood in the loose stools.

32. For the client described in question 31, initial management of symptoms may include:
    a. alosetron
    b. fiber supplements
    c. lubiprostone
    d. trial of elimination of dairy products

33. Black women are at increased risk for:
    a. systemic lupus erythematosus
    b. skin cancer
    c. iron-deficiency anemia
    d. tinea corporis

34. Appendicitis typically presents with:
    a. high fever as the initial symptom
    b. pain beginning in the RLQ
    c. diarrhea as the initial symptom
    d. pain in the periumbilical area followed by localization to the RLQ

35. Peptic ulcer disease associated with the presence of *H. pylori* can be diagnosed by:
    a. visualization of *H. pylori* on Gram-stained preparation
    b. positive urea breath analysis
    c. negative urease assay via endoscopy
    d. serology negative for *H. pylori* antibodies

36. A 42-year-old individual had a diagnosis of acute HBV infection 6 months ago. Expected laboratory test results, if the infection is resolved and the individual is now immune to HBV infection, include a positive:
    a. HBV DNA test
    b. HBV e antigen test
    c. HBV surface antibody test
    d. HBV surface antigen test

37. Which of the following is the most appropriate pharmacologic therapy for chronic hepatitis B?
    a. Recombinant interferon alfa-2b
    b. Antiemetic
    c. Pegylated interferon
    d. Hepatitis B immune globulin

38. Most gallstones are composed of:
    a. precipitated bile salts
    b. precipitated calcium salts
    c. cholesterol
    d. pigments

39. A 45-year-old patient presents with RUQ pain that radiates to the right infrascapular area. The pain is described as colicky and was precipitated by eating pizza. The onset of the symptom was a few hours ago, and the pain is beginning to ease. There was associated nausea and vomiting. The initial study of choice in this patient is:
    a. plain abdominal radiograph
    b. ultrasound
    c. CT
    d. percutaneous transhepatic cholangiogram

40. Among the following causes of viral hepatitis, which is most likely to lead to chronic infection and is the most common reason for liver transplantation?
    a. Hepatitis A
    b. Hepatitis B
    c. Hepatitis C
    d. Hepatitis D

41. Patients with acute cholecystitis should be advised:
    a. to undertake strict weight-reduction diets if they are obese to prevent recurrences
    b. that recurrences are uncommon except in the elderly
    c. that hospital admission and cholecystectomy are the recommended treatment
    d. that lithotripsy is a highly successful treatment done in the outpatient setting

42. A 35-year-old overweight individual presents with intermittent heartburn for several months. The use of Tums antacids provides temporary relief. During the past week, the individual has been awakened during the night with a burning sensation in the chest. The individual is not taking any other medications and has no major health problems. What additional information would support a diagnosis of GERD as the cause of these symptoms?
    a. The individual experiences the presence of occasional nausea and vomiting.
    b. The individual coughs during the night and has a bad taste in their mouth.
    c. The pain is usually relieved by eating.
    d. Constipation has been a chronic problem, and the individual uses laxatives twice a week.

43. The patient in question 42 denies weight loss, dysphagia, and dark, tarry stools. What is your next step?
    a. Order an endoscopic exam.
    b. Start them on H_2-receptor blockers.
    c. Tell them to eat a snack before bedtime.
    d. Refer them to a gastroenterologist.

44. Assuming a diagnosis of GERD for the patient in questions 42 and 43, you would advise that:
    a. the individual probably has a hiatal hernia causing the reflux.
    b. the individual will likely require surgery.
    c. the individual should avoid dairy products.
    d. high-fat foods and chocolate may aggravate the problem.

45. The laboratory diagnosis of diabetes mellitus can be determined by:
    a. fasting plasma glucose ≥126 mg/dL
    b. a 2-hour postprandial glucose ≥126 mg/dL
    c. HbA_{1c} >5.5%
    d. random glucose ≥150 mg/dL

46. A 26-year-old patient presents with the complaint of watery diarrhea and abdominal cramping for the past 2 days that started a few days after returning from a trip to Mexico. No noted blood in the stool and no fever. The physical examination reveals hyperactive bowel sounds and mild, diffuse abdominal tenderness. Initial management for this patient should include:
    a. instructions to take bismuth subsalicylate for 24 to 48 hours
    b. instructions to maintain fluid intake and limit the use of antidiarrheal agents
    c. prescribing metronidazole and ciprofloxacin for 5 days
    d. stool evaluation for bacterial pathogens, ova and parasites, and occult blood

47. The mechanism of action for the drug ezetimibe used in combination with a moderate-intensity statin for treatment of dyslipidemia in some individuals is:
    a. binding cholesterol bile acids to increase excretion
    b. decreasing synthesis of LDL
    c. increasing synthesis of HDL
    d. inhibiting cholesterol absorption

48. The condition accounting for 90% of hyperthyroidism cases is:
    a. Graves' disease
    b. thyroiditis
    c. toxic goiter
    d. adenoma

49. Infiltrative ophthalmopathy (exophthalmos) is unique to:
    a. Graves' disease
    b. Hashimoto's thyroiditis
    c. toxic multinodular goiter
    d. papillary thyroid carcinoma

50. Which of the following test results would be expected with primary hyperthyroidism?
    a. Low serum TSH and elevated free T_4
    b. Low serum TSH and low free T_4
    c. High serum TSH and elevated free T_4
    d. High serum TSH and low free T_4

51. A patient with a history of radioactive iodine treatment for Graves' disease presents with fatigue, weight gain, and dry skin. You would expect this patient to have which one of the following laboratory findings?
    a. Low T_3, low TSH, high total T_4
    b. Low TSH, high total T_4, normal free T_4
    c. High TSH, low free T_4
    d. High TSH, high free T_4

52. A 35-year-old patient was diagnosed with Hashimoto's thyroiditis and placed on 0.1 mg of levothyroxine. After 1 week of treatment, the patient still feels fatigued. How would you manage this patient?
    a. Increase the dose of levothyroxine to 0.125 mg.
    b. Schedule an appointment this week to have a TSH drawn.
    c. Add propranolol to the regimen.
    d. No change in levothyroxine is indicated at this time.

53. A factor associated with exacerbation of facial acne is:
    a. salicylic acid
    b. topical corticosteroids
    c. fried foods
    d. contraceptive pills

54. The most important point to stress with patients using isotretinoin for acne is:
    a. the possibility of hematologic disturbances
    b. the rare occurrence of pseudotumor cerebri
    c. the necessity for highly effective contraception
    d. avoiding alcohol while on this drug

55. An 18-year-old presents with open and closed comedones without inflammation. The most appropriate first-line treatment would be:
    a. topical antibiotics
    b. oral tetracycline

    c. tretinoin cream (Retin-A)
    d. isotretinoin (Accutane)

56. The most common form of skin cancer is:
    a. squamous cell
    b. basal cell
    c. malignant melanoma
    d. basal cell nevus syndrome

57. A 60-year-old presents with a pearly, translucent smooth papule on her forehead with rolled edges and surface telangiectasias. It has been there for at least a year but has recently increased in size. The lesion most likely represents which one of the following?
    a. Squamous cell carcinoma
    b. Basal cell carcinoma
    c. Seborrheic keratosis
    d. Malignant melanoma

58. Education for the individual with SLE should include which of the following?
    a. The individual should not use hormonal contraception.
    b. The individual should receive annual live attenuated influenza vaccine.
    c. If pregnant, a cesarean section will be planned to avoid the stress of labor.
    d. The individual should use sunscreen and sun-protective clothing when outdoors.

59. Which of the following is a risk factor for malignant melanoma?
    a. Hispanic ethnicity
    b. A pigmented nevi
    c. Severe childhood sunburn
    d. Psoraiasis

60. A 20-year-old individual presents with two annular lesions with a scaly border and central clearing on the trunk. The lesions have been present for 1 week and are mildly pruritic. What is the most likely diagnosis?
    a. Psoriasis
    b. Pityriasis rosea
    c. Scabies
    d. Tinea corporis

61. A 20-year-old individual presents with the complaint of itching, and a red eye with a sticky, yellow discharge that started in one eye yesterday afternoon, and this morning is in both eyes. The individual has no fever or other symptoms. The most likely diagnosis is:
    a. allergic conjunctivitis
    b. bacterial conjunctivitis
    c. chemical exposure conjunctivitis
    d. viral conjunctivitis

62. All of the following are known teratogens *except*:
    a. alcohol
    b. methotrexate
    c. opioids
    d. statins

63. A 28-year-old individual presents with complaints of low back pain after helping a friend move 2 days ago. There is no radiation of the pain, numbness, or tingling in the lower extremities or problems with elimination. On

physical exam, mild paravertebral muscle spasm is noted with decreased range of motion of the spine. There are no focal neurologic findings. Appropriate management would include:
a. radiograph of the lumbosacral spine
b. bed rest for 3-4 days
c. NSAIDs
d. referral to a neurologist

64. The frequency of sickle cell crises may be reduced by:
a. activity restrictions
b. oxygen therapy
c. aggressive treatment of infections
d. a high-protein diet

65. Which one of the following is an expected finding in tinea unguium?
a. Hair loss in affected areas
b. Negative KOH slide preparation
c. Yellowish, thickened nails
d. Crusted ulcerations

66. Approximately 10% of all individuals infected with hepatitis B virus become chronic carriers of the disease, a state putting them at risk for:
a. hepatocellular carcinoma
b. mononucleosis
c. gallbladder disease
d. chronic immunocompromised status

67. A patient's blood test returns with a positive hepatitis B surface antigen (HBsAg), which suggests:
a. chronic liver disease
b. previous infection with hepatitis B virus
c. acute or chronic infection with hepatitis B virus
d. recent vaccination

68. An adult with a blood pressure (BP) of 136/84 and a calculated 10-year risk of atherosclerotic cardiovascular disease less than 10% should be:
a. advised this is within normal limits and to have BP checked annually
b. advised on lifestyle modifications and return to have BP checked in 3 to 6 months
c. started on one anti-hypertensive medication and return to have BP checked in 1 month
d. started on two anti-hypertensive medications from different classes and return to have BP checked in 1 month

69. Management of constipation should include:
a. routine use of stool softeners
b. bulk-forming agents for acute constipation
c. hyperosmolar laxatives (sorbitol) as initial treatment for chronic constipation
d. saline laxatives (milk of magnesia) for acute constipation

70. Using the CURB-65 criteria, a 65-year-old individual with community-acquired pneumonia should be hospitalized if the individual develops:
a. blood pressure greater than 140/90 mm Hg
b. confusion or disorientation
c. dyspnea on exertion
d. pleuritic chest pain

71. Appropriate initial management for an otherwise healthy 52-year-old individual with viral community-acquired pneumonia would include:
a. comfort measures with antibiotics if symptoms persist more than 5 days
b. ordering a sputum culture before any antibiotic treatment
c. treatment with azithromycin
d. treatment with levofloxacin

72. Which one of the following most likely suggests a secondary cause of hypertension?
a. Body mass index greater than 30
b. Abdominal bruit
c. Total cholesterol greater than 280 mg/dL
d. Enlarged spleen

73. A 30-year-old woman is taking an ACE inhibitor for hypertension, and her BP today is 130/78 mm Hg. She is sexually active and is not currently using any contraception. Appropriate counseling would include:
a. She should increase the dosage of the ACE inhibitor to better control her BP prior to planning a pregnancy.
b. She should not take any antihypertensive medication if she is planning a pregnancy.
c. The best contraceptive choice would be a combination of hormonal contraception with the transdermal patch.
d. The use of an ACE inhibitor is contraindicated during pregnancy because it is associated with fetal anomalies.

74. A 21-year-old client comes to the clinic with a complaint of amenorrhea. The client also complains of feeling cold all the time. Physical examination reveals an underweight individual with a heart rate of 58 beats per minute and blood pressure of 96/52 mm Hg. A pregnancy test is negative. Which of the following additional findings would contribute to a diagnosis of anorexia nervosa?
a. Currently on probation for shoplifting
b. Fine body hair on extremities
c. Migraine headaches
d. Swollen parotid glands

75. Common physical findings with allergic rhinitis include:
a. facial tenderness
b. inflamed nasal mucosa
c. nasal crease
d. purulent nasal discharge

76. The recommended initial test for DVT in a symptomatic patient is:
a. plasma D-dimer
b. contrast venography
c. antithrombin III
d. duplex ultrasound

77. Which of the following is a recommended treatment for superficial thrombophlebitis?
a. Massage
b. Ice pack
c. Heparin
d. NSAIDs

78. The most likely diagnosis for physical examination findings that include presence of lesions located on the elbows, knees, and scalp that have well-defined borders, an erythematous base, and silvery scales is:
    a. contact dermatitis
    b. psoriasis
    c. scabies
    d. seborrheic keratosis

79. A 44-year-old patient presents with type 2 diabetes and hyperlipidemia. Which of the following should be your main treatment goal?
    a. HDL > 40 mg/dL
    b. LDL cholesterol < 70 mg/dL
    c. Total cholesterol < 200 mg/dL
    d. Triglycerides < 250 mg/dL

80. A 50-year-old patient presents with a complaint of severe pain that started in the upper mid-abdomen and is now worse in the RUQ. The patient also had nausea and vomiting. On deep palpation of the RUQ, the patient momentarily holds their breath on inspiration. You suspect:
    a. appendicitis
    b. acute cholecystitis
    c. pancreatitis
    d. peptic ulcer disease

81. A microcytic anemia with a low serum ferritin is likely secondary to:
    a. anemia of chronic disease
    b. iron deficiency
    c. hypersplenism
    d. thalassemia minor

82. Naloxone is a(n):
    a. alcohol antagonist that creates a toxic response when an individual consumes alcohol
    b. long-acting opioid agonist used to help prevent relapse in individuals with either alcohol or opioid use disorder
    c. opioid antagonist used to reverse the physical effects of opioid overdose
    d. partial opioid receptor agonist used in medication-assisted treatment for opioid use disorder

83. Fibromyalgia most commonly presents with which one of the following signs and symptoms?
    a. Abrupt onset of proximal muscle weakness
    b. Widespread musculoskeletal pain and tender points
    c. Effusion of involved joints with mild local warmth
    d. Subcutaneous nodules

84. Long-term use of corticosteroids may be a secondary cause of:
    a. asthma
    b. dyslipidemia
    c. iron-deficiency anemia
    d. osteoarthritis

85. A systolic click preceding a mid- to late systolic murmur is most likely caused by which one of the following?
    a. Aortic stenosis
    b. Mitral valve prolapse
    c. Mitral valve stenosis
    d. Idiopathic hypertrophic subaortic stenosis

86. Which one of the following is a common finding with an innocent murmur?
    a. Heard best with the patient supine
    b. Decreases with increased cardiac output
    c. Increases with a Valsalva maneuver
    d. Most frequently heard during dyastole

87. The leading killer of women in the United States is:
    a. coronary heart disease
    b. lung cancer
    c. ovarian cancer
    d. violence

88. Virchow's triad defines the clinical origin of most venous thrombi and includes all of the following factors *except*:
    a. stasis
    b. endothelial damage
    c. deposition of cholesterol plaques
    d. hypercoagulability

89. A patient presents with signs and symptoms suggestive of a superficial phlebitis. Physical findings in this patient would include:
    a. tenderness in the area of the involved vein
    b. edema of the involved extremity
    c. pale, cool skin in the area of the involved vein
    d. a palpable venous cord

90. In the United States, the most common cause of community-acquired bacterial pneumonia is:
    a. *Streptococcus pneumoniae*
    b. *Streptococcus pyogenes*
    c. *Haemophilus influenzae*
    d. *Legionella pneumophilia*

91. A 24-year-old individual with asthma classified as mild persistent is considering pregnancy. The individual currently uses an albuterol metered-dose inhaler and the inhaled corticosteroid budesonide. Advice concerning asthma and pregnancy should include which one of the following?
    a. Exacerbations during pregnancy are common but will not harm the fetus/infant.
    b. It is safer to be treated for asthma during pregnancy than to have symptoms and exacerbations.
    c. Oral corticosteroids should be initiated prior to conception so that asthma is well controlled in early pregnancy.
    d. The medications the individual is currently using are contraindicated during pregnancy.

92. The American College of Rheumatology (2010) classification criteria for a diagnosis of RA include:
    a. fever
    b. elevated erythrocyte sedimentation rate
    c. joint erosion on radiography
    d. symmetrical joint involvement

93. Your patient is experiencing three to four migraine headaches per month. You decide to begin prophylactic medication. Which of the following is recommended for migraine headache prophylaxis?
    a. Ergotamine
    b. Propranolol (beta blocker)
    c. Sumatriptan
    d. An SSRI

94. Which of the following is *true* concerning the treatment of RA?
    a. NSAIDs and corticosteroids are important for long-term management.
    b. The main mechanism of action of DMARDs is analgesia.
    c. DMARDs and immunomodulating biologic agents may be combined if monotherapy is not effective.
    d. Methotrexate is the preferred DMARD for use by pregnant people with RA.

95. Metabolic syndrome is defined as having at least three of a set of five risk factors. One of these risk factors for women is:
    a. blood pressure of 150/90 mm Hg or higher
    b. HDL-C of 40 mg/dL or less
    c. triglycerides of 200 mg/dL or higher
    d. waist circumference greater than 35 inches

96. Acute otitis media is characterized by all of the following physical examination findings *except*:
    a. distorted light reflex
    b. obscured bony landmarks
    c. erythema of the ear canal
    d. postauricular lymphadenopathy

97. Physical examination and laboratory test findings expected with a diagnosis of infectious mononucleosis include:
    a. elevated basophils and eosinophils
    b. erythematous rash in the groin and axillary areas
    c. purulent nasal discharge
    d. tonsillar enlargement with exudate

98. A patient presents with a complaint of extremely itchy, dry areas of skin on the wrists, hands, and knees. Physical examination reveals erythematous, dry, scaly, excoriated patches of skin with lichenification in these areas. The most likely diagnosis is:
    a. contact dermatitis
    b. eczema
    c. psoriasis
    d. tinea

99. Which of the following statements about genetic carrier screening is correct?
    a. All genetic carrier screening decisions should be based on family history, ethnicity, or history of a child with a congenital anomaly.
    b. All individuals considering pregnancy should be offered genetic carrier screening for cystic fibrosis and spinal muscular atrophy.
    c. Decisions regarding genetic carrier screening for thalassemia are best based on the individual's race and ethnicity.
    d. There is no benefit to screening the individual's reproductive partner in determining the risk of having an affected child.

100. Macrocytic anemias include:
    a. anemia of chronic disease
    b. vitamin B_{12}–deficiency anemia
    c. iron-deficiency anemia
    d. sickle cell anemia

101. A 65-year-old menopausal individual had a deep vein thrombosis in the leg 2 years ago. The individual has a BMD T-score of –1.75. Which of the following medications would be the most appropriate for this client to prevent osteoporosis?
    a. Alendronate
    b. Calcitonin
    c. Estrogen
    d. Raloxifene

102. Which one of the following statements is correct concerning BMD testing?
    a. Test results are most predictive of bone fracture when done on an annual basis.
    b. The T-score compares the BMD of the client with that of an age-matched normal adult.
    c. BMD T-scores should be combined with bone X-ray to confirm osteoporosis.
    d. Treatment decisions based on T-scores may vary according to risk factors.

103. For which one of the following individuals would VFA with vertebral imaging be most appropriate?
    a. A 40-year-old woman with a history of low-trauma fracture during adulthood
    b. A 40-year-old woman on long-term glucocorticoid treatment
    c. A 60-year-old woman with measured height loss of 2 cm or more
    d. A 60-year-old woman with BMD T-score at or below –1.5

104. Client instructions for taking alendronate should include which one of the following?
    a. Take the medication with breakfast.
    b. Take the medication at bedtime.
    c. Take the medication on an empty stomach.
    d. Take the medication with an antacid.

105. Which one of the following is no longer a criterion for a diagnosis of anorexia nervosa according to the *DSM-5* criteria?
    a. Amenorrhea
    b. Disturbed body image
    c. Intense fear of gaining weight
    d. Significantly low body weight

106. One of the most significant laboratory tests for evaluating an individual for chronic or heavy alcohol use is a(n):
    a. ALP
    b. BUN
    c. CBC
    d. GGT

107. Two months after being raped, a client tells you she cannot concentrate on her schoolwork and is having nightmares about the experience. These symptoms indicate that she:
    a. is still in the acute phase of rape trauma syndrome
    b. is going through normal reorganization following a rape
    c. is experiencing posttraumatic stress disorder
    d. now has a generalized anxiety disorder

108. A client who has been experiencing fatigue, insomnia, difficulty concentrating, and feelings of worthlessness for the past 2 weeks would meet the *DSM-5* criteria for a major depressive disorder if the client also has:
    a. loss of interest in usual activities
    b. psychomotor retardation
    c. psychosomatic complaints
    d. suicidal ideation

109. Contraceptive counseling for a 24-year-old patient with diabetes who has no complications or other health problems should include which one of the following?
    a. Combination hormonal contraceptives are contraindicated.
    b. Progestin-only methods are a better choice than those containing estrogen.
    c. The patient can use any of the long-acting reversible contraceptives.
    d. The patient should complete childbearing by age 30 and consider sterilization.

110. A 24-year-old woman with major depression tells the APRN that she feels as if her life is falling apart with no hope of improving. She recently lost her job, had to move out of her apartment, and now lives with her sister. Her risk factors for a suicide attempt include:
    a. age between 20 and 30 years
    b. female sex
    c. current living situation
    d. sense of hopelessness

111. A client reports experiencing chest tightness, difficulty breathing, and dizziness whenever riding on the city bus. The client has been trying to find other transportation because the client is very fearful about these symptoms recurring. These symptoms best fit the description of:
    a. acute stress disorder
    b. panic disorder with agoraphobia
    c. obsessive–compulsive disorder
    d. social phobia

112. The most common type of anxiety disorder is:
    a. generalized anxiety disorder
    b. specific phobia
    c. panic disorder
    d. post-traumatic stress disorder

113. Which one of the following statements concerning bulimia is correct?
    a. Age of onset is usually early adolescence.
    b. Amenorrhea is usually present.
    c. The mortality rate for bulimia is higher than that for anorexia nervosa.
    d. Impulsive behavior is a common characteristic.

114. Major side effects of selective serotonin reuptake inhibitors include:
    a. anticholinergic effects
    b. nausea
    c. orthostatic hypotension
    d. urinary retention

115. Which of the following medications should be used only for short-term management of generalized anxiety disorder?
    a. Alpraxolam (Xanax)
    b. Buspirone (Buspar)
    c. Duloxetine (Cymbalta)
    d. Paroxetine (Paxil)

116. Physiologic dependence on a substance is defined as evidence of withdrawal symptoms and/or:
    a. craving or strong desire to use the substance
    b. inability to carry out major obligations due to the substance use
    c. markedly increased amounts of the substance needed to achieve intoxication or desired effect
    d. unsuccessful attempts to cut down on or control substance use

117. Physical findings that help the clinician make a diagnosis of bulimia would include:
    a. erosion of tooth enamel
    b. hypotension
    c. presence of lanugo
    d. stress fractures

118. Which one of the following statements concerning rape is *true*?
    a. All U.S. states have now established the same legal definition for rape.
    b. The majority of rapes are committed by acquaintances.
    c. The most common emotional response in the acute phase is anger.
    d. The clinician is responsible for determining whether a rape has actually occurred.

119. Which one of the following drugs decreases hepatic glucose production?
    a. Biguanides (metformin)
    b. Insulin
    c. Meglitinides (repaglinide)
    d. Sulfonylureas (glyburide, glipizide)

120. Severe exacerbations in an individual with intermittent (step 1) asthma are appropriately treated with:
    a. mast-cell stabilizers
    b. short-acting inhaled β_2 agonists
    c. systemic corticosteroids
    d. theophylline

121. Client education concerning the use of bupropion hydrochloride (Zyban) for smoking cessation should include:
    a. discontinue smoking prior to initiation of this medication
    b. the medication should not be used for more than 8 weeks
    c. initiate the medication at least 1 week prior to smoking cessation
    d. side effects may include drowsiness and weight gain

122. Which of the following statements regarding influenza vaccination during pregnancy is true?
    a. Influenza vaccination should be given only if the individual has health problems that place them at high risk for complications with influenza.

b. Influenza vaccination may be safely given in any trimester of pregnancy.

c. Intranasal influenza vaccine is recommended for pregnant individuals to reduce the chances of side effects.

d. Influenza vaccination is contraindicated during pregnancy.

123. When using a three-dose regimen, the second and third doses of the HPV vaccination should be given:
    a. 1 month and 3 months after the initial dose
    b. 1 month and 6 months after the initial dose
    c. 2 months and 6 months after the initial dose
    d. 3 months and 12 months after the initial dose

124. Which one of the following types of vaccinations are contraindicated in pregnancy?
    a. Bacterial vaccines
    b. Inactivated virus vaccines
    c. Live attenuated virus vaccines
    d. Immunoglobulins

125. USPSTF recommendations for routine breast cancer screening include:
    a. biennial mammograms starting at age 50
    b. breast self-examination starting at age 21
    c. clinical breast examination annually starting at age 30
    d. discontinue mammograms after age 65

126. Good dietary sources for folic acid include:
    a. chicken
    b. dried beans
    c. egg yolks
    d. milk

127. A model that can be used by clinicians who are not sex therapists to address sexual concerns and make appropriate referrals is the:
    a. Basson nonlinear model
    b. Cisgender model
    c. Masters and Johnson linear model
    d. PLISSIT model

128. The term that best describes an individual's pattern of emotional, romantic, and sexual attraction to other people is:
    a. gender identity
    b. sexual drive
    c. sexual motivation
    d. sexual orientation

129. An example of secondary prevention is providing:
    a. immunizations
    b. health promotion counseling to reduce risk factors for disease
    c. health care that focuses on restoring optimal function following diagnosis of disease
    d. screening tests for early detection of disease states

130. A 20-year-old sexually active person assigned female at birth presents at the office for an initial visit. Which one of the following screening tests/procedures should be provided?
    a. Cervical cancer screening
    b. Chlamydia test

c. Clinical breast examination
d. Hepatitis B test

131. Hepatitis C screening is recommended for:
    a. all adults aged 40 years and older annually
    b. all adults aged 18 years and older at least once in a lifetime
    c. pregnant individuals if they have risk factors
    d. only for individuals with identified risk factors

132. A BMD test to screen for osteopenia/osteoporosis would be appropriate for all of the following individuals *except*:
    a. a 40-year-old cisgender woman who smokes cigarettes and whose alcohol intake averages three drinks/day
    b. a 55-year-old cisgender woman who has a low BMI, and her mother had a hip fracture at age 70
    c. a 60-year-old cisgender woman who has recently experienced a low-trauma fracture
    d. a 65-year-old transgender woman who has no apparent risk factors associated with increased fracture risk

133. A 45-year-old patient presents with a complaint of lower abdominal pain with urinary urgency and frequency for the past 3 months. The pain is worse during sexual intercourse and relieved somewhat with urination. Physical examination reveals suprapubic tenderness as well as tenderness along the anterior vaginal wall and urethra. The remainder of the exam is normal. What diagnosis best fits these findings?
    a. Chronic urinary tract infection
    b. Interstitial cystitis/painful bladder syndrome
    c. Pelvic inflammatory disease
    d. Pyelonephritis

134. Anticholinergic agents may be used in the treatment of:
    a. stress incontinence
    b. urge incontinence
    c. vestibulitis
    d. vulvodynia

135. First-line prophylaxis for recurrent urinary tract infection/cystitis for the perimenopausal patient may include:
    a. vaginal/local estrogen therapy for vaginal atrophy/genital syndrome of menopause
    b. regular use of barrier contraceptive methods or spermicide
    c. single-dose nitrofurantoin after sexual intercourse
    d. 6-month prophylaxis regimen with oral doxycycline

136. A 63-year-old patient presents for a wellness visit. The patient had a screening mammogram and cervical cancer screening co-testing (cytology and HPV test) at age 60 and a colonoscopy for colorectal cancer screening at age 55. All results were normal with no more recent screenings. The patient smoked a pack a day for 30+ years and discontinued smoking at age 55. The patient's mother was recently diagnosed with colon cancer at age 85. Recommended cancer screening at this visit includes:
    a. cervical cancer screening, colonoscopy, and mammogram
    b. cervical cancer screening, lung cancer screening, and mammogram
    c. colonoscopy, lung cancer screening, and mammogram
    d. lung cancer screening and mammogram

137. Iron requirements are highest for nonpregnant women at:
    a. 14–18 years of age
    b. 19–50 years of age
    c. 51–70 years of age
    d. 71 years of age and older

138. All of the following increase the risk for vitamin D deficiency *except*:
    a. age older than 59 years
    b. dark skin
    c. irritable bowel syndrome
    d. residing in northern areas

139. Which of the following meets the definitions for risky or hazardous alcohol for women?
    a. Any alcohol use during pregnancy
    b. Five or more drinks per week
    c. Three or more drinks on one occasion within a couple of hours
    d. Two or more drinks per day

140. A 48-year-old women presents sick in clinic and reports that she is concerned that she may have contracted SARS CoV-2 as her friend was recently diagnosed with this virus. She is worried that she may be contagious. Which of the following is the most accurate advise with regard to contagion?
    a. You may be contagious 48 hours prior to symptom onset.
    b. Limit close proximity from others to 30 minutes cumulatively in 24 hours.
    c. Getting a booster today will prevent the spread of the virus.
    d. You must quarantine starting immediately for 10 days.

141. A 36-year-old G2P1001 at 23 weeks' gestation reports feeling very tired and having a fever, runny nose, and cough. What differential diagnosis can you strike from your work-up?
    a. Influenza
    b. SARS CoV-2
    c. Adenovirus
    d. Infectious mononucleosis

142. A 20-year-old individual presents to clinic with acute abdominal pain. On exam appears to be midline to right lower quadrant with a positive McBurney's and obturators sign. Which diagnostic imaging would you want to order next?
    a. KUB
    b. CT of the abdomen
    c. Ultrasound
    d. Chest XR

143. You perform a medicine reconciliation for a 55-year-old woman with hypertension, GERD, and plantar fasciitis. Her medications for the last four years have been on lisinopril/hydrochlorothiazide 20 mg/12.5 mg PO QD, Omeprazole 20 mg PO QD, acetaminophen 500 mg PO QD PRN pain, and ibuprofen 200mg PO q8h PRN pain. Which medicine would you be concerned about?
    a. Lisinopril/hydrochlorothiazide 20 mg/12.5 mg PO QD,
    b. Omeprazole 20 mg PO QD
    c. Acetaminophen 500 mg PO QD PRN pain
    d. Ibuprofen 200 mg PO q8h PRN pain

144. A 24-year-old G0P0 at 10 weeks' gestation is heterozygous HgbS. How would you interpret this lab?
    a. This meets the criteria for sickle cell anemia.
    b. This meets the criteria for Beta- thalassemia.
    c. This meets the criteria for alpha- thalassemia.
    d. This meets the criteria for sickle cell trait.

145. In order to meet the criteria for systemic lupus erythematous, a client must meet which of the criteria?
    a. 4 of the 11 criteria and totaling a score of >10
    b. Entry criterion first and then additional clinical/immunologic domains to have a total score ≥10
    c. Entry criterion first and then additional clinical/immunologic domains to have a total score ≥11
    d. 3 of the 11 criteria and totaling a score of >10

146. In pregnancy, how should the APRN manage TSH in hypothyroidism?
    a. Maintain TSH >3.5 mU/L
    b. Unable to monitor as it fluctuates day to day
    c. Maintain levels per trimester-specific levels
    d. Maintain TSH >3.0 mU/L

147. What is the first-line abortive therapy for a moderate to severe migraine?
    a. Tramadol
    b. Acetaminophen
    c. Naproxen with acetaminophen
    d. Sumatriptan

148. Which physical finding is more indicative of a lumbosacral strain?
    a. Radicular pain with a passive straight leg raise
    b. Weakness with dorsiflexion of the great toe
    c. Bladder incontinence
    d. Tenderness to palpation along the paraspinal muscles

149. The World Health Organization (WHO) standard for anemia diagnosis for women is:
    a. ≤12 g/dL
    b. ≤13 g/dL
    c. ≤14 g/dL
    d. ≤15 g/dL

150. Which of the following is a method of recruitment used by human traffickers?
    a. Promises of employment
    b. Convincing poor families to sell their children
    c. Collaborating with storefronts who pretend they are employment agencies
    d. All of the above

Answers with Rationales

1. **c.** a physiologic (innocent) murmur
Pregnant individuals may have grade 1 or 2 systolic murmurs due to physiologic increased cardiac output.

2. **c.** Actinic keratosis
Sixty percent of squamous cell carcinomas occur at the site of previous actinic keratosis.

3. **d.** Diminished lung sounds
Physical respiratory findings in asthma include hyperresonance with percussion, wheezing, prolonged expiratory phase, and diminished breath sounds; tachypnea; and dyspnea.

4. **c.** Symptoms cause mild interference with normal activities
Mild persistent asthma is characterized by daytime symptoms greater than two times per week but not daily; nocturnal symptoms three to four times per month; use of a short-acting beta-agonist inhaler to manage symptoms more frequent than 2 days per week, no more than one time a day and not daily; two or more exacerbations requiring oral corticosteroids over the last year; mild interference with normal activity; FEV_1 greater than 80% predicted (normal FEV_1/FVC ratio for age between exacerbations).

5. **d.** 10%
The asymptomatic state (latent TB infection) may last months to years, with 10% of patients ultimately developing active TB.

6. **a.** A 35-year-old healthy individual with a tuberculin reaction of 5 mm who has been in close contact with a TB-infected person
A 5-mm or greater skin reaction on the PPD test is considered positive in individuals who are HIV positive, immunocompromised, with abnormal chest radiograph findings consistent with healed TB lesions, or in recent close contact with a TB-infected person.

7. **d.** Night sweats
Individuals with active TB may have generalized symptoms of night sweats, fever, malaise, weakness, anorexia and weight loss, and pulmonary symptoms of productive cough, hemoptysis, chest pain, and dyspnea.

8. **d.** side effect that usually abates in a few minutes
Sumatriptan is used for abortive treatment of migraine headaches and may initially cause tightness of the throat/chest, flushing, numbness, tingling, and dizziness. This side effect typically abates in a few minutes and is not a contraindication for future use.

9. **a.** new headaches occur in an individual older than 50
Reasons for referral for neurologic evaluation of headaches include a new type of headache occurring in an individual older than 50 years of age, sudden onset of the worst headache ever experienced, headaches increasing in severity or frequency, headache initiated by exertion, focal neurologic symptoms persisting after headache onset, headache subsequent to head trauma, and any other indicators of a potentially serious secondary cause.

10. **c.** strength-building activity
Nonpharmacologic interventions for managing lower back pain include the continuation of daily activities rather than bed rest, in addition to local application of heat, warm baths, a physical therapy program to improve strength and conditioning, and low-stress aerobic exercise—walking, biking, swimming.

11. **a.** asymmetry of joint involvement
Osteoarthritis often has asymmetrical symptoms. Pain is aggravated by joint use and subsides with rest. Physical findings for the affected joints may include decreased range of motion, crepitus with movement, minimal local warmth without erythema, and enlargement of distal and proximal interphalangeal joints.

12. **a.** nonpharmacologic therapy plan for muscle injuries.
RICE is the mnemonic to remember the initial therapeutic strategy for muscle injuries. It stands for:
*R*est or immobilization of injured part
*I*ce or application of cold
*C*ompression, elastic wrap
*E*levation of affected area

13. **d.** herniated disc involving the S1 root.
A herniated disc is characterized by radicular pain; paresthesias may occur in the distribution of the involved nerve root. The most common disc ruptures involve the L5 or S1 nerve roots. An affected S1 root/L5–S1 disc involves pain in the buttocks, lateral leg, and malleolus and numbness in the lateral foot and posterior calf.

14. **c.** saline gargles
Symptomatic relief measures are appropriate for this individual. A rapid streptococcal antigen test is recommended for an adult with pharyngitis who meets two or more of the following criteria: fever, lack of cough, tonsillar exudates, tender anterior cervical adenopathy.

15. **d.** antiretroviral therapy during pregnancy
The risk of vertical transmission of the HIV virus from an HIV-positive person to the infant may be reduced to less than 1% if the parent receives multiagent antiretroviral therapy and has an undetectable viral load at delivery.

16. **d.** have severe renal function disorders
PrEP is contraindicated for individuals with severe renal function disorders. Laboratory tests for prospective PrEP recipients include renal function tests. Renal function tests should be repeated every 6 months while on PrEP.

17. **c.** response to drug therapy is monitored by HIV RNA levels
HIV RNA levels are useful for predicting progression of disease by indicating viral load and are used to monitor antiretroviral therapy.

18. **d.** AIDS
    PCP is an opportunistic infection that rarely occurs in healthy people. Most opportunistic infections occur in HIV-infected individuals with a CD4$^+$ count less than 200 cells/mm^3. PCP is a major AIDS-defining diagnosis.

19. **a.** 5 mm
    A 5-mm or greater skin reaction on the PPD test is considered positive in individuals who are living with HIV, immunocompromised, with abnormal chest radiograph findings consistent with healed TB lesions, or in recent close contact with a TB-infected person.

20. **a.** female sex, reproductive age group, Hispanic descent
    Risk factors for SLE include being of Black or Hispanic descent or having a first-degree relative with SLE.

21. **b.** presence of at least four combined signs, symptoms, and laboratory findings
    The American College of Rheumatology has set the SLE diagnostic criteria to include the presence of at least 4 of 11 criteria. These criteria include the presence of specific dermatologic symptoms; arthritis; serositis; renal, neurologic, and hematologic conditions; positive ANA test; and other immunologic positive tests.

22. **a.** periods of exacerbation and remission
    SLE is a chronic, inflammatory, multisystem disorder of the immune system characterized by periods of remission and exacerbation, with the course of the disease being unpredictable and highly variable.

23. **b.** Environmental factors
    The exact etiology of RA is unknown, although it is suspected to have an autoimmune component influenced by genetic, environmental, and perhaps hormonal factors.

24. **c.** 12 g/dL
    According to the World Health Organization, anemia is defined as hemoglobin <12 g/dL for women and <13 g/dL for men.

25. **c.** an upper respiratory infection
    Eustachian tube dysfunction secondary to URI (often viral) or allergies causes edema and congestion that impedes the flow of middle ear secretions; accumulation of secretions promotes the growth of pathogens.

26. **b.** comfort measures only
    Viral conjunctivitis usually has an acute onset, mild symptoms in one or both eyes, and a watery discharge. It may be associated with an upper respiratory infection and is self-limited. Cold compresses and liquid tears may offer relief of symptoms.

27. **b.** symptoms present for 10 or more days without clinical improvement
    Antibiotic treatment for acute sinusitis should be initiated if signs and symptoms are present for 10 or more days after the onset of upper respiratory symptoms or if symptoms first improve and then worsen again within 10 days.

28. **c.** Lymphocytic leukocytosis
    The classic triad of symptoms for mononucleosis is fever, sore throat, and swollen lymph nodes (particularly the anterior and posterior cervical chain). A monospot/heterophile antibody test will usually be positive within

1–2 weeks after onset of symptoms. The CBC will show lymphocytic leukocytosis, with 10% of cells being atypical.

29. **d.** people in their teens to early twenties
    Most clinically apparent mononucleosis infections occur in individuals 10–30 years old, with a peak rate in those ages 15–19 years old.

30. **b.** internal hemorrhoids
    Internal hemorrhoids originate above the anorectal line, are covered by a nonsensitive rectal mucosa, and are usually painless. The patient may present with bright red bleeding during defecation.

31. **a.** Abdominal pain is relieved with defecation.
    Abdominal pain and bloating are often relieved at least temporarily with defecation in patients with IBS. IBS is not characterized by symptoms that awaken the patient at night or by blood in the stools.

32. **d.** trial of elimination of dairy products
    A 2-week trial of lactose-free, fructose-free, or sorbitol-free foods (one at a time) may be considered to rule out food intolerance in a patient who has bloating, gas, abdominal distention, and diarrhea. Alosetron should be limited to use in those with severe chronic diarrhea–predominant IBS not responsive to conventional therapy. Lubiprostone and fiber supplements may be appropriate for the patient with constipation-dominant IBS.

33. **a.** systemic lupus erythematosus
    The prevalence of SLE is much higher in Black women (1 in 250) and Hispanic women (100 in 100,000) than in white women (12–39 in 100,000).

34. **d.** pain in the periumbilical area followed by localization to the RLQ
    Pain is the initial symptom in an appendicitis, beginning in the epigastrium or periumbilical area and localizing to the RLQ after several hours.

35. **b.** positive urea breath test
    Positive serology for *H. pylori* antibodies indicates previous exposure, not current/active infection. A serologic ELISA test detects IgG antibodies, indicating current or past infection with *H. pylori*. It may or may not revert to negative after treatment.

36. **c.** HBV surface antibody test
    A positive HBV surface antibody test indicates the resolution of HBV infection and immunity to future infection. The test will also be positive in individuals with immunity as a result of HBV vaccination.

37. **a.** Recombinant interferon alfa-2b
    Recombinant interferon alfa-2b is a medication that inhibits replication of the virus to improve viral load and reduce liver damage.

38. **c.** cholesterol
    Approximately 85%–95% of gallstones are composed primarily of cholesterol.

39. **b.** ultrasound
    This patient's symptoms are consistent with acute cholecystitis. Ultrasound has a 95% sensitivity in detecting

stones in the gallbladder. It is the best noninvasive imaging technique to diagnose acute cholecystitis.

40. **c.** Hepatitis C
As many as 80% of patients with hepatitis C will develop chronic hepatitis; 20%–30% eventually develop cirrhosis or hepatocellular carcinoma.

41. **c.** that hospital admission and cholecystectomy are the recommended treatment
Acute cholecystitis is managed with hospital admission and early cholecystectomy once the patient is stable.

42. **b.** The individual coughs during the night and has a bad taste in their mouth.
Acid regurgitation with GERD is most common when reclining, straining, bending, or stooping. This can cause coughing and a bad taste in the mouth.

43. **b.** Start them on H$_2$-receptor blockers
GI referral and diagnostic evaluation are needed if symptoms are chronic or refractory to therapy; if esophageal complications are suspected; or if the patient has dysphagia, weight loss, or evidence of GI bleeding. H$_2$-receptor blockers inhibit acid secretions and are effective for less severe GERD.

44. **d.** high-fat foods and chocolate may aggravate the problem
High-fat foods, chocolate, and peppermint decrease lower esophageal pressure, making reflux more likely

45. **a.** fasting plasma glucose ≥126 mg/dL
The criteria for diagnosis of diabetes include any of the following: fasting plasma glucose ≥126mg/dL, 2-hour postprandial glucose ≥200 mg/dL, HbA$_{1c}$ ≥6.5%, or random glucose ≥200mg/dL with classic symptoms of hyperglycemia or hyperglycemic crisis.

46. **b.** instructions to maintain fluid intake and limit the use of antidiarrheal agents
The most common causative agent in traveler's diarrhea is *E. coli*. If the patient does not have bloody stools or a fever, and symptoms are self-limiting, no stool evaluation or antibiotic treatment is needed.

47. **d.** inhibiting cholesterol absorption
Ezetimibe is a drug considered for use in combination with a moderate-intensity statin for individuals with dyslipidemia who need but cannot tolerate high-intensity statins. This drug works by inhibiting cholesterol absorption.

48. **a.** Graves' disease
Graves' disease accounts for 90% of hyperthyroidism cases. This autoimmune condition is characterized by excess synthesis and secretion of thyroid hormone caused by antibodies that stimulate TSH receptors.

49. **a.** Graves' disease
Hyperthyroidism caused by Graves' disease is characterized by exophthalmos

50. **a.** Low serum TSH and elevated free T$_4$
Low TSH is a result of excess circulation of thyroid hormone (T$_4$, T$_3$) with hyperthyroidism.

51. **c.** High TSH, low free T$_4$
Radioactive iodine treatment for Graves' disease usually results in long-term hypothyroidism; this outcome occurs in 70% of patients at 10 years.

52. **d.** No change in levothyroxine is indicated at this time. Levothyroxine has a half-life of 6 days and achieves a steady state slowly. Adjust the dose every 6 weeks until TSH normalizes.

53. **b. topical corticosteroids**
Factors that can exacerbate acne include hormonal cycling, use of topical corticosteroids, and contact with irritant oils or cosmetics.

54. **c.** the necessity for highly effective contraception
Isotretinoin is a known teratogen and is contraindicated for use during pregnancy or if the patient could become pregnant, and it should not be used in pregnancy because of its detrimental effects on the fetus.

55. **c.** tretinoin cream (Retin-A)
Tretinoin cream is an effective comedolytic agent for mild, noninflammatory acne that is applied topically to affected areas.

56. **b.** basal cell
Basal cell carcinoma is the most common skin cancer, accounting for approximately 75% of all skin cancers. It affects nearly 1 million people per year in the United States.

57. **b.** Basal cell carcinoma
Basal cell carcinoma has several clinical variants; nodular basal cell is most common. Basal cell carcinoma presents as waxy, semitranslucent nodules with rolled borders that may have central ulcerations and telangiectasias. These nodules are slow-growing lesions.

58. **d.** The individual should use sunscreen and sun-protective clothing when outdoors.
Photosensitivity is a characteristic of systemic lupus erythematosus. Malar skin rash and rash on other exposed body parts may occur with sun exposure. Sun exposure may also exacerbate disease activity.

59. **c.** Severe childhood sunburn
Risk factors for malignant carcinoma include history of changing mole, family and/or personal history of melanoma, history of nonmelanoma skin cancer, atypical nevus syndrome, fair complexion, and tendency to sunburn.

60. **d.** Tinea corporis
The classic presentation of tinea is a lesion with a central clearing surrounded by an advancing, red, scaly, elevated border. If the tinea is found on the body, it is classified as tinea corporis.

61. **b.** bacterial conjunctivitis
Bacterial conjunctivitis has an acute onset with itchy sensation/discomfort and mucopurulent discharge beginning in one eye and spreading to the other eye.

62. **c.** opioids
Alcohol, methotrexate, and statins are known teratogens.

63. **c.** NSAIDs
Lower back pain is located in the back, buttocks, or one or both thighs. Pain is usually aggravated by standing/flexion and relieved with rest/reclining. Increased pain occurs with flexion and negative SLR, with a normal neurologic exam. A radiograph of the lumbosacral spine or a referral to the neurologist is not necessary at this time. Bed rest is not recommended for the treatment of lower

back pain. NSAIDs would be an appropriate management for this patient.

64. **c.** aggressive treatment of infections
Precipitating factors for vaso-occlusive crises include infection, physical or emotional stress, blood loss, pregnancy, surgery, and high altitudes. Aggressive treatment of infections may prevent a crisis for the patient with sickle cell disease.

65. **c.** Yellowish, thickened nails
Tinea unguium is characterized by toenails being more frequently involved than fingernails and nails that are yellowish/thickened.

66. **a.** hepatocellular carcinoma
As many as 10% of hepatitis B–infected adults and 90% of those infected as neonates become chronic carriers, with an increased risk of cirrhosis and hepatocellular carcinoma.

67. **c.** acute or chronic infection with hepatitis B virus
Positive HBsAg indicates acute or chronic infection with hepatitis B virus. Positive IgM anti-HBc indicates acute infection and disappears in 3 to 13 months.

68. **b.** advised on lifestyle modifications and return to have BP checked in 3 to 6 months
An adult with a BP of 136/84 would be classified as having Stage I hypertension (SBP 130–139 and/or DBP 80–9). If this individual has a calculated 10-year risk of atherosclerotic cardiovascular disease less than 10%, lifestyle modifications are recommended as first line therapy with a recheck of BP in 3 to 6 months.

69. **d.** saline laxatives (milk of magnesia) for acute constipation
Saline laxatives draw water into the intestinal lumen, causing fecal mass to soften and swell; swelling stretches the intestinal lumen and simulates peristalsis.

70. **b.** confusion or disorientation
CURB-65 criteria include confusion, uremia (BUN > 19 mg/dL), respiratory rate greater than 30 breaths per minute, blood pressure <90 mm Hg systolic or <60 mm Hg diastolic, and age 65 or older. If an individual meets two or more of the five CURB-65 criteria for community-acquired pneumonia, the patient should be hospitalized for treatment.

71. **c.** treatment with azithromycin
Recommended first-line treatment of community-acquired pneumonia, whether viral or bacterial, is empiric antimicrobial therapy with an advanced-generation macrolide such as azithromycin. If the patient has risk factors for DRSP, the recommended antibiotic is a respiratory fluoroquinolone.

72. **b.** Abdominal bruit
Secondary hypertension may be the result of renal artery stenosis. An abdominal bruit may indicate renal artery stenosis.

73. **d.** The use of an ACE inhibitor is contraindicated during pregnancy because it is associated with fetal anomalies.
ACE inhibitors (e.g., captopril, enalapril) and ARBs (e.g., losartan, valsartan) are both contraindicated during pregnancy because of associated fetal anomalies.

74. **b.** Fine body hair on extremities
Physical examination findings with anorexia nervosa include emaciation, dry skin, fine body hair (lanugo), muscle wasting, peripheral edema, bradycardia, arrhythmias, hypotension, delayed sexual maturation, and stress fractures.

75. **c.** nasal crease
A common physical finding with perennial allergic rhinitis is a horizontal crease along the lower bridge of the nose from the patient pushing the nose upward and backward because of itching and nasal discharge.

76. **d.** duplex ultrasound
Duplex ultrasound has good sensitivity and specificity for the diagnosis of a patient who has an intermediate to high probability of DVT. A negative test, however, does not rule out DVT in the symptomatic patient, so other follow-up tests are needed.

77. **d. NSAIDs**
Treatment for superficial thrombophlebitis includes elevation of the affected limb, compression with an ace wrap, and NSAIDs.

78. **b.** psoriasis
The characteristic lesions of psoriasis are located on the knees, elbows, and scalp; have well-defined borders and an erythematous base; and have silvery scales overlaying the lesions.

79. **b.** LDL cholesterol < 70 mg/dL
Treatment goals for hyperlipidemia are based on risk factors. Diabetes is considered a CHD risk equivalent. The treatment goal for an individual who has hyperlipidemia and clinically manifested CHD or a CHD risk equivalent is an LDL-C of less than 70 mg/dL.

80. **b.** acute cholecystitis
Symptoms of acute cholecystitis include pain that starts in the epigastrium and then moves to the RUQ, accompanied with nausea and vomiting. The patient with acute cholecystitis has a stop in inspiratory effort because of the sharp increase in pain (Murphy's sign) when the RUQ is palpated.

81. **b.** iron deficiency
Diagnostic findings for iron-deficiency anemia include hypochromic microcytic RBCs, MCV less than 80 fL, increased RDW, a low serum ferritin less than 10 mg/L, and decreased reticulocyte count.

82. **c.** opioid antagonist used to reverse the physical effects of opioid overdose
Naloxone is an opioid antagonist used to reverse the physical effects of an opioid overdose. It reverses depression of the CNS and respiratory system.

83. **b.** Widespread musculoskeletal pain and tender points
Fibromyalgia is a syndrome characterized by chronic fatigue and by generalized, widespread musculoskeletal pain and stiffness associated with the finding of characteristic tender points of pain on physical examination.

84. **b.** dyslipidemia
Secondary causes of dyslipidemia include obesity; endocrine and metabolic disorders; obstructive liver disease;

renal disorders; and some medications that include corticosteroids, thiazide diuretics, antipsychotics, and beta blockers.

85. **b.** Mitral valve prolapse
A mid- or late systolic click is usually caused by mitral valve prolapse. A late systolic murmur may be present in case of mitral valve regurgitation.

86. **a.** Heard best when supine
Innocent murmurs are usually soft (grade 1 or 2), medium-pitch, systolic murmurs. They are heard best with the patient supine and disappear with standing or straining. They increase with increased cardiac output—for example, with pregnancy, exercise, or fever.

87. **a.** coronary heart disease
Coronary heart disease is the cause of death for one out of every three women each year.

88. **c.** deposition of cholesterol plaques.
The origin of most venous thrombi lies in Virchow's triad—endothelial damage, stasis, and hypercoagulability.

89. **a.** tenderness in the area of the involved vein
A localized area of edema, erythema, and tenderness of the involved vein in an extremity are suggestive of superficial phlebitis.

90. **a.** *Streptococcus pneumoniae*
The most common cause of bacterial community-acquired pneumonia is *S. pneumoniae*.

91. **b.** It is safer to be treated for asthma during pregnancy than to have symptoms and exacerbations.
Asthma exacerbations during pregnancy increase the risk for perinatal mortality, preterm birth, and low-birth-weight infants. First-line treatment during pregnancy includes the short-acting inhaled β_2 agonist albuterol and the inhaled corticosteroid budesonide.

92. **b.** elevated erythrocyte sedimentation rate
The 2010 American College of Rheumatology classification criteria for diagnosis of RA involves a score-based algorithm that includes joint involvement (stiffness, swelling), serology (RF, anti-citrullinated protein antibody), acute-phase reactants (C-reactive protein, erythrocyte sedimentation rate), and duration of symptoms.

93. **b.** Propranolol (beta blocker)
For patients who experience more than two severe headaches per month, who need acute treatment medication more than two times per week, or who are unable to tolerate abortive agents, consider prophylactic therapy: beta blockers such as propranolol/timolol, calcium channel blockers, or antiepileptic agents.

94. **c.** DMARDs and immunomodulating biologic agents may be combined if monotherapy is not effective.
DMARDs are the preferred therapy for long-term management of RA. Immunomodulating biologic agents are commonly used for individuals with RA who have toxicity and/or intolerance, or who cannot find relief with nonbiologic DMARDs; they may be used as initial therapy for individuals with severe RA, and they may be used in combination with DMARDs.

95. **d.** waist circumference greater than 35 inches
Metabolic syndrome is defined as pthe resence of at least three of five risk factors. For women, these include abdominal adiposity/waist circumference >35 inches, triglycerides ≥150 mg/dL, HDL-C <50 mg/dL, blood pressure ≥130/85, and fasting glucose ≥110 mg/dL.

96. **c.** erythema of the ear canal
Common physical examination findings with otitis media include a full or bulging tympanic membrane with absent or obscured landmarks, distorted light reflex, and postauricular or cervical lymphadenopathy.

97. **d.** tonsillar enlargement with exudate
Physical examination findings with infectious mononucleosis include tonsillar enlargement with exudate; palatal petechiae at the junction of the hard and soft palates (25% of cases); lymphadenopathy, particularly involving the posterior cervical chain; fever compatible with severity of infection; hepatomegaly (25%); and splenomegaly (50%). CBC will reveal lymphocytic leukocytosis with atypical lymphocytes common.

98. **b.** eczema
Symptoms of eczema include extremely itchy, dry patches of skin commonly on the face, wrists, hands, arms, knees, and genitals. Physical examination findings include erythematous, dry, scaly, excoriated patches of skin with lichenification in these areas.

99. **b.** All individuals considering pregnancy should be offered genetic carrier screening for cystic fibrosis and spinal muscular atrophy.
Additional genetic carrier screening decisions may be based on family history (both sides), ethnicity, history of child with a congenital anomaly, or CBC results suggesting a potential hemoglobinopathy. If an individual is found to be a carrier for a specific condition, the individual's reproductive partner should be offered screening to determine risk of having an affected child.

100. **b.** vitamin B_{12}–deficiency anemia
Macrocytic anemia (MCV > 100 fL) is found in people with vitamin B_{12} deficiency, folate deficiency, liver disease, and hypothyroidism.

101. **a.** Alendronate
Alendronate is indicated for prevention and treatment of osteoporosis. Given the patient's history of DVT, the patient should not use estrogen therapy or an estrogen agonist/antagonist because of the possible increased risk of a thromboembolic event. Calcitonin is indicated for treatment only; it is not appropriate for prevention.

102. **d.** Treatment decisions based on T-scores may vary according to risk factors.
Pharmacologic treatment is considered for postmenopausal individuals presenting with any of the following criteria: hip or vertebral fracture; T-score of 2.5 or less at the femoral neck or spine after appropriate evaluation to exclude secondary causes; T-score between 1.0 and 2.5 at femoral neck or spine and 10-year probability of hip fracture of 3% or greater; or a 10-year probability of major osteoporotic-related fracture of 20% or greater based on U.S.-adapted WHO algorithm.

103. **c.** A 60-year-old woman with measured height loss of 2 cm or more
Vertebral imaging for VFA is available on most modern DXA machines. Vertebral fracture is consistent with diagnosis of osteoporosis independent of BMD results; consider VFA for women who are age 70 or older if the BMD T-score is at or below 1.0; those age 65–69 if the BMD T-score is at or below 1.5; and postmenopausal individuals with a low trauma fracture during adulthood, historical height loss of 4 cm or more, prospective height loss of 2 cm or more, and recent or ongoing long-term glucocorticoid treatment.

104. **c.** Take the medication on an empty stomach.
Client instructions for taking alendronate include the following: take the medication with 8 oz of water in the morning at least 30 minutes before any beverage, food, or medication, and avoid lying down for at least 30 minutes and until intake of the first food of the day.

105. **a.** Amenorrhea
DSM-5 criteria for the diagnosis of anorexia nervosa include restriction of intake relative to requirements leading to significantly low body weight in the context of age, sex, and physical health; intense fear of gaining weight and/or persistent behavior that interferes with weight gain, even though the patient is at a significantly low body weight; and disturbed body image.

106. **d.** GGT
An elevated GGT level may indicate heavy or chronic alcohol use.

107. **c.** is experiencing post-traumatic stress disorder
PTSD occurs in 30%–65% of sexual assault survivors. PTSD is persistent anxiety lasting more than 1 month following an extremely traumatic event. Inability to concentrate and nightmares are characteristic of PTSD.

108. **a.** loss of interest in usual activities
Loss of interest in usual activities and/or sad or depressed mood most of the day, every day, are required for diagnosis of major depressive disorder, along with a complex of symptoms that may include fatigue, insomnia, difficulty concentrating, feelings of worthlessness, and others.

109. **c.** The patient can use any of the long-acting reversible contraceptives.
People with uncomplicated diabetes of less than 20 years' duration can use any of the available contraceptive methods, including long-acting reversible contraceptives, such as intrauterine contraception, progestin-only injections, and progestin-only implants. Combination hormonal contraceptives are also acceptable choices.

110. **d.** sense of hopelessness
Risk factors for suicide in the individual with major depressive disorder include, but are not limited to, a sense of hopelessness, substance abuse/family history of substance abuse, prior suicide attempt/family history of suicide attempt, living alone, medical illness, advanced age, and male sex.

111. **b.** panic disorder with agoraphobia
Agoraphobia is an anxiety disorder that includes avoidance of places or situations in which leaving suddenly may be difficult in the event that the individual has a panic attack. The recurrence of these panic attacks and fear related to their possible occurrence are considered panic disorder.

112. **b.** specific phobia
Anxiety is one of the most prevalent psychiatric disorders. Specific phobia is the most common type (25%), followed by social phobia (13%), PTSD (12% in women), general anxiety disorder (5%), and panic disorder (3.5%).

113. **d.** Impulsive behavior is a common characteristic
The typical age of onset for bulimia nervosa is late adolescence to early adulthood. The mortality rate for this eating disorder is lower than that for anorexia nervosa. Impulsive behaviors, such as shoplifting, alcohol and drug use, and unsafe sexual behaviors, are characteristic of bulimia nervosa.

114. **b.** nausea
Side effects of SSRIs include anxiety, insomnia/hypersomnia, headache, nausea, anorexia, and sexual dysfunction.

115. **a.** Alpraxolam (Xanax)
Alpraxolam (Xanax) is a benzodiazepine that should be used only for short-term management of generalized anxiety if needed for severe impairment until acceptable reduction of symptoms is achieved with an appropriate non-benzodiazepine medication, which may include selective serotonin reuptake inhibitors, selective norepinephrine reuptake inhibitors, or buspirone, and/or cognitive-behavioral therapy. Benzodiazepines have a high dependence and misuse potential.

116. **c.** markedly increased amounts of the substance needed to achieve intoxication or desired effect
Physiologic dependence on a substance is defined as evidence of characteristic withdrawal syndrome or use of the substance to avoid withdrawal and/or tolerance in which markedly increased amounts of the substance are needed to achieve intoxication or the desired effect.

117. **a.** erosion of tooth enamel
Erosion of tooth enamel may occur in the individual with bulimia nervosa as a result of frequent induced vomiting that exposes enamel to gastric acid.

118. **b.** The majority of rapes are committed by acquaintances.
The majority of rapes are perpetuated by an acquaintance rather than a stranger. *Rape* is a legal term whose definition may vary in different states, but typically includes the use of force, threat, or coercion and lack of consent in relation to sexual intercourse. The initial response of the individual who has been raped may range from being calm to anxious to angry.

119. **a.** Biguanides (metformin)
Metformin, a biguanide, is an oral hypoglycemic used in the treatment of type 2 diabetes. It works by decreasing hepatic glucose production and intestinal absorption of glucose and by increasing peripheral glucose uptake and utilization.

120. **c.** systemic corticosteroids
Severe exacerbations (peak flow < 60%) of asthma may require the use of a short course of oral steroids for 5–10 days.

121. **c.** initiate the medication at least 1 week prior to smoking cessation
Individuals should initiate bupropion hydrochloride sustained-release tablets (Zyban) 1–2 weeks before they stop smoking. This medication reduces the cravings that people with tobacco use disorder experience.

122. **b.** Influenza vaccination may be safely given in any trimester of pregnancy.
Administration of IIV is recommended for all individuals who will be in the second or third trimester of pregnancy during the influenza season. IIV is considered safe at any stage in pregnancy and during lactation. LAIV given intranasally is contraindicated in pregnancy.

123. **c.** 2 months and 6 months after the initial dose
The recommended schedule for the three-dose series HPV vaccination is initial dose, second dose 2 months after the initial dose, and third dose 6 months after the initial dose.

124. **c.** Live attenuated virus vaccines
Live attenuated virus vaccines are contraindicated during pregnancy. Rubella, measles, mumps, varicella, zoster, and the intranasal form of influenza vaccine (LAIV) are all live attenuated viruses.

125. **a.** biennial mammograms starting at age 50
The USPSTF recommends biennial mammograms for people assigned female at birth with chest tissue from 50 to 74 years of age.

126. **b.** dried beans
Dried beans, leafy green vegetables, citrus fruits and juices, and fortified cereals are good dietary sources of folic acid.

127. **d.** PLISSIT model
The clinician who is not a sex therapist can use the PLISSIT model to address sexual concerns and make appropriate referrals. The PLISSIT model includes permission giving, limited information, and specific suggestions provided by the clinician and referral for more intensive therapy if needed.

128. **d.** sexual orientation
Sexual orientation is a general term used to describe an individual's pattern of emotional, romantic, and sexual attraction to other people. Common variations include heterosexual, homosexual (gay or lesbian), bisexual, pansexual, and asexual. Gender identity is the internal sense that one is female, male, neither, both, or a different gender.

129. **d.** screening tests for early detection of disease states
Secondary prevention is the delivery of healthcare services focused on early detection of disease states as well as interventions that limit severity and morbidity (e.g., identification of risk factors, screening tests, counseling/education).

130. **b.** Chlamydia test
Routine annual screening for chlamydia and gonorrhea is recommended for sexually active people assigned female at birth age ≤25 years and in those >25 years with risk factors (e.g., new sex partner, more than one sex partner, sex partner with concurrent partners, transactional sex or other commercial sex work).

131. **c.** pregnant individuals if they have risk factors
The CDC and USPSTF recommend screening all individuals born between 1945 and 1965 one time if they have no other risk factors. Screen others based on risk factors—current injection or intranasal drug use, blood transfusion prior to 1992, long-term hemodialysis, born to parent with HCV infection, receipt of an unregulated tattoo, other percutaneous exposures, HIV infection.

132. **a.** a 40-year-old cisgender woman who smokes cigarettes and whose alcohol intake averages three drinks/day
Screen all cisgender women and transgender individuals using gender-affirming hormones at 65 years of age or older for osteoporosis/osteopenia with a BMD test. Screen postmenopausal people younger than 65 years of age with risk factors associated with increased fracture risk. Risk factors include low BMI, history of low-trauma fracture, smoking, alcohol intake ≥3 drinks/day, and family history of hip fracture or osteoporosis.

133. **b.** Interstitial cystitis/painful bladder syndrome
Interstitial cystitis/painful bladder syndrome is defined as an unpleasant sensation (pain, pressure, discomfort) perceived to be related to the urinary bladder. It is associated with lower urinary tract symptoms greater than 6 weeks' duration with the absence of infection. The individual may have lower abdominal pain that becomes worse during sexual intercourse and is relieved somewhat with urination. Physical examination findings may include suprapubic tenderness as well as tenderness along the anterior vaginal wall and urethra.

134. **b.** urge incontinence
Management/treatment of urge incontinence includes bladder retraining with scheduled voiding, biofeedback, Kegel exercises, avoidance of bladder irritants, and use of anticholinergic agents (oxybutynin chloride [Ditropan], tolterodine tartrate [Detrol]).

135. **a.** vaginal/local estrogen therapy for vaginal atrophy/genital syndrome of menopause
Vaginal (but not oral) estrogen therapy may be considered for peri/postmenopausal individuals with vaginal atrophy/genital syndrome of menopause to prevent urinary tract infections.

136. **d.** lung cancer screening and mammogram.
The USPSTF and American Cancer Society recommend screening individuals 55–74 (USPSTF up to age 80) annually for lung cancer with a low-dose CT scan if they have a 30+ pack-year smoking history and are still smoking or quit within the last 15 years. At age 63, annual or biennial mammograms are recommended. The patient should plan for another colonoscopy or other colorectal cancer screening and cervical cancer screening with HPV or cytology alone or co-testing at age 65.

137. **b.** 19 to 50 years of age
Iron requirements are highest for nonpregnant individuals in the age group that is most likely to be menstruating regularly.

138. **c.** irritable bowel syndrome
Digestive diseases, such as Crohn's disease, celiac disease, and milk allergy/lactose intolerance, increase the

risk for vitamin D deficiency. Individuals with dark skin, obesity, older that 59 years of age, and residing in northern areas are at increased risk for vitamin D deficiency.

139. **a.** Any alcohol use during pregnancy
There is no safe amount, type, or time to drink alcohol during pregnancy; alcohol is a known teratogen; use during pregnancy is one of the major preventable causes of congenital disabilities and developmental disabilities. To avoid fetal alcohol exposure before a person might be aware of being pregnant, encourage individuals who are trying to conceive to not drink; encourage individuals who are sexually active, drink alcohol, and could become pregnant to consider use of effective contraception.

140. **a.** You may be contagious 48 hours prior to symptom onset
All other options are false related to SARS CoV-2

141. **d.** Infectious mononucleosis
The client does not report a sore throat and the peak rate ages for IM is 15–19 years old. All others would be considered given the symptoms.

142. **c.** Ultrasound
Would recommend an ultrasound first along with a pregnancy test as well. CT would be the next imaging option if unclear; however, 85% of the time, an ultrasound is diagnostic. A KUB would not help nor would a chest XR.

143. **b.** Omeprazole 20 mg PO QD
Since it is a prolonged use of a proton pump inhibitor and puts the patient at risk for further complications of

decreased bone density, pneumonia, etc., all other medications are required and recommended, especially if not having any adverse effects from them.

144. **d.** This meets criteria for sickle cell trait
This patient is a carrier of the trait, and the next step would be to offer testing to the reproductive partner for this fetus. The patient does not meet all of the other criteria for the other answers.

145. **b.** Entry criterion first and then additional clinical/immunologic domains to have a total score ≥10
A positive ANA is the entry criterion and that must be met first. All other clinical and immunological domains to include the entry criterion must total ≥10. All other answers are incorrect.

146. **c.** Maintain levels per trimester-specific levels

147. **d.** Sumatriptan
Triptans are recommended as first-line abortive therapy for moderate to severe migraines.

148. **d.** Tenderness to palpation along the paraspinal muscles
Tenderness to palpation along the paraspinal muscles are classic symptoms of lumbosacral pain. Answers a and b are findings consistent with a herniated disc. Answer c is an emergency and likely cauda equina syndrome.

149. **a.** ≤12 g/dL

150. **d.** All of the above

Bibliography

Abrahami, D., McDonald, E. G., Schnitzer, M. E., Barkun, A. N., Suissa, S., & Azoulay, L. (2022). Proton pump inhibitors and risk of gastric cancer: population-based cohort study. *Gut, 71*(1), 16–24.

Abramson, B., Srivaratharajh, K., Davis, L., & Parapid, B. (2018). *Women and hypertension: Beyond the 2017 guideline for prevention, detection, evaluation, and management of high blood pressure in adults.* American College of Cardiology. https://www.acc.org/latest-in-cardiology/articles/2018/07/27/09/02/women-and-hypertension

Alexander, E. K., Pearce, E. N., Brent, G. A., Brown, R. S., Chen, H., Dosiou, C., Grobman, W. A., Laurberg, P., Lazarus, J. H., Mandel, S. J., Peeters, R. P., & Sullivan, S. (2017). 2017 guidelines of the American Thyroid Association for the diagnosis and management of thyroid disease during pregnancy and the postpartum. *Thyroid, 27*(3), 315–389. https://doi.org/10.1089/thy.2016.0457

American Academy of Dermatology. (n.d.). *Vitiligo: Tips for managing.* https://www.aad.org/public/diseases/color-problems/vitiligo#tips

American College of Cardiology. (2019). *2018 Guideline on the management of blood cholesterol.* https://www.acc.org/~/media/Non-Clinical/Files-PDFs-Excel-MS-Word-etc/Guidelines/2018/Guidelines-Made-Simple-Tool-2018-Cholesterol.pdf

American College of Cardiology & American Heart Association Task Force on Clinical Practice Guidelines. (2018). 2017 AHA/AAPA/ABC/ACPM/AGS/APHA/ASH/ASPC/NMA/PCNA guideline for the prevention, detection, evaluation, and management of high blood pressure in adults. *Journal of American College of Cardiology, 71*(19), e127–e248.

American College of Obstetricians and Gynecologists. (2008, reaffirmed 2019). *Practice bulletin no. 90: Asthma in pregnancy.* Author.

American College of Obstetricians and Gynecologists. (2008, reaffirmed 2016). Practice bulletin 91: Treatment of urinary tract infections in nonpregnant women. *Obstetrics and Gynecology, 111*(3), 785–794.

American College of Obstetricians and Gynecologists' Committee on Practice Bulletins—Obstetrics. (2019). ACOG Practice bulletin 203: Chronic hypertension in pregnancy. *Obstetrics and Gynecology, 133*(1), e26-e50. https://doi.org/10.1097/AOG.0000000000003020

American College of Obstetricians and Gynecologists. (2015). Practice bulletin 155: Urinary incontinence in women. *Obstetrics and Gynecology, 126*, e66–e81.

American College of Obstetricians and Gynecologists. (2016). Practice bulletin 162: Prenatal diagnostic testing for genetic disorders. *Obstetrics and Gynecology, 127*(5), e108–e122.

American College of Obstetricians and Gynecologists. (2019). Committee Opinion No. 762: Prepregnancy counseling. *Obstetrics and Gynecology, 133*(1), e78–e89.

American College of Obstetricians and Gynecologists. (2017, reaffirmed 2019). Practice bulletin 179: Breast cancer risk assessment and screening in average-risk women. *Obstetrics and Gynecology, 130*, e1–e16.

American College of Obstetricians and Gynecologists. (2021). *Updated cervical cancer screening guidelines.* https://www.acog.org/clinical/clinical-guidance/practice-advisory/articles/2021/04/updated-cervical-cancer-screening-guidelines

American College of Obstetricians and Gynecologists. (2022). *COVID-19 Vaccination Considerations for Obstetric-Gynecologic Care* https://www.acog.org/clinical/clinical-guidance/practice-advisory/articles/2020/12/covid-19-vaccination-considerations-for-obstetric-gynecologic-care?utm_source=redirect&utm_medium=web&utm_campaign=int

American College of Obstetricians and Gynecologists & Society for Maternal Fetal Medicine. (2019). Obstetric care consensus: Interpregnancy care. *Obstetrics and Gynecology, 133*(1), e51–e72.

American College of Obstetricians and Gynecologists (2020). Committee opinion no. 807: Tobacco and nicotine cessation during pregnancy. *Obstetrics and Gynecology, 135*(5), e221–e229.

American College of Rheumatology. (2010). *ACR-endorsed criteria for rheumatic diseases.* https://assets.contentstack.io/v3/assets/blte37|abb6b 278ab2c/blte43cd74b071b5873/rheumatoid-arthritis-classification -criteria-complete-article-2010.pdf

American Diabetes Association. (2019). Classification and diagnosis of diabetes mellitus. *Diabetes Care, 42*(suppl 1), S13–S28.

American Diabetes Association. (2021). Standards of medical care in diabetes. *Diabetes Care, 44*(supp.1), S1–232.

American Heart Association. (2019). Heart disease and stroke statistics— 2019 update: A report from the American Heart Association. *Circulation,* 139. https://healthmetrics.heart.org/wp-content/uploads /2019/02/Heart-Disease-and-Stroke-Statistics-%E2%80%93-2019- Update.pdf

American Heart Association Council on Epidemiology and Prevention Statistics Committee and Stroke Statistics Subcommittee (2019). Heart Disease and Stroke Statistics-2019 Update: A Report From the American Heart Association. *Circulation, 139*(10), e56-e528. https:// doi.org/10.1161/CIR.0000000000000659

American Thyroid Association & American Association of Clinical Endocrinologists. (2011). *Hyperthyroidism and other causes of thyrotoxicosis: Management guidelines of the American Thyroid Association and American Association of Clinical Endocrinologists.* http://www.thyroid .org/thyroid-guidelines/hyperthyroidism/

Anger, J., Lee, U., A. Ackerman, L., Chou, R., Chughtai, B., Clemens, J. Q., Chai, T. (2019). Recurrent uncomplicated urinary tract infections in women: American Urologic Association; Canadian Urologic Association; Society of Urodynamics, Female Pelvic Medicine and Urological Reconstruction. *Journal of Urology, 202*(2), 282–289.

Aringer, M., Costenbader, K., Daikh, D., Brinks, R., Mosca, M., Ramsey-Goldman, R., Smolen, J. S., Wofsy, D., Boumpas, D. T., Kamen, D. L., Jayne, D., Cervera, R., Costedoat-Chalumeau, N., Diamond, B., Gladman, D. D., Hahn, B., Hiepe, F., Jacobsen, S., Khanna, D., . . . Johnson, S. R. (2019). 2019 European League Against Rheumatism/American College of Rheumatology classification criteria for systemic lupus erythematosus. *Annals of the Rheumatic Diseases, 78*(9), 1151. https://doi.org/10.1136/annrheumdis-2018 -214819

Arnett, D., Blumenthal, R., Albert, M., Buroker, A., Goldberger, Z., et al. (2019). 2019 ACC/AHA guideline on the primary prevention of cardiovascular disease: Executive summary: A Report of the American College of Cardiology/American Heart Association Task Force on Clinical Practice Guidelines. *Circulation, 140*(11), e563–595.

Arnold, M. J., O'Malley, P. G., & Downs, J. R. (2021). Key recommendations on managing dyslipidemia for cardiovascular risk reduction: Stopping where the evidence does. *American Family Physician, 103*(8), 455–458. https://www.aafp.org/afp/2021/0415/p455.html

American Psychiatric Association. (2023). *Diagnostic and statistical manual of mental disorders* (5th ed. Text Revision). Author.

Auwaerter, P. G. (2022). *Johns Hopkins ABX Guide; Coronavirus COVID-19 (SARS-CoV-2).* https://www.hopkinsguides.com/hopkins /view/Johns_Hopkins_ABX_Guide/540747/all/Coronavirus _COVID_19__SARS_CoV_2_#4.0

Basile, K., Smith, S., Breiding, M., Black, M., & Mahendra, R. (2014). *Sexual violence surveillance: Uniform definitions and recommended data elements, Version 2.0.* National Center for Injury Prevention and Control, Centers for Disease Control and Prevention. https://www.cdc .gov/sexual-violence/communication-resources/sv_surveillance _definitionsl-2009-a.pdf

Basile KC, Smith SG, Friar N, Wang J (2022). Characteristics and impacts of sexual violence and stalking victimization by the same perpetrator using a nationally representative sample. *Journal of Aggression, Maltreatment, and Trauma.* https://doi.org/10.1080/10926771.2022.2 133660.

Basson, R. (2000). The female sexual response: A different model. *Journal of Sex and Marital Therapy,* 26, 51–65.

Basson, R. (2014). Sexuality and sexual disorders. *Clinical Update Women's Health Care, XIII*(2), 1–108.

Beloff, M. S., Greenspan, S. L., Insogna, K. L., Lewiecki, E. M., Saag, K. G., Singer, A. J., & Siris, E. S. (2022). The clinician's guide to prevention and treatment of osteoporosis. *Osteoporosis International, 33:*2049–2102.

Bharucha, A. E., & Wald, A. (2019). Chronic constipation. *Mayo Clinic Proceedings, 94*(11), 2340–2357.

Bharucha, A. E., & Lacy, B. E. (2020). Mechanisms, evaluation, and management of chronic constipation. *Gastroenterology, 158*(5), 1232–1249. https://doi.org/10.1053/j.gastro.2019.12.034

Buttaro, T., Trybulski, J., Polgar-Bailey, P., & Sandberg-Cook, J. (2017). *Primary care: A collaborative approach* (5th ed.). Elsevier.

Cason, P., Cwiak, C., Edelman, A., & Kowal, D. (2023). *Contraceptive technology.* Jones & Bartlett Learning.

CDC. (2014). *Planning and implementing screening and brief intervention for risky alcohol use: A step-by-step guide for primary care practices.* https:// stacks.cdc.gov/view/cdc/26542

CDC. (2015). Viral hepatitis serology training. https://www.cdc.gov /hepatitis/resources/professionals/training/serology/training.htm

CDC. (2018). *Annual surveillance report of drug-related risks and outcomes – United States,* 1–91.

CDC. (n.d.). *Stages of HIV infection.* https://wwwn.cdc.gov/hivrisk/what _is/stages_hiv_infection.html

CDC. (2020). *Influenza virus testing methods.* https://www.cdc.gov/flu /professionals/diagnosis/table-testing-methods.htm

CDC. (2020). *Testing recommendations for hepatitis C virus infection.* https://www.cdc.gov/hepatitis-c/hcp/diagnosis-testing/?CDC_AAref _Val=https://www.cdc.gov/hepatitis/hcv/guidelinesc.htm

CDC. (2021). Sexually transmitted infections treatment guidelines, 2021. *MMWR Recommendations and Reports, 70*(4),1–187.

CDC. (2022). *Influenza antiviral medications: Summary for Clinicians.* https:// www.cdc.gov/flu/professionals/antivirals/summary-clinicians.htm

CDC. (2022). *Key facts about influenza (flu).* https://www.cdc.gov/flu /about/keyfacts.htm

CDC. (2022). *Overview of Testing for SARS-CoV-2, the virus that causes COVID-19.* https://www.cdc.gov/coronavirus/2019-ncov/hcp/testing -overview.html

CDC. (2022). *Adult immunization schedule, United States,* 2022. https:// www.cdc.gov/vaccines/schedules/hcp/imz/adult.html

CDC. (2023). *About micronutrients.* https://www.cdc.gov/nutrition/php /micronutrients/

CDC. (2023). *Child and adolescent immunization schedule by age* (Addendum updated June 27, 2024). https://www.cdc.gov/vaccines/hcp/imz -schedules/child-adolescent-age.html?CDC_AAref_Val=https://www. cdc.gov/vaccines/schedules/hcp/imz/child-adolescent.html

CDC. (2024). *COVID-19 vaccination for people who are pregnant or breastfeeding.* https://www.cdc.gov/covid/vaccines/pregnant-or-breastfeeding .html?s_cid=SEM.GA:PAI:RG_AO_GA_TM_A18_C-CVD-Expectant Parents-Brd:covid%20booster%20breastfeeding:SEM00003&utm_id =SEM.GA:PAI:RG_AO_GA_TM_A18_C-CVD-ExpectantParents -Brd:covid%20booster%20breastfeeding:SEM00003&gad_source=1

CDC. (2024). *Fast facts HIV and women.* https://www.cdc.gov/hiv/data -research/facts-stats/women.html?CDC_AAref_Val=https://www.cdc .gov/hiv/group/gender/women/index.html

CDC. (2024). *Overdose data to action.* https://www.cdc.gov/overdose -prevention/php/od2a/index.html

Centers for Disease Control and Prevention. (2022). *Fact sheets – excessive alcohol use and risks to women's health.* Retrieved from https://www.cdc .gov/alcohol/fact-sheets/womens-health.htm

Centers for Disease Control and Prevention. 2024. *HV Surveillance Supplemental Report: Estimated HIV Incidence and Prevalence in the United States, 2018–2022.* https://stacks.cdc.gov/view/cdc/156513

Clemens JQ, Erickson DR, Varela NP, Lai HH. Diagnosis and treatment of interstitial cystitis/bladder pain syndrome. J Urol. 2022;208(1): 34–42.

Colantonio, L. D., Booth, J. N., Bress, A. P., Whelton, P. K., Shimbo, D., Levitan, E. B., Howard, G., Safford, M. M., & Muntner, P. (2018,

September 11). 2017 ACC/AHA Blood Pressure Treatment Guideline Recommendations and Cardiovascular Risk. *Journal of the American College of Cardiology, 72*(11), 1187–1197. https://doi.org/10.1016/j.jacc.2018.05.074

Colgan, R., Williams, M., & Johnson, J. (2011). *Diagnosis and treatment of acute pyelonephritis in women. American Family Physician, 84*(5), 519–526.

Drugs.com (2022). *Azelastine nasal Pregnancy and Breastfeeding Warnings.* https://www.drugs.com/pregnancy/azelastine-nasal.html

Drugs.com (2022). *Budesonide.* https://www.drugs.com/pro/budesonide-nasal-spray.html

Drugs.com (2022). *Nedocromil pregnancy and breastfeeding warnings.* https://www.drugs.com/pregnancy/nedocromil.html

Drugs.com (2022). *Theophylline pregnancy and breastfeeding warnings.* https://www.drugs.com/pregnancy/theophylline.html

Elsevier Drug Class Overview. (2023). Sodium-glucose cotransporter-2 (SGLT2) inhibitors. https://elsevier.health/en-US/preview/sodium-glucose-co-transporter-2-sglt2-inhibitors

Fontham, E., Wolf, A., & Church, T. (2020). Cervical cancer screening for individuals at average risk: 2020 guideline update from the American Cancer Society. *CA Cancer Journal for Clinicians, 70*(5), 321–346.

Food and Drug Administration. (2019) *Tetrahydrocannabinol (THC)-containing vaping products: Vaping illnesses.* https://www.fda.gov/safety/medical-product-safety-information/tetrahydrocannabinol-thc-containing-vaping-products-vaping-illnesses

Ford, B., Dore, M., & Harris, E. (2021). Outpatient primary care management of headaches: Guidelines from the VA/DoD. *American Family Physician, 104*(2), 316–320. https://www.proquest.com/scholarly-journals/outpatient-primary-care-management-headaches/docview/2572517811/se-2

Gaitonde, D. Y., Moore, F. C., & Morgan, M. K. (2019). Influenza: diagnosis and treatment. *American Family Physician, 100*(12), 751–758.

Galvez-Sánchez, C. M., & Reyes del Paso, G. A. (2020). Diagnostic criteria for fibromyalgia: critical review and future perspectives. *Journal of clinical medicine, 9*(4), 1219. http://doi.org/10.3390/cm9041219.

Garber, J., Cobin, R., Gharib, H, Hennessey, J., Klein, I., Mechanick, J. I.... Woeber, K. (2012). Clinical practice guidelines for hypothyroidism in adults: Cosponsored by the American Association of Clinical Endocrinologists and the American Thyroid Association. *Endocrinology Practice, 18*(6), 989–1028.

Gilbert LK, Zhang X, Basile KC, Breiding M, & Kresnow MJ. (2022). Intimate Partner Violence and Health Conditions Among US Adults—National Intimate Partner Violence Survey, 2010–2012. *Journal of Interpersonal Violence.* https://doi.org/10.1177/08862605221080147.

Greenbaum, J., Crawford-Jakubiak, J. E., & Committee on Child Abuse and Neglect. (2015). Child sex trafficking and commercial sexual exploitation: Health care needs of victims. *Pediatrics, 135,* 566–574.

Guttenplan, M. (2017). The evaluation and office management of hemorrhoids for the gastroenterologist. *Current Gastroenterology Reports, 19*(7), 30. https://doi.org/10.1007/s11894-017-0574-9

Ha, H., & Gonzalez, A. (2019). Migraine headache prophylaxis. *American Family Physician, 99*(1), 17–24.

Headache Classification Committee of the International Headache Society (IHS). (2018). The international classification of headache disorders, 3rd edition. *Cephalalgia: An International Journal of Headache, 38*(1), 1–211. https://doi.org/10.1177/0333102417738202

Institute of Medicine. (2010). *Dietary reference intakes for calcium and vitamin D.* Author.

Jonklaas, J., Bianco, A. C., Bauer, A. J., Burman, K. D., Cappola, A. R., Celi, F. S., Cooper, D. S., Kim, B. W., Peeters, R. P., Rosenthal, M. S., & Sawka, A. M. (2014). Guidelines for the treatment of hypothyroidism: Prepared by the American Thyroid Association Task Force on Thyroid Hormone Replacement. *Thyroid, 24*(12), 1670–1751. https://doi.org/10.1089/thy.2014.0028

Koyyada, A. (2021). Long-term use of proton pump inhibitors as a risk factor for various adverse manifestations. *Therapies, 76*(1), 13–21. https://doi.org/10.1016/j.therap.2020.06.019

Lacy, B. E., & Patel, N. K. (2017). Rome criteria and a diagnostic approach to irritable bowel syndrome. *Journal of Clinical Medicine, 6*(11), 99. https://doi.org/10.3390/jcm6110099

Masters, W., & Johnson, V. (1966). *Human sexual response.* Little Brown.

Meisenheimer, E. S., Epstein, C., & Thiel, D. (2022). Acute diarrhea in adults. *American Family Physician, 106*(1), 72. https://www.proquest.com/scholarly-journals/acute-diarrhea-adults/docview/2689648724/se-2

Menter A, Gelfand JM, et al. "Joint American Academy of Dermatology-National Psoriasis Foundation guidelines of care for the management of psoriasis with systemic nonbiologic therapies." *J Am Acad Dermatol.* 2020 Jun; 82(6),1445–1486.

Metlay, J. P., Waterer, G. W., Long, A. C., Anzueto, A., Brozek, J., Crothers, K., ... & Whitney, C. G. (2019). Diagnosis and treatment of adults with community-acquired pneumonia. An official clinical practice guideline of the American Thoracic Society and Infectious Diseases Society of America. *American Journal of Respiratory and Critical Care Medicine, 200*(7), e45–e67. https://doi.org/10.1164/rccm.201908-1581ST

Mohamadi, J., Ghazanfari, F., & Drikvand, F. M. (2019). Comparison of the effect of dialectical behavior therapy, mindfulness based cognitive therapy and positive psychotherapy on perceived stress and quality of life in patients with irritable bowel syndrome: a pilot randomized controlled trial. *Psychiatric Quarterly, 90*(3), 565–578.

National Heart, Lung, and Blood Institute. (2001). *Third report of the National Cholesterol Education Program Expert Panel on detection, evaluation, and treatment of high cholesterol in adults* (Adult Treatment Panel III). (NIH Publication No. 01 3095). Author.

National Heart, Lung, and Blood Institute. (2007). *Expert panel report 3: Guidelines for the diagnosis and management of asthma.* (NIH Publication No. 08-4051). Author.

National Institute on Alcohol Abuse and Alcoholism. (2019). *Alcohol use disorders.* https://www.niaaa.nih.gov/alcohol-health/overview-alcohol-consumption/alcohol-use-disorders

National Institutes of Health. (2022). *COVID-19 treatment guidelines; Special considerations in pregnancy and after delivery.* https://www.covid19treatmentguidelines.nih.gov/special-populations/pregnancy/

Petri, M. (2005). Review of classification criteria for systemic lupus erythematosus. *Rheumatic Diseases Clinics of North America, 31*(2), 245–254.

Preventive Services Task Force. (2021). Lung cancer: Screening. https://www.preventiveservicestaskforce.org/uspstf/recommendation/lung-cancer-screening

Raisi-Estabragh, Z., Kobo, O., Mieres, J. H., Bullock-Palmer, R. P., Van Spall, H. G. C., Breathett, K., & Mamas, M. A. (2023, September 19). Racial Disparities in Obesity-Related Cardiovascular Mortality in the United States: Temporal Trends from 1999 to 2020. *Journal of the American Heart Association, 12*(18), e028409. https://doi.org/10.1161/JAHA.122.028409

Ross, D. S., Burch, H. B., Cooper, D. S., Greenlee, M. C., Laurberg, P., Maia, A. L., Rivkees, S. A., Samuels, M., Sosa, J. A., Stan, M. N., & Walter, M. A. (2016). 2016 American Thyroid Association Guidelines for diagnosis and management of hyperthyroidism and other causes of thyrotoxicosis. *Thyroid, 26*(10), 1343–1421. https://doi.org/10.1089/thy.2016.0229

Schuiling, K., & Likis, F. (2022). *Gynecologic health: With an introduction to prenatal and postpartum care* (4th ed.). Jones & Bartlett Learning.

Schadewald, D. M., Pritham, U. S., Youngkin, E. Q., Davis, M. S., & Juve, C. (2020). *Women's health: A primary care clinical guide* (5th ed.). Pearson Education, Inc.

Seidman, M. D., Gurgel, R. K., Lin, S. Y., Schwartz, S. R., Baroody, F. M., Bonner, J. R., ... & Nnacheta, L. C. (2015). Clinical practice guideline: Allergic rhinitis. *Otolaryngology—Head and Neck Surgery, 152*(1_suppl), S1–S43.

Smith, R., Andrews, K., Brooks, D., Fedewa, S., Manassaram-Baptiste, D., et al. (2019). Cancer screening in the United States, 2019: A review of current American Cancer Society guidelines and current issues in cancer screening. *CA Cancer Journal for Clinicians, 69*(3), 184–210.

Snyder, M. J., Guthrie, M., & Cagle, S. (2018). Acute appendicitis: Efficient diagnosis and management. *American Family Physician, 98*(1), 25–33.

Sussman, R. D., Syan, R., & Brucker, B. M. (2020). Guideline of guidelines: urinary incontinence in women. *BJU International, 125*(5). Https://doi.org/10.1111/bju.14927

Virani, S. S., Newby, L. K., Arnold, S. V., Bittner, V., Brewer, L. C., ... & Williams, M. S. (2023). 2023 AHA/ACC/ACCP/ASPC/NLA/PCNA guideline for the management of patients with chronic coronary disease: a report of the American Heart Association/American College of Cardiology Joint Committee on Clinical Practice Guidelines. *Journal of the American College of Cardiology, 82*(9), 833-955. https://doi.org/10.1016/j.jacc.2023.04.003

Stevens, A. (2021). Streamlining a carrier screening routine into practice: Proactive prepregnancy planning. *Women's Healthcare, A Clinical Journal for NPs, 9*(4), 20–28, 49.

Substance Abuse and Mental Health Services Administration (SAMHSA). (2015). *Medication and counseling treatment.* http://www.samhsa.gov/medication-assisted-treatment/treatment

Substance Abuse and Mental Health Services Administration (SAMHSA). (2020). 2018 National survey on drug use and health (NSDUH). https://www.samhsa.gov/data/nsduh/reports-detailed-tables-2018-NSDUH

Substance Abuse and Mental Health Services Administration. (2022). *2020 national survey on drug use and health: Lesbian, gay, and bisexual (LGB) adults.* https://www.samhsa.gov/data/report/2020-nsduh-lesbian-gay-bisexual-lgb-adults

Tharpe, N., Farley, C., & Jordan, R. (2022). *Clinical practice guidelines for midwifery and women's health* (6th ed.). Jones & Bartlett Learning.

Trafficking Victim Protection Act. (2017). *Fight slavery now!* https://fightslaverynow.org/why-fight-there-are-27-million-reasons/the-law-and-trafficking/trafficking-victims-protection-act/trafficking-victims-protection-act

The Trevor Project. (2023). U.S. National survey on the mental health of LGBTQ young people. https://www.thetrevorproject.org/survey-2023/assets/static/05_TREVOR05_2023survey.pdf

United Nations Office on Drugs and Crime. (2017). *Human trafficking.* https://www.unodc.org/unodc/en/human-trafficking/what-is-human-trafficking.html

U.S. Department of Health and Human Services, Panel on Antiretroviral Guidelines for Adults and Adolescents. (2024). *Guidelines for the use of antiretroviral agents in HIV-1–infected adults and adolescents.* https://clinicalinfo.hiv.gov/sites/default/files/guidelines/documents/adult-adolescent-arv/guidelines-adult-adolescent-arv.pdf

U.S. Department of Health and Human Services. (2018). *Physical activity guidelines for Americans* (2nd ed.). Author.

U.S. Department of Health and Human Services (2020). *Dietary guidelines for Americans 2020–2025.* Author.

U.S. Preventive Services Task Force. (2016). *Statin use for the primary prevention of cardiovascular disease in adults: Preventive medication.* https://www.uspreventiveservicestaskforce.org/Page/Document/RecommendationStatementFinal/statin-use-in-adults-preventive-medication1

U.S. Preventive Services Task Force. (2016). *Testicular cancer: Screening.* https://www.uspreventiveservicestaskforce.org/Page/Document/RecommendationStatementFinal/testicular-cancer-screening

U.S. Preventive Services Task Force. (2018). *Cervical cancer: Screening.* https://www.uspreventiveservicestaskforce.org/Page/Document/RecommendationStatementFinal/cervical-cancer-screening2

U.S. Preventive Services Task Force. (2018). *Prostate cancer: Screening.* https://www.uspreventiveservicestaskforce.org/uspstf/recommendation/prostate-cancer-screening

U.S. Preventive Services Task Force. (2018). *Unhealthy alcohol use in adolescents and adults: Screening and behavioral counseling interventions.* https://www.uspreventiveservicestaskforce.org/Page/Document/RecommendationStatementFinal/unhealthy-alcohol-use-in-adolescents-and-adults-screening-and-behavioral-counseling-interventions

U.S. Preventive Services Task Force. (2018). *Weight loss to prevent obesity-related morbidity and mortality in adults: Behavioral interventions.* https://www.uspreventiveservicestaskforce.org/Page/Document/RecommendationStatementFinal/obesity-in-adults-interventions1

U.S. Preventive Services Task Force. (2019). *Breast cancer: Screening.* https://www.uspreventiveservicestaskforce.org/Page/Document/RecommendationStatementFinal/breast-cancer-screening1

U.S. Preventive Services Task Force. (2019). *HIV infection: Screening.* https://www.preventiveservicestaskforce.org/uspstf/recommendation/huma-immuno-deficiency-virus-hiv-infection-screening

U.S. Preventive Services Task Force. (2021). *Colorectal cancer: Screening.* https://www.preventiveservicestaskforce.org/uspstf/recommendation/colorectal-cancer-screening

U.S. Preventive Services Task Force. (2021). *Hypertension in adults: Screening.* https://www.preventiveservicestaskforce.org/uspstf/recommendation/hypertension-in-adults-screening

Woo, T., & Robinson, M. (2020). *Pharmacotherapeutics for advanced practice nurse prescribers* (5th ed.). F. A. Davis.

CHAPTER 4

Gynecologic, Reproductive, Sexual, and Menopause Health

Beth M. Kelsey

Sandi Tenfelde

Signey Olson

Female Reproductive Anatomy

- Reproductive organs/structures—breasts, pelvic musculature, bones and joints, external genitalia, internal pelvic organs/structures
  1. Breast (**Figure 4-1**)—a modified sebaceous/mammary gland responsible for lactation; located within the superficial fascia of the anterior chest wall over the pectoral muscles; extends from clavicle and second rib down to the sixth rib and from the sternum across the midaxillary line; a triangle of breast tissue (also known as the tail of Spence) extends laterally across the anterior axillary fold
     a. Breast attached to skin and underlying muscle by fibrous tissue
     b. Suspensory ligaments (also known as Cooper's ligaments) support glandular structures of the breast, allowing mobility on the chest wall
     c. Adipose tissue surrounds superficial and peripheral areas of the breast
     d. Firm transverse ridge of compressed tissue may be present along the lower edge of the breast called the inframammary ridge
     e. Lobes—sections of the breast composed of glandular tissue and surrounded by fatty and connective tissue radiating around the nipple; 15–20 in each breast
     f. Lobules—small branching glands within each lobe containing tiny, hollow sacs called alveoli, which are responsible for milk production
     g. Each lobe empties into a single lactiferous duct that opens out through the nipple; lactiferous ducts enlarge behind the nipple to form small reservoirs called lactiferous sinuses
     h. Unique proliferation occurs under the influence of estrogen during puberty
     i. Nipple—composed of pigmented erectile tissue, areola, and areolar glands (also known as Montgomery's glands); terminus into which lactiferous sinuses secrete milk; multiple duct openings
        (1) Erectile tissue—contains smooth muscle fibers that contract in response to tactile, sensory, or autonomic stimuli

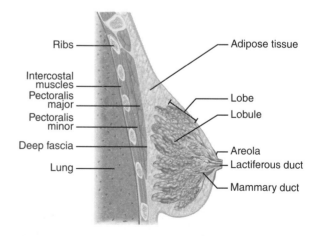

Figure 4-1 Structure of the breast and mammary glands

Ribs, Intercostal muscles, Pectoralis major, Pectoralis minor, Deep fascia, Lung, Adipose tissue, Lobe, Lobule, Areola, Lactiferous duct, Mammary duct

(2) Areola—circular pigmented area that surrounds the nipple

(3) Montgomery's glands—sebaceous glands that circle the nipple located within the areola

(4) Nipples usually are everted—protrude out from the surface of the breast; long-standing inversion is a normal variant; recent or fixed flattening or depression constitutes retraction that may be caused by an underlying cancer

(5) Supernumerary nipples—small amount of breast tissue occasionally found along the embryonic ridge of mammary tissue extending from the axilla, over the breasts, and down toward the groin; no pathologic significance

j. Lymphatics—most drain toward the axilla

(1) Central nodes along chest wall, high in axilla between anterior and posterior axillary folds; most likely to be palpable; pectoral, subscapular, lateral nodes drain into central nodes

(2) Central nodes drain into infraclavicular and supraclavicular nodes; the internal mammary chain also drains into infraclavicular nodes

2. Pelvic musculature, bones, and joints
   a. Perineal muscles
      (1) Bulbocavernosus—surrounds the vagina and acts as the weak sphincter
      (2) Ischiovernosus—surrounds the clitoris; responsible for clitoral erection
      (3) Superficial/deep transverse perineal muscles—converge with urethral sphincter
      (4) External anal sphincter
   b. Pelvic floor muscles
      (1) Levator ani—pubococcygeus, iliococcygeus, and puborectalis muscles
      (2) Pubococcygeus—pubovaginalis, puborectalis, and pubococcygeus proper
      (3) Pelvic floor muscles along with ligaments and fascia support abdominal and pelvic organs, maintain continence, and facilitate passage of the fetus during birth
   c. Pelvic bones and joints
      (1) Pelvis composed of four bones—two innominate bones (hip bones), sacrum, and coccyx
      (2) Each innominate bone has three parts—ilium, ischium, pubis
      (3) Four joints within the bony pelvis—two sacroiliac joints, sacrococcygeal joint, and symphysis pubis; during pregnancy under the influence of relaxin and progesterone, these joints soften and become more elastic, allowing for enlargement of pelvic dimensions

3. External genitalia (**Figure 4-2**)—composed of the vulva and its associated structures
   a. Vulva—visible external structures bordered by symphysis pubis anteriorly, buttocks posteriorly, and thighs laterally; develops as a secondary sex characteristic under the influence of estrogen during puberty
      (1) Mons pubis—fatty tissue prominence overlying symphysis pubis, covered by coarse hair in an inverted triangular pattern

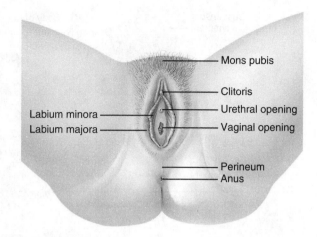

Figure 4-2 Female external genitalia

(2) Labia majora—two longitudinal folds of adipose tissue extending from the mons pubis downward and enclosing four structures:
   (a) Labia minora—thin folds inside/parallel to the labia majora; forms prepuce anteriorly, encloses the vestibule, and terminates in the fourchette above the perineum
   (b) Clitoris—a complex erectile body of tissue composed of an external glans and internal vestibular bulbs and corpus cavernosum; abundant supply of sensory nerve endings; rich vascular supply; important for sexual response
   (c) Vestibule—contains urethral/vaginal openings, hymen, paraurenthral or lesser vestibular glands (also known as Skene's glands) on each side of the urethral meatus, greater vestibular glands (also known as Bartholin's glands) with openings located posteriorly on each side of vaginal orifice
   (d) Perineum—located between the fourchette anteriorly and the anus posteriorly

4. Internal pelvic structures (**Figure 4-3**)—develop primarily because of stimulation by estrogen initiated during puberty; structures reach their adult size/appearance by approximately age 16
   a. Vagina—muscular/membranous canal that connects the external genitalia to the uterus
      (1) Length—approximately 7 cm anterior, 10 cm posterior
      (2) Stratified squamous epithelium
      (3) Rugae—transverse folds in sidewalls; allows for distention during coitus and childbirth
      (4) pH—acidic because of the prevalence of lactobacilli, which in turn is due to the influence of estrogen initiated during puberty
      (5) Upper part of vagina surrounds cervix, creating recessed spaces called fornices—anterior, posterior, lateral; rectovaginal pouch separates posterior fornix and rectum
   b. Uterus—pear-shaped organ that is composed of the following:

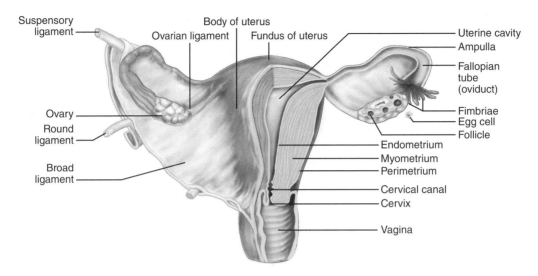

Figure 4-3 Female internal genital anatomy

(1) Cervix—round, firm terminus to the uterus that protrudes into the vagina; approximately 2–3 cm in diameter depending on parity, about 2.5 cm in length
   (a) Surface generally smooth but may have single or multiple translucent nodules (nabothian cysts) of no pathologic significance
   (b) Os—opening in cervix that provides access to the uterine cavity; external os is proximal to the vagina, and internal os is proximal to the uterine cavity; external os small, round or oval if nulliparous, may appear larger and slit-like or stellate after vaginal births
   (c) Squamocolumnar junction—juncture of the squamous epithelium covering the cervical body (ectocervix) and the columnar epithelium lining the endocervix; before puberty, junction may be visible as broad band of columnar epithelium circling external os (ectropion)
   (d) Transformation zone—area around the squamocolumnar junction where squamous metaplasia occurs
   (e) Squamous metaplasia—process whereby columnar cells of the endocervix are replaced by mature squamous epithelium
(2) Uterine body—extends upward from cervix and lies in the pelvic cavity; contains cavity or potential space that can accommodate pregnancy
   (a) Located between the bladder and the rectum
   (b) Approximately 8 cm in length, 5 cm in width, 2.5 cm in thickness
   (c) Composed externally of thick myometrial muscles (myometrium)
   (d) Composed internally of columnar epithelium (endometrium); shed during menstruation

   (e) Fundus—top portion where fallopian tubes insert
   (f) Isthmus (lower uterine segment)—immediately superior to cervix
   (g) Corpus—main body
   (h) Position of the uterus within the pelvis described in terms of the direction in which the corpus is inclined or tilted and flexion between the corpus and the cervix—anteverted, anteflexed, retroverted, retroflexed, midposition (see Figure 2-3 in Chapter 2, *Health Assessment and Diagnostic Tests*)
   (i) Supported by numerous ligaments—broad, round, cardinal, uterosacral, pubocervical; allow for mobility and accommodate increased uterine size during pregnancy
c. Oviducts (also known as Fallopian tubes)—ciliated muscular tubes that transport ova from the ovaries to the uterus
   (1) Length—approximately 10 cm
   (2) Interstitial portion—within the uterus
   (3) Isthmus—main body
   (4) Ampulla—adjacent to the ovary; receives ova at ovulation
   (5) Fimbriated ends/infundibulum
d. Ovaries—pair of endocrine organs located at the end of oviducts
   (1) Responsible for secretion of steroid hormones—estrogen/progesterone
   (2) Approximately 3 cm × 2 cm × 1 cm
   (3) Cyclic release of ovum
   (4) Supported by numerous ligaments—broad ligament, ovarian ligament, suspensory ligament
e. Lymphatics—lymph from the vulva and lower vagina drains into inguinal nodes; lymph from internal genitalia and upper vagina drains into pelvic and abdominal nodes

Female Reproductive Physiology

- Hypothalamic–pituitary–ovarian (H-P-O) axis
  1. Three endocrine organs work together in an intricate and coordinated manner, responding to positive and negative feedback loops to regulate steroid hormone production
  2. Gonadotropin-releasing hormone (GnRH)—released from the hypothalamus in a pulsatile fashion
  3. Gonadotropins—follicle-stimulating hormone (FSH) and luteinizing hormone (LH); released from the anterior pituitary gland in response to GnRH
  4. Steroid hormones—estrogen, progesterone, androgens; primarily produced in ovaries in response to FSH and LH
  5. Negative and positive feedback loops related to estrogen (E) and progesterone (P) levels control FSH and LH secretion
  6. Negative feedback loops—when E and P reach levels above a set point, the hypothalamus decreases secretion of GnRH, which leads to a decrease in secretion of FSH and LH; when E and P levels fall below the set point, the hypothalamus increases secretion of GnRH, which leads to an increase in secretion of FSH and LH
  7. Positive feedback loop—when E reaches a peak just before ovulation, the hypothalamus increases secretion of GnRH, causing a surge of FSH and LH (primarily LH) and subsequent release of mature ovum from the ovary
- Ovarian hormones—see **Table 4-1**
  1. Three major classes of steroid hormones produced primarily by ovaries (follicles, corpus luteum, stroma); also produced by the adrenal gland, peripheral tissues

Table 4-1 Ovarian Hormones

Hormone	Location of Production	Main Functions
Estrogen	Ovaries, adrenal cortex, conversion of androgens in adipose tissue, placenta	Maturation of reproductive organs; development of secondary sex characteristics; closure of long bones; regulation of menstrual cycle; maternal physiologic adaptations of pregnancy; metabolic effects on several other organs
Estradiol—most potent and plentiful estrogen in reproductive years	Ovarian follicles and corpus luteum, small amounts from adrenal cortex	See estrogen for function
Estrone—major source of estrogen after menopause	Ovaries, adrenal cortex, conversion of androgens in peripheral adipose tissue	See estrogen for function
Estriol—least potent estrogen; major source of estrogen during pregnancy	Placenta, small amounts in ovaries as metabolite of estradiol and estrone	See estrogen for function
Progesterone	Ovaries, corpus luteum, small amounts from adrenal cortex	Contributes to mammary gland development; regulation of menstrual cycle; maternal physiologic adaptations in pregnancy
Androgens	Ovaries, adrenal cortex	Contribute to long bone growth; growth of pubic and axillary hair
Testosterone	Ovaries, adrenal cortex, peripheral conversion of other androgens in adipose tissue	Serves as precursor in estradiol synthesis; see androgens for other functions
Androstenedione	Ovaries, adrenal cortex	Weak androgen that serves as precursor for estrogen synthesis
Activin	Ovarian follicular fluid, anterior pituitary gland	Stimulates follicle-stimulating hormone (FSH) secretion
Inhibin	Ovarian follicular fluid	Inhibits FSH secretion by binding to activin
Follistatin	Anterior pituitary gland, found in ovarian follicular fluid	Inhibits FSH secretion by binding to activin
Anti-Müllerian hormone (AMH)	Small, undeveloped (primordial) follicles	Inhibits FSH-dependent follicular growth of primordial follicles; role in selective recruitment of follicles that will continue to grow and develop
Insulin-like growth factors	Liver and ovaries are major sources; multiple sites throughout body	Involved in growth and differentiation in response to growth hormone; promote steroidogenesis by stimulating increase in size and number of FSH and luteinizing hormone (LH) receptors

a. Estrogen—estradiol, estrone, estriol
b. Progesterone
c. Androgens

2. Several nonsteroidal hormones and growth factors contribute to ovarian function
   a. Polypeptide hormones produced by ovaries—activin, inhibin, follistatin
   b. Anti-Müllerian hormone (AMH)
   c. Polypeptides produced in the liver and ovaries—insulin-like growth factors

3. Prostaglandins—group of lipid compounds derived from fatty acids at different sites in the body via enzymatic action (prostaglandin synthetase enzymes) acting at target sites near the area of secretion
   a. Regulate contraction and relaxation of smooth muscle
   b. Peak levels produced by endometrium in the late secretory phase
   c. Stimulate uterine myometrial contractions

4. Sex hormone–binding globulin (SHBG)
   a. Produced in the liver
   b. Serum protein that binds to estrogens and androgens in blood; protein-bound hormones can move through general circulation to target tissues throughout the body; target tissues have receptors specific to a particular hormone
   c. Only a certain number of hormone molecules are released at a time to maintain the equilibrium of bound and unbound molecules
   d. Factors that increase SHBG—hyperthyroidism, pregnancy, estrogen-containing oral contraception
   e. Factors that decrease SHBG—obesity, hyperinsulinemia, androgens
   f. Biological activity of these hormones in a particular tissue depends on the presence of specific receptors, the number of available receptors, and the local concentration of unbound hormone

5. Prolactin
   a. Hormone produced in the anterior pituitary gland
   b. Progressive release during pregnancy
   c. Stimulates synthesis of milk proteins in mammary tissue
   d. Stimulates epithelial growth in the breast during pregnancy

- Puberty/adolescence—*adolescence* means "to grow up"; *puberty* denotes the biology of adolescence, beginning around age 9 years and culminating in the development of regular menstrual cycles; some variations with ethnicity, race, and nutritional status
  1. Hormonal changes—begin as H-P-O axis matures
  2. Physical changes—physical characteristics of breast and pubic hair development and distribution delineate progressive advancement of physiologic maturity
     a. Growth spurt—may grow from 6 to 11 cm taller; greatest height velocity (peak of growth spurt) occurs around age 12 or just prior to onset of menses
     b. Thelarche—breast development; begins with breast budding (elevation of breast and nipple as a small mound) around age 9; progresses to conical shape with further enlargement of elevation but no separation of contours, then projection of areola and nipple to form second mound above level of breast, followed by fully developed breast with round contour and projection of nipple only around age 17
     c. Adrenarche—growth of pubic and axillary hair; results from secretion of adrenal androgens; usually starts after breast development begins; starts with sparse growth of long downy hair along labia; progresses to coarser, curlier hair spreading sparsely over the pubic symphysis, then further spread eventually including the medial surface of the thighs
     d. Menstruation—results from shedding of estrogen-primed endometrium; average age is 12.5 years following peak height velocity
     e. Tanner stages—used to assess progressive sexual maturity changes that occur in breast development (thelarche) and pubic hair growth (adrenarche)
  3. Delayed onset of puberty—secondary sexual characteristics begin development later than average age; usually a normal variant and catch-up occurs; defined as no breast growth by age 14 or no skeletal growth spurt by age 15
  4. Precocious puberty—breast or pubic hair development before age 7 in white females or age 6 in Black females; 75% of cases are idiopathic; evaluate to rule out congenital or neoplastic causes

- Menstrual cycle (**Figure 4-4**)
  1. Cycle length: Timed from day 1 of one menstrual bleed to day 1 of next menstrual bleed; average 28 days, plus or minus 2 days; duration of bleeding 4–6 days, plus or minus 2 days; volume average 40 cc
  2. Ovarian cycle—defined by ovarian changes
     a. Follicular phase
        (1) Begins day 1 of menses
        (2) Variable length (time frame)
        (3) Estradiol (E_2) and progesterone levels are low at the end of the previous cycle
        (4) GnRH stimulates the anterior pituitary gland to release FSH and LH
        (5) Cohort of follicles recruited in ovaries mature and produce E_2
        (6) High levels of E_2 result in a decrease in FSH and LH
        (7) Dominant follicle with the greatest number of E_2 receptors emerges, and other follicles undergo atrophy causing a decrease in E_2
        (8) Drop in E_2 causes the release of high levels of FSH and LH
        (9) Dominant follicle begins producing high levels of E_2
        (10) LH surge begins with ovulation occurring 32–44 hours later
     b. Ovulation
        (1) LH surge peaks 10–12 hours before ovulation
        (2) Prostaglandins and proteolytic enzymes break down the follicular wall
        (3) Dominant follicle ruptures, releasing oocyte

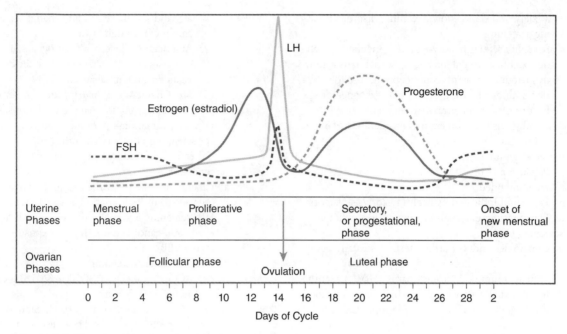

Figure 4-4 Phases of the menstrual cycle

(4) Oocyte can be fertilized for 12–24 hours after released
c. Luteal phase
   (1) Begins after ovulation occurs
   (2) Approximately 14 days plus or minus 2 days in length
   (3) Corpus luteum (CL) formed from a ruptured follicle
   (4) CL produces high levels of progesterone peaking at 7–8 days postovulation
   (5) CL produces moderate levels of estrogen
   (6) If no pregnancy occurs, the CL regresses, and both progesterone and E2 levels drop
   (7) Luteal phase ends with the onset of menses
3. Uterine cycle—defined by endometrial changes
   a. Proliferative phase—estrogen influence
      (1) Endometrium grows/thickens
      (2) Lasts approximately 10 days from end of menses to ovulation
   b. Secretory phase—progesterone influence
      (1) Average 12–16 days
      (2) From ovulation to menses
      (3) Endometrial hypertrophy
      (4) Increased vascularity
      (5) Favorable for implantation of fertilized ovum
   c. Menstruation—declining progesterone from CL
      (1) Endometrium undergoes involution, necrosis, sloughing
      (2) Average 3–6 days
4. Other physical/physiologic changes during the menstrual cycle
   a. Cervical mucus
      (1) After menses in the early follicular phase—scant, thick, cloudy, low elasticity
      (2) Late follicular phase—increasing amount, thin, clear, becomes more elastic

(3) At ovulation—abundant, highly elastic, thin, clear cervical mucus under the influence of estrogen; can stretch mucus between thumb and index fingers (spinnbarkeit); characteristic ferning appearance if mucus observed under microscope
   (4) After ovulation—cervical mucus again becomes thick with low elasticity under the influence of progesterone; impenetrable to sperm
   b. Basal body temperature (BBT)
      (1) BBT is the temperature of the body at rest
      (2) Lowest in follicular phase
      (3) Increases after ovulation under the influence of progesterone
      (4) Remains elevated until 2–4 days before menses

Wellness Visits: The Reproductive Years

- Includes health history, physical examination, screening tests, counseling, and immunizations based on age, risk factors, and individual's concerns
- General health history, physical examination, screening tests, immunizations, and health promotion counseling are covered in other sections of this text
- The focus of this section is reproductive/sexual/gynecologic health
- Adolescent (13–20 years of age)
  1. Health history
     a. Menstrual, gynecologic, and obstetric history
     b. Psychosocial assessment—family and peer relationships; emotional, physical, or sexual abuse by family, peers, or partner; drug/alcohol use;

anxiety and depression screening, disordered eating screening

c. Sexuality/sexual history—sexual orientation, gender identity, sexual practices, sexual satisfaction, dyspareunia, use of contraception, use of condoms, understanding of consent, exchange of sex for drugs or money/transactional sex

d. Conduct risk assessment for consideration of *BRCA 1/2* testing

2. Physical examination
   a. Pelvic and breast examinations not routinely recommended
   b. Perform if indicated by health history/risk factors
   c. May consider external-only genital examination

3. Screening tests
   a. Chlamydia and gonorrhea tests if sexually active (urine or self-collected vaginal specimen)
   b. Human immunodeficiency virus (HIV) screening test if sexually active; yearly if high risk; evaluate if candidate for HIV preexposure prophylaxis (PrEP)
   c. Other as indicated by history/risk factors; see Chapter 3, *Primary Care.*

4. Counseling/education
   a. Expected body changes during puberty
   b. Reproductive life planning—plan for having children, timing, use of contraception, prepregnancy care
   c. Safer sex practices—abstinence, outercourse (stimulation of genitals with no penetration of any kind, including fingers, sex toys, and anal sex), condom use, use of lubricated condoms for receptive anal sex, dental dams for oral sex, limiting partners, sexually transmitted infection (STI) screening; acquaintance rape prevention; Internet/phone safety
   d. Other as indicated by health history/physical examination/risk factors

5. Immunizations—human papillomavirus (HPV) vaccination series for cervical cancer prevention; see Chapter 3, *Primary Care*, for all adolescent immunization recommendations

- Ages 21–29 years
  1. Health history
     a. Menstrual, gynecologic, and obstetric history
     b. Psychosocial assessment—emotional, physical, or sexual abuse by family or partner, current or past; drug/alcohol use; anxiety and depression screening, disordered eating screening
     c. Sexuality/sexual history—sexual orientation, gender identity, sexual practices, sexual satisfaction, dyspareunia, use of contraception, use of condoms, understanding of consent, exchange of sex for drugs or money/transactional sex
     d. Conduct risk assessment for consideration of *BRCA 1/2* testing
  2. Physical examination
     a. Clinical breast examination
        (1) American Cancer Society (ACS, 2024)) not recommended for individuals at average risk for breast cancer; but patients should be familiar with how their breasts normally look and

feel and should report any changes to a health care provider right away.
        (2) American College of Obstetricians and Gynecologists (ACOG, 2017): may offer every 1–3 years for individuals aged 25–39
        (3) See Chapter 3, *Primary Care*, for all clinical breast examination recommendations
     b. Pelvic examination—periodic, if need cervical cancer screening or otherwise indicated
     c. Other as indicated by health history/risk factors
  3. Screening tests
     a. Chlamydia and gonorrhea tests if sexually active (age < 25) or if older and has risk factors
     b. HIV screening if sexually active; yearly if high risk; evaluate if candidate for HIV preexposure prophylaxis (PrEP)
     c. Cervical cancer screening
        (1) ACOG (2021); USPSTF (2018): cytology alone every 3 years
        (2) ACS (Fontham et al., 2022): Start screening at age 25; primary HPV test every 5 years preferred; cytology and HPV co-testing every 5 years or cytology alone every 3 years acceptable
        (3) See Chapter 3, *Primary Care*, for all cervical cancer screening recommendations
     d. Other as indicated by health history/risk factors
  4. Counseling/education
     a. Reproductive life planning—plan for having children, timing, use of contraception, prepregnancy care
     b. Safer sex practices—abstinence, outercourse (stimulation of genitals with no penetration of any kind, including fingers, sex toys, and anal sex), condom use, use of lubricated condoms for receptive anal sex, dental dams for oral sex, limiting partners, STI screening
     c. Breast health—for individuals age 20 years and older educate about breast self-awareness and when to seek further evaluation; it is not recommended to teach routine, systematic breast self-examination for any age group
     d. Purpose of cervical cancer screening and how often to schedule
     e. Other as indicated by health history/physical examination/risk factors
  5. Immunizations—HPV vaccination series for cervical cancer prevention if not done earlier and 26 years of age or younger; may offer to individuals older than 26 years of age; see Chapter 3, *Primary Care*, for all adult immunization recommendations

- Ages 30–49
  1. Health history
     a. Menstrual, gynecologic, and obstetric history; perimenopausal/menopausal symptoms; pelvic prolapse; urinary or fecal incontinence
     b. Psychosocial assessment—emotional, physical, or sexual abuse by family or partner, current or past; drug/alcohol use; anxiety and depression screening, disordered eating screening

c. Sexuality/sexual history—sexual orientation, gender identity, sexual practices, sexual satisfaction, dyspareunia, use of contraception, use of condoms, understanding of consent, exchange of sex for drugs or money/transactional sex

d. Conduct risk assessment for consideration of *BRCA 1/2* testing

2. Physical examination
   a. Clinical breast examination
      (1) ACOG (2017): yearly aged 40 and older
      (2) ACS (Smith et al., 2019), USPSTF (2016): not recommended for individuals at average risk for breast cancer
      (3) See Chapter 3, *Primary Care*, for all clinical breast examination recommendations
   b. Pelvic examination—if need cervical cancer screening or otherwise indicated
   c. Other as indicated by health history/risk factors

3. Screening tests
   a. Cervical cancer screening
      (1) ACOG (2021); USPSTF (2018): Primary HPV test every 5 years or cytology and HPV co-testing every 5 years or cytology alone every 3 years
      (2) ACS (Fontham et al., 2022): Primary HPV test every 5 years preferred; cytology and HPV co-testing every 5 years or cytology alone every 3 years acceptable
      (3) See Chapter 3, *Primary Care*, for all cervical cancer screening recommendations
   b. Mammogram
      (1) ACS (Smith et al., 2019): yearly beginning at age 45 years if at average risk; individuals aged 55 and older can transition to biennial screening or continue annual screening if they prefer; individuals should have the opportunity to begin mammograms between age 40 and 44 years
      (2) ACOG (2017): offer starting at age 40 years; initiate at ages 40–49 years after counseling, if individual desires; recommend no later than age 50 years if not already initiated; annual or biennial interval
      (3) USPSTF (2016): biennial screening from age 50 to 74 years (Grade B)
      (4) See Chapter 3, *Primary Care*, for all breast cancer screening recommendations
   c. HIV screening if sexually active; yearly if high risk; evaluate if candidate for HIV preexposure prophylaxis (PrEP)
   d. Other as indicated by health history/risk factors

4. Counseling/education
   a. Reproductive life planning—plan for having or not having children, timing, use of contraception, prepregnancy care
   b. Safer sex practices—abstinence, outercourse (stimulation of genitals with no penetration of any kind, including fingers, sex toys, and anal sex), condom use, use of lubricated condoms for receptive anal sex, dental dams for oral sex, limiting partners, STI screening

   c. Breast health—breast self-awareness, purpose of screening mammograms
   d. Purpose of cervical cancer screening, how often to schedule
   e. Expected physical and hormonal changes during perimenopause
   f. Management of perimenopausal/menopausal symptoms—see information later in this chapter
   g. Other as indicated by health history/physical examination/risk factors

- Fertility/infertility
  1. Fertility—approximate time required for conception for a couple having unprotected coitus is 57% within 3 months, 72% within 6 months; 85% within 1 year; 93% within 2 years
  2. Infertility—no conception after 1 year of unprotected coitus if younger than age 35; after 6 months if 35 years of age or older; inability to carry a pregnancy to live birth; estimated infertility rate in the United States is 6%–15% of women
  3. Anatomy and physiology of the female reproductive system covered earlier in this chapter
  4. Anatomy and physiology of the male reproductive system
     a. Anatomic components of the male reproductive system—penis, urethra, seminal vesicles, prostate gland, vas deferens, epididymis, testes, bulbourethral (Cowper's) glands
     b. Sperm production relies on a functioning hypothalamic–pituitary–testicular axis
     c. Anterior pituitary gland produces FSH and LH (named for their effects in the female reproductive system) in response to the secretion of GnRH
     d. FSH and LH initiate testicular production of sperm and testosterone
     e. Process of spermatogenesis takes approximately 72 days
     f. Sperm matures in the epididymis and travels through the vas deferens and out of the urethra during ejaculation
     g. Healthy sperm can survive in the female reproductive tract and retain the ability to fertilize an egg for 3–5 days
  5. See Chapter 5, *Gynecologic, Reproductive, and Sexual Disorders,* for details on infertility etiology/incidence, assessment, diagnostic tests, and management/treatment

Contraception

- Contraceptive efficacy
  1. Risk of pregnancy—unintended pregnancy in the first year of use
  2. Perfect use—pregnancy rate when used consistently and correctly
  3. Typical use—pregnancy rate during actual use; includes inconsistent and incorrect use
  4. User characteristics that influence efficacy—frequency of intercourse, age, regularity of menstrual cycles

5. How to choose a contraceptive method
   a. Determine the need for reversible contraception (One Key Question and PATH questions) with every pregnancy-capable person
   b. Assess for contraindications (Use CDC Medical Eligibility Criteria [MEC] criteria)
   c. Elicit patient preferences
6. Long-acting reversible contraceptive methods (e.g., IUC and progestin-only contraceptive implants) are highly effective without concerns of inconsistent or incorrect use; consider as first-line options for pregnancy-capable persons
7. Typical use of effectiveness comparisons
   a. Less than one pregnancy per 100 method users in 1 year—progestin-only contraceptive implant, IUC, sterilization
   b. Between 6 and 12 pregnancies per 100 method users in 1 year—depot medroxyprogesterone acetate (DMPA), combination hormonal contraceptives (CHCs; pills, patch, vaginal ring), progestin-only contraceptive pills, diaphragm
   c. Eighteen or more pregnancies per 100 method users in 1 year—internal/vulvovaginal condom and external/penis condom, sponge, withdrawal, spermicides, fertility awareness methods
8. Drug interactions that may decrease contraceptive efficacy
   a. Drugs that increase production of liver enzyme cytochrome P-450 may cause more rapid clearance of other drugs metabolized by this enzyme
   b. Drugs that increase cytochrome P-450—rifampin, rifapentine, some anticonvulsants, some antiretrovirals, griseofulvin, St. John's wort
   c. Contraceptives that may have decreased efficacy when used concomitantly with a drug that increases production of cytochrome P-450—all CHC methods, progestin-only contraceptive pills, progestin-only contraceptive implants
   d. DMPA and LNG IUD efficacy is not affected
9. Maintaining efficacy when switching methods
   a. Use quick-start method—if switching among different CHC, progestin-only methods, or intrauterine contraceptives (IUC), start the new method the same day as discontinuing the other method
      (1) Start the new method the same day that an IUC or progestin-only implant is removed
      (2) Continue the current method until the day that IUC or progestin-only implant is placed
      (3) Start the new method at the time that progestin-only injection is due
      (4) Follow backup contraception instructions for the new method just as if not using the quick-start method
   b. If a gap of time between stopping one method/starting another method and unprotected intercourse occurs
      (1) Offer emergency contraception
      (2) Start the new method no later than the next day; exception: ideally do not start a hormonal method any sooner than 5 days after taking

ulipristal acetate (UPA) because of concern may decrease the effectiveness of UPA; use a barrier method or abstinence
      (3) Use the backup method for 7 days
      (4) Advise individual to have urine pregnancy test if no withdrawal bleed within 3 weeks

- Initiating a Method of Contraception
  1. Reasonably certain the patient is not pregnant
     a. A urine pregnancy test alone is not sufficient to exclude pregnancy
     b. NO symptoms or signs of pregnancy and meets any one of the following criteria:
        (1) Is 7 days or less after the start of normal menses
        (2) Has not had sexual intercourse since the start of last normal menses
        (3) Has correctly and consistently used a reliable method of contraception
        (4) Is 7 days or less after a spontaneous or induced abortion

- Safety of contraceptive methods
  1. Major health risks associated with contraceptive use are uncommon; the risk of death extremely low
  2. Most major health risks occur in individuals with underlying medical conditions
  3. Thorough health assessment for potential increase in risk with the selected method is key
  4. Educate individuals about risks and danger signs
  5. Centers for Disease Control and Prevention (CDC) Medical Eligibility Criteria (MEC) for Contraceptive Use (2016)—individual characteristics or known preexisting medical/pathologic condition affecting eligibility for use of a contraceptive method classified under one of four categories
     a. Category 1—condition for which there is no restriction on the use of the method
     b. Category 2—condition for which advantages of using the method generally outweigh theoretical or proven risks
     c. Category 3—condition for which theoretical or proven risks usually outweigh advantages of using the method
     d. Category 4—condition that represents an unacceptable health risk if the method is used

- Intrauterine contraception (IUC)
  1. Description—device placed in uterus for purpose of long-acting contraception
     a. Copper-releasing IUC (Copper T 380A)
        (1) T-shaped plastic device with copper wrapped around both vertical stem and horizontal arms
        (2) Primary action is spermicidal and direct effects of copper salts on endometrial inflammation
        (3) Effective for at least 10 years
        (4) Typical pregnancy rates are 1% per year
        (5) No effect on HPO axis and ovulation and menstrual cyclicity continues
        (6) Can increase the amount, duration, and discomfort of menses during the first 3–6 months
     b. Levonorgestrel intrauterine system (LNG-IUS)—four types available

(1) T-shaped plastic frame with steroid reservoir in vertical stem that contains levonorgestrel

(2) Skyla (13.5 mg LNG) is effective for 3 years; Kyleena (19.5 mg LNG) is effective for 5 years, and Liletta and Mirena (52 mg LNG) are effective for 8 years

2. Mechanism of action
   a. Copper T 380A
      (1) Copper may inhibit sperm capacitation
      (2) Alters tubal/uterine transport of ovum
      (3) Enzymatic influence on endometrium
   b. LNG-IUS—progestin influence
      (1) Thickens cervical mucus
      (2) Produces atrophic endometrium
      (3) Slows ovum transport through tube
      (4) Inhibits sperm motility and function
3. Effectiveness/first-year failure rate
   a. Perfect use
      (1) Copper T—0.6%
      (2) LNG-IUS—0.2%
   b. Typical use
      (1) Copper T—0.8%
      (2) LNG-IUS—0.2%
4. Advantages
   a. Ease of use
   b. Not coitally dependent
   c. Effective
   d. Reversible
   e. Cost-effective (if used longer than 1 year)
   f. LNG-IUS can decrease blood loss and dysmenorrhea during menses
   g. Effective choice for individuals who cannot use estrogen-containing methods
   h. Can be used during lactation and immediately postpartum
5. Disadvantages and side effects
   a. Altered menstrual bleeding patterns
      (1) Increased amount and length of menstrual bleeding—Copper T
      (2) Increased dysmenorrhea in first few months of use—Copper T
      (3) Irregular bleeding and spotting first few months of use—LNG-IUS
      (4) Absence or decrease of bleeding—LNG-IUS
   b. Risk of pelvic inflammatory disease (PID)—increased risk in first 20 days following insertion
   c. Risk of spontaneous expulsion
      (1) May go undetected by the individual
      (2) More likely at the time of menses
6. Contraindications (CDC categories 3 and 4)
   a. Category 4 for IUC use (**Box 4-1**)—do not use the method if the conditions in Box 4-3 exist
   b. Category 3 for IUC use (Box 4-2)—use of the method not generally recommended for the conditions in **Box 4-2** unless other, more appropriate methods are not available or acceptable
7. Management
   a. Health assessment prior to initiation of method
      (1) History to include:
         (a) Menstrual history

Box 4-1 Category 4 for IUC Use

- Known/suspected pregnancy
- Postpartum or postabortion sepsis
- Unexplained vaginal bleeding prior to insertion and before evaluation
- Gestational trophoblastic disease with persistently elevated hCG levels or malignant disease with evidence or suspicion of intrauterine disease—initiation but not continuation
- Cervical cancer prior to insertion and awaiting treatment
- Current breast cancer within past 5 years—LNG-IUS only
- Any uterine anatomic abnormalities distorting the uterine cavity and incompatible with IUC insertion
- Current PID, purulent cervicitis, chlamydia, or gonorrhea—initiation but not continuation
- Endometrial cancer—initiation but not continuation
- Known pelvic tuberculosis—initiation but not continuation

Jones & Bartlett Learning

Box 4-2 Category 3 for IUC Use

- Ischemic heart disease occurring after insertion—LNG-IUS only
- History of breast cancer with no evidence of disease for 5 years—LNG-IUS only
- High likelihood of exposure to chlamydia or gonorrhea—initiation but not continuation
- Acquired immunodeficiency syndrome (AIDS; unless clinically well on antiretroviral therapy)—initiation but not continuation
- Severe cirrhosis, benign hepatocellular adenoma, or malignant hepatoma—LNG-IUS only
- Systemic lupus erythematosus (SLE) with positive or unknown antiphospholipid antibodies—LNG-IUS only
- SLE with severe thrombocytopenia—initiation of Copper T IUC only
- Solid organ transplantation with complications—initiation but not continuation
- Pelvic tuberculosis—continuation

Jones & Bartlett Learning

         (b) Heavy menses/ history of anemia
         (c) STI/PID, vaginitis symptoms
         (d) STI risk factors
         (e) HIV status/exposure
         (f) Cervical cancer screening history of abnormal results
      (2) Physical examination to include:
         (a) Pregnancy test
         (b) Speculum examination to assess for possible vaginal/cervical infection
         (c) Chlamydia and gonorrhea (GC) tests/wet prep (if history/physical examination indicates)
         (d) Bimanual examination—contour, size, consistency, mobility, position of uterus
      (3) Placement technique
         (a) Insert speculum, visualize cervix

    (b) Wash cervix and vagina with antiseptic

    (c) Apply the tenaculum to the anterior or posterior lip of the cervix and apply gentle traction to straighten the axis of the uterus

    (d) Sound uterus prior to placing IUC— should sound to the length of 6–9 cm for best placement

    (e) Place IUC per manufacturer's instructions

    (f) Trim IUC threads to 3–4 cm

    (g) Have the client remain supine until the client feels well—then monitor as the client sits up, because the client may have vasovagal reaction from instrumentation of cervical os

    (h) An ultrasound to assess for correct placement is not routinely necessary

  b. Follow-up

    (1) Advise to return at any time to discuss side effects, other problems, desire to change method, and when time to remove or replace the IUC

    (2) No routine follow-up is required

    (3) At other routine visits, assess satisfaction with the method, any concerns, any changes in health status or medications that might affect IUC use

  c. Special considerations

    (1) Timing of placement

      (a) Not necessary to wait for menses if can be reasonably certain that the patient is not pregnant

      (b) May be placed within 48 hours after delivery (vaginal) or prior to uterine closure (cesarean)

      (c) May be placed 4 or more weeks postpartum

      (d) Placement after 48 hours and before 4 weeks postpartum is associated with increased risk of uterine perforation

      (e) May be placed immediately following first- or second-trimester abortion

      (f) Use backup method for 7 days after LNG-IUS placement; backup method not needed after placement of CU-IUD

    (2) Irregular bleeding (spotting/light bleeding/ heavy bleeding/prolonged bleeding)

      (a) Common first 3–6 months of CU-IUD use; irregular spotting/bleeding for several months and then amenorrhea common with LNG-IUS

      (b) Short-term (5–7 days) nonsteroidal anti-inflammatory drugs (NSAIDs) may reduce bleeding when occurs

      (c) Assess for other causes if persistent abnormal bleeding or bleeding associated with pain—cervicitis; pregnancy, including ectopic; pelvic infection

      (d) Remove IUC if patient desires and provide alternative contraception; may consider switching to LNG-IUS if having excessive bleeding with CU-IUD and patient wants to continue IUC as method

    (3) Cramping and pain

      (a) If severe—rule out perforation

      (b) If mild—NSAID/other analgesic or remove IUC

      (c) May indicate infection, pregnancy

    (4) Expulsion—2% to 10% within the first year

      (a) Symptoms—cramping, spotting, dyspareunia, lengthening or absence of threads

      (b) Partial expulsion

        ∘ Remove IUC

        ∘ Rule out pregnancy/infection

        ∘ Replace IUC if patient desires

        ∘ Doxycycline for 5–7 days

      (c) Complete expulsion

        ∘ Pregnancy test

        ∘ Replace IUC if patient desires

    (5) Pregnancy

      (a) Ultrasound evaluation to rule out ectopic pregnancy

      (b) Remove IUC promptly regardless of plans for pregnancy—reduces risk for spontaneous abortion and preterm delivery

      (c) Spontaneous abortion—treat with doxycycline/ampicillin for 7 days

      (d) Patient wants to continue pregnancy

        ∘ Advise concerning risk for spontaneous septic abortion if IUC not removed

        ∘ If threads not visible, use ultrasound to see if IUC is still present

        ∘ If unable to remove IUC, monitor closely for infection during pregnancy

    (6) Perforation, embedding

      (a) Perforation occurs 1 in 1,000 insertions

        ∘ May or may not be associated with severe pain at time of insertion

        ∘ Ultrasound to determine location— may require laparoscopic removal

        ∘ If protrusion through cervix, can be removed in office with local anesthetic

      (b) Embedding

        ∘ Can remove IUC from uterus with forceps if visualized

        ∘ May need to be removed with dilation and curettage (D&C)

    (7) Pelvic Inflammatory Disease (PID)

      (a) No evidence supporting the use of prophylactic antibiotics to reduce postinsertion infection

      (b) Most IUC-related PID occurs within the first 20 days after insertion

      (c) Treat PID with appropriate antibiotics

      (d) Not necessary to remove IUC unless has current high risk for STI or no clinical improvement within 48–72 hours of antibiotic initiation

    (8) *Actinomyces*-like organisms on cervical cytology

      (a) Cervical cytology test does not diagnose actinomycosis infection

(b) *Actinomyces* are normal female genital tract organisms

(c) Colonization of *Actinomyces* more likely in IUC user

(d) Pelvic actinomycosis is very rare but serious infection

(e) Asymptomatic—inform IUC user of cervical cytology report; no treatment necessary; advise to contact healthcare provider if has infection symptoms

(f) Symptomatic—endometritis
    i. Treat with antibiotics—sensitive to penicillin and several other antibiotics
    ii. Remove IUC—*Actinomyces* preferentially grows on foreign bodies

8. Instructions for using the method
   a. Check IUD threads
      (1) After each menses; not all resources recommend this as a routine
      (2) If increased cramping
      (3) If absent—use backup birth control and notify healthcare provider
      (4) If longer—may be in the process of expulsion; use backup birth control and notify healthcare provider
   b. Signs of infection—notify healthcare provider if any of the following:
      (1) Pelvic pain
      (2) Increased or malodorous vaginal discharge
      (3) Unexplained vaginal bleeding
   c. Monitor menses—notify healthcare provider if any of the following:
      (1) Heavy, irregular bleeding
      (2) Missed menses—may have amenorrhea with LNG-IUS
      (3) Increased cramping
      (4) Management of unscheduled bleeding
          (a) Anticipatory guidance is important
          (b) If abrupt change in bleeding pattern, rule out pregnancy
          (c) Exogenous estrogen, such as estradiol patch 0.1 mg weekly × 12 weeks
   d. Warning signs (PAINS)
      (1) *Period* late/missed; abnormal spotting or bleeding
      (2) *Abdominal* pain
      (3) *Infection*—vaginal discharge
      (4) *Not* feeling well—fever, aches, chills
      (5) *String* missing, shorter or longer

• Progestin-only implant—etonogestrel (Nexplanon)
1. Description—long-term (3 years) contraceptive; single rod-shaped implant placed subdermally on inner side of upper arm; provides low-dose sustained release of the progestin etonogestrel; rod is radiopaque
2. Mechanism of action
   a. Suppresses LH—ovulation inhibited in almost all users
   b. Produces atrophic endometrium
   c. Thickens cervical mucus

3. Effectiveness/first-year failure rate
   a. Perfect use—0.05%
   b. Typical use—0.05%
   c. Cumulative evidence supports that obesity does not reduce efficacy
4. Advantages
   a. Ease of use
   b. Effective
   c. Reversible—most users ovulate within 6 weeks after removal of the implant
   d. Contains no estrogen for individuals with contraindications to estrogen or who cannot tolerate estrogenic side effects
   e. Can be used during lactation and immediately postpartum
   f. Affords long-term contraception (3 years)
   g. Reduced dysmenorrhea and pain from endometriosis
5. Disadvantages and side effects
   a. Requires clinician insertion and removal; removal requires a minor surgical procedure
   b. Specific information on drug interactions is not available; very low-dose progestin; potential for reduced efficacy with same drugs as listed for combination oral contraceptives
   c. Pain, bruising, infection (potential) at the insertion site
   d. Irregular, prolonged, more frequent uterine bleeding especially in the first few months; may have amenorrhea
   e. No protection against STIs/HIV
   f. Implant may be visible or palpable
   g. Nonpalpable devices require imaging for localization prior to removal (Nexplanon is radiopaque and can be imaged by 2-dimensional x-ray views)
   h. Possible side effects include:
      (1) Increased incidence of functional ovarian cysts
      (2) Headache
      (3) Emotional lability
      (4) Breast tenderness
      (5) Loss of libido
      (6) Vaginal secretion changes—dryness, leukorrhea
      (7) Acne
      (8) Serious neurovascular injury can complicate insertion or removal—may need removal by a surgeon with the understanding of upper arm anatomy
6. Contraindications (CDC categories 3 and 4)
   a. Category 4 for etonogestrel implant use—do not use the method if breast cancer within the past 5 years
   b. Category 3 for use etonogestrel implant—use of the method not generally recommended for the conditions in **Box 4-3** unless other, more appropriate methods are not available or acceptable
7. Management
   a. Health assessment prior to initiation of method
      (1) Elicit information from thorough history concerning any contraindications, risks, and specific noncontraceptive benefits for the use of progestin-only implant

---

Box 4-3 Category 3 for Use of Etonogestrel Implant

- Ischemic heart disease or stroke occurring while using the method
- Unexplained vaginal bleeding before evaluation
- History of breast cancer with no evidence of disease for 5 years
- Severe cirrhosis, benign hepatocellular adenoma, malignant hepatoma
- SLE with positive or unknown antiphospholipid antibodies

Jones & Bartlett Learning

---

    (2) Breast examination, pelvic examination, cervical cytology, STI tests are not needed prior to insertion of progestin-only implant but may be indicated for other reasons

  b. Placement technique

    (1) Inserted subdermally in the inner side of the upper nondominant arm

    (2) Identify the bicep groove, which lies between the biceps and the triceps muscle

    (3) Near this groove, the medial antebrachial cutaneous nerve, medial brachial cutaneous nerve, ulnar nerve, and basilica vein typically run. These are structures to avoid with placement.

    (4) Select a site that lies closer to the posterior arm, inserting 8–10 cm proximal to the humerus' medial condyl and 3–5 cm posterior to the groove between the biceps and triceps muscles

    (5) A second mark is placed 4 cm proximal to the first and serves as a guide for the insertion path along the arm's long axis

    (6) Remove the implant from the packaging and hold the applicator between the thumb and forefingers, remove the transparent protection cap by sliding it horizontally away from the device, and check that the implant is loaded inside of the device

    (7) With free hand, counter traction the skin while inserting the needle at a 30-degree angle

    (8) Once the needle has punctured the skin, hold the applicator horizontal to the skin, and tent the skin upward as the entirety of the needle is slid into the subdermal space

    (9) While holding the applicator in place, the purple slider is unlocked with the clinician's index finger by pushing the slider downward and backward until it locks

    (10) The needle inside the applicator and the applicator can be removed from the field

    (11) Place a small adhesive dressing or steristrips and immediately palpate the implant to ensure proper placement and have the patient to palpate the implant

    (12) Place a pressure dressing

  c. Follow-up

    (1) Advise client to return at any time to discuss side effects or other problems, or if the patient wants to change method

    (2) The pressure dressing may be removed in 24 hours and the small adhesive bandage or steristrips in 3–5 days

    (3) No routine follow-up required

    (4) At other routine visits, assess satisfaction with the method, any concerns, any changes in health status, or medications that might affect progestin-only implant use

8. Instructions for using the method

  a. Discuss possible bleeding changes prior to insertion

  b. Inform client must be replaced every 3 years for effective contraception

  c. Insert within days 1–5 of menses; no backup method needed

  d. If irregular menses, rule out pregnancy with menstrual and coital history and pregnancy test

  e. If inserted other than days 1–5 of menses, use the backup method for 7 days

  f. Discuss the use of condoms for STI prevention

  g. Management of unscheduled bleeding

    (1) Anticipatory guidance is important

    (2) If abrupt change in bleeding pattern, rule out pregnancy

    (3) Exogenous estrogen

      (a) Ethinyl estradiol 50 mcg for 20 days

      (b) Ethinyl estradiol 20 mcg for 10 days

      (c) COCs for 1–3 cycles

      (d) Estradiol patch 0.1mg/d × 6 weeks

  h. Warning signs to report

    (1) Abdominal pain (severe)

    (2) Arm pain or signs of infection

    (3) Heavy vaginal bleeding

    (4) Missed menses after a period of regularity

    (5) Onset of severe headaches

- Combination oral contraceptives (COCs)

1. Description—pill taken daily for contraception; combination of estrogen and progestin; also has noncontraceptive applications

  a. Monophasic pills—deliver a constant amount of estrogen/progestin throughout the cycle

  b. Multiphasic pills—vary amount of estrogen and/or progestin delivered throughout the cycle

  c. Patterns of use—monthly cycling (21/7, 24/3), extended cycle, continuous use

2. Mechanism of action

  a. Estrogen—inhibits ovulation through suppression of FSH, potentiates action of progestin, stabilizes endometrium for less unscheduled bleeding and spotting

    (1) Ethinyl estradiol (E_2)—most prevalent synthetic estrogen in COCs

    (2) Estradiol valerate (E_2V)—newer synthetic estrogen available in one brand of COC

  b. Progestin—provides most of the contraceptive effect; inhibits ovulation through suppression of LH surge; inhibits sperm penetration by thickening cervical mucus; progestins available vary in bioavailability, dose needed for ovulation inhibition, and half-life

    (1) One method of categorizing progestins is by historical generation of introduction in COCs available in the United States

(2) First three generations include progestins that are derivatives of testosterone, designated as 19-nortestosterones with class names of estranes and gonanes

(3) First-generation progestins (norethindrone, norethindrone acetate, ethynodiol diacetate)—lowest potency, short half-life; lower doses more likely to have unscheduled bleeding and spotting

(4) Second-generation progestins (norgestrel, levonorgestrel)—more potent and longer half-life designed to decrease unscheduled bleeding and spotting, associated with more androgen-related side effects

(5) Third-generation progestins (desogestrel, norgestimate, gestodene [not available in United States])—designed to maintain the potency of second-generation progestins but with less androgenic side effects

(6) Fourth-generation progestins

  (a) Drospirenone—analogue of spironolactone, a potassium-sparing diuretic; progestogenic effect, antiandrogenic properties

  (b) Dienogest—a 19-nortestosterone with a slightly different structure to maintain a strong progestin effect and exert an antiandrogenic effect

3. Effectiveness/first-year failure rate
   a. Perfect use—0.3%
   b. Typical use—9%
4. Advantages
   a. Ease of use
   b. Reversible
   c. Effective
   d. May reduce the incidence of/afford protection against
      (1) Acne
      (2) Dysmenorrhea
      (3) PID
      (4) Endometriosis
      (5) Iron-deficiency anemia
      (6) Osteoporosis
      (7) Benign breast conditions
      (8) Functional ovarian cysts
      (9) Ovarian cancer, endometrial cancer, colorectal cancer
      (10) Menstrual migraine headaches—extended-cycle or continuous-use regimens
      (11) Premenstrual syndrome/premenstrual dysphoric disorder
   e. May be used as emergency contraception
5. Disadvantages/side effects
   a. Does not prevent transmission of STIs/HIV
   b. Requires user compliance/daily dosing schedule
   c. Side effects/adverse effects
      (1) Possible estrogenic effects
         (a) Nausea
         (b) Increased breast size/breast tenderness
         (c) Chloasma
         (d) Telangiectasia
         (e) Cervical eversion/ectopy
         (f) Increased blood pressure
         (g) Increased cholesterol concentration in gallbladder bile
         (h) Migraine headaches
         (i) Increased triglycerides
         (j) Hepatocellular adenoma
         (k) Arterial thrombosis
         (l) Venous thromboembolism (VTE)
      (2) Possible progestogenic side effects/adverse effects
         (a) Breast tenderness
         (b) Fatigue
         (c) Depressive symptoms
         (d) Increased insulin resistance
         (e) Constipation/bloating
         (f) Precipitation of gallbladder sludge or stones
         (g) Cyclic weight gain
      (3) Possible androgenic side effects/adverse effects
         (a) Increased appetite/weight gain
         (b) Hirsutism
         (c) Acne, oily skin
         (d) Increased low-density lipoprotein cholesterol (LDL-C)
6. Contraindications (CDC categories 3 and 4)
   a. Category 4 for COC use—do not use the method if conditions in **Box 4-4** exist

---

Box 4-4 Category 4 for COC Use

- Smokers 35 years of age or older, 15 or more cigarettes/day
- Multiple risk factors for arterial cardiovascular disease
- Hypertension (160/100 mm Hg) or hypertension with vascular disease
- Acute deep vein thrombosis (DVT) or pulmonary embolism (PE)
- History of DVT or PE and one or more risk factors for recurrence
- Major surgery with prolonged immobilization
- Known thrombogenic mutations
- History of or current ischemic heart disease, stroke, complicated valvular heart disease
- Migraine headaches with aura at any age
- Breast cancer within the past 5 years
- Diabetes with nephropathy, retinopathy, neuropathy, other vascular disease; diabetes longer than 20 years' duration
- Active viral hepatitis, severe cirrhosis, hepatocellular adenoma, malignant hepatoma
- SLE with positive or unknown antiphospholipid antibodies
- Peripartum cardiomyopathy—moderately or severely impaired cardiac function or less than 6 months postpartum
- Solid organ transplantation with complications
- Less than 21 days postpartum (breastfeeding/chestfeeding and nonbreastfeeding/chestfeeding)

Box 4-5 Category 3 for COC Use

- Twenty-one to 42 days postpartum, nonbreastfeeding/chestfeeding, with other risk factors for VTE
- Twenty-one to <30 days postpartum, breastfeeding/chestfeeding, with or without other risk factors for VTE
- Thirty to 42 days postpartum, breastfeeding/chestfeeding, with other risk factors for VTE
- Smokers 35 years of age or older, fewer than 15 cigarettes/day
- Hypertension—adequately controlled or less than 160/100 mm Hg
- Known hyperlipidemia—consider type, severity, and other cardiovascular risk factors
- History of breast cancer with no evidence of disease for 5 years
- Symptomatic gallbladder disease; history of cholestasis related to past COC use
- Mild cirrhosis
- History of bariatric surgery with malabsorptive procedure
- History of DVT or PE with no risk factors for recurrence
- Peripartum cardiomyopathy with normal or mildly impaired cardiac function and 6 or more months postpartum
- Moderate or severe inflammatory bowel disease with associated risks for DVT or PE

Jones & Bartlett Learning

    b. Category 3 for COC use—use of the method not generally recommended for the conditions in **Box 4-5** unless other, more appropriate methods are not available or acceptable

7. Management
    a. Health assessment prior to initiation of method
       (1) Elicit information from thorough history concerning any contraindications, risks, specific noncontraceptive benefits for the use of COCs
       (2) Blood pressure
       (3) Breast examination, pelvic examination, cervical cytology, STI tests are not needed prior to starting COC but may be indicated for other reasons
    b. Follow-up
       (1) Advise client to return at any time to discuss side effects or other problems, or if the client wants to change method
       (2) No routine follow-up required
       (3) At other routine visits, measure blood pressure; assess satisfaction with the method, any concerns, any changes in health status, or medications that might affect COC use
    c. Special considerations
       (1) Drug interactions
          (a) Most broad-spectrum antibiotics (e.g., ampicillin, metronidazole, doxycycline, fluconazole) do *not* lower hormone levels or reduce COC effectiveness
          (b) A few broad-spectrum antibiotics (e.g., rifampin, rifapentine, griseofulvin) do induce cytochrome P-450 enzyme activity and may reduce COC effectiveness

          (c) Some anticonvulsants (carbamazepine, felbamate, oxcarbazepine, primidone, phenobarbital, phenytoin, topiramate) induce cytochrome P-450 enzyme activity
          (d) Other anticonvulsants (clonazepam, gabapentin, pregabalin, valproic acid) do not induce cytochrome P-450 enzyme and do not affect COC efficacy
          (e) Anticonvulsants may be used for the treatment of other conditions: neuropathic pain, bipolar disease, schizophrenia, migraine headaches
          (f) Some antiretroviral drugs (protease inhibitors) induce cytochrome P-450 enzyme and may affect COC efficacy
          (g) St. John's wort is a cytochrome P-450 enzyme inducer that may increase the hepatic metabolism of COC
          (h) Orlistat—blocks fat absorption and may reduce intestinal absorption of COCs, as well as induce diarrhea
       (2) Drug interactions—COCs may potentiate the effect of some drugs
          (a) Benzodiazepines—diazepam and chlordiazepoxide
          (b) Tricyclic antidepressants
          (c) Theophylline
          (d) The following potassium-sparing drugs may interact with drospirenone-containing COCs and cause hyperkalemia: angiotensin-converting enzyme (ACE) inhibitors, angiotensin II antagonists, potassium-sparing diuretics, heparin, aldosterone antagonists, chronic daily use of NSAIDs; if taking any of these medications, check potassium level after first cycle of COC
       (3) Management of unscheduled bleeding/spotting
          (a) Common side effect first 3 months of use; usually decreases over time
          (b) Reinforce to take pills daily at the same time
          (c) May consider timing of unscheduled bleeding in cycle to decide on pill formulation change if persists
          (d) Spotting/bleeding before complete active pills—increase progestin content for more endometrial support
          (e) Continued spotting/bleeding following scheduled bleeding—increase estrogen content of first pills in pack or decrease progestin content of first pills for more estrogen to proliferate endometrium
          (f) Unscheduled spotting/bleeding with extended cycle or continuous use—take at least 21 active pills, take 3–4 days off for withdrawal bleed to start, restart active pills, and take for at least 21 days before stops again

(g) If the problem persists, consider another cause for bleeding (e.g., infection, polyps)

(4) Management of absence of withdrawal bleeding

(a) Occurs in about 5% of women after several years of COC use

(b) Rule out pregnancy or other potential causes of amenorrhea

(c) No intervention required if the woman is okay with no menses

(d) Change to 30–35 mcg estrogen if on 20-mcg COC or triphasic formulation with lower levels of progestin in early pills

8. Instructions for use

a. General instructions

(1) Quick-start method—reasonably certain not pregnant, take the first pill on the day of office visit; backup method for 7 days if more than 5 days since last menstrual period (LMP)

(2) First-day start—take the first pill on the first day of menses; no backup method needed

(3) Take the pill at approximately the same time each day

(4) If nausea occurs, take pill with meals or at bedtime

(5) Use a backup method (condoms) if efficacy/absorbency compromised by severe vomiting and/or diarrhea

(6) Emergency contraception instructions

(7) Use condoms for the prevention of STIs/HIV

b. Recommended actions after late or missed COCs—see **Figure 4-5**

c. Warning signs (ACHES)

(1) *Abdominal pain (severe)*

(2) *Chest pain (sharp, severe, shortness of breath)*

(3) *Headache (severe, dizziness, unilateral)*

(4) *Eye problems (scotoma, blurred vision, blind spots)*

(5) *Severe leg pain (calf or thigh)*

- Transdermal contraceptive system

1. Description—patch applied to skin; delivers continuous daily systemic dose of progestin (norelgestromin) and estrogen (ethinyl estradiol) or progestin (levonorgestrel) and estrogen (ethinyl estradiol) (Twirla)

2. New patch applied each week for 3 weeks, followed by 1 week without a patch to induce withdrawal bleeding

3. Mechanism of action—same as COCs

4. Effectiveness/first-year failure rate

a. Perfect use—0.3%

b. Typical use—9%

5. Advantages

a. Ease of use—no daily dosing regimen

b. Reversible

c. Effective

d. Good menstrual cycle control

6. Disadvantages and side effects

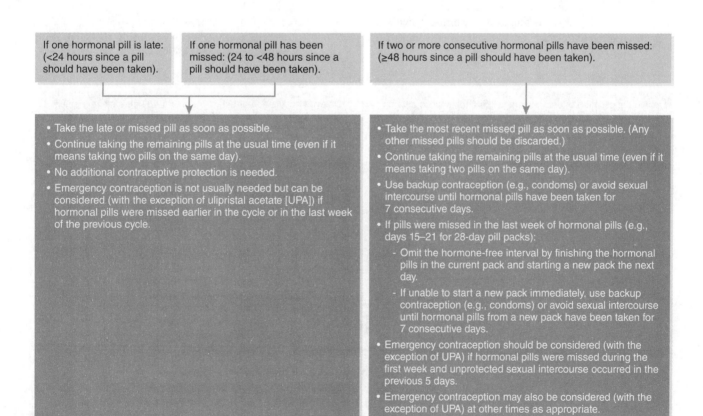

Figure 4-5 Recommended actions after late or missed combination oral contraceptives

Reproduced from Curtis, K. M., Jatlaoui, T. C., Tepper, N. K., Zapata, L. B., Horton, L. G., Jamieson, D. J., & Whiteman, M. K. (2016). U.S. selected practice recommendations for contraceptive use, 2016. *Morbidity and Mortality Weekly Report, 65*(4), 1–66. http://dx.doi .org/10.15585/mmwr.rr6504a1

a. Does not prevent transmission of STIs/HIV
b. Skin irritation at the application site
c. Other side effects similar to those of COCs

7. Contraindications (CDC categories 3 and 4)—same as with COCs except history of bariatric surgery not relevant

8. Management
   a. Health assessment prior to initiation—same as with COCs
   b. Follow-up—same as with COCs
   c. Special considerations
      (1) May be less effective in women who weigh 90 kg (198 lb) or more
      (2) Not recommended for users with a BMI greater than or equal to 30
      (3) Probably same drug interactions as with COCs

9. Instructions for using the method
   a. Quick-start method—reasonably certain not pregnant, apply patch on day of office visit; if more than 5 days since LMP, use backup method for 7 days
   b. First-day start—apply patch on first day of menses; no backup method needed
   c. Apply patch to buttocks, abdomen, upper torso front or back (excluding breasts), upper outer arm—rotate application site
   d. Apply a new patch on the same day each week for a total of 3 weeks
   e. Do not wear a patch on week 4; withdrawal bleeding will occur
   f. Use condoms for STI/HIV prevention
   g. May be worn in saunas and whirlpools without decreased efficacy (Twirla swimming is limited to 30 minutes)

h. Recommended actions after delayed application or detachment with contraceptive patch—see **Figure 4-6**
i. Contact healthcare provider if warning signs occur—same as COC warning signs

- Contraceptive vaginal ring (NuvaRing)
   1. Description—soft, malleable, clear plastic ring; delivers continuous, systemic dose of estrogen (ethinyl estradiol) and progestin (etonogestrel); worn in vagina for 3 weeks, followed by 1 week without ring to induce withdrawal bleeding
   2. Mechanism of action—same as COCs
   3. Effectiveness/first-year failure rate
      a. Perfect use—0.3%
      b. Typical use—9%
   4. Advantages
      a. Ease of use—no daily dosing regimen
      b. Reversible
      c. Effective
      d. Good menstrual cycle control
   5. Disadvantages and side effects
      a. Does not prevent transmission of STIs/HIV
      b. Side effects similar to those of COCs
      c. Vaginal discharge/vaginal irritation
   6. Contraindications (CDC categories 3 and 4)—same as with COCs except history of bariatric surgery not relevant
   7. Management
      a. Health assessment prior to initiation—same as with COCs
      b. Follow-up—same as with COCs
      c. Special considerations—probably the same drug interactions as with COCs

---

Delayed application or detachment for <48 hours since a patch should have been applied or reattached.

↓

- Apply a new patch as soon as possible. (If detachment occurred < 24 hours since the patch was applied, try to reapply the patch or replace with a new patch.)
- Keep the same patch change day.
- No additional contraceptive protection is needed.
- Emergency contraception is not usually needed but can be considered (with the exception of ulipristal acetate [UPA]) if delayed application or detachment occurred earlier in the cycle or in the last week of the previous cycle.

Delayed application or detachment for ≥48 hours since a patch should have been applied or reattached.

↓

- Apply a new patch as soon as possible.
- Keep the same patch change day.
- Use backup contraception (e.g., condoms) or avoid sexual intercourse until a patch has been worn for 7 consecutive days.
- If the delayed application or detachment occurred in the third patch week:
  - Omit the hormone-free week by finishing the third week of patch use (keeping the same patch change day) and starting a new patch immediately.
  - If unable to start a new patch immediately, use backup contraception (e.g., condoms) or avoid sexual intercourse until a new patch has been worn for 7 consecutive days.
- Emergency contraception should be considered (with the exception of UPA) if the delayed application or detachment occurred within the first week of patch use and unprotected sexual intercourse occurred in the previous 5 days.
- Emergency contraception may also be considered (with the exception of UPA) at other times as appropriate.

Figure 4-6 Recommended actions after delayed application or detachment with contraceptive patch

Reproduced from Curtis, K. M., Jatlaoui, T. C., Tepper, N. K., Zapata, L. B., Horton, L. G., Jamieson, D. J., & Whiteman, M. K. (2016). U.S. selected practice recommendations for contraceptive use, 2016. *Morbidity and Mortality Weekly Report, 65*(4), 1–66. http://dx.doi.org/10.15585/mmwr.rr6504a1

8. Instructions for using the method
   a. Quick-start method—reasonably certain not pregnant, insert ring on day of office visit; if more than 5 days since LMP, use backup method for 7 days
   b. First-day start—insert ring on first day of menses; no backup method needed
   c. Wash hands before inserting
   d. Fold ring and gently insert into the vagina
   e. Exact position of the ring in the vagina is not important
   f. May be worn during vaginal penetrative intercourse
   g. If desires to remove the ring, should be replaced within 3 hours to maintain efficacy
   h. Insert ring for 3 weeks of use, remove for one week to allow withdrawal bleeding
   i. NuvaRing is single use—after 3 weeks of use and 1-week withdrawal bleed, a new ring is placed (possible for continuous use, a new ring is inserted immediately after removal of the old ring at 3-week intervals)
   j. Recommended actions after delayed insertion or reinsertion of contraceptive vaginal ring—see **Figure 4-7**
   k. If the ring is left in the vagina for more than 3 weeks but less than 4 weeks, it should be removed; insert a new ring after a ring-free period of 1 week
   l. If the ring is left in the vagina more than 4 weeks, it may not protect from pregnancy; use a backup method until new ring in the vagina for 7 days
   m. Use condoms for the prevention of STIs/HIV
   n. Contact healthcare provider if warning signs occur—same as COC warning signs

- Contraceptive vaginal ring (Annovera)—extended use
  1. Description—soft, malleable, white plastic ring; same diameter as NuvaRing but twice as thick; delivers continuous, systemic dose of estrogen (ethinyl estradiol) and progestin (segesterone acetate); one ring used for 13 28-day cycles; inserted and left in place for 21 days, removed for 7 days to allow withdrawal bleed, then reinserted (more studies are needed to determine safety and efficacy for extended use)
  2. Mechanism of action—same as COCs
  3. Effectiveness/first-year failure rate
     a. Perfect use—3.0%
     b. Typical use—not available
  4. Advantages
     a. Ease of use—no daily dosing regimen
     b. Reversible
     c. Effective
     d. Good menstrual cycle control
  5. Disadvantages and side effects
     a. Does not prevent transmission of STIs/HIV
     b. Side effects similar to those of COCs
     c. Vaginal discharge/vaginal irritation
  6. Contraindications (CDC categories 3 and 4)
     a. Same as with COCs except history of bariatric surgery not relevant
     b. Not recommended if using hepatitis C drug combinations containing ombitasvir/paritaprevir/ritonavir, with or without dasabuvir, due to the potential for alanine transaminase (ALT) elevations
     c. Has not been studied for use with body mass index of more than $29 kg/m^2$
  7. Management

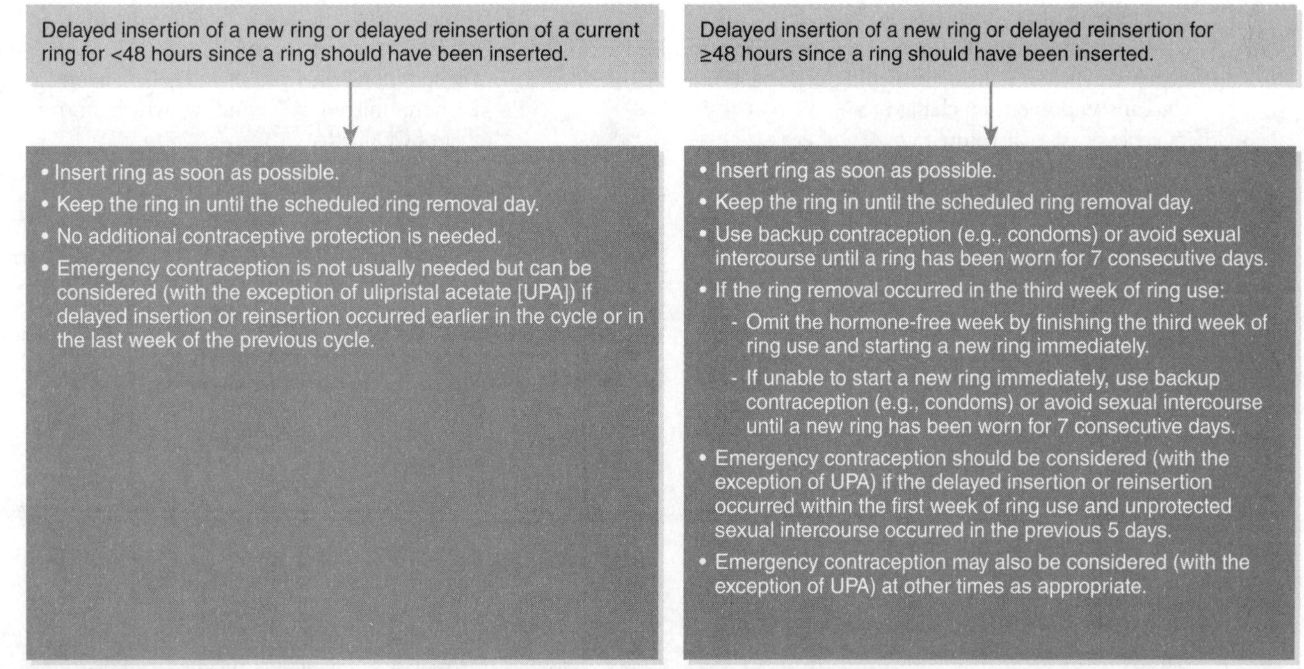

Delayed insertion of a new ring or delayed reinsertion of a current ring for <48 hours since a ring should have been inserted.

- Insert ring as soon as possible.
- Keep the ring in until the scheduled ring removal day.
- No additional contraceptive protection is needed.
- Emergency contraception is not usually needed but can be considered (with the exception of ulipristal acetate [UPA]) if delayed insertion or reinsertion occurred earlier in the cycle or in the last week of the previous cycle.

Delayed insertion of a new ring or delayed reinsertion for ≥48 hours since a ring should have been inserted.

- Insert ring as soon as possible.
- Keep the ring in until the scheduled ring removal day.
- Use backup contraception (e.g., condoms) or avoid sexual intercourse until a ring has been worn for 7 consecutive days.
- If the ring removal occurred in the third week of ring use:
  - Omit the hormone-free week by finishing the third week of ring use and starting a new ring immediately.
  - If unable to start a new ring immediately, use backup contraception (e.g., condoms) or avoid sexual intercourse until a new ring has been worn for 7 consecutive days.
- Emergency contraception should be considered (with the exception of UPA) if the delayed insertion or reinsertion occurred within the first week of ring use and unprotected sexual intercourse occurred in the previous 5 days.
- Emergency contraception may also be considered (with the exception of UPA) at other times as appropriate.

Figure 4-7 Recommended actions after delayed insertion or reinsertion of contraceptive vaginal ring

Reproduced from Curtis, K. M., Jatlaoui, T. C., Tepper, N. K., Zapata, L. B., Horton, L. G., Jamieson, D. J., & Whiteman, M. K. (2016). U.S. selected practice recommendations for contraceptive use, 2016. *Morbidity and Mortality Weekly Report, 65*(4), 1–66. http://dx.doi.org/10.15585/mmwr.rr6504a1

a. Health assessment prior to initiation—same as with COCs

b. Follow-up—same as with COCs

c. Special considerations—probably the same drug interactions as with COCs

d. Ring may be used concurrently with tampon or vaginal medications

e. The concurrent use of a miconazole suppository increases systemic hormone concentrations (not altered by miconazole cream)

8. Instructions for using the method

a. Quick-start method—reasonably certain not pregnant, insert ring on day of office visit; if more than 5 days since LMP, use backup method for 7 days

b. First-day start—insert ring on first day of menses; no backup method needed

c. Wash hands before inserting

d. Fold ring and gently insert into the vagina so it is placed behind the pelvic bone

e. May be worn during vaginal penetrative intercourse

f. If desires to remove the ring, should be replaced within 2 hours to maintain efficacy

g. Leave ring in vagina for 3 weeks, then remove; clean with mild soap and water, pat dry and place in provided case during 1-week dose-free interval, then reinsert for 3 weeks

h. More studies are needed to determine the efficacy of continuous use

- Progestin-only pills (POPs)

1. Description—pill taken daily for purposes of contraception; contains synthetic progestins in lower doses than those used in COCs

2. Mechanism of action

a. Thickens cervical mucus

b. Produces atrophic endometrium

c. Inhibits ovulation—inconsistent; variable

d. Drospirenone-only pill (Slynd) reliably inhibits ovulation in addition to thickening cervical mucous and endometrium changes

3. Effectiveness/first-year failure rate

a. Perfect use—0.3%

b. Typical use—9%

4. Advantages

a. Ease of use

b. Reversible

c. Effective

d. Contains no estrogen for individuals in whom it is contraindicated or who cannot tolerate estrogenic side effects

e. Can be used during lactation and immediately postpartum

5. Disadvantages and side effects

a. Effectiveness may be compromised by the same drug interactions as COCs because of low-dose formulation

b. Decreased availability/increased expense compared to COCs

c. Strict daily dosing schedule; serum progestin levels peak shortly after taking POP, then decline to nearly undetectable levels 24 hours later

d. Drospirenone-only pill (Slynd) offers a longer, 24-hour missed pill window, which mirrors that of COC pills

e. Possible side effects

(1) Increased incidence of functional follicular cysts

(2) Menstrual cycle irregularities

(3) Mastalgia

(4) Depression

(5) No protection against STIs/HIV

6. Contraindications (CDC categories 3 and 4)

a. Category 4 for POP use—do not use the method if breast cancer within the past 5 years

b. Category 3 for POP use—use of the method not generally recommended for the conditions in **Box 4-6** unless other, more appropriate methods are not available or acceptable

c. Drospironone-only pill (Slynd) contraindication renal or adrenal insufficiency

7. Management

a. Health assessment prior to initiation of method—same as with COCs

b. Follow-up—same as with COCs

c. Special considerations—ectopic pregnancy more likely if pregnancy occurs

8. Instructions for using POPs

a. General instruction

(1) Quick-start method—reasonably certain not pregnant, take first pill on day of office visit; backup method for 48 hours if more than 5 days since LMP

(2) First-day start—take first pill on first day of menses; no backup method needed

(3) Take the pill at the same time each day, every day; no placebo/off week

(4) If more than 3 hours late taking the pill, use the backup method for 48 hours

(5) Drospirenone-only pill (Slynd) offers a longer, 24-hour missed pill window, which mirrors that of COC pills

(6) Advise may have irregular periods or may have amenorrhea

Box 4-6 Category 3 for POP Use

- History of breast cancer with no evidence of disease for 5 years
- Severe cirrhosis, benign hepatocellular adenoma, malignant hepatoma
- History of bariatric surgery with malabsorptive procedure
- Ischemic heart disease or stroke occurring while on POP
- SLE and positive or unknown antiphospholipid antibodies
- Taking ritonavir-boosted protease inhibitors as part of HIV/AIDS treatment; some anticonvulsants; rifampin or rifabutin

Jones & Bartlett Learning

b. Warning signs
   (1) Severe low abdominal pain
   (2) No bleeding after a series of regular cycles
   (3) Severe headache

- Progestin-only injectable contraception (DMPA)
  1. Description—intramuscular (IM) or subcutaneous (SC); injectable progestin administered in 3-month intervals for contraception
  2. Mechanism of action
     a. Inhibits ovulation through suppression of FSH and LH
     b. Produces atrophic endometrium
     c. Thickens cervical mucus
  3. Effectiveness/first-year failure rate
     a. Perfect use—0.2%
     b. Typical use—6%
  4. Advantages
     a. Ease of use
     b. Effective
     c. Long-term contraceptive option
     d. Does not require compliance with daily/event regimen
     e. Minimal drug interaction profile—only drug that may decrease effectiveness is aminoglutethimide (used to treat Cushing's disease)
     f. Results in absence of menstrual bleeding in as many as 50% of individuals by end of first year of use (four injections); by end of second year, 70% are amenorrheic
     g. Contains no estrogen for individuals in whom it is contraindicated or who cannot tolerate estrogenic side effects
     h. Can be used during lactation and immediately postpartum
     i. May decrease the following:
        (1) Intravascular sickling in patients with sickle cell disease
        (2) Incidence of seizures in affected individuals
        (3) Pain from endometriosis; SC formulation approved for treatment of pain associated with endometriosis
        (4) Risk for PID
        (5) Risk for endometrial cancer
  5. Disadvantages/side effects
     a. Menstrual cycle irregularities
     b. Mastalgia
     c. Depression
     d. No protection against STIs/HIV
     e. Not immediately reversible—requires 3 months to be eliminated
     f. Requires routine 3-month injection schedule
     g. Weight gain
        (1) Average 5.4 lb first year
        (2) 13.8 lb after 4 years
     h. In some individuals, 6- to 12-month delayed return to fertility
     i. Decreased bone density in long-term (greater than 5 years) user—returned to normal following discontinuance; no data indicating association between temporary decreased bone density and fracture risk

j. May decrease HDL-C; may increase LDL-C and total cholesterol

6. Contraindications (CDC categories 3 and 4)
   a. Category 4 for DMPA use—do not use the method if breast cancer within the past 5 years
   b. Category 3 for DMPA use—use of the method not generally recommended for the conditions in **Box 4-7** unless other, more appropriate methods are not available or acceptable

7. Management
   a. Health assessment prior to initiation of method—same as with COCs
   b. Follow-up
      (1) Return every 3 months for injection
      (2) Determine LMP; ask about any concerns with bleeding pattern
      (3) Assess for side effects/problems
      (4) Consider assessing weight and counseling if an individual concerned about weight change perceived to be associated with DMPA

8. Instructions for using the method
   a. Explain the importance of adherence to a 3-month (13 weeks) injection schedule—contraceptive efficacy maintained for at least 14 weeks after injection
   b. Quick-start method—Administer first injection at any time if reasonably certain not pregnant; if more than 5 days since LMP, use backup method for 7 days
   c. First-day start—administer injection on first day of menses; no backup method needed
   d. Counsel patients regarding the possibility of irregular bleeding; |use of backup contraception if more than 3 months between injections; use of condoms for STI/HIV prevention
   e. Late for injection
      (1) Can be given up to 2 weeks late (15 weeks from last injection) without needing additional contraceptive protection

---

Box 4-7 Category 3 for DMPA Use

- Multiple risk factors for arterial cardiovascular disease
- Hypertension (160/100 mm Hg) or with vascular disease
- Current/history of ischemic heart disease or stroke
- History of breast cancer with no evidence of disease for 5 years
- Unexplained vaginal bleeding before evaluation
- Diabetes with nephropathy, retinopathy, neuropathy, other vascular disease; diabetes longer than 20 years' duration
- Severe cirrhosis, benign hepatocellular adenoma, malignant hepatoma
- SLE with positive or unknown antiphospholipid antibodies
- SLE with severe thrombocytopenia—initiation category 3, continuation category 2
- Rheumatoid arthritis or long-term corticosteroid therapy with a history of or risk factors for nontraumatic fractures

(2) If more than 2 weeks late (more than 15 weeks from last injection), give injection if reasonably certain patient is not pregnant; use backup method or abstain for seven days after injection

(3) Might consider the use of EC (except for UPA) if appropriate

f. Procedure for injection

   (1) IM formulation—deep intramuscular injection in deltoid or gluteal muscle

   (2) SC formulation—anterior thigh or abdominal wall

   (3) Do not massage the injection site (alters absorption/efficacy)

   (4) Observe the patient for 20 minutes following the first injection to rule out an allergic reaction

g. Management of unscheduled bleeding

   (1) Anticipatory guidance is important

   (2) If abrupt change in bleeding pattern, rule out pregnancy

   (3) Nonsteroidal anti-inflammatory (NSAID) medication inhibits cyclooxygenase with an anti-prostaglandin effect

     (a) Mefenamic acid 500 mg 2 times per day × 5 days

     (b) Valdecoxib 40 mg daily × 5 days

   (4) Exogenous estrogen, such as ethinyl estradiol 50 mcg daily for 14 days

h. Warning signs

   (1) Frequent intense headache

   (2) Heavy bleeding

   (3) Depression

   (4) Abdominal pain (severe)

   (5) Signs of infection at injection site (prolonged redness, bleeding, pain, discharge)

- Emergency contraception

1. Definition—method used to prevent conception after unprotected coitus; levonorgestrel pill (Plan B or generic), UPA pill (ella), combination of ethinyl estradiol and norgestrel or levonorgestrel pills (COC), or copper-releasing IUC

2. Mechanism of action

a. Emergency contraception pill (ECP)

   (1) Inhibits or delays ovulation

   (2) Will not disrupt an established pregnancy—minimal endometrial effect

b. Copper-releasing IUC

   (1) Prevents fertilization

   (2) Interferes with implantation

3. Effectiveness

a. ECP

   (1) Depends on preexisting fertility, timing of intercourse during the cycle, timing of taking ECP

   (2) Studies have compared the estimated pregnancy rate from one act of unprotected intercourse (5.5%–8%) to the observed pregnancy rate after using either UPA or levonorgestrel ECP (1%–2.2%)

   (3) Some studies have shown higher pregnancy rates for individuals who are "overweight or obese" than for individuals who are "normal weight" taking UPA and levonorgestrel ECP (more significant with levonorgestrel ECP)

   (4) Some studies have shown that levonorgestrel ECP may be less effective if treatment is delayed beyond 72 hours; moderate effectiveness if taken between 72 and 120 hours after sexual intercourse

   (5) Studies with UPA have shown no significant decrease in effectiveness up to 120 hours after sexual intercourse

b. Copper-releasing IUC—reduces the risk of pregnancy by more than 99%

4. Advantages

a. Provides means of emergency contraception in the event of any of the following:

   (1) Unplanned intercourse

   (2) Sexual assault

   (3) Method failure—condom breaks/leaks; IUC expelled; cap or diaphragm dislodged or improperly placed

   (4) Missed pills

   (5) Late using contraceptive method—injection, patch, vaginal ring, pills

b. ECP may be provided with instructions for use by individuals using any contraceptive method or not using a contraceptive method

c. Levonorgestrel ECP available without prescription

d. IUC can provide ongoing contraception

5. Disadvantages and side effects

a. ECP

   (1) Nausea/vomiting—less common with levonorgestrel or UPA than with COCs

   (2) Change in next menses—timing, length, intermenstrual bleeding

b. Copper-releasing IUC

   (1) Irregular, heavy bleeding

   (2) Uterine cramping/abdominal pain

   (3) Refer to the intrauterine contraception section earlier in this chapter

6. Precautions and risks

a. Contraindications for ECP—no CDC category 3 or 4 conditions

b. Contraindications for copper-releasing IUC—see the intrauterine contraception section earlier in this chapter

7. Management

a. Health assessment prior to initiation of method

   (1) Individuals may purchase levonorgestrel ECP over the counter; clinicians may provide a prescription or advance supply of any of the ECPs so the individual can begin taking it as soon as possible after unprotected sex

   (2) If the clinician sees an individual needing ECP, may obtain health history—menstrual; first episode of unprotected sex in cycle to determine if should consider pregnancy test; last

episode of unprotected sex to ensure within time frame for emergency contraception

    (3) If using IUC—see the intrauterine contraception section earlier in this chapter for required history and examination

    (4) Discuss/provide ongoing contraception

  b. Follow-up—no routine follow-up visit required

8. Instructions for using emergency contraception

  a. ECP

    (1) Take as soon as possible after unprotected sex and within 120 hours for maximum effectiveness

    (2) If using COC for emergency contraception, take in two doses 12 hours apart

    (3) If using COC for emergency contraception, consider taking antinausea medicine 1 hour before the first dose

    (4) If individual vomits within 2 hours of taking pills, may need a repeat dose

    (5) ECP will not provide any ongoing protection from pregnancy

    (6) Levonorgestrel ECPs or COCs—resume current method or begin new method immediately; wait until next day to start or restart oral contraceptives to prevent nausea/vomiting; abstain from sexual intercourse or use additional contraception with any hormonal method for 7 days.

    (7) UPA—start hormonal method no sooner than 5 days after UPA, as may reduce effectiveness of EC; use additional contraception with any hormonal method for 7 days.

    (8) Advise patient to have a pregnancy test if no withdrawal bleed within 3 weeks of ECP

  b. Copper-releasing IUC (Copper T 380A)

    (1) Can be inserted up to 5 days after first unprotected sex since LMP

    (2) Minimal evidence that progestin-releasing IUC offers effective emergency contraception

- Vaginal spermicides

1. Description—cream, foam, suppository, tablet, film, gel, or other preparation that destroys sperm when placed in vagina

2. Mechanism of action

  a. Traditional—Nonoxynol-9 is active ingredient

  b. Destroys sperm cell membrane

  c. Duration of effectiveness is usually no more than 1 hour

  d. Vaginal contraceptive gel containing lactic acid, citric acid, and potassium bitartrate (Phexxi)

  e. Mechanism of action—acidifying agent, it resists the buffering effect of semen, which is alkaline

3. Effectiveness/first-year failure rate

  a. Traditional—Perfect use—18%

  b. Traditional—Typical use—28%

  c. Phexxi—typical use 86%

4. Advantages

  a. Accessible

  b. Inexpensive

  c. Readily available backup method

  d. No systemic effects

5. Disadvantages and side effects

  a. Coitally dependent

  b. Does not protect against STIs/HIV

  c. Potential for allergy, sensitivity, irritation

  d. Must follow instructions carefully for effective use

6. Contraindications (CDC categories 3 and 4)

  a. Category 4—do not use the method if the patient at a high risk for HIV (relates to frequent spermicide use two or more times a day, vulvovaginal epithelium disruption, and theoretically increased susceptibility to HIV infection)

  b. Category 3—use of method not generally recommended for patients diagnosed with HIV/AIDS unless other, more appropriate methods are not available or acceptable (relates to frequent spermicide use, disruption of cervical mucosa, potential increased viral shedding, and HIV transmission)

7. Management

  a. No health assessment needed prior to the initiation of the method

  b. Individuals with skin sensitivities may want to test first or avoid use altogether

  c. Vaginal abnormalities (septa, prolapse) may preclude use

8. Instructions for using the method

  a. Use spermicide with each act of intercourse, must be reinserted before repeated intercourse

  b. Read all instructions carefully

  c. Follow instructions regarding how long prior to intercourse the spermicide may be inserted—if too much time has lapsed, pregnancy may occur

  d. Place spermicide deep within the vagina

  e. Allow adequate time for spermicide to dissolve (if film, tablets, or suppositories)

  f. With foam use—shake canister well, as directed, prior to filling the applicator

  g. Use with condom for increased effectiveness

  h. Leave spermicide in place (no douching) for at least 6 hours following last intercourse

- External condom

1. Description—latex/polyurethane/natural membranous sleeve placed over erect penis prior to intercourse to prevent transmission of semen/sperm into vaginal vault

2. Mechanism of action—barrier; prevents transmission of semen/sperm into the vagina

3. Effectiveness/first-year failure rate

  a. Perfect use—2%

  b. Typical use—18%

4. Advantages

  a. Accessible

  b. Cost-effective

  c. Prevents/reduces transmission of STIs (except with membrane condoms)

  d. Portable—can be easily and discretely carried with individual

  e. Prevents allergic reaction to semen

  f. Arrests development of anti-sperm antibodies in infertility patients

g. May help prevent premature ejaculation
h. Does not require a visit to a healthcare provider
5. Disadvantages
   a. Decreased penile sensitivity
   b. Interrupts act of coitus
   c. Some individuals cannot maintain an erection during condom use
   d. Requires active involvement of partner with penis
   e. Possibility of condom rupture
6. Contraindications—latex allergy; can use polyurethane
7. Management—no health assessment needed prior to initiation of the method
8. Instructions for using the method
   a. Natural membrane condoms may not protect against STIs/HIV
   b. Use water-soluble lubricants (e.g., K-Y Jelly, Astroglide, egg whites) or silicone lubricants (e.g. Uber Lube, Pjur); avoid oil-based lubricants with latex condoms (e.g., baby oil, vegetable or mineral oils, petroleum jelly)
   c. Use a new condom with each act of intercourse
   d. Unroll condom over penis completely (to the base) prior to any genital contact
   e. Immediately after ejaculation, hold the rim of the condom and withdraw the penis from vagina while it is still erect
   f. If the condom slips or breaks
      (1) Before ejaculation—apply a new condom
      (2) After ejaculation—consider emergency contraception
- Internal condom
   1. Description—nitrile sheath placed in the vagina that acts as a barrier to prevent direct contact with seminal fluid during intercourse; smaller ring at closed end lies inside vagina and wider ring at open end of sheath remains outside the vagina; has silicone-based lubricant on inside
   2. Mechanism of action—barrier, protects vagina/vulva from direct contact with penis/seminal fluid
   3. Effectiveness/first-year failure rate
      a. Perfect use—5%
      b. Typical use—21%
   4. Advantages
      a. Prevents/reduces transmission of STIs
      b. Does not require the use of spermicide
      c. Stronger than latex and less likely to tear or break
      d. Does not require a visit to a healthcare provider
   5. Disadvantages and side effects
      a. Coitally dependent
      b. Requires active involvement of partner with vagina
      c. May be aesthetically unappealing
      d. Expensive
      e. No longer available over the counter, requires a prescription
   6. Contraindications—nitrile allergy
   7. Management
      a. No health assessment needed prior to the initiation of the method
      b. Individuals with vaginal anatomic abnormalities may not be able to use this method

8. Instructions for using the method
   a. Hold the pouch with the open end down—inner ring should be at the bottom of the pouch
   b. Squeeze inner ring together and insert inner ring and pouch into the vagina
   c. Push inner ring deep into the vagina
   d. Outer ring should rest outside the vulva
   e. Remove the condom immediately after intercourse
   f. Squeeze the outer ring together and twist to prevent spillage
   g. Discard the whole condom
   h. Use a new condom with each act of intercourse
   i. Do not use external condoms when using internal condoms—may adhere together causing dislodgement
- Caya diaphragm—the Caya diaphragm has essentially replaced earlier dome-shaped fitted diaphragms in the United States
   1. Description—reusable silicone device with two cup-like structures; larger cup fits over cervix and holds spermicide in place over cervical os, smaller everted cup tucks behind symphysis pubis and facilitates removal; 75 mm in length, 67 mm in maximum width; circular nylon spring enables use for a variety of cervical sizes and degrees of vaginal muscle support
   2. Mechanism of action
      a. Barrier—prevents direct cervical contact with seminal fluid
      b. Used with spermicide—destroys sperm cell membrane
   3. Effectiveness/first-year failure rate
      a. Perfect use—14%
      b. Typical use—17.4%
   4. Advantages
      a. Cost-effective—may be used for 1–2 years
      b. Affords some protection against STIs—possible decreased incidence of PID
      c. No systemic effects
      d. May use with external condom for increased effectiveness
   5. Disadvantages
      a. Requires visit to clinician for examination to ensure proper fitting
      b. May have sensitivity to spermicide
      c. Potential risk of toxic shock
   6. Contraindications (CDC categories 3 and 4)
      a. Category 4 for diaphragm use—do not use method if high risk for HIV, related to concerns about frequent spermicide use disrupting vaginal epithelium rather than diaphragm
      b. Category 3 for diaphragm use—use of method not generally recommended for the following conditions unless other, more appropriate methods are not available or acceptable:
         (1) History of toxic shock syndrome
         (2) HIV/AIDS—related to concerns about frequent spermicide use disrupting vaginal epithelium rather than diaphragm
   7. Management
      a. Health assessment prior to initiation of method

(1) Health history to determine any special circumstances or contraindications

(2) Vaginal examination to determine any abnormal anatomy (prolapse, cystocele, rectocele, vaginal septum) that may preclude proper fit and retention

(3) Clinician should ensure proper fit and confirm the client's ability to place and remove correctly

(4) Wait until 6 weeks postpartum or until uterine involution complete and 6 weeks after second-trimester abortion to use

b. Follow-up—no routine follow-up required

8. Instructions for using the method

a. Insert just prior to intercourse or up to 2 hours before

b. Place 1 teaspoon of spermicidal gel into each fold of the diaphragm and a small amount around the rim

c. Insert the diaphragm so the cervix is completely covered and positioned behind the symphysis pubis

d. If repeated intercourse, insert another application of spermicide in the vagina; do not remove the diaphragm

e. Leave the diaphragm in place for at least 6 hours following last intercourse

f. Do not leave in place for more than 24 hours

g. After each use, wash the diaphragm with plain soap and water and store in the provided case

h. Replace diaphragm every 2 years

i. Assess for holes and tears periodically by filling with water and inspecting for leaks

j. Consider emergency contraception if the diaphragm is dislodged during or less than 6 hours after sex

k. Warning signs (toxic shock)

(1) High fever

(2) Nausea, vomiting, diarrhea

(3) Syncope, weakness

(4) Joint/muscle aches

(5) Rash resembling sunburn

- Cervical cap (FemCap)

1. Description—reusable silicone cap, fits over cervix, providing barrier contraception; spermicide placed in dome affords additional contraceptive efficacy; three sizes—22 mm, 26 mm, 30 mm; strap on convex side of cap aids in removal

2. Mechanism of action

a. Barrier—prevents direct cervical contact with seminal fluid

b. Spermicide—destroys sperm cell membrane

3. Effectiveness/first-year failure rate

a. Perfect use

(1) Parous women—21%

(2) Nulliparous women—10%

b. Typical use

(1) Parous women—40%

(2) Nulliparous women—20%

4. Advantages

a. Cost-effective—may be used for 1–2 years

b. Affords some protection against STIs

c. Possible decreased incidence of PID

d. Possible decreased incidence of cervical dysplasia/neoplasia

e. No systemic effects

f. May be left in place for 48 hours

g. Does not require insertion of more spermicide with repeat intercourse

h. Does not increase the incidence of bladder infection

i. May use with condoms to increase effectiveness

5. Disadvantages

a. Requires trained clinician for sizing

b. May have sensitivity to silicone or spermicide

c. Not every patient can be fitted appropriately—short cervix, asymmetry

d. May become dislodged during intercourse

6. Contraindications (CDC categories 3 and 4)

a. Category 4 for cervical cap use—do not use the method if high risk for HIV exists, related to concerns about frequent spermicide use disrupting vaginal epithelium rather than the cervical cap

b. Category 3 for cervical cap use—use of method not generally recommended for the following conditions unless other, more appropriate methods are not available or acceptable:

(1) HIV/AIDS—related to concerns about frequent spermicide use disrupting vaginal epithelium rather than the cervical cap

(2) History of toxic shock syndrome

7. Management

a. Health assessment prior to initiation of method

(1) Visualization of cervix to rule out abnormalities/anatomy that may prevent proper fit—extensive lacerations, asymmetry, short cervix

(2) Palpation of cervix—length, position, symmetry

(3) Size generally determined by obstetric history—smallest size if never pregnant, middle size if miscarried or had cesarean section, largest size if had vaginally delivered full-term baby

(4) Wait until 6 weeks postpartum or until uterine involution complete and 6 weeks after second-trimester abortion to fit and use

b. Follow-up—no routine follow-up required; reevaluate cap fit if patient complains of dislodgement during intercourse

c. Special considerations—do not use if less than 6 weeks postpartum, immediately postabortion, or during menses

8. Instructions for using the method

a. Insert cap at least 15 minutes prior to intercourse to create suction

b. Fill one-third of the cap with spermicide

c. Compress rim prior to insertion

d. Advance into the vagina so rim can slide over the cervix

e. Check that cap covers the cervix

f. Not necessary to reinsert spermicide with repeated intercourse

g. Leave in place for at least 6 hours and no more than 48 hours after sex

h. Warning signs (toxic shock)—refer to the Diaphragm section earlier in this chapter

i. Do not use after a recent spontaneous or induced abortion

j. Do not use during menses or any other vaginal bleeding

- Contraceptive sponge
  1. Description—small, pillow-shaped polyurethane sponge containing 1 g of nonoxynol-9 spermicide; concave side fits over cervix; polyester loop facilitates removal; one size
  2. Mechanism of action
     a. Barrier—prevents direct cervical contact with seminal fluid
     b. Spermicide—destroys sperm cell membrane
  3. Effectiveness/first-year failure rate
     a. Perfect use
        (1) Nulliparous—9%
        (2) Parous—20%
     b. Typical use
        (1) Nulliparous—12%
        (2) Parous—24%
  4. Advantages
     a. No prescription required
     b. No systemic effects
     c. May be used with a male condom for additional contraceptive and STI protection
     d. Protects up to 24 hours regardless of how many times intercourse occurs
  5. Disadvantages
     a. Significant decrease in efficacy for parous women versus nulliparous woman
     b. Potential risk of toxic shock—same as with diaphragm
     c. May have sensitivity to polyurethane or spermicide
     d. Abnormal vaginal anatomy (prolapse, cystocele, rectocele) may prevent proper placement
  6. Contraindications (CDC recommendations not specifically provided)—consider same as for diaphragm and cervical cap
  7. Management
     a. No health assessment needed prior to the initiation of the method
     b. Wait until 6 weeks postpartum to use
  8. Instructions for using the method
     a. Moisten sponge with tap water prior to use
     b. Insert deep into the vagina
     c. Check to be sure the cervix is covered by the sponge
     d. Leave in place for at least 6 hours after last intercourse
     e. If repeated intercourse, no additional spermicide needed
     f. Do not wear the sponge for more than 24–30 hours
     g. Discard sponge after use
     h. Do not use after a recent spontaneous or induced abortion
     i. Do not use during menses or any other vaginal bleeding

j. Warning signs (toxic shock)—refer to the Diaphragm section earlier in this chapter

- Fertility awareness-based methods (FABMs)
  1. Description—method of contraception using abstinence during the estimated fertile period based on all or some of the following indicators
     a. Menstrual cycle pattern (calendar method)
     b. Basal body temperature (BBT)—determines ovulation
     c. Evaluation of cervical mucus (ovulation/Billings method)—determines ovulation
     d. Sympto-thermal method—combines BBT with evaluation of cervical mucus and cervical position/consistency
     e. Standard days method—consider fertile days 8 through 19 of each menstrual cycle
  2. Mechanism of action—intercourse is avoided during the fertile period
     a. Ovum remains fertile for 24 hours
     b. Sperm viability approximately 72 hours
     c. Most pregnancies occur when intercourse occurs before ovulation
  3. Effectiveness/first-year failure rate
     a. Perfect use
        (1) Calendar method—9%
        (2) BBT—2%
        (3) Ovulation method—3%
        (4) Sympto-thermal—0.4%
        (5) Standard days method—5%
     b. Typical use for all methods—24%
  4. Advantages
     a. Minimal cost
     b. Natural
     c. No systemic effects
     d. No localized side effects—for example, latex allergy
     e. Can be utilized for contraception and conception planning
  5. Disadvantages
     a. Requires motivation from both partners
     b. Requires periodic abstinence
     c. No protection against STIs/HIV
  6. Precautions and risks
     a. Not reliable for individuals with the following conditions:
        (1) Irregular menses (consider sympto-thermal and ovulation methods)
        (2) Perimenopausal
        (3) Recently postpartum
        (4) Have had recent menarche
     b. Not a suitable method for individuals with the following conditions:
        (1) Individuals who cannot accurately evaluate their fertile period
           (a) Inability to use/read thermometer
           (b) Inability to understand cervical mucus/changes
           (c) Inability to time intercourse based on calendar evaluation
        (2) Couples unwilling to abstain during fertile time period
        (3) If nonconsensual coitus is likely to occur

7. Management
   a. Health assessment prior to initiation of method
      (1) History to reflect pattern of menses
      (2) Evaluation of client's willingness/ability to check cervical mucus/consistency/position
   b. Follow-up—BBT/sympto-thermal chart evaluation
8. Instructions for using the method
   a. Calendar method
      (1) Keep a record of menstrual cycle intervals for several months
      (2) From the shortest cycle length, subtract 18 days—this determines the first fertile day
      (3) From the longest cycle length, subtract 11 days—this determines the last fertile day
      (4) Use these numbers to determine days of abstinence for every cycle
   b. BBT method
      (1) Take temperature each morning before rising
         (a) BBT thermometer
         (b) Temperature can be oral, vaginal, or rectal (maintain same route)
      (2) Record on BBT chart
      (3) Temperature increase of 0.4°F or higher at ovulation—remains elevated for at least 3 days
      (4) Abstain from intercourse until a 3-day temperature increase occurs
   c. Ovulation method
      (1) Inspect cervical mucus/secretions on underwear, toilet tissue, with fingers, beginning the day after menses
      (2) Determine consistency—elastic, slippery, wet by touch indicates preovulatory
         (a) Amount increases; becomes thinner and more elastic around the time of ovulation
         (b) After ovulation, mucus becomes thick, tacky, and cloudy
      (3) Abstain from intercourse during "wet days" at the onset of increased, slippery, thin mucus discharge until 4 days past the peak day (last day of clear, stretchy, slippery secretions)
      (4) Abstain from intercourse during menses because of inability to assess mucus
   d. Sympto-thermal method—combines cervical mucus evaluation, BBT, and assessment of consistency/position of cervix in vagina
      (1) May also use the calendar method and other symptoms such as ovulatory pain ("mittelschmerz") as additional indicators
      (2) Abstain until the last combined method indicates a "safe" time
   e. Standard days method
      (1) Abstain from intercourse on days 8 through 19 of each menstrual cycle
      (2) CycleBeads are a color-coded string of beads to help individuals keep track of cycle days; there is also a CycleBeads app
      (3) FABM apps—use embedded predictive algorithms; Natural Cycles is an FDA-approved app for contraception, which relies on cycle patterns and BBT

- Lactational amenorrhea method (LAM)
   1. Description—method of contraception for individuals who are breastfeeding/chestfeeding without supplementation or with minimal supplementation, have not had a postpartum menstrual cycle, and are less than 6 months postpartum
   2. Mechanism of action—high prolactin
      a. FSH normal; LH decreased—no ovarian follicular development
      b. Inhibits pulsatile GnRH
      c. Results in anovulation
   3. Effectiveness/first-year failure rate
      a. Perfect use—0.5% to 1.5% (if amenorrheic)
      b. Typical use—data not available
   4. Advantages
      a. Requires no pills or other devices
      b. No cost
      c. Not coitally dependent
      d. Advantageous for infant
         (1) Nutritional
         (2) Bonding
   5. Disadvantages
      a. Individuals must breastfeed/chestfeed completely or with minimal supplementation—may lead to exhaustion
      b. Decreased estrogen due to the absence of follicular development
         (1) Atrophic vaginitis
         (2) Decreased vaginal lubrication
         (3) Dyspareunia
      c. Affords no protection against STIs/HIV
   6. Management
      a. No health assessment needed prior to the initiation of the method
      b. Special considerations—should not use vaginal estrogen cream to treat atrophic vaginitis
         (1) Absorption can inhibit milk production
         (2) Recommend use of vaginal lubricants
   7. Instructions for using the method
      a. Use no or only minimal supplementation
      b. Choose an alternative contraceptive method when any of the following occurs:
         (1) Menses
         (2) Regular supplementation is being used
         (3) Long periods without breastfeeding/chestfeeding (e.g., baby sleeping through the night)
         (4) Baby is 6 months old
      c. Ovulation may occur before the onset of menses
      d. Milk expression by hand or pump does not have the same fertility-inhibiting effect as breastfeeding/chestfeeding
      e. Do not use vaginal estrogen cream for atrophic vaginitis—absorption may inhibit milk production
      f. Use vaginal lubricants as needed
- Coitus interruptus (withdrawal)
   1. Description—contraceptive method whereby partner withdraws penis from vagina prior to ejaculation
   2. Mechanism of action—sperm not introduced into the vagina

3. Effectiveness/first-year failure rate
   a. Perfect use—4%
   b. Typical use—22%
4. Advantages
   a. Requires no devices
   b. No systemic effects
   c. No expense
   d. May result in decreased transmission of HIV if semen does not enter the vagina
5. Disadvantages and side effects
   a. Requires self-control on the part of sperm-producing partner
   b. Requires the ability to predict the time of ejaculation
   c. Does not afford protection from STIs
6. Precautions and risks—should not be used by individuals with premature ejaculatory disorder
7. Management—no health assessment needed prior to initiation of the method
8. Instructions for using the method
   a. Partner should void prior to intercourse
   b. Withdraw penis prior to ejaculation; do not ejaculate near partner's external genital area
   c. If intercourse will be repeated in a short period of time, the sperm-producing partner should urinate again and wipe the tip of penis to remove any sperm remaining from previous intercourse
   d. Although preejaculate itself contains little or no sperm, repeated intercourse may result in increased amounts of sperm in the preejaculatory fluid

- Abstinence
  1. Description—contraception based on abstaining from penile–vaginal intercourse
  2. Mechanism of action—sperm not introduced into the vagina
  3. Effectiveness/first-year failure rate
     a. Perfect use—0%
     b. Typical use—data not available
  4. Advantages
     a. No cost
     b. Prevention of STIs
  5. Disadvantages—requires motivation and acceptance by both partners
  6. Management—no health assessment needed prior to initiation of the method
  7. Instructions for using the method
     a. Avoid any penile–vaginal contact
     b. Consider alternative means of intimacy/sexual expression (e.g., mutual masturbation, massage, kissing)
     c. Penile–anal intercourse may result in some sperm entering vagina during withdrawal
     d. Penile–anal, oral–genital, and digital–genital contact may result in STI/HIV transmission
     e. Avoid alcohol or drug use; may affect commitment to the method

- Sterilization—fallopian tube occlusion
  1. Description—permanent contraception achieved through surgical means; commonly performed on an outpatient basis or postpartum prior to discharge

2. Mechanism of action
   a. Fallopian tubes are obstructed to prevent the union of sperm and ovum
   b. Transabdominal occlusion methods—laparoscopy or suprapubic mini-laparoscopy approach; general or local anesthesia
      (1) Surgical ligation—Pomeroy procedure
      (2) Surgical ligation and attachment to uterine body—Irving procedure
      (3) Electrocauterization
      (4) Section of tube excised
         (a) Pritchard procedure
         (b) Fimbriectomy
      (5) Occluded—compressed with silastic band (Falope Ring) or clip (Filshie)
3. Effectiveness/first-year failure rate
   a. Perfect use—0.5%
   b. Typical use—0.5%
4. Advantages
   a. Affords permanent contraception
   b. Highly effective
   c. Cost-effective over the long term
   d. Not coitally dependent
5. Disadvantages
   a. Invasive surgical procedure requiring anesthesia
   b. Reversal is difficult, expensive, and often unsuccessful
   c. No protection against STIs/HIV
   d. Initially expensive
   e. Probability of pregnancy being ectopic is higher if the method fails
6. Precautions and risks
   a. Surgical procedure
      (1) Operative complications—bladder/uterine/intestinal injury may occur
      (2) Anesthetic complications—death (rare)
   b. Wound infection
   c. If pregnancy occurs following the procedure, increased risk of the pregnancy being ectopic
7. Management
   a. Health assessment prior to initiation of method
      (1) Assess if the client is a candidate for surgery
      (2) Assess psychological readiness for permanent contraceptive method
      (3) Follow federal and state regulations regarding the informed consent process
   b. Follow-up—assess for appropriate healing and signs and symptoms of infection 1–2 weeks after the procedure
8. Instructions for using the method
   a. Nothing by mouth at least 8 hours prior to the procedure
   b. Need transportation assistance from hospital or clinic to home
   c. Rest for at least 24 hours recommended following the procedure
   d. Avoid strenuous physical activity and intercourse for 1 week
   e. Notify healthcare provider of any signs and/or symptoms of infection

f. If pregnancy suspected, see a healthcare provider as soon as possible to evaluate for possible ectopic pregnancy

- Sterilization—vas deferens surgery
 1. Description—permanent contraception involving occlusion of vas deferens, preventing transmission of sperm through semen
    a. Approaches to vas deferens
       (1) Conventional vasectomy—local anesthesia; skin and muscle overlying vas deferens is incised with scalpel, vas deferens is occluded, and incisions are closed with absorbable suture
       (2) No-scalpel vasectomy—local anesthesia; ringed clamp secures vas deferens, midline puncture of scrotum with dissecting forceps rather than incision; vas deferens occluded; sutures not needed; less risk of infection, hematoma, pain than conventional method
    b. Methods of occlusion
       (1) Ligation with sutures and excision of section of vas deferens—most common
       (2) Other methods—electrosurgical or thermal cautery, application of clips, combination of methods
 2. Mechanism of action—sperm not present in ejaculate
 3. Effectiveness/first-year failure rate
    a. Perfect use—0.10%
    b. Typical use—0.15%
 4. Advantages
    a. Cost-effective
    b. Highly effective
    c. Affords permanent contraception
    d. Not coitally dependent
    e. No systemic effects/artificial devices
 5. Disadvantages
    a. Initial expense
    b. Should be considered irreversible
    c. Invasive surgical procedure
    d. No protection against STIs/HIV
 6. Precautions and risks
    a. Surgical procedure
    b. Wound infection
    c. Extensive research has identified no significant long-term physical or mental health effects with vas surgery
 7. Management
    a. Health assessment prior to initiation of procedure
       (1) Assess psychological readiness for permanent contraceptive method
       (2) Assess general health and inguinal area, scrotum, and testicles
       (3) Follow federal and state regulations regarding informed consent process
    b. Follow-up—confirm vasectomy success with semen analysis 3 months after the procedure
 8. Instructions for using the method
    a. Use scrotal support (e.g., wearing brief-style underwear) for at least 2 days to reduce pain
    b. Apply ice pack to scrotum for minimum of 4 hours after procedure

c. Notify healthcare provider if signs and/or symptoms of infection appear
   (1) Fever greater than 100.4°F
   (2) Increasing pain not relieved by analgesics
   (3) Redness, inflammation, swelling, drainage, or discharge at incision site
   (4) Stitches causing extreme pulling sensation
d. Avoid ejaculation for 1 week
e. Avoid strenuous exercise or heavy lifting for 1 week
f. Continue using other contraception for at least 3 months; obtain semen analysis to confirm azoospermia (no sperm)

- Special considerations in contraceptive management
 1. Postpartum contraception
    a. On average, the first ovulation occurs 45 days postpartum in nonlactating individuals; however, it may occur as early as 25 days postpartum
    b. LAM is a highly effective temporary method of contraception up to 6 months postpartum if individual follows recommended parameters
    c. VTE risk is increased for first few weeks postpartum, generally declining to baseline levels by 42 days postpartum
    d. Initiation of CHC methods in lactating individuals
       (1) Less than 21 days postpartum (CDC category 4)
       (2) Twenty-one to <30 days postpartum (CDC category 3)—regardless of other VTE risk factors
       (3) Thirty to 42 days postpartum—with other VTE risk factors (CDC category 3), without other VTE risk factors (CDC category 2)
       (4) Greater than 42 days postpartum (CDC category 2)
    e. Initiation of CHC methods for nonlactating individuals who have recently given birth
       (1) Less than 21 days postpartum (CDC category 4)
       (2) Twenty-one to 42 days postpartum with other VTE risk factors (CDC category 3), without other VTE risk factors (category 2)
       (3) Greater than 42 days postpartum (CDC category 1)
    f. Initiation of progestin-only contraceptive methods for lactating individuals
       (1) Less than 21 days postpartum (CDC category 2)
       (2) Twenty-one to <30 days postpartum (CDC category 2) regardless of other VTE risk factors
       (3) Thirty or greater days postpartum (CDC category 1)
    g. Initiation of progestin-only contraceptive methods for nonlactating individuals who have recently given birth (CDC category 1)—may initiate immediately postpartum
    h. Initiation of IUC—lactating, nonlactating, including post-cesarean delivery
       (1) Less than 10 minutes after delivery of placenta—LNG-IUS (CDC category 2), copper-releasing IUC (CDC category 1)

(2) Ten minutes after delivery of placenta to less than 4 weeks (both CDC category 2)

(3) Four weeks or greater postpartum (both CDC category 1)

2. Contraception for individuals older than 40 years

a. Most contraceptive options safe for individuals older than 40 without category 3 or 4 contraindications

b. Combination hormonal contraception (CHC)—pills, patch, vaginal ring

(1) Safe option for individuals who are nonsmoking, nonobese, and healthy perimenopausal

(2) Noncontraceptive benefits may be especially attractive to perimenopausal individuals—relief of vasomotor symptoms, menstrual regulation

(3) May reduce the risk of endometrial hyperplasia/cancer associated with anovulatory cycles during perimenopausal years

c. Progestin-only methods (DMPA, POPs, implants)

(1) No specific age-related contraindications

(2) May provide some relief from vasomotor symptoms

(3) May reduce the risk of endometrial hyperplasia/cancer

(4) DMPA may diminish bone mineral density in perimenopausal individuals; however, these individuals do not undergo the typical rapid loss of bone mineral density following menopause

d. Intrauterine contraceptives

(1) Long-acting reversible method option as effective as sterilization

(2) LNG-IUS may also be therapeutic for perimenopausal individuals with heavy bleeding

e. Barrier methods—safe option

f. Sterilization—most prevalent contraceptive method among married women in the United States

g. Fertility awareness methods—may be less effective during perimenopause because of irregular ovulation and menstrual cycles

h. Approaches used in deciding when to discontinue contraception

(1) There are no definitive answers for when to discontinue contraception

(2) North American Menopause Society states that 90% of patients will reach menopause by age 55 and recommends continuing contraception until mid-50s

(3) CHC

(a) Two methods

i. Stop method for 6 weeks to eliminate effect on FSH and estradiol levels; if no menses, check FSH twice 1–2 months apart; if elevated > 30 IU/l both times contraception can be discontinued

ii. Stop method for 7–14 days starting at age 50; check FSH on two occasions

6–8 weeks apart; if elevated >30 IU/l both times contraception can be discontinued

(b) Use a backup method while not on CHC

(4) Progestin-only methods

(5) DMPA

i. FSH levels are not always impacted

ii. For women ages 50–55, FSH can be checked on the day of injection and repeated 13 weeks later prior to the next injection; if both levels are ≥ 30 mIU/mL, contraception can be discontinued

iii. At age 50, providers can consider switching to an alternative method if significant risk factors for osteoporosis exist and menopause cannot be confirmed

iv. DMPA can be stopped at age 55 without checking hormonal levels

(6) LNG-IUS, POP, progestin implant—two options

i. At age 50–54, check FSH once, if level is ≥ 30 mIU/mL, method should be continued for one more year and then stopped

ii. These methods can be stopped at age 55 without checking hormonal levels

(7) Nonhormonal methods—copper-releasing IUC and barrier methods are two options

(a) Continue until amenorrhea for 1 year

(b) If younger than age 50, continue until amenorrhea for 2 years or 1 year of amenorrhea and two FSH levels ≥30 mIU/mL at least 1–2 months apart

3. Contraception for transgender men

a. Gender-affirming testosterone therapy (and sometimes GnRH analogues in adolescents) may suppress ovarian function but cannot be relied on for contraceptive protection

b. Testosterone—a teratogen contraindicated in pregnancy

c. Transgender men who have a uterus and ovaries and who have vaginal sex with a risk of pregnancy who do not wish to conceive can use any contraceptive method not otherwise contraindicated

d. The estrogen component of CHC methods may counteract the masculinizing effects of testosterone

e. Copper IUDs and progestin-only contraceptive methods do not interfere with masculinizing effects of testosterone

Unintended Pregnancy

- Definition—a pregnancy that is mistimed or unplanned at the time of conception
- Approximately 50% of pregnancies in the United States are unintended

- Unintended or mistimed does not necessarily mean unwanted
- Options counseling
  1. Definition—process of providing a pregnant individual who is undecided about available choices with information about all available options
  2. Options—maintaining pregnancy with intention to parent, maintaining pregnancy and placing infant for adoption, choosing medical or surgical abortion
  3. Follow principles of informed choice and right to self-determination when providing options counseling
  4. Provide information in a nondirective manner and withhold personal judgment concerning the individual's situation and decision
  5. If own conscience does not allow for the provision of abortion counseling or treatment, let the client know and facilitate access to a provider who will offer counseling on all options in a timely manner
  6. If an individual chooses to maintain pregnancy—initiate prenatal care, arrange for ongoing prenatal care, provide information about available resources
  7. If an individual chooses to place infant for adoption—connect with resources to assist in creating an adoption plan
  8. If an individual chooses to seek abortion—provide information on abortion method-specific risks and benefits, gestational age limits, and provide referrals as needed
- Abortion
  1. Medication abortion—FDA approved up to 70 days (10 weeks) of gestation
     a. Access to medication abortion reduces the number of second-trimester abortions
     b. Most medication abortion care can be provided based on LMP and without ultrasound examination; consider reserving ultrasound for unknown LMP or history of irregular menses
     c. Mifepristone plus misoprostol
        (1) Mifepristone—19-norsteroid, progesterone antagonist
            (a) Blocks action of progesterone needed to establish and maintain placental attachment(b) Softens cervix
            (b) Stimulates prostaglandin synthesis by cells of early decidua
            (c) Restricted access by FDA under the risk evaluation and mitigation strategy (REMS) program
            (d) Can be administered vaginally, sublingually, or buccally
            (e) Should not be administered orally due to lowered efficacy
            (f) Similar safety and efficacy between vaginal, sublingual, and buccal
        (2) Misoprostol—prostaglandin analogue
            (a) Softens cervix
            (b) Stimulates uterine contractions
            (c) Common short-term side effects—nausea, vomiting, diarrhea, temporary elevation of body temperature

            (d) Prenatal exposure to misoprostol associated with major congenital anomalies, absolute risk low (about 1%)
        (3) € Low risk of excessive bleeding (<1%) and need for blood transfusion (0.1%)
        (4) Combination of oral mifepristone 200 mg and misoprostol 800 mcg is 92%–99% effective through 10 weeks of gestation
        (5) If mifepristone is unavailable, may use misoprostol-only protocol with lower efficacy noted
        (6) Contraindications
            (a) Known or suspected ectopic pregnancy
            (b) IUC in place; remove prior to giving medication
            (c) Hypersensitivity to either medication
            (d) Hemorrhagic disorders
            (e) Anticoagulant therapy
            (f) Chronic renal failure
            (g) Long-term systemic corticosteroid therapy
            (h) Inherited porphyrias
        (7) Method can be conducted via telemedicine and mail delivery system or in-person visit
            (a) Mifepristone orally at the initial visit or as instructed with mail delivery
            (b) Misoprostol at home—administered vaginally in 6–48 hours, buccal or sublingual in 24–48 hours after mifepristone
            (c) When possible, recommend 1- to 2-week follow-up appointment to assess for complete abortion
            (d) May repeat misoprostol or provide aspiration if abortion is not complete
            (e) Aspiration abortion if pregnancy persists 2–3 weeks after initiation of medication abortion
     d. Methotrexate plus misoprostol—less commonly used
        (1) Methotrexate—folic acid analogue
            (a) Inhibits enzyme necessary for DNA synthesis
            (b) Acts on rapidly dividing cells of the placenta
        (2) Ninety-two percent to 96% effective through 49 days of gestation
        (3) More gradual action, may take up to 1 month for expulsion of gestational sac
        (4) Precautions
            (a) Known teratogen when taken in large doses
            (b) Discontinue breastfeeding/chestfeeding for 72 hours after methotrexate administration
            (c) Avoid use of folic acid supplements for 1 week after procedure—may inhibit action of methotrexate
        (5) Contraindications—same as mifepristone plus misoprostol; acute inflammatory bowel disease; uncontrolled seizure disorder
        (6) Two clinic visits
            (a) Methotrexate IM or orally at the initial visit

(b) Misoprostol vaginally at home 3–7 days later

(c) Follow-up appointment same as with mifepristone–misoprostol regimen

2. Surgical methods: Shorter amount of time to complete abortion and slightly more effective than medication abortion

    (1) Vacuum aspiration (first trimester)

        (a) Suction curettage

        (b) Local anesthetic

    (2) Dilation and evacuation (D&E)— performed between 13 and 20 weeks' gestation

        (a) Pre-abortion health assessment and counseling

        (b) History

        (c) LMP and menstrual history

        (d) Surgical history including gynecologic surgeries

        (e) Contraceptive history

        (f) Medical history, assess for history of anemia

        (g) Current medications/history of allergic responses

3. Physical examination

    (a) Pelvic examination—uterine size, position, presence of uterine/cervical/adnexal abnormalities prior to surgical abortion; confirm gestational age based on LMP if no ultrasound done

    (b) Laboratory tests

        (1) Pregnancy test—urine

        (2) Hemoglobin (Hgb)/hematocrit (Hct)

        (3) Blood type and Rh

        (4) STI evaluation if indicated

4. Counseling

  a. Discuss all pregnancy options and avenues/ability to access care

  b. Discuss options for abortion—medical and surgical

5. Postabortion health assessment and counseling

  a. Contraceptive counseling

  b. Discuss Rh status—research supports that there is unlikely a need for Rh immunization after a first trimester abortion if client is Rh negative because the concentration of fetal red blood cells in the first trimester is below threshold for Rh sensitization—if Rh immunization given, can be administered at time of surgical procedure or first visit with medication abortion

  c. Prophylactic antibiotics may be given to surgical clients

  d. Client education regarding possible complications

  e. Tissue examined to rule out molar pregnancy

6. Potential postabortion complications

  a. Infection

  b. Retained products of conception

  c. Trauma to uterus/cervix

  d. Excessive bleeding

  e. Warning signs

    (1) Fever

    (2) Persistent/increasing lower abdominal pain

    (3) Prolonged/excessive vaginal bleeding

    (4) Purulent vaginal discharge

    (5) No return of menses within 6 weeks

Menopause

- Demographics
  1. An estimated 6,000 U.S. individuals reach menopause every day; more than 2 million per year
  2. With life expectancy of U.S. women estimated at 81.2 years, they can expect to live about one-third of their lives beyond menopause
- Definitions
  1. Menopause—permanent cessation of ovulation and menses; average age in United States is 52 years; genetically predetermined; confirmed after 12 consecutive months without a period
  2. Menopause transition—span of time when menstrual cycle and endocrine changes begin to occur and ending with the final menstrual period (FMP)
  3. Perimenopause—extends from beginning of menopause transition until 12 months after FMP
  4. Postmenopause—refers to the years following menopause
  5. Premature menopause—cessation of ovulation and menses before age 40; spontaneous or induced
  6. STRAW reproductive-aging continuum (North American Menopause Society, 2019)
     a. Standardized definition of reproductive aging based on specific clinical criteria, endocrine parameters, and characteristic markers
     b. Menstrual cycle changes are considered the principal clinical criteria
     c. Characteristic markers—vasomotor symptoms and symptoms of urogenital atrophy
     d. Endocrine parameters, including FSH, are considered supportive criteria; not typically measured for purposes of staging reproductive aging or menopause
        (1) AMH—produced exclusively by granulosa cells of preantral/small ovarian follicles; inhibits FSH-dependent follicular growth; may play a role in follicle recruitment and selection; marker of ovarian reserve; AMH begins to decrease as early as late 20s and 30s; undetectable about 5 years after menopause
        (2) Inhibin B—major ovarian peptide; rises and falls in first half of follicular phase, peaks midcycle, falls to lowest level in luteal phase; forms negative feedback loop to fine-tune pituitary FSH regulation; as number of ovarian follicles declines, inhibin B levels fall and FSH levels rise
        (3) Antral follicle count—determined by ultrasound evaluation of ovary; used primarily as factor in fertility counseling
     e. Stages—reproductive (early, peak, late), menopausal transition (early, late), and postmenopause (early, late)

   f. Menopausal transition (early)—duration variable; menstrual cycle length varies (persistent difference of 7 or more days in length of consecutive cycles); FSH in early follicular phase elevated but variable; AMH low; inhibin B low; antral follicle count low

   g. Menopausal transition (late)—duration 1–3 years; intervals of amenorrhea ≥ 60 days; may have extreme fluctuations in hormone levels; FSH fluctuates between postmenopausal levels and those consistent with reproductive stages; AMH low; inhibin B low; antral follicle count low; vasomotor symptoms likely

   h. Postmenopause (early)—divided into two phases

     (1) First 12 months after FMP—FSH elevated but variable; AMH low; inhibin B low; antral follicle count very low; vasomotor symptoms most likely

     (2) Second postmenopausal year until point in time when high FSH and low estradiol levels begin to stabilize—duration 3–6 years; FSH stabilizes; AMH very low; inhibin B very low; antral follicle count very low

   i. Postmenopause (late)—duration remaining lifespan; increasing symptoms related to atrophic changes in urogenital tissues may occur

   j. Criteria may vary in relation to factors such as body size, lifestyle characteristics, and health status

- Physiology—see **Box 4-8**
- Laboratory findings
  1. FSH—greater than 40 mIU/mL
  2. LH—threefold elevation after menopause (20–100 mIU/mL)
  3. E_2—less than 20 pg/mL
- Physical changes
  1. Some related to hormonal changes; some related to normal changes with aging; some related to combination of both
  2. Body weight and fat distribution
     a. No data to support that menopause hormonal changes are responsible for weight gain; more likely the result of aging and lifestyle
     b. Some evidence that changes in body composition and fat distribution may be related to menopause; change in fat distribution from subcutaneous stores to visceral abdominal fat
  3. Skin
     a. Skin has a significant number of estrogen receptors
     b. Declines in skin collagen and skin thickness correlate with years since menopause
     c. Scalp, pubic, and axillary hair becomes thinner and drier
  4. Bone integrity—increased bone loss associated with decrease in estrogen; greatest loss in first few years after menopause, then slows but continues
  5. External and internal genitalia
     a. Labia—decrease in subcutaneous fat and tissue elasticity
     b. Vagina
        (1) Decrease in estrogen and concomitant change in vaginal microbes increases vaginal pH from acidic to alkaline environment; pH ≥ 5.0

Box 4-8 Physiology of Menopause

- Reproductive aging results in changes in the hypothalamic–pituitary–ovarian axis
- Ovarian aging with follicular atresia is predominant event leading to menopause
- Decrease in number of responsive follicles → decrease in production of estradiol (E_2)
- Decrease in E_2 and inhibin B → rise in FSH through negative feedback system
- Variable hormone secretion and inconsistent ovulation during menopause transition
- Measurement of E_2 and/or FSH levels is not a reliable way to determine menopause
  - Elevated E_2 levels may occur in some cycles during menopause transition because of a luteal out-of-phase (LOOP) event—elevated FSH level is adequate to recruit a second follicle in luteal phase of a cycle, resulting in a rise in E_2 secretion
  - Elevated E_2 levels may also occur with conversion of androgen to estrogen through aromatization, which also increases with age and body weight
- Early menopause transition—menstrual cycle length typically begins to vary
- Late menopause transition—episodes of amenorrhea of 60 consecutive days or more
- Menstrual change patterns vary with individuals
- The hallmark for the end of menopause transition and initiation of the postmenopause is the FMP
- Generally rely on cessation of menses, hypoestrogenic symptoms, and age for diagnosis of menopause
- Elevated FSH and luteinizing hormone (LH) levels and low E_2 levels stabilize after the first 1–2 years postmenopause
- After menopause, estrone becomes the predominant circulating estrogen
- Estrone is derived primarily through peripheral conversion in adipose tissue (i.e., aromatization) of androstenedione, an androgen produced by adrenal cortex and ovarian stroma

     (2) Decrease in estrogen results in vaginal epithelium with higher proportion of parabasal cells than mature superficial cells

      (a) Epithelium becomes thinner, less vascular, and less elastic

      (b) Vaginal walls appear thin, smooth, and pale

      (c) Vaginal walls may have small petechiae and be friable to touch

   c. Cervix—decrease in size; os may become flush with vaginal walls; may become stenotic

   d. Uterus and ovaries—decrease in size; ovaries usually not palpable

  6. Urinary tract
     a. Urethra and trigone of the bladder have high concentration of estrogen receptors; as with the vulva and vagina, decreased estrogen may result in atrophic changes
     b. Urethral meatus may become more prominent as labia minora thin and introitus retracts, urethral caruncles are common.

- Mood changes and cognitive function
  1. Majority of individuals do not have psychological problems attributable to menopause
  2. Individuals with history of previous clinical depression, premenstrual syndrome, or postpartum depression may be more vulnerable to recurrent depression during perimenopause
  3. Perimenopausal depression may be an interplay between hormonal fluctuations, stressful events, lifestyle factors, psychosocial support
  4. About one-fourth of individuals do report some mood changes during menopause transition
  5. Individual characteristics and self-perception appear to be important determinants of each individual's experience of perimenopause
  6. No evidence that memory or cognitive skills decline directly as a result of normal menopause transition
  7. Ability to concentrate may be reduced by sleep disturbances and fatigue related to hot flashes
  8. Women's Health Initiative Memory Study (WHIMS)—risk of dementia increased in healthy women aged 65–79 years using estrogen with progesterone therapy
  9. Unclear how estrogen or estrogen with progesterone therapy affects cognitive function in younger menopausal individuals
- Cardiovascular system effects
  1. Increase in LDL-C, very-low-density lipoprotein cholesterol (VLDL-C), triglycerides; possible decrease in HDL-C
  2. Increase in certain fibrinolytic and procoagulation factors that regulate clotting processes
  3. Increase in endothelin and decrease in ACE (vasoconstrictors); increase in nitric oxide and decrease in prostacyclin (vasodilators)
  4. Extent of impact of decreased estrogen levels on cardiovascular disease not definitively established
- Wellness visit ages 40–64
  1. Comprehensive health history
     a. Identify disease risk factors, health-promoting behaviors, symptoms of disease, current status of diagnosed conditions, medications used
     b. Identify psychological and social concerns—emotional, physical, sexual abuse by family or partner, current or past; drug/alcohol use; anxiety; depression
     c. Discuss sexuality/sexual history—sexual orientation, gender identity, sexual practices, sexual satisfaction, dyspareunia, use of contraception if needed; use of condoms
     d. Ask about perimenopausal/menopausal symptoms, symptoms of pelvic prolapse, urinary and fecal incontinence
     e. Conduct risk assessment for consideration of *BRCA 1/2* testing
     f. Learn what is most important to the individual client as it relates to health and quality of life moving through perimenopause and beyond
  2. Physical examination
     a. Height—yearly; height loss greater than 1.5 in. (3.8 cm) may be associated with vertebral compression fractures and osteoporosis
     b. Weight/BMI—yearly
     c. Blood pressure—yearly
     d. Clinical breast examination—ACS (Smith et al., 2019); USPSTF (2016): not recommended among individuals at average-risk at any age; ACOG (2017): annually for individuals aged 40 and older; see Chapter 3, *Primary Care*, for breast cancer screening recommendations
     e. Pelvic examination—if need cervical cancer screening or otherwise indicated; performing routine pelvic exam (external genitalia, speculum, bimanual) should be a shared, informed decision between patient and healthcare provider
     f. Other, as indicated by history and/or risk factors
  3. Screening tests
     a. Cervical cancer screening
        (1) ACOG (2021), USPSTF (2018): Primary HPV test every 5 years or cytology and HPV co-testing every 5 years or cytology alone every 3 years
        (2) ACS (Fontham, 2020: Primary HPV test every 5 years preferred; cytology and HPV co-testing every 5 years or cytology alone every 3 years acceptable
        (3) See Chapter 3, *Primary Care*, for all cervical cancer screening recommendations
     b. Mammography
        (1) ACS (Smith et al., 2019)—yearly beginning at age 45 if at average risk; individuals 55 and older can transition to biennial screening or continue annual screening if they prefer; individuals should have the opportunity to begin mammograms at ages 40–44
        (2) ACOG (2017)—offer starting at age 40; initiate at ages 40–49 after counseling, if individual desires; recommend no later than age 50 if not already initiated; annual or biennial interval
        (3) USPSTF (2016)—biennial screening from age 50 to 74 years (Grade B); individualize decision to begin screening before age 50 according to patient's circumstances and values
        (4) See Chapter 3, *Primary Care*, for all breast cancer screening recommendations
     c. Colorectal cancer screening ACS (Smith et al., 2019); USPSTF (2021)
        (1) Adults aged 45–75 should have a colonoscopy every 10 years, fecal immunochemical test or highly sensitive guaiac-based fecal occult blood test annually, or multi-targeted stool test every 3 years
        (2) See Chapter 3, *Primary Care*, for all colorectal cancer screening recommendations
     d. HIV screening if sexually active—yearly if high risk
     e. Diabetes screening—every 3 years starting age 45 (American Diabetes Association, 2021)
     f. Lipid screening—Check cholesterol and other risk factors every 4–6 years as long as risk remains low; use equation to calculate 10-year risk of having heart attack or stroke (American College of

Cardiologists/American Heart Association [Arnett et al., 2019])

  g. Other, as indicated by health history and risk factors

4. Immunizations—see Chapter 3, *Primary Care*, for all adult immunization recommendations

5. Counseling/education

  a. Lifestyle modifications to reduce disease risk factors/promote health—nutrition, physical activity, safer sex practices, smoking cessation, avoiding unhealthy alcohol and other substance use, stress management

  b. Contraception if needed—see Contraception section of this chapter for information about contraception for individuals older than 40 years; hormonal contraception may alleviate some menopause transition symptoms

  c. Breast self-awareness

  d. Recommended screening tests schedule

  e. Expected hormonal and menstrual changes during perimenopause

  f. Management of perimenopause symptoms

  g. Other, as indicated by health history/physical examination findings/risk factors

- Wellness visit age 65 and beyond

1. Comprehensive health history

  a. Identify disease risk factors/health-promoting behaviors, symptoms of disease, current status of diagnosed conditions, medications used

  b. Identify psychological and social concerns—social support systems; isolation; emotional, physical, sexual, financial abuse or neglect by family or partner; drug/alcohol use; anxiety; depression

  c. Discuss sexuality/sexual history—sexual orientation, gender identity, sexual practices, sexual satisfaction, dyspareunia, use of condoms

  d. Ask about menopausal symptoms, symptoms of pelvic prolapse, urinary and fecal incontinence

  e. Conduct risk assessment for consideration of *BRCA 1/2* testing

  f. Learn what is most important to the individual as it relates to health and quality of life

2. Physical examination

  a. Height—yearly; height loss greater than 1.5 in. (3.8 cm) may be associated with vertebral compression fractures (VCFs) and osteoporosis

  b. Weight/BMI—yearly

  c. Blood pressure—yearly

  d. Clinical breast examination—ACS (Smith et al., 2019); USPSTF (2016): not recommended if average risk at any age; ACOG (2017): annually; see Chapter 3, *Primary Care*, for breast cancer screening recommendations

  e. Pelvic examination—if need cervical cancer screening or otherwise indicated; performing routine pelvic exam (external genitalia, speculum, bimanual) should be a shared, informed decision between patient and healthcare provider

  f. Other, as indicated by history and/or risk factors

3. Functional assessment

  a. Evaluation of individual's ability to carry out basic tasks for self-care (activities of daily living [ADLs]) and tasks needed to support independent living (instrumental activities of daily living [IADLs])

  b. ADLs—ability to eat, bathe, dress, groom, ambulate, toilet

  c. IADLs—ability to use phone, get to appointments, shop, prepare meals, take medications, manage money

  d. Provides information for healthcare provider to:

    (1) Identify specific areas in which help is needed/not needed

    (2) Identify changes in abilities from one period of time to another

    (3) Determine need for any special services

    (4) Assess safety of a particular living situation

  e. Includes assessment of physical, cognitive, emotional, and social functions

  f. Affected by medical conditions, sensory deficits, resources, support system

4. Screening tests

  a. Cervical cancer screening (ACS [Fontham et al., 2021]); ACOG [2021]; USPSTF [2018])

    (1) Stop screening at age 65 if adequate prior negative screening results—defined as three consecutive negative cytology results or two consecutive co-testing results within previous 10 years and most recent test within past 5 years

    (2) If history of cervical intraepithelial neoplasia 2 (CIN2) or higher, continue screening for 20 years after spontaneous regression or appropriate management

    (3) Once screening has stopped, do not resume even if individual reports a new sexual partner

    (4) See Chapter 3, *Primary Care*, for all cervical cancer screening recommendations

  b. Mammography

    (1) ACS (Smith et al., 2019) and ACOG (2017)—annual or biennial interval; no definitive age to discontinue screening; base on individual's health and whether would be candidate for treatment of breast cancer

    (2) USPSTF (2016)—biennial screening from age 50 to 74 (Grade B)

    (3) See Chapter 3, *Primary Care*, for all breast cancer screening recommendations

  c. Colorectal cancer screening—ACS (Smith et al., 2019); USPSTF (2021)

    (1) Adults aged 45–75 should have colonoscopy every 10 years, fecal immunochemical test or highly sensitive guaiac-based fecal occult blood test annually, or multi-targeted stool test every 3 years

    (2) See Chapter 3, *Primary Care*, for all colorectal cancer screening recommendations

  d. HIV screening if sexually active—yearly if high risk; evaluate if candidate for HIV preexposure prophylaxis (PrEP)

    (1) Diabetes screening—every 3 years starting age 45 (American Diabetes Association, 2021)

(2) Lipid screening—check cholesterol and other risk factors every 4–6 years as long as risk remains low; use equation to calculate 10-year risk of having heart attack or stroke (American College of Cardiologists/American Heart Association [Arnett et al., 2019])

(3) Bone mineral density (BMD)—National Osteoporosis Foundation (Beloff et al., 2022)

    (a) Screen all women 65 and older for osteoporosis/osteopenia with BMD test

    (b) No available specific recommendations on frequency of screening or when to discontinue

    (c) See Chapter 3, *Primary Care*, for more information on BMD screening recommendations

(4) Other, as indicated by health history/risk factors

5. Immunizations—see Chapter 3, *Primary Care*, for all adult immunization recommendations

6. Counseling/education

  a. Lifestyle modifications to reduce disease risk factors and promote health—nutrition, physical activity, safer sex practices, smoking cessation, avoiding unhealthy alcohol or other substance use, stress management, fall prevention

  b. Breast self-awareness

  c. Recommended screening tests schedule

  d. Discussion about establishing advance directives, living wills, durable power of attorney for health care

  e. Other, as indicated by health history/physical examination findings/risk factors

• Vasomotor symptoms (VMS)

1. Definition—recurrent, transient episodes of flushing accompanied by sensation of warmth to intense heat on upper body and face

2. May include profuse sweating and palpitations

3. May awaken during night, leading to insomnia, sleep disturbance, cognitive (memory) and affective (anxiety) disruptions with loss of REM sleep

4. Demographics/prevalence

  a. About 75% of U.S. women experience VMS during perimenopause

  b. Usually begins in late menopause transition, with greatest frequency and severity within first 2 years after FMP

  c. VMS typically last 5–7 years but may continue longer than 10–15 years

  d. Induced menopause (surgical, chemotherapy) may result in more frequent and severe VMS

  e. Greater proportion of individuals who are overweight or obese report VMS compared with individuals of normal weight

5. Etiology—specific mechanism unknown; gonadotropin-related effect on the central thermoregulatory function of the hypothalamus (measurable increase in core body temperature; increase in body surface temperature, peripheral vasodilation, then decrease in core temperature)

6. Management—nonpharmacologic (North American Menopause Society, 2019)

  a. Level I evidence (high-quality randomized controlled trials [RCTs], systematic review of level I studies) supports the following strategies for managing mild–moderate VMS, although data on long-term use are limited: cognitive behavioral therapy—group or self-guided; clinical hypnosis

  b. Level II evidence (lesser-quality RCTs, systematic review of level II studies, level I studies with inconsistent results) suggests the following strategies may be beneficial but additional studies are warranted: weight loss for individuals with obesity or overweight, mindfulness-based stress reduction, use of derivatives of soy isoflavones

  c. Level I evidence shows the following strategies are unlikely to alleviate VMS: exercise, yoga, paced respiration, acupuncture

  d. Level II or lower studies show that the following over-the-counter and herbal therapies are unlikely to be beneficial in alleviating VMS: black cohosh, dong quai, evening primrose, and several others

  e. Insufficient or inconclusive data are available regarding some of the commonly recommended lifestyle change strategies for managing VMS: cooling techniques, avoiding triggers

  f. Clinicians should provide individuals with VMS with information about evidence-based nonpharmacologic therapies so that they can make informed decisions

7. Management—pharmacologic (hormonal therapy [HT])

  a. Terminology

    (1) Estrogen therapy (ET)—unopposed estrogen prescribed for individual without uterus

    (2) Estrogen–progesterone therapy (EPT)—combination of estrogen and progestogen (either progesterone or progestin, a synthetic form of progesterone); progestogen's main purpose is to reduce risk of endometrial cancer in individual with a uterus associated with unopposed estrogen

    (3) Estrogen types

      (a) Micronized 17β-estradiol—identical to the structure of estradiol produced by the ovaries

      (b) Conjugated equine estrogen (CEE)—mixture of estrogens isolated from urine of pregnant mares

      (c) Synthetic estrogens—esterified estrogen, synthetic conjugated estrogen, ethinyl estradiol, estropipate

    (4) Progestogen types

      (a) Micronized progesterone—compound identical to endogenous steroid hormone produced by corpus luteum

      (b) Progestin—synthetic product that has progesterone-like activity but is not identical to endogenous progesterone (medroxyprogesterone acetate [MPA], norethindrone acetate, levonorgestrel)

(5) Selective estrogen-receptor modulators (SERMs), also known as estrogen receptor agonists/antagonists (ERAAs)—estrogen-like compounds that act as estrogen agonists or antagonists depending on the SERM and target tissue

    (a) Bazedoxifene (BZA)—SERM with estrogen antagonist effects on endometrial and breast tissue and estrogen agonist effects on bone

    (b) BZA combined with CEE (BZA/CEE)—alternative to adding a progestogen to prevent endometrial hyperplasia

    (c) Study data indicate less unscheduled uterine bleeding and less breast tenderness is seen with CEE combined with MPA (CEE/MPA) and similar prevention of bone loss, vasomotor symptoms, and vulvovaginal atrophy compared with CEE/MPA

(6) Bioidentical hormones

    (a) Hormones chemically identical to hormones produced during the reproductive years (17β-estradiol, estrone, estradiol, progesterone, testosterone)

    (b) Bioidentical hormone therapy (BHT) provides one or more of these hormones as active ingredients

    (c) 17β-estradiol—available in several FDA-approved ET products in oral, transdermal, and vaginal preparations

    (d) Progesterone—available in an FDA-approved oral capsule and vaginal gels

    (e) Custom-compounded BHT—uses commercially available hormones with the type and amount prescribed by the clinician

    (f) Custom-compounded BHT products are *not* FDA approved; there is no evidence that they are safer than conventional HT; the same contraindications apply to their use

    (g) No evidence that saliva or urine testing is effective for customizing hormone dosing regimens

b. Indications for HT

(1) Treatment of moderate to severe VMS due to menopause

(2) Treatment of moderate–severe vulvar and vaginal atrophy due to menopause

(3) Prevention of postmenopausal osteoporosis

(4) Treatment of premature hypoestrogenism resulting from hypogonadism, bilateral oophorectomy, or primary ovarian insufficiency

(5) HT should *not* be used to prevent coronary heart disease, stroke, or dementia

c. Contraindications

(1) See **Box 4-9**

(2) For survivors of breast cancer with bothersome genitourinary syndrome of menopause not relieved by nonhormonal therapies, low-dose vaginal ET with minimal systemic

---

Box 4-9 Contraindications to Use of Hormone Therapy

1. Undiagnosed abnormal genital bleeding
2. Known, suspected, or history of breast cancer
3. Known or suspected estrogen-dependent neoplasia
4. Active or history of DVT or PE
5. Active or history of arterial thromboembolic disease (e.g., stroke, myocardial infarction)
6. Known liver dysfunction or disease
7. Known protein C, protein S, or antithrombin deficiency, or other known thrombophilic disorders
8. Known or suspected pregnancy

---

absorption may be considered in consultation with oncologist

d. Potential risks

(1) Overall, the increased absolute risks associated with EPT and ET are rare (< 10 in 10,000/y)

(2) Use of lowest, effective dose that provides benefits and minimize risks for the individual should be the therapeutic goal

(3) Endometrial hyperplasia/cancer—increased risk with inadequately opposed estrogen

(4) Breast cancer—possible increased risk with EPT use that may be duration dependent; possible decreased risk with ET use

(5) Thromboembolic disorders—coronary heart disease, stroke, VTE

    (a) Relationship with HT inconclusive

    (b) Individuals who start HT at age younger than 60 or within 10 years of menopause do not incur the same risks as those who start several years after menopause

    (c) Oral ET affects cardiovascular markers—positive effects are increase in HDL-C and decrease in LDL-C levels; negative effects are increase in triglycerides and C-reactive protein levels

    (d) Transdermal ET has no effect on cardiovascular markers

    (e) VTE risk is lower with transdermal ET than with oral ET

    (f) No HT regimen should be used for primary or secondary prevention of cardiovascular disease or stroke

(6) Gallbladder disease—increased risk with ET and EPT

(7) Dementia

    (a) Several large clinical trials indicate EPT does not improve memory or other cognitive abilities and may be harmful for memory when initiated at age older than 65; ET alone did not significantly increase risk of dementia

    (b) In the absence of more definitive findings, HT is not recommended at any age to prevent or treat a decline in cognitive function or dementia.

(8) The absolute risks are reduced for all-cause mortality, fracture, diabetes mellitus (EPT and ET), and breast cancer (ET) in individuals aged younger than 60 years

(9) Well-designed clinical trials are still needed to establish the effect of different types of progestogens, different estrogen doses and administration routes, timing of initiation, and length of use on risks associated with HT

e. Assessment and education prior to initiation of HT
  (1) Safety profile is most favorable when HT is initiated prior to age 60 and within 10 years of menopause onset
  (2) Health history with attention to specific contraindications and precautions
  (3) General physical examination, cervical cancer screening per recommended schedule
  (4) Clinical breast examination and screening mammogram per recommended schedule
  (5) Informed and shared decision-making concerning HT use based on individual's symptoms, treatment goals, risk–benefit analysis
  (6) Provide anticipatory guidance on possible need to adjust type and amount of HT for symptom relief or to alleviate possible side effects (e.g., breast tenderness, headaches, bloating, mood changes); expected bleeding patterns and what to report

f. Routine follow-up after HT initiation
  (1) Evaluate continuing need for HT at annual wellness visits and discontinue as appropriate
  (2) No data available regarding choice of abrupt cessation versus tapering to avoid resumption of menopausal symptoms
  (3) Approximately 50% of individuals experience recurrence of VMS with discontinuation regardless of age or length of time HT was used
  (4) Decision to continue HT should be individualized based on the severity of symptoms and risk–benefit ratio
  (5) Consider low-dose vaginal ET for symptoms of genital syndrome of menopause (GSM) not relieved by nonhormonal therapies
  (6) Consider nonhormonal therapies for prevention of osteoporosis if long-term therapy needed

g. Routes of administration
  (1) Oral
    (a) ET, EPT, CEE/BZA
    (b) First-pass metabolism determines bioavailability
    (c) Increased HDL-C and decreased LDL-C
    (d) Increased triglycerides, C-reactive protein
  (2) Transdermal/topical
    (a) Systemic absorption
    (b) Patch—estrogen and progestogen combined or estrogen only
    (c) Topical sprays, gels, and emulsions—17β-estradiol
    (d) May use lower doses as not dependent on GI absorption and no first-pass hepatic metabolism

    (e) No significant impact on HDL-C, LDL-C, triglycerides, C-reactive protein
    (f) May have less adverse effects on gallbladder and coagulation factors than oral estrogen
    (g) Need added progestogen with intact uterus
    (h) Topical progesterone preparations may not provide sufficient endometrial protection
  (3) Estrogen vaginal ring (Femring)
    (a) Systemic absorption
    (b) Approved for treatment of VMS and vulvovaginal atrophy/GSM
    (c) 90-day duration
    (d) Need added progestogen if have intact uterus
  (4) Estrogen vaginal ring (Estring)
    (a) Low dose with little or no systemic absorption
    (b) Used for treatment of vulvovaginal atrophy/GSM
    (c) Will not provide relief from VMS
    (d) 90-day duration
    (e) Progestogen does not need to be added with low-dose vaginal ring
  (5) Vaginal estrogen creams and tablets
    (a) Used for treatment of vulvovaginal atrophy/GSM
    (b) Little or no systemic absorption
    (c) Will not provide relief from VMS
    (d) Progestogen does not need to be added with low-dose vaginal estrogens
  (6) Progestogens
    (a) Oral—medroxyprogesterone acetate (MPA), norethindrone acetate, micronized progesterone
    (b) Transdermal in EPT patches—norethindrone acetate, levonorgestrel
    (c) Intrauterine—LNG-IUS
    (d) Vaginal—progesterone gel, micronized progesterone insert

h. Regimen options
  (1) Recommendations for progestogen use for endometrial protection with standard estrogen dosing
    (a) 12–14 days each month of 5 mg of MPA or equivalent
    (b) Daily doses of 2.5 mg MPA or equivalent
    (c) LNG-IUS
    (d) Vaginal progesterone gel 45 mg daily or 12–14 days each month
  (2) Continuous-cyclic EPT
    (a) Estrogen every day
    (b) Progestogen added 12–14 days each month
    (c) No estrogen-free period during which vasomotor symptoms can occur
    (d) Withdrawal bleeding when progestogen withdrawn each month; may start 1–2 days earlier depending on dose and type of progestogen used

(3) Continuous-combined EPT
  (a) Estrogen and progestogen every day
  (b) Lower cumulative dose of progestogen than with cyclic regimens
  (c) May initially have unpredictable bleeding
  (d) After several months endometrium atrophies and amenorrhea usually results
  (e) No estrogen-free period during which vasomotor symptoms can occur
(4) Combination CEE/BZA—FDA approved for treatment of moderate–severe vasomotor symptoms and prevention of osteoporosis
(5) Continuous unopposed estrogen—for individual without uterus

8. Side effects of HT
   a. Breast tenderness—estrogen or progestogen (usually subsides after first few weeks)
   b. Nausea—estrogen (relieved if taken at mealtime or bedtime)
   c. Skin irritation with transdermal patches
   d. Fluid retention and bloating—estrogen or progestogen
   e. Alterations in mood—progestogen
9. Management of side effects
   a. Lowering dose
   b. Altering route of administration
   c. Changing to different formulation
10. Management of bleeding during HT
    a. Continuous-cyclic regimen—usually experience some uterine bleeding; starts last few days of progestogen administration or during progestogen-free days; earlier bleeding, heavy or persistent bleeding may indicate endometrial hyperplasia and warrants endometrial evaluation
    b. Continuous-combined regimen—erratic spotting and light bleeding of 1–5 days duration in first 3–6 months; need endometrial evaluation if bleeding heavier or longer than usual or if resumes after several months of amenorrhea
    c. Use of LNG-IUS for progestogen may result in less bleeding
    d. CEE/BZA—data indicate less unscheduled uterine bleeding than CEE/MPA
11. Management—pharmacologic (nonhormonal)
    a. Selective serotonin reuptake inhibitor (SSRI)—paroxetine 7.5 mg taken once daily at bedtime is only nonhormonal prescription medication approved by FDA for treatment of VMS
    b. Other SSRIs and serotonin–norepinephrine reuptake inhibitors (SNRIs) have demonstrated positive results in treatment of hot flashes
    c. Gabapentin, an anticonvulsant medication, has been shown to be effective in reduction of severity and frequency of hot flashes

• Genitourinary syndrome of menopause (GSM)
  1. Definition—collection of symptoms and physical findings associated with decreased estrogen and other sex steroids involving changes to the labia majora/minora, vestibule/introitus, clitoris, vagina, urethra, and bladder (North American Menopause Society, 2019)
     a. Genital dryness, burning, irritation
     b. Sexual symptoms of lack of lubrication, discomfort or pain, impaired function
     c. Urinary symptoms of frequency, nocturia, urgency, dysuria, and recurrent urinary tract infections
  2. Demographics—affects as many as 50% of perimenopausal individuals and up to .% of older menopausal individuals
  3. Etiology
     a. Signs and symptoms associated with GSM are related to reduced circulating estrogen and aging
     b. High concentration of estrogen receptors in vagina, vestibule, urethra, and bladder trigone modulates cell proliferation and maturation
     c. Low circulating levels of estrogen result in anatomic and physiologic changes in urogenital tissues
  4. Reduced collagen, decreased elastin, epithelium thinning, and fewer blood vessels
  5. Decreased vaginal blood flow, diminished lubrication, decreased elasticity and flexibility of vaginal vault, decreased vaginal tissue strength
  6. Thinning and regression of labia minora, retraction of introitus, more prominent urethral meatus
  7. Decreased vaginal lactobacilli and increased vaginal pH
  8. Management/treatment
     a. Symptoms of GSM can have a negative effect on quality of life that may extend to activities of daily living, exercise, sexual function, interpersonal relationships
     b. Rule out other causes of symptoms—e.g., allergic or inflammatory conditions, vaginal infections, trauma, malignancy, vulvodynia
     c. Unlike VMS that typically improve with time, GSM symptoms often worsen in the absence of treatment with symptoms likely to return upon discontinuation of treatment
     d. Nonhormonal therapies
        (1) Vaginal lubricants—effects immediate; intended to reduce friction on atrophic vulvovaginal structures during sex; may be water-, silicone-, or oil-based
        (2) Vaginal moisturizers—applied several times weekly for longer-term relief of vaginal dryness; help to maintain vaginal moisture and lower vaginal pH
        (3) Regular sexual activity—promotes blood flow to genital area
        (4) Noncoital methods of sexual expression if penetration is painful—massage, oral stimulation, mutual masturbation
     e. Hormonal therapies
        (1) Low-dose vaginal estrogen—consider if nonhormonal therapies do not relieve symptoms or if have severe GSM symptoms
           (a) Available as cream, slow-release estradiol intravaginal ring, and estradiol vaginal tablet
           (b) Creams, tablets, and inserts generally used 2–3 times each week although may use daily for 2 weeks at initiation; estradiol vaginal ring changed every 3 months

(c) FDA labeling notes the same risks associated with systemic estrogen; however, there is minimal systemic absorption

(d) Concomitant use of a progestogen is not routinely recommended, if high risk for endometrial cancer consider endometrial surveillance with transvaginal ultrasound or intermittent progestogen therapy

(e) Contraindication—abnormal genital bleeding of unknown cause

(f) Use in individuals with history of breast or endometrial cancer should consider individual's preference, symptom severity, and understanding of potential risks after consultation with oncologist

(2) Ospemifene—SERM approved for treatment of vaginal dryness and moderate–severe dyspareunia related to GSM; daily oral dose

(a) Estrogen agonist effect on vaginal tissue to thicken and make less fragile; decrease in vaginal pH; may take several weeks for full relief of symptoms

(b) No FDA indication for bone health protection listed

(c) Weak estrogen agonist effect on uterus and breasts—FDA requires listing of same contraindications as those for use of estrogen

(d) Should not be used with estrogen or another SERM

(e) Use of progestogen with ospemifene has not been evaluated in clinical trials

(f) Most common side effects—hot flashes, vaginal discharge, muscle spasm, increased sweating

(3) Prasterone/dehydroepiandrosterone (DHEA)—approved for treatment of moderate–severe dyspareunia related to GSM; once-daily vaginal dose at bedtime

(a) Inactive endogenous steroid prohormone converted into active androgen and estrogens locally in vaginal cells, improves vaginal epithelium maturation index and lowers vaginal pH

(b) Contraindication—abnormal genital bleeding of unknown cause

(c) Precaution—prasterone has not been studied in individuals with a history of breast cancer

(d) Most common side effect is vaginal discharge

(4) Systemic ET/EPT—only if also using for relief of moderate to severe VMS

Questions

Select the best answer.

1. Which of the following actions does the estrogen in COCs include?
   a. Inhibits ovulation through suppression of the LH surge
   b. Inhibits sperm penetration by thickening the cervical mucus
   c. Provides most of the contraceptive effect for COCs
   d. Stabilizes the endometrium for less unscheduled bleeding

2. A 58-year-old patient with vaginal dryness causing irritation and dyspareunia has no problem with hot flashes. Of the following treatment choices, the best for this patient would be:
   a. continuous-combined regimen hormone therapy (HT)
   b. continuous-cyclic HT with added testosterone
   c. low-dose estrogen vaginal ring
   d. progestin-only therapy

3. The most prevalent contraceptive method among married couples in the United States is:
   a. COCs
   b. condoms
   c. sterilization
   d. withdrawal

4. A client taking UPA for emergency contraception because the client was late starting a new pack of COC and had unprotected sex should be advised to:
   a. Abstain from sex or use a barrier method for 5 days and then restart COCs.
   b. Abstain from sex or use a barrier method until menses and then restart COCs.
   c. Restart COCs the next day; no backup method is needed.
   d. Restart COCs the next day and use a backup method for 7 days.

5. A 51-year-old patient asks you about taking estrogen to help with memory because of occasional forgetfulness and difficulty concentrating. The patient's mother developed dementia at age 65. The best initial response would be to:
   a. Advise the patient that there may be a benefit from taking estrogen for about 5 years.
   b. Ask about other menopausal symptoms, such as hot flashes and night sweats.
   c. Tell the patient the WHIMS study showed an increase in dementia for individuals in their 50s who took estrogen.
   d. Tell the patient that memory changes are likely caused by depression.

6. The polypeptide hormone produced by the ovaries that stimulates FSH production is:
   a. activin
   b. follistatin
   c. inhibin
   d. prolactin

7. Sex hormone binding globulin (SHBG) is produced in the:
   a. adrenal glands
   b. anterior pituitary gland
   c. liver
   d. ovaries

8. The lymph nodes that drain directly into the infraclavicular nodes are the:
   a. central nodes
   b. lateral nodes
   c. subscapular nodes
   d. supraclavicular nodes

9. A vaginal pH less than 4.5 is an expected finding in a:
   a. healthy reproductive-age individual
   b. menopausal individual with atrophic vaginitis
   c. Individual using the lactational amenorrhea method of contraception
   d. healthy prepubertal-age individual

10. The predominant vaginal organism responsible for an acidic pH is:
    a. *Doderlein bacillus*
    b. *Gardnerella*
    c. *Haemophilus*
    d. *Lactobacillus*

11. Squamous metaplasia of the cervix occurs within the:
    a. columnar epithelium
    b. internal cervical os
    c. squamous epithelium
    d. transformation zone

12. Which of the following statements is true concerning the luteal phase of the menstrual cycle?
    a. It begins at the time of the LH surge.
    b. It corresponds with the uterine proliferative phase.
    c. There is thickened cervical mucus.
    d. It lasts an average of 10 days from the time of ovulation to menses.

13. Estrogen is released by the ovary in response to:
    a. FSH
    b. GnRH
    c. hCG
    d. LH

14. The predominant estrogen after menopause is:
    a. estradiol
    b. estriol
    c. estrone
    d. estropipate

15. Which of the following androgens can be converted to estradiol?
    a. Androstenedione
    b. Cortisol
    c. DHA
    d. Testosterone

16. Which phase of the menstrual cycle is the most variable?
    a. Follicular
    b. Luteal
    c. Ovarian
    d. Secretory

17. Which hormone is dominant during the proliferative phase of the menstrual cycle?
    a. Estrogen
    b. LH
    c. Progesterone
    d. Prolactin

18. Which of the following lab values would be expected with menopause?
    a. Decreased FSH, increased LH, decreased estradiol
    b. Decreased LH, increased FSH, increased estradiol
    c. Increased FSH, increased LH, decreased estradiol
    d. Increased LH, decreased FSH, increased estradiol

19. Urine ovulation tests detect:
    a. estrogen levels
    b. FSH surge
    c. LH surge
    d. progesterone levels

20. Which of the following statements about prolactin is correct?
    a. It is produced by the placenta during pregnancy.
    b. It is secreted by the posterior pituitary gland.
    c. It stimulates the breast milk ejection reflex with suckling.
    d. It stimulates the synthesis of milk proteins in mammary glands.

21. A 52-year-old individual who had a hysterectomy 2 years ago for uterine bleeding caused by fibroids presents with a complaint of severe hot flashes and night sweats for the past few months. Of the following treatment choices, the most appropriate for the client's vasomotor symptoms at this time would be:
    a. continuous-combined oral HT
    b. ospemifene (estrogen agonist/antagonist)
    c. transdermal estrogen patch
    d. vaginal estrogen cream

22. Which of the following is *not* an FDA-approved indication for the use of HT?
    a. Prevention of cardiovascular disease
    b. Prevention of osteoporosis
    c. Relief of moderate to severe symptoms of vulvovaginal atrophy
    d. Relief of moderate to severe vasomotor symptom

23. Which of the following would *not* be an expected pelvic examination finding in a 70-year-old patient?
    a. Narrow vaginal canal
    b. Palpable ovaries
    c. Small uterus
    d. Thin vaginal walls

24. The ACS recommends yearly mammogram screening beginning at age:
    a. 40
    b. 45
    c. 50
    d. 55

25. When comparing conjugated estrogen combined with bazedoxifene (CEE/BZA) to conjugated estrogen combined with medroxyprogesterone acetate (CEE/MPA), data have shown:
    a. better prevention of bone loss with CEE/BZA
    b. less prevention of hot flashes with CEE/BZA
    c. less unscheduled bleeding with CEE/BZA
    d. more breast tenderness with CEE/BZA

26. When evaluating cervical mucus, the term *spinnbarkeit* refers to:
    a. amount
    b. cellularity
    c. clarity
    d. elasticity

27. A 24-year-old patient presents to your office with a request for COCs. The patient's current medications include a bronchodilator for asthma. Management for this patient should include providing advice that:
    a. COCs are not recommended for individuals with asthma.
    b. COCs may potentiate the action of a bronchodilator.
    c. The patient should use a backup method if using the bronchodilator several days in a row.
    d. Progestin-only contraceptive injections may reduce the occurrence of asthma attacks.

28. Which of the following contraceptive methods would be best for an individual with a seizure disorder who is taking phenytoin?
    a. COCs
    b. Transdermal contraceptive patch
    c. Progestin-only oral contraceptives
    d. Progestin-only contraceptive injections

29. A client calls the clinic on Monday morning. The client had unprotected sex Friday night and is interested in emergency contraception. Appropriate information for this client would include which of the following statements?
    a. Emergency contraception pills are very effective for a medication abortion in early pregnancy.
    b. If the client is not mid-cycle when the client had sex, the client does not need emergency contraception.
    c. It is too late for emergency contraceptive pills, but insertion of an IUC is an option.
    d. The client can use emergency contraception pills even if there has been other unprotected sex since the last period.

30. The levonorgestrel-releasing IUC may be a better choice than the copper-releasing IUC for the individual who:
    a. has never been pregnant
    b. has dysmenorrhea
    c. is currently breastfeeding/chestfeeding
    d. does not want more children

31. A 25-year-old patient who has had an IUC for 2 years has a cervical cytology showing actinomycosis. The patient has no symptoms of infection. Appropriate management would include:
    a. removing the IUC and repeating the cervical cytology in 6 months

b. removing the IUC, treating with doxycycline, and repeating the cervical cytology in 1 year
    c. keeping the IUC and repeating the cervical cytology in 3 years
    d. keeping the IUC, treating with doxycycline, and repeating the cervical cytology in 3 months

32. An advantage of continuous-combined HT over continuous-cyclic HT regimens is:
    a. no estrogen-free period during which vasomotor symptoms can occur
    b. predictable withdrawal bleeding each month
    c. lower cumulative dose of progestin
    d. less negative impact on triglyceride levels

33. Level I evidence (i.e., high-quality randomized controlled trials, systematic review of level I studies) supports the use of which of the following strategies for managing mild-moderate vasomotor symptoms related to menopause?
    a. Acupuncture
    b. Cognitive behavior therapy
    c. Exercise
    d. Yoga

34. Advantages of the cervical cap over the diaphragm include which of the following?
    a. It has a lower failure rate.
    b. It is easier to insert.
    c. It can remain in place for 48 hours.
    d. Spermicide is not needed.

35. The term for the anatomic abnormality in which an individual has a tight foreskin that cannot be retracted is:
    a. hypospadias.
    b. Peyronie's disease
    c. phimosis
    d. varicocele

36. The main mechanism of action of misoprostol in medically induced abortion is:
    a. blocking the action of progesterone
    b. inhibiting enzymes necessary for DNA synthesis
    c. stimulating synthesis of prostaglandin by cells of the early decidua
    d. stimulating uterine contractions

37. Potential disadvantages of progestin-only implants include which of the following?
    a. Side effects may be increased in individuals who are underweight.
    b. They may cause a significant decrease in bone mineral density.
    c. They may cause irregular bleeding and spotting.
    d. Return to fertility after discontinuation may take several months.

38. An advantage of the transdermal patch over oral delivery of estrogen for the individual experiencing menopausal symptoms is that the transdermal delivery method:
    a. does not require the addition of a progestogen
    b. has fewer adverse effects on coagulation factors
    c. improves vulvovaginal symptoms more quickly
    d. increases HDL-C levels and decreases LDL-C levels

39. Which endogenous estrogen is known as the "estrogen of pregnancy"?
    a. Estradiol
    b. Estriol
    c. Estrone
    d. Estropipate

40. Increased production of _____ is associated with primary dysmenorrhea.
    a. androstenedione
    b. arachidonic acid
    c. cortisol
    d. prostaglandin

41. Which of the following individuals should have an endometrial biopsy/evaluation?
    a. Individual on continuous-cyclic HT regimen with amenorrhea
    b. Individual on continuous-cyclic HT regimen with bleeding starting on the last few days of progestogen administration each month
    c. Individual on continuous-combined HT regimen with irregular bleeding in the first year of use
    d. Individual on continuous-combined HT regimen with spotting that occurs after several months of amenorrhea

42. An individual who had an IUC placed 3 months ago returns to the office with complaints of cramping and states the IUC thread feels longer. You determine that the individual likely has a partial IUC expulsion. Appropriate management if the individual wants to continue with an IUC for contraception includes the following steps:
    a. Remove the IUC, place a new IUC at the current visit, and start doxycycline for 5–7 days.
    b. Remove the IUC and instruct the client to return at the next menses to place a new one.
    c. Start doxycycline and have the client return in 1 week to remove the IUC and replace with a new IUC.
    d. Use sterile forceps to move the IUC, so it is back at the fundus of the uterus.

43. A client calls the office to ask what to do because the client's contraceptive patch had come off, although it was easily reapplied. The client knows it was fully attached last evening before having sex. Appropriate advice would include:
    a. Remove the current patch, apply a new one, and use a backup method for 7 days.
    b. Keep the current patch on if it adheres well and consider emergency contraception.
    c. Remove the current patch, start the patch-free week now, and then apply a new patch.
    d. Keep the current patch on if it adheres well and keep the same patch-change day.

44. A client who is requesting contraception and who also wants to get pregnant in 1 year should avoid using:
    a. COCs
    b. fertility awareness methods
    c. progestin-only oral contraceptives
    d. progestin-only contraceptive injections

45. A client plans to use the calendar method for contraception. The client has charted menstrual cycles for several months and has noted the longest cycle to be 30 days and the shortest cycle to be 27 days. The client should abstain from sexual intercourse each cycle from day _____ through day _____.
    a. 9; 19
    b. 10; 15
    c. 11; 18
    d. 12; 16

46. Which of the following statements by a client indicates the need for the clinician to provide additional information about the use of the contraceptive vaginal ring?
    a. "I should insert a new ring every 7 days."
    b. "I should expect to have regular periods while using the ring."
    c. "My partner can use a male condom while I am wearing the ring."
    d. "The exact position of the ring in the vagina is not important."

47. According to the CDC, initiating progestin-only contraceptive injections (DMPA) is a category 3 when which of the following conditions exists?
    a. Age 35 years or older and smoking more than 15 cigarettes daily
    b. History of DVT or pulmonary emboli
    c. Unexplained vaginal bleeding prior to evaluation
    d. Use of drugs that alter liver enzymes

48. A 4-week-postpartum individual who is breastfeeding/chestfeeding on demand without supplements presents in your office to discuss contraceptive options. The client plans to continue breastfeeding/chestfeeding for at least 6 months. Information for this client concerning the lactational amenorrhea method of contraception should include which of the following statements?
    a. The expected failure rate for this method of contraception is about 20%.
    b. This method is considered effective for only 3 months postpartum.
    c. The patient can rely on this method as long as a period has not occurred.
    d. Another method of contraception should be considered when the infant begins sleeping through the night.

49. A 4-week-postpartum individual who is breastfeeding/chestfeeding now and plans to start weaning the baby in the next month is in your office to discuss contraceptive options. The individual has a BMI of 35 (obese). Of the following, the best contraceptive choice for the individual at this time would be:
    a. COCs
    b. fertility awareness method
    c. lactational amenorrhea method
    d. progestin-only pills

50. An individual using a diaphragm for contraception has sexual intercourse at 8:00 p.m. on Friday, at 2:00 a.m. on Saturday, and again at 8:00 a.m. on Saturday. When can the individual safely remove the diaphragm for effective

contraception while minimizing problems related to leaving the diaphragm in for extended periods of time?
a. 10:00 a.m. on Saturday
b. 2:00 p.m. on Saturday
c. 10:00 p.m. on Saturday
d. 8:00 a.m. on Sunday

51. Individuals who are going to take ospemifene for treatment of dyspareunia related to vulvovaginal atrophy should be advised that they:
a. will need to take a progestogen in addition to prevent endometrial hyperplasia
b. may also use vaginal estrogen to further enhance the medication's effect
c. may experience hot flashes as a side effect of this medication
d. should take the medication 2–3 hours before having sexual intercourse

52. The area located between the fourchette anteriorly and the anus posteriorly is the:
a. levator ani
b. perineum
c. prepuce
d. vestibule

53. A 68-year-old individual had cervical cancer screening done at age 65, and the results were normal. The individual has no history of abnormal screenings. The individual has recently started having sexual intercourse with a new partner and asks if it would be advisable to start having cervical cancer screening again. An appropriate answer would be that the individual:
a. does not need cervical cytology but should have HPV testing every 5 years
b. does not need to resume either cervical cytology or HPV testing
c. should have a cervical cytology with HPV co-testing in 5 years and, if it is negative, can stop screening
d. should resume cervical cytology with HPV co-testing every 5 years

54. According to USPSTF recommendations, an 80-year-old female should have:
a. a clinical breast examination and a screening mammogram annually
b. a clinical breast examination annually but no screening mammogram
c. neither a clinical breast examination nor a screening mammogram
d. a screening mammogram biennially but no clinical breast examination

55. The anatomic area that contains the urethral/vaginal openings, hymen, Skene's glands, and Bartholin's glands is called the:
a. labia majora
b. perineum
c. vestibule
d. vulva

56. Findings on a pelvic examination of a 25-year-old nulliparous patient include a uterus 8 cm in length, a right ovary 3 cm × 2 cm, and a left ovary not palpable. These findings indicate a(n):

a. normal uterus and normal ovaries
b. normal uterus and enlarged right ovary
c. enlarged uterus and normal ovaries
d. enlarged uterus and enlarged right ovary

57. Which of the following occurs first during female puberty?
a. Beginning breast development
b. Beginning pubic hair development
c. Growth spurt peak
d. Menstruation

58. Which of the following structures produces GnRH?
a. Anterior pituitary gland
b. Hypothalamus
c. Posterior pituitary gland
d. Ovaries

59. Which of the following list of events is in the correct chronological order?
a. LH surge, ovulation, rise in BBT, thickened cervical mucus
b. Ovulation, LH surge, thickened cervical mucus, rise in BBT
c. Rise in BBT, thickened cervical mucus, ovulation, LH surge
d. Thickened cervical mucus, rise in BBT, LH surge, ovulation

60. According to CDC recommendations, which of the following would be considered a category 4 condition for the indicated contraceptive method?
a. Levonorgestrel IUC for individuals with endometriosis
b. Copper IUC for individuals with a history of breast cancer
c. Progestin-only pills for individuals with a history of DVT
d. Vaginal contraceptive ring for individual older than 35 years of age who smokes one pack of cigarettes per day

61. An advantage of the internal condom is that it:
a. can be used with an external condom for added protection
b. can be used for repeated acts of intercourse
c. may be used by individuals with latex allergy
d. has a lower failure rate than the external condom does

62. Which is a noncontraceptive benefit of COCs?
a. Decrease in risk for benign breast disease
b. Decrease in risk for cervical cancer
c. Decrease in risk for lung cancer
d. Decrease in risk for obesity

63. For which of the contraceptive methods is there the *least* difference between the perfect use and typical use failure rates?
a. COCs
b. Diaphragm
c. Intrauterine contraceptive
d. External condom

64. An individual who weighs 200 lbs or more may have decreased effectiveness with which of the following contraceptive methods?
a. Progestin-only injectable contraception
b. Contraceptive vaginal ring
c. Levonorgestrel intrauterine system
d. Transdermal contraceptive system

65. Drugs that increase the production of cytochrome P-450 may decrease the effectiveness of COCs by which of the following mechanisms?
    a. Decrease in absorption in the gastrointestinal tract
    b. Decrease in enterohepatic recirculation
    c. Increase in first-pass metabolism in the liver
    d. Increase in protein binding at receptor sites

66. A 20-year-old individual who has a BMI of 38 (obese) presents for the individual's first DMPA injection. Concerns in administering DMPA to this client include which of the following?
    a. The client may need a larger dose than the usual 150 mg.
    b. The client should return for repeat injections every 2 months.
    c. You should massage the injection site well to ensure absorption.
    d. You should choose a site that ensures deep IM injection.

67. Instructions for progestin-only oral contraceptive users should include which of the following statements?
    a. If you are more than 3 hours late taking a pill, use a backup method for 48 hours.
    b. If you miss taking two pills in the third week of the pack, throw away the pack and start a new one.
    c. If you miss pills in the fourth week of the pack, you do not have to use a backup method.
    d. If you miss two pills in the first week of the pack, make them up and use a backup method for 7 days.

68. Which of the following estrogen therapy options is considered safe to use without aprogestogen in an individual with an intact uterus?
    a. Bioidentical oral estrogen formulation
    b. Estring vaginal ring
    c. Plant-based (estriol) oral estrogen
    d. Transdermal estrogen patch

69. The structure in the breast that is responsible for milk production is the:
    a. areola
    b. alveoli
    c. lobule
    d. lactiferous sinus

70. The hormone that stimulates synthesis of milk is:
    a. aldosterone.
    b. estrogen.
    c. progesterone.
    d. prolactin.

71. Which of the following is a contraindication to a medication abortion using mifepristone and misoprostol:
    a. current use of an NSAID
    b. fewer than 7 weeks' gestation
    c. known or suspected ectopic pregnancy
    d. use of long-term antidepressant therapy

72. Which of the following contraceptive choices should *not* be recommended for the perimenopausal individual who is having irregular menses?
    a. COCs
    b. Diaphragm

c. Fertility awareness methods
d. LNG-IUS

73. A 53-year-old patient asks you if increasing soy product intake or taking an isoflavone supplement has any benefit now that she is menopausal. Information you would want to provide would include evidence showing that increasing soy product intake may help:
    a. improve memory and concentration in menopausal individuals
    b. prevent osteoporosis in menopausal individuals
    c. prevent the skin changes that typically occur with aging
    d. reduce hot flash frequency and severity for some individuals

74. A client is planning to use the measurement of basal body temperatures as a means of contraception. Which of the following statements would indicate the need for further instruction about this method?
    a. "I will take my temperature at the same time each day before getting out of bed."
    b. "I know that I am about to ovulate when my temperature rises at least 0.4°F."
    c. "I will need to use a special thermometer to take my basal body temperature."
    d. "A rise of 0.4°F above my baseline for 3 days indicates that it is safe to have sex."

75. A client who has been using a copper-releasing IUC presents with a positive pregnancy test. After determining that the pregnancy is intrauterine and the IUC is in place, the client should be informed that:
    a. Removing the IUC may increase the chance of a spontaneous abortion.
    b. The fetus is at risk for congenital anomalies related to copper exposure.
    c. The IUC should be removed promptly regardless of the client's plans for the pregnancy.
    d. There is no risk to the fetus if the client leaves the IUC in place until birth.

76. Instructions and/or information for a new user of COCs should include:
    a. COCs may decrease the effectiveness of some antibiotics.
    b. Discontinue your pills immediately if you miss a period.
    c. Start the first pack of pills on the last day of your next period.
    d. Sunday starters should use a backup method for the first week of the first pack of pills.

77. A menopausal client experiencing discomfort with sexual intercourse related to vaginal dryness wants to know whether it would be more advisable to use a vaginal lubricant or a vaginal moisturizer. Which of the following statements would be incorrect?
    a. Lubricants are intended to reduce friction during sex.
    b. Lubricants may take several weeks of use before becoming effective.
    c. Moisturizers provide longer-term relief of vaginal dryness than do lubricants.
    d. Moisturizers are typically applied several times weekly.

78. Instructions for the use of nonoxynol-9 spermicide should include which of the following?
    a. Place the spermicide close to the opening of the vagina for maximal effectiveness.
    b. Remove excess spermicide from the vagina within 6 hours to reduce vaginal irritation.
    c. When used with a condom, spermicide will further decrease the risk of STIs.
    d. Frequent use of spermicide may cause vaginal changes, making you more susceptible to HIV infection.

79. According to CDC recommendations, which of the following is a category 4 condition for the use of the indicated contraceptive method?
    a. Use of emergency contraceptive pills by an individual who has a history of DVT
    b. Insertion of an IUC in a client with a history of PID
    c. Use of COC by a 40-year-old individual who has migraine headaches without aura
    d. Use of progestin-only pills by an individual who has type 2 diabetes

80. Which of the following statements concerning coitus interruptus is *false*?
    a. It has a lower perfect use failure rate than the cervical cap.
    b. It may result in a decreased risk for HIV transmission to partners with vaginas.
    c. Individuals are typically not able to predict the timing of their ejaculation.
    d. There is a decreased chance for the presence of preejaculatory sperm with repeat acts of intercourse.

81. Healthy sperm can survive in the female reproductive tract and retain the ability to fertilize an egg for:
    a. 12–24 hours
    b. 24–48 hours
    c. 3–5 days
    d. up to 7 days

82. Which of the following factors may increase levels of sex hormone-binding globulin (SHBG)?
    a. Estrogen-containing oral contraceptives
    b. Hyperinsulinemia
    c. Increased androgen levels
    d. Adipose tissue

83. A 53-year-old patient is sexually active and wants to continue to prevent pregnancy. The patient has been using injectable medroxyprogesterone acetate (Depo-Provera). Of the following, which reflects appropriate clinical decision-making for safely discontinuing contraception while preventing pregnancy?
    a. Because the patient is over 52 years old, contraception may be discontinued at this time.
    b. After two FSH levels in a series—on the day of injection and repeated 13 weeks later prior to the next injection—are >30 mIU/mL, the method can be stopped immediately.
    c. After achieving two FSH levels of >30 mIU/mL at least 1–2 months apart, the method should be continued for an additional year.
    d. After stopping all contraception, if menses returns within 6 months, restart contraceptive method.

84. Which statement regarding extended cycling of combined hormonal contraception is correct?
    a. Patients who are using NuvaRing can insert a new ring every 3 weeks, avoiding withdrawal bleeding.
    b. Patients who are using Annovera can reinsert the ring every 3 weeks, avoiding withdrawal bleeding.
    c. Only combined hormonal contraceptive pills designated for extended cycling can be used to avoid withdrawal bleeding.
    d. Patients should be encouraged to have withdrawal bleeding as it is physiologically necessary for the contraception to work effectively.

85. Which progesterone is a potassium-sparing diuretic and has anti-androgenic properties?
    a. Norethindrone
    b. Norgestrel
    c. Desogestrel
    d. Drospirenone

86. Which statement about lactational amenorrhea is correct?
    a. Patients who are exclusively breastfeeding/chestfeeding, have not had a menstrual cycle, and are less than 6 months postpartum are not likely to ovulate.
    b. Patients who are exclusively breastfeeding/chestfeeding, have not had a menstrual cycle, and are less than 6 months postpartum have estrogen concentrations that are higher in the breasts and minimal development of the endometrial lining, making implantation of a fertilized zygote unlikely.
    c. Patients who are exclusively breastfeeding/chestfeeding, have not had a menstrual cycle, and are less than 6 months postpartum may have decreased estrogen resulting in atrophic changes in the vagina, which can be treated with local vaginal estrogen.
    d. Patients who are combination feeding (breastfeeding/chestfeeding and bottle feeding), are less than 6 months postpartum, and who have not resumed menstruation are not likely to ovulate.

87. Which statement is most accurate about pelvic inflammatory disease and intrauterine devices?
    a. Prophylactic antibiotics should be administered prior to the insertion of an intrauterine device to reduce pelvic inflammatory disease.
    b. A negative test for sexually transmitted infections is required prior to the insertion of an intrauterine device to reduce pelvic inflammatory disease.
    c. Most cases of pelvic inflammatory disease occur within 20 days after insertion.
    d. It is necessary to remove the intrauterine device immediately with the diagnosis of pelvic inflammatory disease.

88. As a component of a wellness visit for a 19-year-old patient, which of the following should routinely be included?
    a. Clinical breast examination
    b. HPV testing alone for cervical cancer screening every 3 years
    c. Risk assessment for HIV preexposure prophylaxis (PrEP)
    d. Syphilis test

89. As a component of a wellness visit for a 26-year-old patient, which of the following components should be routinely included?
    a. Clinical breast examination
    b. HPV/cytology co-testing for cervical cancer screening every 3 years
    c. HPV vaccination if series not previously completed
    d. Tests for chlamydia and gonorrhea if sexually active

90. As a component of a wellness visit for a 35-year-old patient, which of the following should routinely be included?
    a. Hereditary breast cancer risk assessment
    b. HPV/cytology co-testing for cervical cancer screening every 3 years
    c. Screening mammogram
    d. Tests for chlamydia and gonorrhea if sexually active

91. Anti-Müllerian hormone (AMH):
    a. begins to decrease after menopause
    b. is a marker of ovarian reserve
    c. is produced by the corpus luteum
    d. promotes the growth of primordial follicles

92. A 53-year-old patient has signs and symptoms indicative of genital syndrome of menopause (GSM) that is significantly affecting sexual functioning. Appropriate information to provide includes:
    a. GSM symptoms start to get better within 3–5 years after menopause.
    b. treatment for 1–2 years is usually sufficient to permanently stop symptoms.
    c. oral estrogen is more effective than vaginal estrogen in relief of symptoms.
    d. nonhormonal and hormonal therapies are options for long-term treatment.

Answers with Rationales

1. **d.** Stabilizes the endometrium for less unscheduled bleeding
   The estrogen in COCs stabilizes the endometrium, so less unscheduled bleeding occurs. Estrogen contributes to the inhibition of ovulation through suppression of FSH; however, it mainly potentiates the action of progestin, which has the most contraceptive effect.

2. **c.** low-dose estrogen vaginal ring
   The menopausal individual who has symptoms related to vulvovaginal atrophy and no vasomotor symptoms is best treated with local low-dose vaginal estrogen.

3. **c.** sterilization
   The most prevalent contraceptive method among married couples in the United States is sterilization (female and male).

4. **a.** Abstain from sex or use a barrier method for 5 days and then restart COCs.
   There is theoretical concern that hormonal contraception may reduce the effectiveness of UPA as emergency contraception. The individual should be advised not to start hormonal contraception for at least 5 days after taking UPA. The individual should also use a backup method for the first 7 days after restarting her COCs.

5. **b.** Ask about other menopausal symptoms, such as hot flashes and night sweats.
   Although more history and a physical examination may be warranted, the best answer choice is to initially ask about other menopausal symptoms, such as hot flashes and night sweats. These vasomotor symptoms can contribute to memory impairment and difficulty concentrating due to sleep disturbance. If the client has vasomotor symptoms, short-term HT may be an option.

6. **a.** activin
   Activin is a polypeptide hormone produced by the ovaries that stimulates FSH production. Inhibin, which is also a polypeptide hormone, inhibits FSH production. Follistatin binds with activin to inactivate it, thereby inhibiting FSH production.

7. **c.** liver
   Sex hormone binding globulin is produced in the liver. It is a serum protein that binds to estrogens and androgens in blood. Because it is protein-bound it can move through the general circulation to target tissues throughout the body that have specific receptors.

8. **a.** central nodes
   The pectoral, subscapular, and lateral axillary lymph nodes drain into the central nodes that are located high in the axilla between the anterior and posterior axillary nodes and are the most likely to be palpable. The central nodes drain into the infraclavicular and supraclavicular nodes.

9. **a.** healthy reproductive-age individual
   An acidic vagina pH (<4.5) is an expected finding in a healthy reproductive-age individual. This acidic pH is the result of the prevalence of *lactobacilli*, which in turn reflects the influence of estrogen initiated during puberty. Menopausal individuals and individuals who are using the lactational amenorrhea method of contraception may have a more alkaline pH as a result of decreased estrogen levels.

10. **d.** *Lactobacillus*
    Lactobacillus is the predominant vaginal organism responsible for an acidic pH in the reproductive-age individual.

11. **d.** transformation zone
    Squamous metaplasia is the process whereby columnar cells of the endocervix are replaced by mature squamous epithelium. The transformation zone is the area around the junction of squamous and columnar cells (squamocolumnar junction) where squamous metaplasia occurs.

12. **c.** There is thickened cervical mucus.
    The luteal phase of the menstrual cycle begins after ovulation occurs, lasts approximately 14 days (± 2 days), and ends with the first day of menses. Progesterone secreted from the corpus luteum causes thickened cervical mucus. The luteal phase corresponds with the uterine secretory phase.

13. **a.** FSH
    FSH is released by the anterior pituitary gland in response to GnRH from the hypothalamus. FSH stimulates ovarian follicular growth, resulting in increased levels of the estradiol.

14. **c.** estrone

The predominant estrogen after menopause is estrone. Estrone is converted from androstenedione produced by the adrenal gland and ovarian stroma.

15. **d.** Testosterone

Testosterone is produced in the adrenal gland, in the ovarian stroma, and through the conversion of androstenedione and DHA in peripheral tissues. Testosterone is aromatized to estradiol in peripheral tissues.

16. **a.** Follicular

The follicular phase begins day 1 of menses and ends with ovulation. This phase is more variable in terms of time frame than the luteal phase, which is normally 14 days (± 2 days).

17. **a.** Estrogen

Estrogen is the predominant hormone during the uterine proliferative phase of the menstrual cycle, which correlates with the ovarian follicular phase. Under the influence of estrogen, the endometrium grows/thickens in the proliferative phase.

18. **c.** Increased FSH, increased LH, decreased estradiol

During the menopausal transition, production of estradiol decreases as the number of responsive ovarian follicles decreases. This decrease in estradiol triggers the increased release of FSH and LH from the anterior pituitary gland.

19. **c.** LH surge

Urine ovulation prediction tests detect an LH surge. Ovulation occurs within 32–44 hours after LH surge begins.

20. **d.** It stimulates the synthesis of milk proteins in mammary glands.

The anterior pituitary gland secretes prolactin, which stimulates the synthesis of milk proteins in the mammary glands during pregnancy. The posterior pituitary gland secretes oxytocin in response to suckling and stimulates the breast milk ejection reflex.

21. **c.** transdermal estrogen patch

HT is indicated for the treatment of moderate to severe vasomotor symptoms. The individual who has had a hysterectomy does not need a progestogen, so estrogen only is appropriate. The estrogen agonist/antagonist (ospemifene) and vaginal estrogen cream are indicated for vulvovaginal atrophy and related symptoms but will not relieve vasomotor symptoms.

22. **a.** Prevention of cardiovascular disease

The FDA-approved indications for HT include relief of moderate to severe menopausal symptoms related to estrogen deficiency (vasomotor instability, vulvar/vaginal atrophy), and prevention of osteoporosis.

23. **b.** Palpable ovaries

Three to 5 years after menopause, ovaries are atrophic and are usually not palpable.

24. **b.** 45

The ACS recommends yearly mammograms for women starting at age 45.

25. **c.** less unscheduled bleeding with CEE/BZA

Data indicate less unscheduled bleeding and less breast tenderness with CEE/BZA than with CEE/MPA.

26. **d.** elasticity

Spinnbarkeit refers to the elasticity of cervical mucus (ability to be stretched between two fingers) seen at ovulation and under the influence of estrogen.

27. **b.** COCs may potentiate the action of a bronchodilator.

COCs may potentiate the action of some drugs, including benzodiazepines, tricyclic antidepressants, and theophylline.

28. **d.** Progestin-only contraceptive injections

Some anticonvulsant medications, including phenytoin, induce cytochrome P-450 enzyme activity and can cause increased first-pass metabolism of COCs as well as progestin-only pills. Although no first-pass metabolism occurs with the transdermal contraceptive patch, the FDA applies the same warning about possible reduced efficacy. The effectiveness of DMPA injections is not affected by anticonvulsant medications and may decrease the incidence of seizures in affected individuals.

29. **d.** The client can use emergency contraception pills even if there has been other unprotected sex since the last period.

Emergency contraception pills should be taken as soon as possible after unprotected sex and within 120 hours for maximum effectiveness. If the individual has had previous unprotected sex since the last period and more than 120 hours ago, obtain a urine pregnancy test to rule out an existing pregnancy.

30. **b.** has dysmenorrhea

The levonorgestrel-releasing IUC may cause reduced menstrual bleeding or amenorrhea and reduce dysmenorrhea. The copper-releasing IUC may increase dysmenorrhea.

31. **c.** keeping the IUC and repeating the cervical cytology in 3 years

Actinomyces is a normal genital tract organism in individuals with vaginas. IUC users are more likely to have colonization. Pelvic infection from *Actinomyces* is very rare, although it is a serious infection if it occurs. The cervical cytology does not diagnose actinomycosis infection. The asymptomatic IUC user should be informed of the cervical cytology result and should be advised that the IUC does not need to be removed and that she does not need any antibiotic treatment unless an infection occurs.

32. **c.** lower cumulative dose of progestin

Estrogen and progestogen are taken every day with a continuous-combined HT regimen with lower cumulative dose of progestogen than continuous-cyclic HT regimen in which estrogen is taken every day and larger doses of progestogen are added 10–14 days each month.

33. **b.** Cognitive behavior therapy

Level I evidence (i.e., high quality randomized controlled trials, systematic review of level I studies) supports the use of cognitive behavioral therapy—group or self-guided and clinical hypnosis for managing mild-moderate vasomotor symptoms related to menopause. Data on long-term use are limited.

34. **c.** It can remain in place for 48 hours.

The diaphragm should not be left in place for more than 24 hours. The cervical cap may be left in place for up to 48 hours.

35. **c.** phimosis
The term for the anatomic abnormality in which an individual has a tight foreskin that cannot be retracted is phimosis. Phimosis may contribute to male infertility in individuals with a penis.

36. **d.** stimulating uterine contractions.
Misoprostol is commonly used in conjunction with mifepristone or methotrexate for medical abortions. Misoprostol, a prostaglandin analogue, softens the cervix and stimulates uterine contractions.

37. **c.** They may cause irregular bleeding and spotting.
Users of progestin-only implants may experience irregular, prolonged, and more frequent bleeding, especially in the first few months of use. Progestin-only implants do not cause any decrease in bone mineral density. Most users ovulate within 6 weeks after removal.

38. **b.** has fewer adverse effects on coagulation factors
Estrogen delivered via a transdermal patch has no effect on cardiovascular markers (HDL-C, LDL-C, triglycerides, C-reactive protein). There is less effect on coagulation factors and a lower risk of venous thromboembolism with transdermal estrogen compared with oral estrogen in menopausal individuals.

39. **b.** Estriol
Estriol is the least potent of the estrogens. It is derived from the conversion of estrone and estradiol in the liver, uterus, placenta, and fetal adrenal gland.

40. **d.** prostaglandin
Prostaglandins act at target sites near areas of secretion. They regulate contraction and relaxation of smooth muscle. Prostaglandins are produced by the endometrium, with peak levels occurring in the late secretory phase. They stimulate uterine myometrial contractions.

41. **d.** Individual on continuous-combined HT regimen with spotting that occurs after several months of amenorrhea
Individuals using continuous-combined HT may initially have some unpredictable spotting and bleeding. After several months of use, the endometrium atrophies, and amenorrhea usually results. If spotting or bleeding recurs after several months of amenorrhea, endometrial evaluation is warranted.

42. **a.** remove the IUC, place a new IUC at the current visit, and start doxycycline for 5–7 days.
A partially expelled IUC should be removed. If the individual wants another IUC, it can be placed that same day after ruling out pregnancy. Doxycycline can be prescribed for 5–7 days to reduce the risk of infection.

43. **d.** Keep the current patch on if it adheres well and keep the same patch-change day.
If a contraceptive patch is detached for less than 24 hours, it can be reattached if it adheres well, or a new patch can be applied. The client should keep the same patch-change day. If it has been less than 48 hours since the patch detached, the individual does not need to use emergency contraception or a backup method.

44. **d.** progestin-only contraceptive injections
Return to fertility after discontinuing progestin-only injections (DMPA) may take 6–12 months.

45. **a.** 9; 19
Individuals who plan to use the calendar method for contraception should chart their menstrual cycles for several months. They should subtract 11 days from their longest recorded cycle and 18 days from their shortest cycle to estimate when they would be fertile and infertile. The individual with 27- to 30-day cycles should abstain from sexual intercourse from day 9 (27 minus 18) through day 19 (30 minus 11).

46. **a.** "I should insert a new ring every 7 days."
The contraceptive vaginal ring is worn in the vagina for 3 weeks, followed by 1 week without the ring, when the individual will have a withdrawal bleed. The exact position of the ring in the vagina is not important to effectiveness. The male (external) condom can be used with the contraceptive vaginal ring.

47. **c.** Unexplained vaginal bleeding prior to evaluation
Unexplained vaginal bleeding prior to evaluation is a CDC category 3 condition for initiation of DMPA. Current and/or history of DVT or pulmonary emboli is a category 2 condition; drugs that alter liver enzymes do not influence effectiveness of DMPA, and smoking at any age is a category 1 condition for use of DMPA.

48. **d.** Another method of contraception should be considered when the infant begins sleeping through the night.
Alternative contraception should be considered when any of the following occur—menses, regular supplementation, long periods without breastfeeding/chestfeeding, baby is 6 months old.

49. **d.** progestin-only pills
Progestin-only methods are classified as CDC category 1 for lactating individuals 30 or more days postpartum. CHCs are classified as CDC category 3 for the first 42 days postpartum for individuals with other venous thromboembolism risk factors, which include obesity. Fertility awareness methods are not recommended until the individual has resumed regular menses. When weaning a baby, the individual will not be able to rely on the lactational amenorrhea method for contraception.

50. **b.** 2:00 p.m. on Saturday
The diaphragm should be left in place for at least 6 hours after sexual intercourse and no longer than 24 hours.

51. **c.** may experience hot flashes as a side effect of this medication
Ospemifene is a SERM taken as a daily oral dose to treat moderate to severe dyspareunia related to vulvovaginal atrophy. Hot flashes are a common side effect. Estrogen should not be used in combination with ospemifene. No studies have looked at using a progestogen with ospemifene.

52. **b.** perineum
The area located between the fourchette anteriorly and the anus posteriorly is the perineum.

53. **b.** does not need to resume either cervical cytology or HPV testing

The ACS, ACOG, and USPSTF recommend no further cervical cancer screening in individuals aged 65 and older following adequate negative prior screening and no history of CIN2 or more serious diagnosis. Screening should not be resumed even if the individual reports a new sexual partner.

54. **c.** neither a clinical breast examination nor a screening mammogram

The USPSTF recommends against routine clinical breast examination at any age and recommends biennial mammograms from age 50–74.

55. **c.** vestibule

The vestibule is enclosed by the labia minora. This area contains the urethral and vaginal openings; hymen; Skene's glands on each side of the urethral meatus; and Bartholin's glands, with openings located posteriorly on either side of the vaginal orifice.

56. **a.** normal uterus and normal ovaries

In a reproductive-age individual, the uterus is approximately 8 cm in length, 5 cm in width, and 2.5 cm in thickness, with slightly larger dimensions in the multiparous woman than in the nulliparous individual. Ovaries are approximately 3 cm × 2 cm × 1 cm.

57. **a.** Beginning breast development

Breast development begins with breast budding around age 9; the growth of pubic and axillary hair usually starts after breast development begins; and the peak growth spurt occurs around age 12, just prior to onset of menses.

58. **b.** Hypothalamus

GnRH is released from the hypothalamus in a pulsatile fashion. GnRH stimulates the anterior pituitary gland to release FSH and LH.

59. **a.** LH surge, ovulation, rise in BBT, thickened cervical mucus

The LH surge occurs in the follicular phase and peaks about 10–12 hours before ovulation occurs. BBT increases at the time of ovulation. After ovulation, the corpus luteum formed from the ruptured follicle secretes progesterone, which causes thickening of cervical mucus and a sustained increase in BBT.

60. **d.** Vaginal contraceptive ring for individual older than 35 years of age who smokes one pack of cigarettes per day

Smoking 15 or more cigarettes a day at age 35 years or older is a CDC category 4 condition for all of the CHCs.

61. **c.** may be used by individuals with latex allergy

The vaginal condom is made of nitrile and previously was made of polyurethane, so it may be used by individuals with a latex allergy.

62. **b.** Decrease in risk for cervical cancer

Noncontraceptive benefits of COCs include decreased risks for benign breast disease, endometrial cancer, and ovarian cancer.

63. **c.** Intrauterine contraceptive

The perfect use and typical use failure rates are the same or very close to the same for both levonorgestrel-releasing and copper-releasing intrauterine contraceptives. These methods do not require the individual to remember to do something each day or to have supplies available and use them at the time of sexual intercourse.

64. **d.** Transdermal contraceptive system

The transdermal contraceptive patch may be less effective in individuals who weigh 90 kg (198 lb) or more.

65. **c.** Increase in first-pass metabolism in the liver

Drugs that increase production of the liver enzyme cytochrome P-450 may cause more rapid clearance of COCs during first-pass metabolism in the liver.

66. **d.** You should choose a site that ensures deep IM injection.

The IM formulation of DMPA must be given as a deep injection in the deltoid or gluteal muscle. For individuals with obesity, the deltoid may be preferable.

67. **a.** If you are more than 3 hours late taking a pill, use a backup method for 48 hours.

The major mechanism of action of progestin-only pills is the thickening of cervical mucus. Progestin-only pills must be taken at the same time each day to maintain adequate progestin for this effect. Progestin levels peak shortly after taking a pill and decline to nearly undetectable levels 24 hours later.

68. **b.** Estring vaginal ring

The Estring vaginal ring has little or no systemic absorption and does not require opposition by a progestogen.

69. **b.** alveoli

Alveoli within the breast lobules are responsible for milk production.

70. **d.** prolactin

Prolactin is released from the anterior pituitary gland in increasing amounts during pregnancy. Prolactin stimulates the synthesis of milk proteins in mammary tissue.

71. **c.** known or suspected ectopic pregnancy

Antidepressant and NSAID use do not interfere with medication abortions. The FDA has approved the use of mifepristone and misoprostol for medication abortion for up to 70 days after an LMP. Medication abortion is contraindicated when there is a known or suspected ectopic pregnancy.

72. **c.** Fertility awareness methods

The perimenopausal individual who is having irregular menses may have unpredictable ovulation, so should not rely on fertility awareness methods for contraception.

73. **d.** reduce hot flash frequency and severity for some individuals

Data from a meta-analysis of 17 small randomized controlled trials support the efficacy of soy products in reducing hot flash frequency and severity for some individuals. Inform patients that soy products vary in composition and concentration.

74. **b.** "I know that I am about to ovulate when my temperature rises at least 0.4°F."

The rise in BBT occurs at the time of ovulation. BBT cannot be used to predict ovulation, but it can be used to determine whether ovulation has occurred.

75. **c.** The IUC should be removed promptly regardless of the client's plans for the pregnancy.

Removing the IUC reduces the risk of spontaneous abortion. There is no risk of congenital anomalies from copper exposure. If the IUC is left in place, the individual is at risk for spontaneous septic abortion as well as preterm delivery.

76. **d.** Sunday starters should use a backup method for the first week of the first pack of pills.
A first day of menses start does not require backup contraception. The quick-start method for COCs requires backup contraception for 7 days except if switching directly from one hormonal method to another. A Sunday start requires 7 days of backup method unless it corresponds with the first day of menses.

77. **b.** Lubricants may take several weeks of use before becoming effective.
Vaginal lubricants have an immediate effect and are intended to reduce friction on atrophic vulvovaginal structures during sex. Vaginal moisturizers are applied several times weekly for longer-term relief of vaginal dryness. Moisturizers help maintain vaginal moisture and lower vaginal pH.

78. **d.** Frequent use of spermicide may cause vaginal changes, making you more susceptible to HIV infection.
Frequent spermicide use (two or more times per day) may cause vulvovaginal epithelium disruption and, theoretically, increase susceptibility to HIV infection. Spermicide should be placed deep in the vagina close to the cervix and left there for at least 6 hours after sexual intercourse. When spermicide is used along with a condom, there is an increased contraceptive efficacy, but it will not further decrease the risk for STIs.

79. **c.** Use of COC by a 40-year-old individual who has migraine headaches without aura
The use of COCs by an individual who is 35 years or older and who has migraine headaches with or without aura is a CDC category 4 condition. The use of COCs by an individual of any age who has migraine headaches with aura is also a CDC category 4 condition.

80. **d.** There is a decreased chance for the presence of preejaculatory sperm with repeat acts of intercourse.
This statement is false. In itself, preejaculatory fluid contains no sperm. However, with repeat acts of intercourse close together, subsequent preejaculatory fluid may have "carryover" sperm from the previous ejaculation.

81. **c.** 3–5 days
Healthy sperm can survive in the reproductive tract and retain ability to fertilize an egg for 3–5 days. An egg can be fertilized for 12–24 hours after release from the ovary.

82. **a.** Estrogen-containing oral contraceptives
Factors that increase SHBG include hyperthyroidism, pregnancy, and use of estrogen-containing oral contraceptives. Factors that decrease SHBG include increased adiposity, hyperinsulinemia, and androgens.

83. **b.** After two FSH levels in a series—on the day of injection and repeated 13 weeks later prior to the next injection—are >30 mIU/mL, the method can be stopped immediately.

For individuals using DMPA, FSH levels are not always impacted. In perimenopausal individuals, if FSH is suppressed, the levels generally return to normal baseline prior to the next injection. Elevated FSH levels >30 mIU/mL 13 weeks apart is indicative of menopausal status and the contraception can be discontinued.

84. **a.** Patients who are using NuvaRing can insert a new ring every 3 weeks, avoiding withdrawal bleeding
NuvaRing has been studied for safety and efficacy for extended cycling, whereas Annovera does not have the evidence to support extended cycling. All COC pills can be used for extended cycling, although some formulations have been especially created to support this. Withdrawal bleeding is not necessary for contraception to work effectively.

85. **d.** Drospirenone
Drospirenone is a fourth-generation progestin, which is an analog of spironolactone, a potassium-sparing diuretic with progestogenic effect and antiandrogenic properties.

86. **a.** Patients who are exclusively breastfeeding/chestfeeding, have not had a menstrual cycle, and are less than 6 months postpartum are not likely to ovulate.
Exclusive breastfeeding/chestfeeding patients who are less than 6 months postpartum and have not resumed menstruation have increased prolactin, which inhibits pulsatile GnRH. While FSH remains normal, LH is decreased, and no ovarian follicular development occurs resulting in anovulation.

87. **c.** Most cases of pelvic inflammatory disease occur within 20 days after insertion.
Prophylactic antibiotics and negative STI testing are not necessary prior to IUD insertion. It is not necessary to remove an IUD with a diagnosis of PID unless there is no clinical improvement following appropriate antibiotic therapy within 48–72 hours.

88. **c.** Risk assessment for HIV preexposure prophylaxis (PrEP)
All sexually active patients should be routinely assessed for risk factors that make them candidates for PrEP.

89. **c.** HPV vaccination if series not previously completed
HPV vaccination series is recommended for cervical cancer prevention if not done earlier and 26 years of age or younger; may offer to individuals older than 26 years of age.

90. **a.** Hereditary breast cancer risk assessment
American College of Obstetricians and Gynecologists recommend performing a hereditary breast cancer risk assessment. The Women's Preventive Services Initiative recommends regular risk assessment for BRCA 1/2 testing starting at age 18.

91. **b.** is a marker of ovarian reserve
AMH is produced exclusively by the granulosa cells or preantral/small ovarian follicles, inhibits FSH-dependent follicular growth, may play a role in follicular recruitment and selection, and is a marker of ovarian reserve. AMH begins to decrease as early as the late 20s and 30s and is undetectable about 5 years after menopause.

92. **d.** nonhormonal and hormonal therapies are options for long-term treatment.

Symptoms of GSM, when untreated, will persist and worsen over time. Symptoms are likely to return after discontinuing treatment. Nonhormonal and hormonal therapies are available for long-term treatment.

Bibliography

American Cancer Society (ACS). (2024). American Cancer Society Recommendations for the Early Detection of Breast Cancer. Retrieved from: https://www.cancer.org/cancer/types/breast-cancer/screening-tests-and-early-detection/american-cancer-society-recommendations-for-the-early-detection-of-breast-cancer.html

American College of Obstetricians and Gynecologists (ACOG). (2017, re-affirmed 2019). Practice bulletin 179: Breast cancer risk assessment and screening in average-risk women. *Obstetrics and Gynecology, 130*, e1–e16.

American College of Obstetricians and Gynecologists. (2020). Practice Bulletin 225: Medication abortion up to 70 days of gestation. *Obstetrics and Gynecology*, 136, e31–e47.

American College of Obstetricians and Gynecologists. (2021). *Updated cervical cancer screening guidelines.* www.acog.org/clinical/clinical-guidance/practice-advisory/articles/2021/04/updated-cervical-cancer-screening-guidelines

American Diabetes Association. (2021). Standards of medical care in diabetes. *Diabetes Care, 44*(supp.1), S1–232.

Arnett, D., Blumenthal, R., Albert, M., Buroker, A., Goldberger, Z., et al. (2019). 2019 ACC/AHA guideline on the primary prevention of cardiovascular disease: executive summary: A report of the American College of Cardiology/American Heart Association Task Force on Clinical Practice Guidelines. *Circulation, 140*(11), e563–595.

Bahamondes, L., Fernandes, A., Monteiro, I., & Bahamondes, M. V. (2020). Long-acting reversible contraceptive (LARCs) methods. *Best practice & research. Clinical Obstetrics & Gynaecology, 66*, 28–40. https://www.sciencedirect.com/science/article/abs/pii/S1521693419301786?via%3Dihub

Ball, J., Dains, J., Flynn, J., Solomon, B., & Stewart, R. (2019). *Seidel's guide to physical examination* (9th ed.). Mosby.

Beloff, M. S., Greenspan, S. L., Insogna, K. L., Lewiecki, E. M., Saag, K. G., Singer, A. J., & Siris, E. S. (2022). The clinician's guide to prevention and treatment of osteoporosis. *Osteoporosis International, 33*, 2049–2102.

Carcio, H. & Secor, M. (2019). *Advanced health assessment of women: Clinical skills and procedures* (4th ed.). Springer.

Cason, P., Cwiak, C., Edelman, A., Kowal, D., Marrazzo, J. M., Nelson, A. L., & Policar, M. S. (2024). *Contraceptive technology* (22nd ed.). Jones & Bartlett Learning.

Centers for Disease Control and Prevention. (2016). U.S. medical eligibility criteria for contraceptive use, 2016. *Morbidity and Mortality Weekly Report, 65*(3), 1–103.

Centers for Disease Control and Prevention. (2022a). *Recommended immunization schedule for children and adolescents aged 18 years and younger, United States, 2022.* https://www.cdc.gov/vaccines/schedules/hcp/child-adolescent.html

Centers for Disease Control and Prevention. (2022b). *Adult immunization schedule, United States,* 2022. https://www.cdc.gov/vaccines/schedules/hcp/imz/adult.html

Curtis, K. M., Jatlaoui, T. C., Tepper, N. K., Zapata, L. B., Horton, L. G., Jamieson, D. J., & Whiteman, M. K. (2016). U.S. selected practice recommendations for contraceptive use, 2016. *Morbidity and Mortality Weekly Report, 65*(4), 1–66. http://dx.doi.org/10.15585/mmwr.rr6504a1

Faculty of Sexual & Reproductive Healthcare of the Royal College of Obstetricians and Gynecologists. (2017). *Clinical effectiveness unit statement: Contraceptive choices and sexual health for transgender and non-binary people.* https://www.fsrh.org/documents/fsrh-ceu-statement-contraceptive-choices-and-sexual-health-for/

Fontham, E., Wolf, A., & Church, T. (2020). Cervical cancer screening for individuals at average risk: 2020 guideline update from the American Cancer Society. *CA Cancer Journal for Clinicians, 70*(5), 321–346.

Gilbert, A. L., & Hoffman, B. L. (2021). Contraceptive technology: Present and future. *Obstetrics and Gynecology Clinics of North America, 48*(4), 723–735. https://doi.org/10.1016/j.ogc.2021.07.001

Lindh, I., Othman, J., Hansson, M., Ekelund, A. C., Svanberg, T., & Strandell, A. (2021). New types of diaphragms and cervical caps versus older types of diaphragms and different gels for contraception: A systematic review. *BMJ Sexual & Reproductive Health, 47*(3), e12. https://doi.org/10.1136/bmjsrh-2020-200632

North American Menopause Society. (2019). *Menopause practice: A clinician's guide* (6th ed.). NAMS.

North American Menopause Society. (2020). The 2020 genitourinary syndrome of menopause position statement of the North American Menopause Society. *Menopause, 27*(9), 976–992.

North American Menopause Society. (2022). The 2022 hormone therapy position statement of the North American Menopause Society. *Menopause, 29*(7), 767–794.

Phillippi, J. & Kantrowitz-Gordon, I. (Eds.). (2025). *Varney's midwifery* (7th ed.). Jones & Bartlett Learning.

Schadewald, D. M., Pritham, U. A., Youngkin. E. Q., Davis, M. S., & Juve, C. (2020). *Women's health: A primary care clinical guide* (5th ed.). Pearson Education, Inc.

Schuiling, K., & Likis, F. (2022). *Gynecologic health care* (4th ed.). Jones & Bartlett Learning.

Sehnal, B., Beneš, J., Kolářovigure á, Z., Mojhová, M., & Zikán, M. (2018). Pelvic actinomycosis and IUD. Pánevní aktinomykóza a IUD. *Ceska Gynekologie, 83*(5), 386–390.

Smith, R., Andrews, K., Brooks, D., Fedewa, S., Manassaramf-Baptiste, D., et al. (2019). Cancer screening in the United States, 2019: A review of current American Cancer Society guidelines and current issues in cancer screening. *CA Cancer Journal for Clinicians, 69*(3), 184–210.

Teal, S., & Edelman, A. (2021). Contraception selection, effectiveness, and adverse effects: A review. *JAMA, 326*(24), 2507–2518. https://doi.org/10.1001/jama.2021.21392

U.S. Preventive Services Task Force (USPSTF). (2018). *Cervical cancer: Screening.* https://www.uspreventiveservicestaskforce.org/Page/Document/RecommendationStatementFinal/cervical-cancer-screening2

U.S. Preventive Services Task Force (USPSTF). (2021a). *Colorectal cancer: Screening.* https://www.uspreventiveservicestaskforce.org/uspstf/recommendation/colorectal-cancer-screening

Voedisch, A. J., & Ariel, D. (2020). Perimenopausal contraception. *Current Opinion in Obstetrics & Gynecology, 32*(6), 399–407. https://doi.org/10.1097/GCO.0000000000000667

Women's Preventive Services Initiative. (2022). *Recommendations for well-woman care.* https://www.womenspreventivehealth.org/recommendations/

Zigler, R. E., & McNicholas, C. (2017). Unscheduled vaginal bleeding with progestin-only contraceptive use. *American Journal of Obstetrics and Gynecology, 216*(5), 443–450. https://doi.org/10.1016/j.ajog.2016.12.008

CHAPTER 5

Gynecologic, Reproductive, and Sexual Disorders

Beth M. Kelsey

Heather C. Quaile

Signey Olson

Menstrual and Endocrine Disorders

Premenstrual Syndrome (PMS)

- Definition—the cyclic occurrence, in the luteal phase, of a group of distressing physical and psychological symptoms that begin about 5–7 days before menses and resolve within about 4 days after onset of menses. These symptoms typically disrupt normal activities and interpersonal relationships to a mild to moderate degree and may not occur in all cycles.
- Etiology/incidence
  1. Unknown etiology; multifactorial and multiorgan disorder; suggested causes include metabolic and endocrine disorders, sensitivity to alterations in estrogen or progesterone levels, withdrawal of endogenous endorphins, fluid imbalance, vitamin and mineral deficiencies, and altered carbohydrate metabolism
  2. Prevalence may be greater than 50%, with most individuals not requiring treatment; severe cases occur in 3%–10% of individuals with PMS, typically resulting in a premenstrual dysphoric disorder (PMDD) diagnosis
- Signs and symptoms
  1. Symptoms recur cyclically in the luteal phase with a symptom-free period in the follicular phase
  2. Range from mild to severe; result in interference with normal activities and personal relationships
     a. Physical
        (1) Headache
        (2) Breast changes
        (3) Fluid retention
        (4) Swelling
        (5) Abdominal bloating
        (6) Nausea/vomiting
        (7) Alterations in appetite
        (8) Food cravings
        (9) Lethargy/fatigue
        (10) Exacerbations of preexisting conditions, such as asthma
     b. Psychological
        (1) Irritability
        (2) Depression
        (3) Anxiety
        (4) Sleep alterations
        (5) Inability to concentrate
        (6) Anger
        (7) Violent behavior
        (8) Crying
        (9) Confusion
        (10) Changes in libido
- Physical findings—no specific physical findings on exam
- Differential diagnosis
  1. A diagnosis of exclusion; all others must be ruled out
  2. Depression and/or anxiety
  3. Bipolar affective disorder
  4. Alcohol or substance use disorder
  5. Personality disorders
  6. Chronic fatigue syndrome
  7. Fibromyalgia
  8. Diabetes
  9. Brain tumor
  10. Thyroid disease
  11. Hyperprolactinemia
  12. Perimenopause
  13. PMDD

- Diagnostic tests/findings
  1. Documentation of symptoms in a diary fashion for 2–3 months to evaluate for cyclic symptom patterns consistent with ovulation and menses; retrospective recall less accurate
  2. Individualized testing, based on symptoms, may include glucose tolerance test and thyroid profile; hormone levels of little value
- Management/treatment
  1. Nonmedical management
     a. Treatment should be individualized; goals are to isolate symptom groups from history and diary and to treat symptomatically
     b. Options for treatment
        (1) Self-help strategies recommended as first-line therapy; help the client understand the possible causes of the symptoms, reassuring the client that no serious health threats exist. Review that there are no immediate cures; patience and team effort are key
        (2) Little evidence to support the helpfulness of dietary revisions such as restriction of salt and refined sugar or limiting caffeine, though individualized reactions should be considered
        (3) Vitamin B_6 (50–150 mg/day) may be beneficial—continuous use, not intermittent
        (4) Calcium carbonate supplementation of 1,200–1,600 mg/day shown in randomized placebo-controlled trial to reduce PMS symptoms
        (5) Chaste tree berry (Vitex) extract shown in placebo-controlled trial to reduce PMS symptoms
        (6) Aerobic exercise 20–30 minutes at least four times a week
        (7) Avoidance of known physical or emotional triggers
        (8) Cognitive therapy, group therapy, relaxation therapy, mindfulness training may improve physical and psychological symptoms
        (9) Self-help, support groups, biofeedback, acupuncture/acupressure, massage to reduce stress levels and discomfort especially if low back pain, and light therapy may help some individuals
  2. Medical management
     a. Selection of medications based on type and intensity of symptoms
     b. Spironolactone during luteal phase to reduce swelling and bloating
     c. Nonsteroidal anti-inflammatory drugs (NSAIDs; antiprostaglandins) given before and during menstruation may reduce fluid retention and breast, lower back, abdominal, pelvic pain
     d. Combined oral contraceptives (consider continuous or extended-use regimens), other combination or progestin-only contraceptive methods may be helpful in decreasing physical symptoms by suppressing ovulation, thus minimizing hormonal fluctuations in the luteal phase. Methods may also reduce menstrual bleeding and pain.
     e. Selective serotonin reuptake inhibitors (SSRIs) have been shown to alleviate severe PMS and become effective much quicker than when treating other mood disorders; equally effective when taken continuously or only in luteal phase each month.
     f. Gonadotropin-releasing hormone (GnRH) agonists to inhibit cyclic gonadotropin release; have significant menopause-like side effects; long-term therapy may predispose individual to heart disease or osteoporosis; limit use to 4–6 months unless combined with combination hormonal therapy

- PMDD
  1. At least five PMS-type symptoms severe enough to disrupt normal functioning markedly in most, if not all, menstrual cycles
  2. Occurs in the luteal phase and resolves within 1 week after onset of menses
  3. Must include at least one of these symptoms: markedly depressed mood, marked anxiety, marked affective lability, persistent and marked anger
  4. Prevalence—3% to 10% of reproductive-age women
  5. Treatment
     a. Same therapeutic interventions as for PMS
     b. Medications with Food and Drug Administration (FDA) approval for the treatment of PMDD include drospirenone-containing combination hormonal contraceptives (CHCs) and the SSRIs fluoxetine, paroxetine, sertraline
     c. Anxiolytic drugs (alprazolam, buspirone)—mixed results in PMDD treatment studies; high potential for drug dependence; reserve for short-term use

Dysmenorrhea

- Definition
  1. Painful menstruation—a sensation of cramping in the lower abdomen during or beginning just before menses; may radiate to the back and thighs
  2. Primary—dysmenorrhea unassociated with underlying pelvic pathology; rarely begins after age 20 years; associated with ovulatory cycles; stimulated by prostaglandin release and typically most severe on first day and likely to last 1–3 days. Pain tends to improve over time. Increased prostaglandin release may also induce GI symptoms, such as diarrhea.
  3. Secondary—dysmenorrhea associated with an underlying pelvic pathologic condition; may occur at any age in menstruating individuals. Pain tends to worsen over time, though may be present from menarche, and may occur more prominently if discontinuing a hormonal contraceptive method that masked symptoms.
- Etiology/incidence
  1. Primary—seen in 50%–75% of all menstruating individuals, with 10%–20% having severe dysmenorrhea; prostaglandins stimulate contractile response on smooth muscles
  2. Secondary—onset may occur many years after menarche; most often in individuals older than age 20 years
- Signs and symptoms
  1. Primary
     a. Pain begins shortly before the onset of menses and usually lasts no longer than 2 days

b. Described as colicky, crampy, and spasmodic pain in the lower abdomen, sometimes radiating to the lower back and thighs

c. May interfere with work or school (15%–29%)

2. Secondary

a. Pain may occur near or during menstruation but may also occur at any time during the cycle, depending on the underlying etiology

b. Depending on etiology, may be accompanied by dyspareunia, GI symptoms, heavy bleeding

c. Unlikely to be adequately relieved by over-the-counter measures

d. Symptoms often persist longer and with more intensity than with primary dysmenorrhea

e. More likely to interfere with work, school, sexual relationships

- Physical findings
  1. Primary—characterized by no abnormalities found on examination or imaging
  2. Secondary—has findings consistent with pathologic condition, imaging may or may not present obvious pathology

- Differential diagnosis
  1. Endometriosis
  2. Adenomyosis
  3. Pelvic congestion syndrome
  4. Leiomyomas
  5. Pelvic floor dysfunction
  6. Uterine abnormalities
  7. Pelvic infection
  8. Ovarian or adnexal mass
  9. Idiopathic chronic pelvic pain
  10. Uterine or pelvic adhesions
  11. Sexually transmitted infections (STIs)
  12. Urinary tract infections (UTIs)
  13. Vaginismus
  14. Interstitial cystitis

- Diagnostic tests/findings
  1. Primary—no specific tests are ordered
  2. Secondary
     a. Analyze pain description and timing to help determine the etiology
     b. Tests based on history and physical examination findings
        (1) Transvaginal ultrasound to evaluate the uterus, ovaries, and adnexa
        (2) Saline infusion sonohysterogram (SIS or SHG) to evaluate endometrial cavity
        (3) Hysteroscopy to evaluate endometrial cavity
        (4) Laparoscopy to evaluate pelvic cavity
        (5) Cultures to evaluate infections
        (6) Lower GI evaluation

- Management/treatment
  1. Primary
     a. Prostaglandin synthetase inhibitors, NSAIDs are treatment of choice; best if initiated 2 days prior to expected menses or at the onset of menses and continuing for 48–72 hours; choices shown to be effective are mefenamic acid, naproxen sodium, ibuprofen, and indomethacin

b. CHCs are good choices if contraception is needed; act by reducing prostaglandins and menstrual flow; may consider extended or continuous dosing regimens

c. Progestin-only contraceptives may relieve symptoms by decreasing or eliminating menstrual bleeding—depot medroxyprogesterone acetate (DMPA), progestin implant, levonorgestrel-releasing intrauterine system (LNG-IUS)

d. Self-help measures include regular exercise, warm heat, relaxation exercises, stress-reduction measures, massage therapy if back involvement

2. Secondary treatment consistent with pathology

Amenorrhea

- Definition
  1. Absence of menses during reproductive years
  2. Primary—no menstruation previously; no menstruation by age 14 years in the absence of development of secondary sex characteristics; no menstruation by age 16 years regardless of secondary sex characteristics
  3. Secondary—absence of menses in a previously menstruating individual; no menses for 3–6 months in an individual who usually has normal periods or for a length of time equivalent to three cycles
  4. A symptom, not a diagnosis

- Etiology/incidence
  1. Incidence is approximately 5% in individuals assigned female at birth who are not pregnant, lactating, or menopausal
  2. Disorders of genital outflow tract—for example, vaginal agenesis, imperforate hymen, cervical stenosis, female genital mutilation
  3. Endocrine disorders—for example, hyperthyroidism, hypothyroidism, hyperprolactinemia, hyperandrogenism, primary ovarian insufficiency/early menopause, polycystic ovary syndrome
  4. Congenital and chromosomal abnormalities—for example, Turner syndrome, androgen insensitivity/resistance syndrome, congenital adrenal hyperplasia
  5. Disordered eating, particularly restrictive types, such as anorexia nervosa
  6. Excessive exercise/competitive sports training
  7. Malnutrition, chronic dieting
  8. Medications—for example, hormones, hormonal contraception, antipsychotics, cancer chemotherapeutic agents
  9. Chronic illness—for example, tuberculosis, alcohol or other substance use disorders, type 1 or 2 diabetes mellitus, disorders of adrenal glands
  10. Asherman's syndrome—irradiation or surgery resulting in destruction of endometrium such as ablation
  11. Sheehan syndrome—condition that may occur with massive hemorrhage during or after delivery, causing severe hypotension and pituitary necrosis resulting in hypopituitarism
  12. Excessive or chronic stress, trauma

- Symptoms—absence of menses at the expected time; other related to etiology

- Physical findings
  1. Abnormal vital signs may indicate chronic illness
  2. Low weight or body mass index (BMI) may indicate malnutrition, restrictive eating disorder, and/or excessive exercise
  3. Galactorrhea may indicate hyperprolactinemia
  4. Abnormal visual fields and/or galactorrhea may indicate pituitary tumor
  5. Enlarged or nodular thyroid may indicate thyroid disorder
  6. Delay in Tanner stage progression (breast development, pubic hair development) may indicate altered pubertal development
  7. Hirsutism, acne, acanthosis nigricans, clitoral enlargement may indicate androgen excess
  8. Vaginal atrophy may indicate lack of estrogen, ovarian insufficiency/premature menopause
  9. Imperforate hymen, cervical stenosis, and female genital cutting may be causes of outflow tract disorder
  10. Enlarged uterus may indicate pregnancy
- Differential diagnosis
  1. Pregnancy
  2. Menopause or perimenopause
  3. Anorexia nervosa or restrictive eating disorder
  4. Excessive physical activity/athletic training
  5. Disorders of the ovary, uterus, anterior pituitary, and/or hypothalamus
  6. Other endocrine disorders
  7. Congenital or acquired anatomic disorders
  8. Chronic illness
  9. Medication effects
- Diagnostic tests/findings
  1. Pregnancy test
  2. Serum prolactin level
  3. Serum thyroid-stimulating hormone (TSH)
  4. If these tests are normal, may evaluate the bioavailability of estrogen with a progestin challenge test
     a. Progestin each day for 10–14 days—wait for bleeding, which should occur within 7–14 days; will indicate adequate estrogen production and stimulation as well as no problem with outflow tract
     b. If no withdrawal bleed in 2 weeks, order follicle-stimulating hormone (FSH)/luteinizing hormone (LH) tests
     c. If FSH and LH are low, the cause is likely hypothalamic or pituitary dysfunction
     d. If FSH and LH are high, the cause is likely ovarian insufficiency/menopause
  5. Determine karyotype if suspect ovarian insufficiency due to chromosomal difference
- Management/treatment
  1. Primary amenorrhea—refer to an endocrinologist
  2. Treat thyroid abnormalities or refer
  3. If prolactin and TSH are normal and bleeding occurs after the progestin challenge, initiate treatment for anovulation based on age, contraceptive needs, and lifestyle
  4. Treatment may include CHCs or cyclic progestins
  5. Evaluate relationship with food, exercise/movement, and body image; consider referral to dietician as needed
  6. Referral for complicated secondary amenorrhea cause or undetermined etiology
  7. Referral for ovulation induction if patient desires pregnancy

Infrequent Menstrual Bleeding

- Definition—infrequent uterine bleeding characterized by one or two bleeding episodes in a 90-day period; previously referred to as oligomenorrhea
- Etiology/incidence
  1. Occurs frequently in perimenopause
  2. Ovarian–pituitary–hypothalamus abnormalities
  3. Endocrine disorders, such as thyroid or adrenal problems
  4. Systemic causes, such as chronic illness, weight loss or gain, extreme stress, excessive exercise
  5. Heavy substance use or substance use disorder
- Signs and symptoms
  1. May alternate with episodes of amenorrhea or heavy uterine bleeding
  2. May present as a menstrual pattern during the first year of menstruation or for several years before menopause
- Differential diagnosis
  1. Pregnancy
  2. Other disturbances with hypothalamic–pituitary–ovarian axis
  3. Menopause or perimenopause
  4. Anorexia nervosa or restrictive eating disorder
  5. Excessive physical activity/athletic training
  6. Disorders of the ovary, uterus, anterior pituitary, and/or hypothalamus
  7. Congenital or acquired anatomic disorders
  8. Chronic illness
  9. Medication effects
- Physical findings—consistent with pathology outlined in the Differential Diagnosis section
- Diagnostic tests/findings
  1. Pregnancy test
  2. Tests to evaluate the function of the thyroid, ovaries, pituitary, or hypothalamus (e.g., TSH, prolactin level, FSH/LH levels)
  3. Transvaginal ultrasound
  4. Pituitary MRI
- Management/treatment
  1. If pregnant, proceed with options counseling
  2. Identify and treat underlying cause (consider referral or collaborative care with an endocrinologist)
  3. Prevent unopposed estrogen resulting in endometrial hyperplasia by prescribing progestin therapy—medroxyprogesterone acetate (MPA) 10 days each month or for 10 days every 3 months or CHCs

Heavy and/or Prolonged Menstrual Bleeding

- Definition—heavy menstrual bleeding (HMB) is characterized by monthly uterine blood loss volume of greater than 80 mL; prolonged menstrual bleeding (PMB) is characterized by bleeding episodes lasting more than 8 days;

heavy and/or prolonged menstrual bleeding previously referred to as menorrhagia
- Etiology/incidence
  1. Often occurs at extremes of the reproductive window—adolescence and perimenopause
  2. Gynecologic causes—leiomyoma, adenomyosis, endometrial and endocervical polyps, endometrial hyperplasia, cervical and endometrial cancers
  3. Inherited and acquired bleeding disorders—von Willebrand disease, idiopathic thrombocytopenia purpura, aplastic anemia, platelet dysfunction
  4. Disturbances of hypothalamic–pituitary–ovarian axis causing continuous endometrial stimulation
  5. Imbalance of prostaglandins, favoring those that cause vasodilation over those that cause vasoconstriction
  6. Systemic diseases—hepatic disease, early renal failure, adrenal hyperplasia, thyroid dysfunction
  7. Medications—anticoagulants, some anticonvulsants, digitalis, nonhormonal intrauterine contraception, chronic aspirin or NSAID use
  8. Other—physical trauma, extreme stress
  9. PALM-COEIN is a pneumonic created by the International Federation of Gynecology and Obstetrics (FIGO) to classify common causes of abnormal uterine bleeding (AUB) in reproductive-aged individuals into structural and nonstructural etiologies (**Box 5-1**)

Box 5-1 PALM-COEIN

PALM—structural causes of AUB

Polyp—endometrial and endocervical, may cause intermenstrual bleeding

Adenomyosis—may cause HMB and/or PMB

Leiomyoma (fibroids)—may cause HMB and/or PMB

Malignancy/hyperplasia—AUB is the most common symptom of endometrial cancer, bleeding patterns are variable

COEIN—nonstructural causes of AUB

Coagulopathy—spectrum of systemic disorders of hemostasis associated with HMB and/or PMB (e.g., clotting factor deficiencies, platelet dysfunction, von Willebrand disease)

Ovulatory dysfunction—includes a variety of endocrine disorders (e.g., polycystic ovarian syndrome, other androgen excess, thyroid disorders), may have irregular menses, HMB, and/or PMB

Endometrial—likely due to vasoconstriction disorders, inflammation, infection, HMB associated with predictable ovulatory cycles

Iatrogenic—a variety of medications and devices that act on the endometrium can cause AUB (e.g., IUDs, hormonal contraception, tamoxifen, some antipsychotics)

Not yet classified—poorly understood conditions and rare disorders (e.g., arteriovenous malformations)

Data from Marnach, M. L., & Laughlin-Tommaso, S. K. (2019). Evaluation and management of abnormal uterine bleeding. *Mayo Clinic Proceedings*, 94(2), 326–335; Munro, M. G., Critchley, H. O., Broder, M. S., & Fraser, I. S. (2011). FIGO classification system (PALM-COEIN) for causes of abnormal uterine bleeding in nongravid women of reproductive age. FIGO Working Group on Menstrual Disorders. *International Journal Gynaecology and Obstetrics, 113*, 3–13.

- Symptoms
  1. Individuals may have different definitions of excessive bleeding; bleeding is relevant if it disrupts the individual's life
  2. Symptoms vary with the cause of bleeding
- Physical findings—depend on the cause of bleeding, see Etiology/Incidence section
- Differential diagnoses
  1. Pregnancy (ectopic or intrauterine)
  2. Gynecologic disorders
  3. Disturbances of hypothalamic–pituitary–ovarian axis
  4. Acquired or inherited bleeding disorders
  5. Systemic diseases
  6. Medication related
- Diagnostic tests/findings
  1. Pregnancy test
  2. Cervical cancer screening if no recent normal screening
  3. Complete blood count (CBC)
  4. FSH and LH to evaluate estrogen stimulation—rarely indicated
  5. TSH
  6. STI testing as indicated
  7. Endometrial evaluation as indicated—consider endometrial biopsy, transvaginal ultrasound, saline infusion sonohysteroscopy
  8. Coagulation studies if indicated
- Management/treatment
  1. Hormonal
     a. Acute excessive bleeding—IV estrogen or high-dose oral estrogen gradually tapered, then MPA added last 10 days to initiate withdrawal bleeding; high-dose oral progestin therapy gradually tapered
     b. Moderate bleeding and maintenance control—LNG-IUS is FDA approved for the treatment of HMB; CHCs cyclic, extended, or continuous regimens; DMPA; cyclic oral MPA
  2. Nonhormonal
     a. Treat anemia
     b. NSAIDs—start at menses onset and continue for 5 days or until cessation of menstruation; increases ratio of vasoconstrictive prostaglandins to vasodilating prostaglandins
     c. Tranexamic acid—antifibrinolytic agent that blocks lysis of fibrin clots; takes up to the first 5 days of menses; decreases blood loss in individuals who have increased endometrial plasminogen activity; side effects include nausea, leg cramps; contraindicated in individuals with history of or at risk for thrombosis
  3. Surgical management
     a. Endometrial ablation
     b. Dilation and curettage (D&C) is diagnostic and therapeutic
     c. Hysterectomy

Polycystic Ovary Syndrome (PCOS)

- Definition—a symptom complex associated with menstrual irregularity due to oligo-ovulation or anovulation and clinical or biochemical signs of hyperandrogenism

- Etiology/incidence
  1. Etiology is unclear
  2. Possible contributing factors
     a. Genetic factors—autosomal dominant transmission
     b. Endocrine factors—increased LH:FSH ratio; increased androgen concentrations; decreased sex-hormone-binding globulin (SHBG) with resultant increase in free testosterone
     c. Metabolic factors—hyperinsulinemia associated with increased insulin resistance; insulin has effects at both the ovarian stroma and the follicle; can have a significant impact on promoting or disrupting follicles
  3. Approximately 25% of individuals without PCOS demonstrate ultrasonographic evidence typical of polycystic ovaries
  4. Prevalence in reproductive-age individuals assigned female at birth is approximately 6%–7% (most common endocrine disorder in this population)
  5. Individuals with PCOS are at risk for future development of endometrial cancer, diabetes mellitus, heart disease, eating disorders; increased adiposity may increase the risk of metabolic complications
- Symptoms
  1. Irregular menses (amenorrhea or infrequent menstrual bleeding)—more than 90%
  2. Gradual onset of hirsutism around puberty or in early 20s—50% to 70%
  3. Other signs of androgen excess (acne, acanthosis nigricans, deep voice, male pattern baldness)—15% to 25%
  4. Anovulation-related infertility
- Physical findings
  1. Physical findings may be normal
  2. Ovaries may not always be palpable—50% will have enlarged ovaries
  3. Virilization—hirsutism, increased muscle mass, frontal balding, enlargement of clitoris, deepening of voice, and decreased breast size
  4. Increased abdominal adiposity—50% to 60%
  5. Acne
  6. Acanthosis nigricans and skin tags, usually in the neck area
- Differential diagnosis
  1. High BMI/larger body
  2. Hypothalamic amenorrhea
  3. Idiopathic hyperandrogenism
  4. Hyperprolactinemia
  5. Thyroid dysfunction
  6. Cushing's disease
  7. Adrenal or ovarian tumors
- Diagnostic tests/findings
  1. Pregnancy test
  2. Prolactin
  3. TSH level
  4. Determinants of biochemical hyperandrogenism—serum total testosterone and SHBG or bioavailable and free testosterone; mild to moderate elevation; controversy over need for such testing if adult patient has clinical signs of hyperandrogenism unless rapid progression or severe; consider for adolescent patients, as they may have acne with normal androgen levels
  5. Serum 17-hydroxyprogesterone (17-OHP)—elevated in PCOS and congenital adrenal hyperplasia
  6. Endometrial biopsy—to rule out hyperplasia if indicated
  7. Assess ovaries and adnexa with ultrasonography
  8. Glucose and lipid levels
- Rotterdam criteria for diagnosis of PCOS—at least two of three of the following in adults; all three present in adolescents to include biochemical confirmation of hyperandrogenism
  1. Oligo-ovulation/anovulation
  2. Clinical or biochemical hyperandrogenism
  3. Polycystic ovaries
- Management/treatment
  1. Goal is to lower androgen levels, treat current clinical manifestations, and decrease the risk of long-term effects of hyperandrogenism
  2. May be determined by the desire for pregnancy and symptom patterns
  3. Spironolactone—blocks androgen receptors to reduce clinical signs of hyperandrogenism; diuretic properties and gradual dosage increase should be considered for those who are normotensive
  4. If pregnancy is desired—recommend referral to a reproductive endocrinologist when available; in lower resource setting, consider the use of letrozole (Femara) as the first-line option, and clomiphene citrate (Clomid) if letrozole is ineffective
  5. If pregnancy is not desired and the patient wants contraception, direct therapy toward preventing endometrial hyperplasia and pregnancy
     a. No hormonal methods contraindicated, consider method selection by patient priorities
     b. Low-dose combined hormonal contraception with low androgenicity—inhibits LH secretion and LH-dependent ovarian androgen production, increases SHBG binding of free testosterone, regulates menstrual cycles, protects from endometrial cancer
     c. Progestin contraceptives—protect from endometrial cancer
  6. If the patient does not desire and is not at risk for pregnancy, and does not want to use hormonal contraception, focus on preventing endometrial hyperplasia
     a. Endometrial biopsy may be indicated
     b. MPA for 10 days per month induces withdrawal bleeding—can be used every month or every 2–3 months with the goal of 4 episodes of withdrawal bleeding per year
  7. Monitor for diabetes and hyperlipidemia
  8. Consider the relationship with food, exercise/movement, and body image; discuss the common recommendations for weight loss and review the risks associated with the pursuit of weight loss, including weight cycling, development of disordered eating, and long-term endocrine damage
  9. Insulin-sensitizing agents—metformin
  10. Excess hair removal—mechanical or eflornithine HCl topical cream for facial hair

Endometriosis

- Definition—Chronic inflammatory condition characterized by the presence of tissue closely resembling endometrial stroma and glands, which occur outside the uterine cavity; occur in the form of adhesions, fibrosis, singular lesions, or endometrioma (only ovarian mass); may adhere to bowel, bladder, outside of uterus, ovaries, rectum, peritoneal cavity
- Endometrioma—benign, enclosed ovarian mass consisting of macerated endometrial cells/blood, described as "chocolate cyst"; represents only type of endometriosis often able to be visualized on imaging (transvaginal ultrasound and pelvic MRI)
- Etiology/incidence
  1. Etiology is not clearly understood
  2. Possible causes
     a. Retrograde menstruation (Sampson's theory)
     b. Immunologic factors
     c. Genetics
     d. Hormonal factors
  3. Found in 5%–15% of surgeries performed on reproductive-age individuals assigned female at birth and as many as 30% of individuals assigned female at birth experiencing infertility
  4. Symptoms may begin in adolescence, common for diagnosis to be delayed into early and middle adulthood; most often occurs in nulliparous individuals
  5. Occurs in all races—most diagnoses occur in White individuals, though racial incidence likely equal, and any difference is theorized to be due to systemic racism and sexism related to pain disorders
  6. Approximately 7%–10% of premenopausal individuals are affected, though true prevalence difficult to ascertain; most common cause of chronic pelvic pain
  7. Endometriosis has been found in areas other than the pelvis, such as the lungs, nose, and spinal column; most common sites are the cul-de-sac, ovary, posterior uterus, and uterosacral ligaments
  8. Most individuals with endometriosis have a positive family history
  9. Positive correlation with high adverse childhood experiences (ACE) scores and reported history of trauma
- Symptoms
  1. Wide range of clinical symptoms; severity does not correlate with the extent of lesions/adhesions. Symptoms classically occur before or during menses, though may increase in frequency as the disease progresses; pain may be localized to the involved area or radiate to other areas of the abdomen
  2. Most common symptoms
     a. Dysmenorrhea, typically severe, debilitating
     b. Pain flares may vary in severity between cycles
     c. Premenstrual spotting
     d. Pelvic fullness
     e. Abdominal bloating, often mistaken for GI symptoms
     f. Dyspareunia, most commonly with deep penetration
     g. Menorrhagia
     h. Chronic pelvic pain, may be dull, sharp, or throbbing
     i. Infertility, often unexplained and theorized to be secondary to chronic inflammation
  3. Symptoms seen less often
     a. Atypical symptoms often correlated with less common lesion locations, such as the bladder, GI tract, peritoneal cavity, and so on.
     b. Low back pain
     c. Diarrhea, constipation
     d. Dysuria
     e. Hematuria
     f. Difficult or painful defecation
     g. Rectal bleeding
- Physical findings
  1. Uterus with limited mobility, though mobility may be present with nonadhesion-type lesions
  2. Tender adnexal masses if endometrioma(s) present
  3. Nodularity and tenderness of uterosacral ligaments and cul-de-sac
  4. Tenderness, thickening, and nodularity of rectal–vaginal septum
  5. Lesions may be visible on laparoscopy or laparotomy
  6. Cervical motion tenderness associated with menses
- Differential diagnosis
  1. Chronic pelvic inflammatory infection
  2. Acute salpingitis
  3. Adenomyosis
  4. Ectopic pregnancy
  5. Ovarian torsion
  6. Benign or malignant ovarian mass
  7. Other causes for pelvic pain and/or dyspareunia
  8. GI disorders, IBS
- Diagnostic tests/findings
  1. Direct visualization with laparoscopy or laparotomy reveals classic implants; classified as Stage I: minimal, Stage II: mild, Stage III: moderate, Stage IV: severe
  2. Transvaginal ultrasound shows no specific pattern regarding lesions or adhesions but may help to differentiate solid and cystic lesions and help distinguish an endometrioma from other adnexal abnormalities
  3. Computed tomography (CT) and magnetic resonance imaging (MRI) provide only presumptive evidence
  4. CA-125 levels may be elevated with endometriosis and diagnosis should be considered along with ovarian malignancy; level typically correlated with the degree of disease and response to therapy; cannot be used for diagnosis because of low sensitivity and specificity
  5. Laparoscopy considered the only definitive way of diagnosing, though a thorough history may lead the clinician to a presumptive diagnosis
- Management/treatment
  1. No medical management provides a universal cure; the goal is to relieve pain, restore fertility, and prevent progression
  2. Medical management
     a. Analgesics (NSAIDs are the first choice), often inadequate
     b. GnRH agonists induce regression of endometrial implants by reducing hormonal production but are accompanied by significant menopause-like symptoms

   c. Progestins—subcutaneous 104 DMPA is FDA approved for treatment; intramuscular DMPA also effective

   d. Continuous use of combined oral contraceptive pills produces atrophy of implants and acyclic hormone environment

3. Surgical management

   a. Laparoscopic excision of endometriosis lesions considered the gold standard, as medical options will suppress symptoms but not remove the source of inflammation/pain

   b. Hysterectomy with bilateral salpingo-ophorectomy may reduce or eliminate symptoms for some individuals but is not considered curative, especially if microscopic lesions are still present in the pelvis.

   c. Many patients find symptom improvement with the use of combined surgical and medication interventions.

4. Key points

   a. May need long-term emotional support as a result of severe chronic pain and possibly infertility

   b. Delayed childbirth may lead to worsening endometriosis over time when exposed to endogenous estrogen contributing to lesion growth; symptoms typically suppressed during pregnancy and lactation; pain flare may occur if the individual has reached the end of back-to-back pregnancies and is no longer suppressing disease

   c. Treatment is considered long term, typically symptoms reduce in perimenopause/menopause; may become a chronic illness

   d. Counsel regarding the risk of infertility, IVF usually shown to be the most effective treatment

Adenomyosis

- Definition—benign condition in which ectopic endometrium or endometrium-like tissue is found within the myometrium; generally considered a type of endometriosis
- Etiology/incidence
  1. May be related to the breakdown of the endometrium during labor and delivery; the cells of the endometrial basal layer grow downward, losing connection with the endometrium
  2. Incidence varies widely, with from 10% to 90% of hysterectomies revealing adenomyosis
  3. Diagnosis most common in parous individuals between ages 40 and 50 years
- Symptoms
  1. Increasingly severe dysmenorrhea and heavy bleeding during menses are common
  2. Dyspareunia
  3. Infertility
- Physical findings
  1. Boggy, tender uterus
  2. Diffuse, globular enlargement—may be 8 to 10 weeks' gestation size
  3. May see evidence of anemia
- Differential diagnosis
  1. Endometriosis

   2. Leiomyoma
   3. Pregnancy
   4. Adhesions

- Diagnostic tests/findings
  1. Ultrasonography or MRI may rule out other pathology
  2. Endometrial biopsy for abnormal bleeding
- Management/treatment
  1. Symptomatic relief may be the only priority
  2. Hysterectomy may be indicated and is more likely to be curative when compared to endometriosis, as abnormal tissue only occurs within the myometrium, not outside of the uterine cavity
  3. NSAIDs for pain
  4. Hormone suppression—symptoms usually subside after hormone production ceases

Hyperprolactinemia, Galactorrhea, and Pituitary Adenoma

- Definitions
  1. Hyperprolactinemia—elevated levels of prolactin
  2. Galactorrhea—secretion of a nonphysiologic, milky fluid from the breast, unrelated to pregnancy
  3. Pituitary adenoma—benign tumor of the pituitary; most common type secretes prolactin
- Etiology/incidence
  1. Etiology and incidence of pituitary adenoma unknown; rarely malignant; can grow for years
  2. Prolactin-secreting adenomas account for 50% of all identified at autopsy
  3. Most pituitary adenomas occur in individuals younger than 40 years of age
  4. High prolactin levels found in approximately one-third of individuals with amenorrhea of unknown origin; one-third of individuals with secondary amenorrhea have pituitary adenoma; one-third of individuals with high levels of prolactin have galactorrhea
  5. Galactorrhea should be evaluated in a nulliparous individual or in a nonlactating parous individual if 12 months have passed since the last pregnancy
- Symptoms
  1. Hyperprolactinemia/galactorrhea
     a. Spontaneous clear or milky bilateral or unilateral breast secretions from multiple ducts
     b. Normal or irregular menses; secondary amenorrhea may occur
     c. Disturbances of vision and headaches may be present (if adenoma is the cause)
  2. Pituitary adenoma
     a. Breast secretions
     b. Menstrual changes as described
     c. Severe vascular headaches and blurred vision
- Physical findings
  1. Normal funduscopic examination—if no adenoma
  2. Funduscopic examination may show papilledema if adenoma present
  3. Normal physical and gynecologic examination
- Differential diagnosis
  1. Pregnancy or breastfeeding/chestfeeding
  2. Breast cancer

3. Hypothyroidism, hyperthyroidism
4. Pituitary adenoma
5. Excessive breast stimulation
6. Disorders or injury of the chest wall
7. Medication effect (e.g., opioids, cannabis, antidepressants)
8. Disturbances of ovarian function
9. Benign and malignant brain neoplasm
- Diagnostic tests/findings
  1. TSH
  2. Serum prolactin—refer if more than 20 ng/mL; if in 100 to 300 ng/mL range, very suspicious for adenoma; always repeat a second serum prolactin if first is elevated
  3. Pregnancy test
  4. Microscopy of breast secretions—milk indicated by fat globules
  5. CT or MRI of the sella turcica to rule out adenoma
- Management/treatment
  1. Management may be accomplished best by referral to a reproductive endocrinologist
  2. If the prolactin level is less than 20 ng/mL and the patient is not amenorrheic, may follow with yearly prolactin levels
  3. Pharmacologic
     a. Dopamine agonist (e.g., bromocriptine, which inhibits prolactin, provides symptomatic relief, decreases or stops galactorrhea); treatment of choice with the highest cure rate
     b. Treat hypothyroidism/hyperthyroidism
  4. Surgical
     a. If medical management has failed to relieve symptoms of adenoma, transsphenoidal neurosurgery may be indicated
     b. Recurrence rate is 10%–70%; requires close follow-up
  5. Radiation
     a. Results are less satisfactory than with surgery
     b. May take several years for prolactin level to fall
     c. Should be reserved for recurrences or patients who do not respond to medical management
  6. Patient education
     a. Discontinue breast stimulation
     b. Disclose all drugs and medications being used

Benign and Malignant Tumors/Neoplasms

Cervical Polyps
- Definition—pedunculated growths arising from the mucosal surface of the endocervix
- Etiology/incidence
  1. Inflammation
  2. Trauma
  3. Pregnancy
  4. Abnormal local response to hypoestrogenic state
  5. Occurs in 4% of all gynecologic patients; change occurs in up to 10% of women

  6. Most common benign neoplasm of the cervix; most often seen in perimenopausal and multigravida individuals between ages 30 and 50 years
  7. Malignant changes are rare
- Symptoms
  1. May be asymptomatic, rarely associated with pain
  2. Leukorrhea
  3. Abnormal vaginal bleeding—intermenstrual, postcoital
- Physical findings
  1. Single or multiple, painless polypoid lesions at the cervix
  2. Size ranges from a few millimeters to 2 to 3 cm
  3. Reddish-purple to cherry red in color; smooth and soft; bleeds easily
  4. Polyps with vascular congestion appear moist, red, glandular
  5. Polyp with atypical appearance biopsied (necrosis, contact bleeding, change in color)
  6. Otherwise, normal pelvic examination
- Differential diagnosis
  1. Adenocarcinoma
  2. Cervical carcinoma
  3. Prolapsed myoma
  4. Squamous papilloma
  5. Retained products of conception
  6. Sarcoma
- Diagnostic tests/findings
  1. Cervical cancer screening to rule out premalignant cervical lesions or cancer
  2. Histologic evaluation of removed polyp to rule out cancer
- Management/treatment
  1. Removal of the polyp is usually curative—avoid removal during pregnancy
  2. Recur frequently

Leiomyomata Uteri (Fibroid, Myoma)
- Definition—nodular, discrete tumors varying in size from microscopic to large multiple, nodular masses; classified according to location
  1. Submucosal—protrudes into the uterine cavity
  2. Subserosal—bulges through the outer uterine wall
  3. Intraligamentous—within the broad ligament
  4. Interstitial (intramural)—stays within the uterine wall as it grows; most common form of myoma
  5. Pedunculated—on a thin pedicle or stalk attached to the uterus
- Etiology/incidence
  1. Etiology unknown
  2. May arise from smooth muscle cells in the myometrium; often benign growths that arise from smooth muscle of the uterus (myomas or leiomyomas)
  3. Most common benign gynecologic pelvic neoplasm
  4. Affects approximately 20% of individuals with a uterus in their reproductive years
  5. Occurs more frequently in Black individuals than in White individuals
  6. Asymptomatic fibroids may be seen in 40%–50% of individuals with a uterus older than age 40; increases with age prior to menopause
  7. Increased incidence with family history

- Symptoms
  1. Usually asymptomatic
  2. Heavy or prolonged menstrual bleeding
  3. Pelvic pain presents as dysmenorrhea, pelvic pressure, or dyspareunia; if pedunculated, twisted, and infarcted, may cause acute pain
  4. Large fibroids may cause constipation; intestinal obstruction may result from compression; venous stasis may occur from pressure; pressure on the bladder may result in urinary retention or overflow incontinence
- Physical findings
  1. Abdominal enlargement
  2. Enlarged, irregularly shaped, firm uterus; may be displaced
  3. Pedunculated tumor may protrude from the cervix
  4. Tumors usually painless on palpation
  5. Wide variance in size (3 to 4 mm, up to 15 lb)
  6. Potential complications
     a. Spontaneous abortion
     b. Premature labor
     c. Anemia
     d. Infertility
- Differential diagnosis
  1. Ovarian mass (benign or malignant)
  2. Pregnancy
  3. Leiomyosarcoma
  4. Uterine malignancy
  5. Adenomyosis
  6. Endometriosis
  7. Colon or rectal tumor (benign or malignant)
- Diagnostic tests/findings
  1. Cervical cytology to rule out cervical cancer
  2. Pregnancy test
  3. CBC if anemia suspected
  4. Occult blood test if rectal or colon symptoms or GI problems
  5. Endometrial biopsy or D&C when abnormal bleeding present
  6. Ultrasound, sonohysterogram, CT, MRI confirm the diagnosis
  7. Hysteroscopy to provide visualization of uterine cavity
- Management/treatment
  1. May require no treatment if asymptomatic
  2. Periodic observation and follow-up with bimanual examination may be indicated to ensure that tumors are not growing or undergoing abnormal changes
  3. Pharmacologic
     a. GnRH agonist results in 40%–60% reduction in volume; regrowth occurs about half the time; may be used to reduce volume preoperatively, before attempting pregnancy, when surgery is contraindicated, or in perimenopausal patients to avoid surgery
     b. Progestational agents, such as MPA, may decrease fibroid size and bleeding
     c. Progestin-containing intrauterine devices (IUDs) with 52 mg of levonorgestrel may reduce heavy bleeding and decrease dysmenorrhea but will not decrease fibroid size; if the uterine cavity is distorted by fibroids, the expulsion rate may be higher

     d. CHCs may help with heavy bleeding but will not decrease fibroid size
     e. Treat anemia if indicated
  4. Surgical
     a. Indications for surgery
        (1) Abnormal bleeding
        (2) Rapid growth
        (3) Definitive diagnosis concerning mass if otherwise uncertain
        (4) Encroachment of organs
        (5) Symptoms not managed with pharmacologic therapies
     b. Myomectomy through laparoscopic resection can preserve fertility; up to 30% recurrence with this method
     c. Uterine artery embolization—fertility may not be preserved; increased rates of intrauterine growth restriction, preterm birth, and miscarriage have been reported; up to 40% recurrence rate with this method
     d. Hysterectomy

Ovarian Cysts

- Definition
  1. Functional—cysts of the ovary that occur secondary to hormonal stimulation
     a. Follicular—simple, fluid-filled cyst occurring in the follicular phase of the menstrual cycle, when continued hormonal stimulation prevents fluid resorption, develops from an unruptured follicle; torsion or rupture increases with the size of cyst
        (1) Sometimes normal follicle (fluid-filled sac that contains an egg) may be mistaken for a follicular cyst
     b. Corpus luteum—occurs in the luteal phase, when the corpus luteum fails to degenerate
  2. Dermoid (benign cystic teratoma)—most common ovarian germ cell tumor
- Etiology/incidence
  1. Follicular cysts
     a. Rare before menarche or after menopause
     b. Account for 20%–50% of ovarian cysts; most common adnexal mass in reproductive years
     c. Often found incidentally during routine pelvic examination or ultrasound
     d. Usually resolves in two to three menstrual cycles; may rupture or undergo torsion, causing pain
  2. Corpus luteum cysts
     a. Form following the failure of the corpus luteum to degenerate after 14 days
     b. May hemorrhage into the cystic cavity, forming a hemorrhagic cyst
  3. Dermoid cysts (benign cystic teratoma)
     a. One of the most common neoplasms of the ovary (10%–20%)
     b. Occur during the reproductive years
     c. Composed usually of well-differentiated tissue from all three germ layers
     d. Usually measure 5–10 cm in diameter; 10%–15% are bilateral

- Symptoms
  1. Functional cysts
     a. Usually asymptomatic
     b. May cause temporary irregular menses
     c. Acute pain if the cyst ruptures or if torsion occurs
     d. Large cysts may cause pelvic pressure, the feeling of fullness or heaviness, and a dull ache on the affected side that may radiate to the lower back
  2. Dermoid (benign cystic teratoma)
     a. Usually asymptomatic and often remain stable over time
     b. May cause acute pain if twists or ruptures; may experience peritonitis
     c. May cause vague feelings of local pelvic pressure if large
     d. AUB (rare)
  3. Signs of rupture include severe, sudden abdominal pain; mimics ruptured ectopic
- Physical findings
  1. Functional cysts are usually 5 cm or less in diameter; cystic to firm, mobile, sometimes tender, usually unilateral
  2. Dermoid cysts may measure 5 to 10 cm; usually unilateral, firm to cystic, often anterior to the uterus
- Differential diagnosis
  1. Pregnancy; ectopic pregnancy
  2. Ovarian torsion
  3. Uterine fibroid; endometrioma
  4. Tubo-ovarian abscess
  5. Diverticulitis/abscess
  6. Distended bladder
  7. Congenital anomaly (pelvic kidney)
  8. Lymphadenopathy
  9. Malignant neoplasm (most often in older women)
- Diagnostic tests/findings
  1. Pregnancy test
  2. Transvaginal ultrasound—to evaluate mass: cystic or solid, complex or simple, bilateral or unilateral; to rule out ectopic pregnancy
  3. CA-125—best drawn in the context of ovarian cysts found in postmenopausal individuals; not diagnostic
     a. Tumor-associated antigens most commonly used to monitor the clinical status of patients with ovarian cancer
     b. Not routinely used for evaluation of adnexal mass in premenopausal individuals because of low specificity for ovarian cancer; several other conditions may cause elevated levels, including endometriosis
     c. Specificity and predictive value are consistently higher in postmenopausal individuals
  4. MRI may be useful if dermoid cyst is suspected
- Management/treatment
  1. Functional cyst
     a. In reproductive years, less than 10 cm in diameter, and ultrasound findings of simple cyst—examine after next menses and/or serial ultrasounds every 4 to 12 weeks
     b. CHCs will not help in resolution but may be used to suppress gonadotropin levels to prevent recurrence

     c. Refer if mass greater than 10 cm, ultrasound findings of solid tumor or complex cyst, concerning symptoms, or persists greater than 12 weeks
     d. Postmenopause—if mass less than 10 cm, ultrasound findings of simple cyst, no concerning symptoms or risk factors for ovarian cancer, and CA-125 < 35 U/mL, perform serial ultrasound every 4 to 12 weeks
     e. Postmenopause—refer if mass is greater than 10 cm, ultrasound findings of solid or complex cyst, concerning symptoms or risk factors, persists greater than 12 weeks, or CA-125 > 35 U/mL
  2. Dermoid cyst—if does not resolve on its own, consider laparoscopic removal

Gynecologic Cancers

- Definition—cancers of the vulva, vagina, cervix, uterus, ovaries, and uterine (also called fallopian) tubes
- Etiology/incidence—varies with type of cancer, age, personal and family history, and other modifiable and nonmodifiable risk factors
- Symptoms—vary with the type and stage of cancer (**Table 5-1**)

Cervical Carcinoma

- Definition—slow penetration of the basement membrane and infiltration of malignant cells into the uterine cervix; characterized by histologically definable stages
- Etiology/incidence
  1. Approximately 14,500 new cases diagnosed annually, with 4,000 to 5,000 deaths
  2. Highest incidence in Hispanic individuals, followed by Black individuals, and then White individuals
  3. Peak incidence between 45 and 55 years of age; increasing in young individuals
  4. Human papillomavirus (HPV) is the primary agent in the development of cervical intraepithelial neoplasia (CIN) and cervical cancer
  5. Risk factors
     a. Smoking
     b. Presence of HPV types with malignant potential (types 16, 18, and 31 most common)
     c. First coitus at early age (< 18 years)
     d. Multiple sexual partners or sexual partners with multiple partners
     e. Nonbarrier method of contraception
     f. Immunosuppression
     g. Long-term oral contraceptive use
     h. Never had cervical cancer screening or infrequent screening
- Symptoms
  1. May be asymptomatic
  2. Postcoital or irregular, painless bleeding
  3. Odorous bloody or purulent discharge
  4. Late symptoms
     a. Pelvic or epigastric pain
     b. Urinary or rectal symptoms

Table 5-1 Gynecologic Cancer Symptoms

Symptoms	Cervical Cancer	Ovarian Cancer	Endometrial Cancer	Vaginal Cancer	Vulvar Cancer
Abnormal vaginal bleeding or discharge	X	X	X	X	
Pelvic pain or pressure		X	X		
Abdominal or back pain		X			
Bloating		X			
Changes in bowel or bladder function		X		X	
Itching or burning of the vulva					X
Changes in vulvar color or changes in skin, such as rash, sores, or warts					X

Modified from Centers for Disease Control and Prevention. (2016). Gynecologic cancer symptoms. (CDC publication #22-0099). Retrieved from http://www.cdc.gov/cancer/knowledge/publications/symptoms_diaries.htm

- Physical findings
  1. Appearance of the cervix ranges from normal to severely ulcerated, necrotic, or large bulky lesions filling the vagina
  2. Cervix may be firm or rocklike to soft and spongy
  3. Sanguineous or purulent, odorous vaginal discharge
  4. Anemia if bleeding is heavy
- Differential diagnosis
  1. Metastasis from another primary site
  2. Cervicitis/STI
  3. Cervical polyp
  4. Cervical ectopy
  5. Preinvasive lesion of cervix
  6. Condyloma acuminata
- Diagnostic tests/findings
  1. Cervical cytology
  2. Biopsy of gross lesions
  3. If malignancy is suspected but no gross lesion is visible, colposcopy is suggested with a biopsy
  4. Colposcopic evaluation of vulva and vagina to rule out other lesions
  5. CT, MRI, cystoscopy, sigmoidoscopy, and barium enema may be indicated
- Management/treatment
  1. Management should be by a gynecologic oncologist involving staging, appropriate treatment, and follow-up
  2. Treatment may consist of surgery, radiation, chemotherapy, or a combination

Endometrial Carcinoma

- Definition—carcinoma of the body of the uterus; malignant transformation of endometrial glands and/or stroma
- Etiology/incidence
  1. Most common gynecologic malignancy—accounts for 90%–95% of malignancies of the uterine corpus
  2. Approximately 30,000 new cases and 6,000 deaths annually; American Cancer Society estimated 4,900 new cases and 8,000 deaths annually
  3. Median age is 63 years at onset; 5% occur prior to age 40
  4. Several risk factors are linked to increased length of time or amount of exposure to estrogen, especially unopposed estrogen, either endogenous or exogenous
     a. Early menarche; late menopause
     b. Unopposed estrogen therapy
     c. Oligo-ovulation, anovulation
     d. High BMI/High adiposity
     e. Estrogen-secreting tumors (granulosa cell)
     f. Use of tamoxifen therapy as a treatment for breast cancer
     g. Endometrial hyperplasia or endometrial polyps
  5. Other risk factors
     a. Family history of endometrial or colorectal cancer
     b. Personal history of colorectal cancer, diabetes, or hypertension
     c. Higher incidence in Black and Hispanic individuals
  6. Protective factors—multiparity, use of oral contraceptive pills, use of DMPA
- Symptoms
  1. Painless vaginal bleeding is typically the first symptom—heavy menses, intermenstrual bleeding, or frequent menstruation
  2. Serous, odorous discharge (watery leukorrhea); soon replaced by bloody discharge; intermittent spotting; spotting to steady, painless bleeding; then hemorrhage
  3. Lower abdominal pain (10%)
- Physical findings
  1. Blood may be present in the vaginal vault
  2. Advanced disease may have pelvic mass present, ascites
  3. Anemia may be present
  4. Uterus may be enlarged and soft
- Differential diagnosis
  1. Atrophic vaginitis
  2. Cervical or endometrial polyps
  3. Benign endometrial pathology (hyperplasia)
  4. Anovulatory uterine bleeding
  5. Bleeding related to hormone therapy

6. Leiomyomas
7. Other genital/gynecologic cancers
- Diagnostic tests/findings
1. Cervical cytology may show glandular abnormalities
2. Endometrial aspiration biopsy
3. Ultrasound to measure endometrial stripe; if less than 5 mm thick, the likelihood of endometrial cancer is rare
4. Fractional D&C is the gold standard for diagnosis
5. Hysteroscopy may be useful in identifying lesions/polyps not found on biopsy
- Management/treatment
1. Refer to a gynecologist or oncologist
2. Hysterectomy
3. Surgical staging to determine treatment
4. Radiation, chemotherapy, steroids (progesterone), or combination

Ovarian Carcinoma

- Definition—malignant neoplasm of the ovary that may arise from ovarian epithelial, stromal, or germ cells
- Etiology/incidence
1. Epithelial ovarian carcinoma is the most common type (80%–85%)
2. Ovary may be the site for metastasis from nonovarian cancers
3. Eighth most common cancer in individuals assigned female at birth; fifth leading cause of cancer-related death in individuals assigned female at birth
4. Highest mortality rate of all gynecologic cancers
5. Approximately 22,530 new cases of ovarian cancer diagnosed and 13,980 deaths from ovarian cancer in 2019
6. Ovarian cancer rates are highest among individuals aged 55 to 64
7. Risk factors
   a. Lifetime risk in the general population—1% to 2%
   b. Family history in one first-degree relative—5% lifetime risk; risk increases with the number of affected first- or second-degree relatives
   c. Inherited gene mutations are responsible for approximately 20%–25% of ovarian cancers, with most common mutations occurring in *BRCA1* or *BRCA2* genes; lifetime risk associated with *BRCA1* mutation is 39%–46%, lifetime risk associated with *BRCA2* mutation is 12%–20%
   d. Other hereditary cancer syndromes associated with ovarian cancer—Lynch syndrome, Peutz-Jeghers syndrome; gene mutations in these syndromes often result in cancers that affect multiple organs
   e. History of breast, colon, or endometrial cancer
   f. Early menarche; late menopause
   g. Nulliparity or birth of first child after age 30
   h. Infertility
   i. Endometriosis
   j. High BMI/high adiposity
   k. Postmenopausal hormonal estrogen therapy
8. Use of oral contraceptives reduces risk—protection lasts up to 2 decades after last use

9. Breastfeeding/chestfeeding is associated with reduced risk
- Symptoms
1. Early
   a. Often asymptomatic
   b. Symptoms are often mild, vague, and inconsistent
   c. Abdominal discomfort or pain
   d. Pressure sensation on the bladder or rectum
   e. Pelvic fullness or bloating
   f. Vague GI symptoms
2. Late
   a. Increasing abdominal girth
   b. Abdominal pain
   c. Abnormal vaginal bleeding
   d. GI symptoms—nausea, loss of appetite, dyspepsia
- Physical findings
1. Fixed, irregular, nontender adnexal mass—usually bilateral
2. Ascites
3. Pleural effusion and subclavicular lymphadenopathy if advanced
- Differential diagnosis
1. Primary peritoneal cancer
2. Benign ovarian tumor
3. Endometriosis
4. Functional ovarian cyst
5. Ovarian torsion
6. Pelvic kidney
7. Pedunculated uterine fibroid
- Diagnostic tests/findings
1. Pelvic ultrasonography/CT/MRI
2. CA-125—elevated levels not diagnostic for ovarian cancers (elevations can occur with endometriosis, leiomyomata, pelvic inflammatory infection, hepatitis, and other malignancies); helpful to follow response to treatment with chemotherapy and subsequent follow-up
3. Definitive diagnosis is made with laparotomy
- Management/treatment
1. Surgical
   a. Total hysterectomy with bilateral salpingo-oophorectomy and omentectomy—establishes histologic staging and grading of tumor
   b. Goal is the removal of as much of the tumor as possible
2. Chemotherapy and/or radiation
3. Rule out metastasis with diagnostic evaluation of other organ systems
4. Consider genetic counseling and genetic testing if indicated for individuals with an ovarian cancer diagnosis to determine if family members may be at increased risk because of pathogenic gene variants (previously called mutations); counseling and consideration of genetic testing for at-risk relatives
5. Consider genetic counseling and genetic testing if indicated for individuals assessed to be at high risk for hereditary breast and ovarian cancer syndrome because of personal or family cancer history; results may guide discussion of risk-reducing surgeries or increased monitoring

Vaginal Carcinoma

- Definition—the abnormal proliferation of the vaginal epithelium with malignant cells extending below the basement membrane
- Etiology/incidence
  1. Accounts for approximately 2% of gynecologic malignancies—vaginal cancer is the rarest gynecologic cancer
  2. Mean age of diagnosis—65 years, with a range from 30 to 90 years
  3. Etiology is multifactorial—risk factors include the presence of persistent HPV infection with high-risk types, other genital cancers, diethylstilbestrol (DES) exposure, prior radiation
  4. Vaginal intraepithelial neoplasm is thought to be a precursor
  5. 5-year survival ranges from 80% for stage I to 17% for stage V
- Symptoms
  1. May present with vaginal bleeding or odorous blood-tinged discharge—may cause pruritus
  2. May have palpable or visible mass or lesion
  3. Urinary problems if the bladder involved
- Physical findings
  1. Early lesions are raised and granular, and may be white
  2. Late lesions are friable, granular, and cauliflower-like and may be palpable; ulceration may be superficial or deep
  3. Most common site is the upper one-third of the vagina
  4. If lesion darkly pigmented, suspect melanoma
- Differential diagnosis
  1. Malignancy of another site if cancer is extended or metastatic to the vagina
  2. Vaginitis
  3. Bleeding from uterus
  4. Ulceration from foreign object (pessary, tampon)
- Diagnostic tests/findings
  1. Cervical cytology to evaluate for cervical cancer
  2. Colposcopy and biopsy of lesions
  3. For staging, use cystoscopy, proctosigmoidoscopy, IV urography, chest radiography, barium enema
  4. CT scan and MRI are used to evaluate metastasis
- Management/treatment
  1. Treatment managed by a gynecologic oncologist
  2. Accurate diagnosis and stage must be determined before treatment is planned
  3. If the lesion is precancerous (VAIN I, II, III), laser is appropriate
  4. Local excision (partial vaginectomy) may be appropriate for early lesions
  5. Radiation is the mainstay of treatment
  6. Radical surgery may be followed with radiation

Vulvar Carcinoma

- Definition—the proliferation of malignant cells of the vulva
- Etiology/incidence
  1. Multifactorial
  2. Risk factors
     a. HPV infection with high-risk types; seen in 30%–50% of cases
     b. Multiple sexual partners
     c. Cigarette smoking, especially if history of HPV
     d. Chronic irritation
     e. Vulvar dermatoses
  3. May be associated with other urogenital cancers
  4. Accounts for 1%–2% of all gynecologic cancer deaths per year
  5. Vulvar malignancies arise from squamous cell carcinoma, melanoma, adenocarcinoma, basal cell carcinoma, and sarcomas
  6. Mean age—65 years, with a range from 30 to 90 years; incidence in young individuals is rising
  7. Fourth most common malignant tumor of the female genital tract
- Symptoms
  1. May be asymptomatic
  2. Lesion on vulva
  3. Pruritus (most common), pain, burning, bleeding
  4. Odorous discharge; may be blood tinged
- Physical findings
  1. White, red, or irregularly pigmented; ulcerated, flat, or wartlike; single or multiple lesion(s)
  2. Hyperkeratotic patches (leukoplakia)
  3. Excoriation and erythema
  4. Most common sites are labia majora and minora
  5. Bartholin's gland enlargement
  6. Inguinal lymphadenopathy
- Differential diagnosis
  1. Vulvar dermatoses
  2. Atrophy
  3. Condyloma acuminata
  4. Vulvar infection/inflammation
  5. Lymphogranuloma inguinale
  6. Paget's disease
- Diagnostic tests/findings
  1. Cervical cytology, colposcopy to rule out other sites of disease
  2. Biopsy/wide resection to make a definitive diagnosis
  3. CT and MRI, chest radiography to evaluate for metastasis
- Management/treatment
  1. Appropriate evaluation by a gynecologic oncologist
  2. Local excision
  3. Simple or radical vulvectomy
  4. Topical treatment—immunologic agents, chemotherapy
  5. Careful follow-up—recurrence is common

Choriocarcinoma

- Definition—a frankly malignant form of gestational trophoblastic disease or may be primary in the ovary
- Etiology/incidence
  1. Gestational trophoblastic disease
     a. May follow any gestational event—intrauterine or ectopic pregnancy, abortion (50%); hydatidiform mole (50%)
     b. Malignant transformation occurs in the chorion
     c. One of the few metastatic tumors that is curable

2. Nongestational—mixed germ cell tumor of the ovary occurring in childhood or early adolescence; unusual in ages 20 to 30 years
3. Disseminated by blood to the lungs, vagina, brain, liver, kidneys, and GI tract
- Symptoms—often masquerade as other diseases as a result of metastasis to other organs
   1. Irregular vaginal bleeding—intermittent to hemorrhage; continuing after immediate postpartum period; uterine subinvolution
   2. Amenorrhea (from gonadotropin secretion)
   3. Hemoptysis, cough, dyspnea with lung metastasis
   4. Evidence of central nervous system (CNS) metastasis—headache, dizziness, fainting
   5. GI—rectal bleeding/tarry stools
   6. Abdominal pain
   7. Hematuria from renal metastasis
- Physical findings
   1. Abdominal mass/ascites
   2. Blood in the vaginal vault
   3. Vaginal or vulvar lesion may indicate metastasis
   4. Enlarged, soft uterus
   5. Abnormalities of multiple organs if metastatic
- Differential diagnosis
   1. May imitate other diseases—suspect strongly if follows a pregnancy event
   2. Intrauterine pregnancy
   3. Invasive mole
   4. Benign ovarian tumor
   5. Other gynecologic malignancies
- Diagnostic tests/findings
   1. Quantitative human chorionic gonadotropin (hCG)
   2. Abnormal beta hCG regression titers following molar pregnancy
   3. CT scan of the abdomen, pelvis, and head
   4. Lumbar puncture may be necessary
   5. Chest radiography
- Management/treatment
   1. Should be managed by a gynecologic oncologist
   2. Treatment usually consists of surgery and chemotherapy or chemotherapy alone
   3. Appropriate follow-up to monitor side effects, disease improvement, and recurrence
   4. Nonmetastatic: good prognosis; metastatic: good to poor prognosis

Vaginal Infections

Bacterial Vaginosis (BV)

- Definition—an alteration of the normal flora of the vagina (*Lactobacillus* species) with dominance of anaerobic bacteria
- Etiology/incidence
   1. Most common vaginal infection in the United States in individuals ages 15 to 44
   2. Occurs twice as frequently as candidiasis
   3. Loss of lactobacilli (hydrogen peroxide–producing strains) results in elevated pH and subsequent

overgrowth of bacteria; bacteria concentrations are increased 100- to 1,000-fold
4. No single offending organism—*Gardnerella vaginalis, Mycoplasma hominis, Bacteroides* species, *Haemophilus, Mobiluncus, Corynebacterium* are among the anaerobes
5. Not sexually transmitted; however, more common in individuals with new or multiple partners; increased risk associated with shared sex toys and douching
6. BV infection may increase the risk of acquiring STIs, such as human immunodeficiency virus (HIV) and herpes simplex virus 2
7. May be associated with intra-amniotic infection, postpartum and postoperative infection, premature labor, complications after gynecologic surgery, endometritis, pelvic inflammatory disease
- Symptoms
   1. Most often asymptomatic, 50% of patients have no symptoms
   2. Pruritus occasionally
   3. Heavy grayish/yellowish/whitish malodorous discharge
   4. Rancid or fishy odor during menses and after sex
- Physical findings
   1. Homogenous, adherent, whitish-gray vaginal discharge
   2. Normal-appearing vulva and vaginal mucosa
   3. Discharge may coat vaginal walls and vulva
   4. Presence of foul odor
   5. Mild erythema
- Differential diagnosis
   1. Trichomoniasis
   2. Candidiasis
- Diagnostic tests/findings
   1. Wet mount of vaginal secretions
   2. Presence of three of the following Amsel criteria is diagnostic
      a. Vaginal pH ≥ 4.5
      b. Clue cells on saline wet mount (epithelial cells with borders obscured as a result of stippling with bacteria); ≥20% of epithelial cells
      c. Homogeneous discharge, white, smoothly coating vaginal wall
      d. Positive "whiff test"—fishy amine odor of vaginal discharge before or after addition of 10% potassium hydroxide (KOH; caused when anaerobic bacteria combined with KOH); may also have positive whiff test in the presence of blood, semen, and *Trichomonas*
   3. No increase in the number of white blood cells (WBCs) on the wet mount is expected, as BV is not an inflammatory infection
   4. Commercially available card tests for detection of elevated pH, presence of amine
   5. Gram stain reveals true clue cells, numerous abnormal bacteria
   6. Cultures for anaerobes are unnecessary
- Management/treatment
   1. Treatment is recommended for individuals with symptoms
   2. Metronidazole 500 mg orally BID for 7 days

3. Metronidazole gel 0.75%, one full applicator (5 g) intravaginally at bedtime for 5 days
4. Clindamycin cream 2%, one full applicator (5 g) intravaginally at bedtime for 7 days
5. Alternative regimens
   a. Clindamycin 300 mg orally BID for 7 days
   b. Clindamycin ovules 100 mg intravaginally at bedtime for 3 days
   c. secnidazole 2 g orally in a single dose
   d. tinidazole 2 g orally 1×/day for 2 days
   e. tinidazole 1 g orally 1×/day for 5 days
6. Treatment of sexual partner does not change the course of disease or prevent recurrences
7. BV may be transferred between sexual partners who both have vulvas
8. Metronidazole may cause a disulfiram effect (flushing, vomiting) if taken when alcohol is consumed; counsel patient to avoid alcohol use during and for 24 hours after completion of metronidazole
9. Side effects—metallic taste, nausea, headache, dry mouth, dark-colored urine
10. Clindamycin cream is oil-based and might weaken latex condoms and diaphragms for 5 days after use; if using these methods for contraception, counsel the patient to refrain from sexual intercourse until the conclusion of the treatment regimen
11. Avoid douching, as it may increase the risk of relapse
12. Vitamin D 2000 IU daily for 15 weeks to eliminate asymptomatic bacterial vaginosis
13. Treatment in pregnancy—see Chapter 7, *High-Risk Pregnancy Care*

Trichomoniasis

- Definition—vaginal infection caused by an anaerobic, flagellated protozoan parasite
- Etiology/incidence
  1. Pathogenesis unknown; humans are the only host
  2. Caused by the *Trichomonas* organism; survives best in a pH of 5.6 to 7.5
  3. Almost exclusively sexually transmitted; theoretically possible fomite spread, but unlikely
  4. Affects 3.7 million people in the United States; responsible for 25% of vaginal infections
  5. Many infections are asymptomatic, especially in older patients
  6. Risk factors
     a. Multiple sexual partners
     b. Presence of another STI
     c. Lack of condom use
     d. Individuals who engage in transactional sex
     e. People who use injectable drugs are at a higher risk
  7. Use of barrier contraceptive methods may decrease prevalence
  8. May be associated with premature rupture of the membranes and preterm labor
  9. Infection may be found in endocervix, vagina, bladder, Bartholin's glands, and periurethral glands

- Symptoms
  1. Symptoms variable; most people infected with trichomoniasis are asymptomatic
  2. Copious, malodorous, yellowish-green discharge; vulva irritation; pruritus; and occasionally dysuria, urgency, frequency of urination, postcoital and intermenstrual bleeding
  3. Onset of symptoms often occurs after menses
- Physical findings
  1. Erythema, edema, excoriation of vulva may be seen
  2. Red speckles ("strawberry spots") on vagina and cervix (punctate lesions)
  3. Homogeneous, watery, yellowish-green, grayish, frothy vaginal discharge
  4. pH ≥ 5.0
  5. Cervix may bleed easily when touched
- Differential diagnosis
  1. BV
  2. Candidiasis
  3. Trauma from foreign body
- Diagnostic tests/findings
  1. Saline wet mount (60%–70% sensitive), higher sensitivity with immediate evaluation of wet preparation slide of vaginal secretions—motile trichomonads; increased number of WBC
  2. Rapid tests (results in 10–45 minutes) on vaginal secretions (>82% sensitivity, >97% specificity)
  3. Definitive test—culture
  4. Urine microscopic examination may reveal live trichomonads
  5. Detection on cervical cytology—40% positive predictive value
- Management/treatment—Vaginal regimen—metronidazole 500 mg orally 2×/day for 7 days OR tinidazole 2 g orally in a single dose; Penile regimen—metronidazole 2 g orally in a single dose OR tinidazole 2 g orally in a single dose
  1. May cause a disulfiram effect (flushing, vomiting) if metronidazole or tinidazole is taken when alcohol is consumed; counsel patient to avoid alcohol use for 24 hours after completion of metronidazole or 72 hours after completion of tinidazole
  2. All sexual partners should be treated
  3. Repeat testing in women in 3 months for detection of reinfection
  4. For treatment failures—exclude reinfection; consider treatment with metronidazole or tinidazole 2 g orally for 7 days
  5. Screen for other STIs as indicated
  6. Encourage safer sex practices to reduce reinfection and the chance of other STIs
  7. Treatment in pregnancy
     a. Metronidazole crosses the placenta, but no teratogenicity or mutagenic effects have been found in infants
  8. Treatment during lactation
     a. Metronidazole is secreted in human milk, but no evidence of adverse effects in infants
     b. Some clinicians recommend deferring breastfeeding/chestfeeding for 12 to 24 hours after treatment of 2 g of metronidazole in one dose

Vulvovaginal Candidiasis (VVC)

- Definition—inflammatory vulvovaginal process caused by a yeast organism, *Candida*, which superficially invades the epithelium cells
- Etiology/incidence
  1. Second most common vulvovaginal infection—caused by *Candida*, a dimorphic fungus
  2. Approximately 75% of women will have at least one episode in their reproductive years; 45% will have a second episode; 5% or less will have recurrent or intractable episodes
  3. *C. albicans* species is responsible 85%–90% of the time; *C. glabrata* and *C. tropicalis* are responsible for the majority of the remaining infections and are more resistant to therapy
  4. Predisposing factors to candidal overgrowth—pregnancy, reproductive age, uncontrolled diabetes, immunosuppressive disorders, frequent intercourse, antibiotic use, high-dose corticosteroids
- Symptoms
  1. Irritation of vulva, pruritus, soreness, external dysuria
  2. Discharge may be thick, curdy, thin, or watery, with yeast odor
  3. Dyspareunia (upon penetration)
- Physical findings
  1. Discharge is usually adherent to the vaginal wall
  2. Erythema of vulva and vagina
  3. Cervix appears normal on speculum examination
  4. Vulvar scabbing possible from the itch/scratch cycle
- Differential diagnosis
  1. Trichomoniasis
  2. BV
  3. Vulvar dermatoses
  4. Allergic reaction
  5. Urethritis/cystitis
  6. Cytolytic Vaginosis
- Diagnostic tests/findings
  1. Wet mount of vaginal secretions with 10% KOH will reveal mycelia, spores, and pseudohyphae
  2. Vaginal pH usually normal (< 4.5); amine test negative
  3. Increased number of WBCs on wet mount
  4. Fungal culture confirms diagnosis—most often used with frequent recurrences or intractable episodes to determine *Candida* species
- Management/treatment
  1. Treatment indicated if:
     a. Symptomatic
     b. Patient desires
     c. Is immunosuppressed
  2. Azole family of antifungals—usual treatment; more effective than nystatin
  3. Recommended regimens
     a. Over-the-counter intravaginal agents
        (1) Clotrimazole 1% cream, 5 g intravaginally daily for 7 to 14 days
        (2) Clotrimazole 2% cream, 5 g intravaginally for 3 days
        (3) Miconazole 2% cream, 5 g intravaginally for 7 days

        (4) Miconazole 4% cream, 5 g intravaginally for 3 days
        (5) Miconazole 100 mg vaginal suppository, one suppository daily for 7 days
        (6) Miconazole 200 mg vaginal suppository, one suppository for 3 days
        (7) Miconazole 1,200 mg vaginal suppository, one suppository for 1 day
        (8) Tioconazole 6.5% ointment, 5 g intravaginally in a single application
     b. Prescription intravaginal agents
        (1) Butoconazole 2% cream (single-dose bioadhesive product), 5 g intravaginally in a single application
        (2) Terconazole 0.4% cream, 5 g intravaginally daily for 7 days
        (3) Terconazole 0.8% cream, 5 g intravaginally daily for 3 days
        (4) Terconazole 80 mg vaginal suppository, one suppository daily for 3 days
     c. Oral agent—fluconazole 150 mg orally in a single dose
  4. Treatment for recurrent VVC—if four or more symptomatic episodes in 1 year; usually no apparent predisposing factor; culture to determine if non-*albicans Candida* species; consider longer-duration therapy and maintenance regimens (several regimens suggested with both topical azoles and oral fluconazole); consider use of intravaginal probiotics
  5. Key points
     a. Azole creams and suppositories are oil-based and may weaken latex condoms and diaphragms
     b. Treatment of partner is not recommended unless the male has balanitis
     c. Severe VVC (extensive erythema, edema, fissure formation) usually requires a 7- to 14-day topical azole regimen or a repeat dose of fluconazole 72 hours after the initial dose
     d. Individuals with uncontrolled diabetes or receiving corticosteroid therapy who have VVC may require a 7- to 14-day treatment regimen
     e. Encourage the use of cotton underwear
     f. Treatment in pregnancy
        (1) VVC occurs frequently in pregnancy
        (2) Topical azole therapies applied for 7 days may be used
        (3) Avoid oral agent

Cytolytic Vaginosis(VVC)

- Definition—a vaginal condition that involves an overgrowth of lactobacillus bacteria. Lactobacilli are a normal part of the vaginal environment. Cytolytic vaginosis is not an infection. It is also *not* a sexually transmitted illness.
- Etiology/incidence
  1. Unknown
  2. Appears to be a pH problem that causes a disruption in the natural balance of bacteria found in the vagina. This leads to an overgrowth of lactobacilli, which produce acids that cause vaginal irritation.

- Symptoms
  1. Itching of the vagina or skin outside the vagina (the vulva)
  2. Burning of the vulva. Symptoms may worsen with urination and mimic the burning associated with a urinary tract infection.
  3. White or yellowish vaginal discharge, which can vary in consistency.
  4. Pain with sex or soreness following sex.
  5. The symptoms of cytolytic vaginosis are often confused with those of a yeast infection or bacterial vaginosis. However, cytolytic vaginosis symptoms tend to be worse before a menstrual period and relieved during menstrual flow (this is because menstrual blood is more alkaline, which helps to neutralize the overly acidic vaginal environment).
- Physical findings
  1. The presence of characteristic cellular changes and excessive lactobacilli help to confirm the diagnosis
  2. Testing will also show a low vaginal pH
  3. There should also be no signs of yeast or bacterial vaginosis
- Differential diagnosis
  1. BV
  2. Vulvar dermatoses
  3. Allergic reaction
  4. Urethritis/cystitis
  5. Candidiasis
  6. Trauma from foreign body
- Diagnostic tests/findings
  1. Vaginal pH usually low (> 4.5); amine test negative
  2. Increased number of lactobacilli on wet mount
  3. No signs of bacteria or yeast
- Management/treatment
  1. Treatment indicated if:
     a. Symptomatic
     b. Goal of treatment is to increase the vaginal pH and restore lactobacilli numbers back to normal.
  2. Baking soda treatments (over the counter)
     a. Baking soda douche: Dissolve 1 rounded teaspoon of baking soda in 600 mL of warm water, and douche once daily for 7–14 days. Alternatively, you can dissolve 1–2 tablespoons of baking soda in 4 cups of water, and douche twice a week for 2 weeks. A douchebag can be purchased at most pharmacies. Over-the-counter baking soda douches are also available.
     b. Baking soda vaginal suppository: Fill empty gelatin capsules with baking soda. Insert 1 capsule into the vagina twice weekly for 2 weeks. Gelatin capsules can be purchased at health food stores.
     c. Baking soda paste: This can be helpful if you are experiencing irritation of the skin outside the vagina. Make a watery paste with baking soda and apply it daily to irritated skin.
     d. Baking soda sitz bath: Dissolve 2–4 tablespoons of baking soda in 2 inches of warm water in a tub. Soak for 15–20 minutes twice daily to a few times a week. Then decrease to once or twice per week to prevent recurrences.

- Lifestyle Changes
  1. Use pads instead of tampons (because menstrual flow increases vaginal pH)
  2. Avoid soap in the genital area. Wash with plain water. If you need soap, use a pH-balanced unscented bar soap, such as Olay or Dove. Avoid liquid soaps as they are more concentrated
  3. Avoid scented hygiene products, like vaginal sprays, powders, toilet paper, pads, etc.
  4. Change out of wet clothing (e.g., swimsuits, exercise clothing) as soon as possible
  5. Avoid tight clothing
  6. Wear cotton underwear. Sleeping without underwear may also help
  7. Consider avoiding sex until symptoms have improved

Sexually Transmitted Infections

Chlamydia

- Definition—infection of epithelial cells of the genital tract; may cause pneumonia and/or conjunctivitis in neonates
- Etiology/incidence
  1. Caused by an intracellular organism, *Chlamydia trachomatis,* which replicates in the host, causing inclusions in stained cells
  2. Most common reportable STI in the United States—approximately 4 million acquired infections annually (reporting not required in all states)
  3. Chlamydia infection may be the etiology of 50% of pelvic infections
  4. May be transmitted vertically to the neonate in as many as 70% of untreated women (conjunctival infection or pneumonia)
  5. Sequelae of chlamydia—cervicitis, endometritis, PID, pelvic pain, ectopic pregnancy, infertility, acute urethral syndrome, postpartum infections, premature labor and delivery, premature rupture of the membranes, and perinatal morbidity
  6. Risk factors
     a. Sexually active females younger than age 25
     b. Multiple partners or partners with multiple sexual partners
     c. Nonuse of barrier methods of contraception
- Symptoms
  1. May be asymptomatic
  2. Postcoital bleeding; intermenstrual bleeding or spotting
  3. Symptoms of urinary tract infection—dysuria, frequency
  4. Vaginal discharge
  5. Abdominal pain
  6. Individuals with male anatomy—usually asymptomatic; may have dysuria, urethral discharge, pruritus
- Physical findings
  1. Mucopurulent endocervical discharge; edematous, tender cervix with easily induced bleeding
  2. Suprapubic pain or slight tenderness upon palpation

3. Individuals with male anatomy—mucoid to mucopurulent urethral discharge
- Differential diagnosis
  1. Gonococcal infection
  2. Urethritis or urinary tract infection
  3. Salpingitis
- Diagnostic tests/findings (see Chapter 2, *Health Assessment and Diagnostic Tests*, for more information)
  1. Culture—expensive
  2. Nonculture methods—nucleic acid amplification test (NAAT) recommended by CDC, 2021.
     a. Specimen source for individuals with female anatomy—vaginal (preferred; patient or provider collected), endocervix, urine (slightly less sensitive)
     b. Specimen source for individuals with male anatomy—first-catch urine (preferred)
     c. Other—anatomic site of exposure; rectal, oropharyngeal
  3. Gonococcal culture or nonculture test to rule out concomitant gonorrhea
  4. Serologic testing for syphilis; wet-mount testing for vaginal infection; consider HIV screen
- Management/treatment
  1. CDC (2021) recommendations
     a. Doxycycline 100 mg PO BID for 7 days
  2. Alternative regimens
     a. Azithromycin 1 g PO, single dose
     b. Levofloxacin 500 mg PO daily for 7 days
  3. Treatment in pregnancy
     a. Recommended regimen—azithromycin 1 g PO in a single dose
     b. Alternative regimens
        (1) Amoxicillin 500 mg PO TID for 7 days
     c. Doxycycline should not be used in pregnancy; may cause discoloration of teeth in children
     d. Erythromycin estolate is contraindicated in pregnancy because of drug-related hepatotoxicity
     e. Quinolones (ofloxacin, levofloxacin) are contraindicated in pregnancy
  4. Managing sex partners
     a. Sex partners should be evaluated, tested, and treated if they had sexual contact with the patient during the 60 days preceding the onset of symptoms in the patient or diagnosis of chlamydia
     b. The most recent sex partner should be evaluated and treated even if the time of the last sexual contact was more than 60 days before symptom onset or diagnosis
     c. Consider expedited partner treatment (EPT) if cannot ensure that the patient's sex partner(s) in the past 60 days will otherwise receive treatment
     d. EPT entails treatment of the sex partner(s) of the patient with chlamydia or gonorrhea by providing the patient with medication or a prescription to give to the partner without the clinician examining the partner
     e. Clinicians must follow any state regulations or laws regarding EPT
     f. Partner treatment is essential for decreasing the risk of reinfection of the patient
     g. Intercourse should be avoided for 7 days after single-dose treatment, or until a 7-day regimen is completed
     h. Retesting for reinfection 3 months posttreatment is recommended
  5. Test of cure
     a. Not recommended if treated with CDC-recommended or alternative regimens and not pregnant
     b. Consider a test of cure if suspect noncompliance with treatment or if symptoms persist
     c. Wait at least 3 weeks after treatment to do a test of cure; before 3 weeks, may get a false negative

Condyloma Acuminata, Anogenital Warts

- Definition—a sexually transmitted, viral disease affecting the vulva, vagina, cervix, penis, and perianal area
- Etiology/incidence
  1. Caused by HPV
  2. The most common STI with the highest incidence among young populations
  3. Approximately 100 species of HPV; more than 30 types infect anogenital mucosal surfaces; patient may be infected with multiple types simultaneously; 90% of anogenital warts caused by HPV types with low risk for malignancy (types 6, 11)
  4. Sexually transmitted by skin-to-skin contact through viral shedding; fomite spread is possible but rare
  5. Highly contagious—25% to 65% of partners will have HPV
  6. Incubation period—4 to 6 weeks
     Risk factors
     a. Previous or current other STI
     b. First intercourse at an early age (< 16 years); multiple sexual partners
     c. Partner who has (or has had) multiple partners
     d. Factors that suppress the immune system—diabetes, pregnancy, steroid hormones, folate deficiencies, immunosuppressive diseases
- Symptoms
  1. Wartlike lesions—pedunculated conical or cauliflower appearance; whitish to pinkish gray; granular, rough texture to skin
  2. Lesions may be singular, multiple, or in clusters on the perineum, vulva, vagina, cervix, the shaft of the penis, under the foreskin of the uncircumcised penis, and perianal area
  3. Perianal area may bleed easily and may be painful, odorous, and pruritic
- Physical findings
  1. Wartlike lesions—conical, cauliflower appearance; may be multiple lesions present anywhere on the perineum, perianal area, vagina, cervix, or penis
  2. May appear granular, macular, or cobblestone
  3. Color varies from pink to gray; darkly pigmented—have high suspicion for malignancy
- Differential diagnosis
  1. Verrucous carcinoma
  2. Normal variants of skin tags

3. *Molluscum contagiosum*
4. Condyloma lata
5. Seborrheic keratosis or other benign skin disorders

- Diagnostic tests/findings
  1. Diagnosis is made by visual inspection
  2. Biopsy if diagnosis is uncertain; no response to or worsening during standard therapy; patient immunocompromised; warts darkly pigmented, indurated, bleeding, ulcerated
  3. Serologic testing for syphilis; testing for other STIs; wet-mount testing for vaginal infections; consider HIV testing
- Management/treatment
  1. Goal of treatment is to eliminate visible disease and improve symptoms
  2. If untreated, may resolve on its own, persist, remain unchanged, or increase in size or number
  3. As no treatment has been proven to be better than another, treatment depends on patient preference, availability of resources, and provider experience
  4. Keep the area dry and clean
  5. Advise condom use
  6. Patient-applied treatment
     a. External anogenital warts
        (1) imiquimod 3.75% or 5% cream13
        (2) podofilox 0.5% solution or gel
        (3) sinecatechins 15%
     b. Provider–administered cryotherapy with liquid nitrogen or cryoprobe OR surgical removal either by tangential scissor excision, tangential shave excision, curettage, laser, or electrosurgery OR trichloroacetic acid (TCA) or bichloroacetic acid (BCA) 80%–90% solution apply small amount carefully to wart, allow to dry; will turn white; apply sodium bicarbonate or talc to neutralize or remove unreacted acid; may reapply weekly; safe in pregnancy
     c. If lesions are not resolved at the end of 6 weeks of treatment, reevaluate, change treatment, or refer
     d. Urethral meatus warts
        (1) cryotherapy with liquid nitrogen OR surgical removal
     e. Vaginal warts, Cervical warts, Intra-anal warts
        (1) cryotherapy with liquid nitrogen OR surgical removal OR TCA or BCA 80%–90% solution
  7. Immunotherapy—interferon
  8. Combination therapy may be useful, especially in single-treatment failures
  9. Refer if treatment fails or if lesions are darkly pigmented, indurated, ulcerated, suspicious, or biopsy positive for HPV type with malignant potential
  10. Rule out high-grade squamous intraepithelial lesion (HSIL) before treating cervical condyloma
  11. Emphasize the importance of cervical cytology per screening recommendations; HPV strains responsible for genital warts are not the same strains responsible for cervical pathology
  12. HPV vaccination of all young girls and women (recommended for ages 11–26 years), boys and young men (recommended for ages 9–26 years); adults ages 27–45 years, public health benefits minimal; adults not adequately vaccinated might benefit so shared clinical decision-making is recommended
  13. Treatment in pregnancy
     a. Podofilox, podophyllin, sinecatechins should be avoided during pregnancy
     b. Imiquimod appears low risk in pregnancy but should be avoided given data are scarce
     c. Wart removal may be considered in pregnancy, but complete resolution may not occur until after completion of pregnancy
     d. HPV types 6 and 11 can cause respiratory papillomatosis in infants and children; although the potential risk is low, counsel women with anogenital warts about this possibility

Gonorrhea (GC)

- Definition—a sexually transmitted bacterial infection with an affinity for columnar and transitional epithelium
- Etiology/incidence
  1. *Neisseria gonorrhoeae*—gram-negative, intracellular diplococcus requiring carbon dioxide environment to survive
  2. Sites for uncomplicated GC may be the urethra, endocervix, greater vestibular and lesser vestibular glands (also known as Bartholin's or Skene's gland), pharynx, and/or anus
  3. Most commonly sexually transmitted; neonate may become infected during birth
  4. Incubation period—3 to 5 days
  5. More than 1 million cases reported annually; may be as many as 2 million
  6. Occurs in individuals younger than age 30 approximately 80% of the time
  7. Male-to-female transmission estimated at 50%–90%; female-to-male transmission 20%–25%; little data available regarding male-to-male and female-to-female transmission rates
  8. Since 1976, penicillinase-producing strains have been present; some are now resistant to tetracycline, spectinomycin, or quinolones
  9. Sequelae include PID, infertility, ectopic pregnancy, septic arthritis, bacteremia, infections of the greater vestibular and lesser vestibular glands, epididymitis, proctitis, perihepatitis, gonorrhea ophthalmia neonatorum in neonates, premature rupture of the membranes, chorioamnionitis, and prematurity
  10. Risk factors
     a. Sexually active individuals with female anatomy younger than age 25
     b. Multiple sexual partners or partners with multiple partners
     c. History of STIs
     d. Inconsistent condom use
     e. Commercial sex work
     f. Illicit drug use
- Symptoms
  1. May be asymptomatic
  2. Individuals with female anatomy—vaginal discharge; postcoital bleeding; dysuria; vulvar pain with greater

vestibular and lesser vestibular glands infections; pelvic pain with PID
3. Individuals with male anatomy—penile discharge; dysuria; severe testicular/scrotal pain and swelling with epididymitis
4. Anal bleeding—proctitis
5. Sore throat—pharyngitis
6. Joint pain; erythema and inflammation of joints—septic arthritis, bacteremia
- Physical findings
  1. Mucopurulent endocervical or penile discharge; inflamed greater or lesser vestibular glands; easily induced bleeding of cervix
  2. Invades uterus after menses in 20% of patients, leading to signs of endometritis, salpingitis, or pelvic peritonitis
  3. Epididymitis—most common causes are gonorrhea and chlamydia; low-grade fever; red, swollen, extremely tender scrotum; enlarged, tender epididymis
  4. Signs associated with infection at other sites or septic arthritis
- Differential diagnosis
  1. Nongonococcal mucopurulent cervicitis (MPC)
  2. Chlamydia
  3. Vaginitis
  4. Males—nongonococcal urethritis (NGU); torsion of spermatic cord
- Diagnostic tests/findings
  1. Gram stain of penile discharge; no value in examining vaginal or cervical discharge (60%–70% false negative)
  2. Culture on the Thayer–Martin medium—allows for susceptibility testing if treatment failure is suspected
  3. Nonculture methods—NAAT recommended by CDC (2015)
  4. Serologic testing for syphilis; chlamydia testing; consider HIV screen
- Management/treatment
  1. CDC (2021) recommendations for uncomplicated infections of the cervix, urethra, and rectum
     a. Ceftriaxone 500 mg intramuscularly in one single dose and azithromycin 1 g orally as a single dose
     b. A coinfection with *C. trachomatis* is frequently found with *N. gonorrhoeae*; CDC recommendation is for patients to be treated routinely for uncomplicated genital *C. trachomatis* infection when treating for *N. gonorrhoeae*
     c. Dual therapy also recommended because of growing concern about antibiotic resistance
  2. Treatment in pregnancy—ceftriaxone 500 mg intramuscularly in one single dose
  3. Key points
     a. A test of cure is not needed if uncomplicated gonorrhea was treated with the recommended regimen
     b. Avoid sexual intercourse until all partners are treated and no longer have symptoms
     c. Patient's sexual partner or partners within 60 days before the onset of symptoms or diagnosis of infection should be evaluated and treated

d. Consider EPT if cannot ensure that the patient's sex partner(s) in the past 60 days will otherwise receive treatment
e. If the patient's last sexual encounter was > 60 days, treatment for the patient's most recent sexual partner is recommended
f. Retesting 3 months after treatment is recommended to detect reinfection

Herpes Simplex (Genital Herpes Simplex, HSV)

- Definition—a common, incurable, chronic, recurrent viral disease
- Etiology/incidence
  1. Causative organism—two serotypes of the herpes simplex virus (HSV)
     a. Type I (HSV-1)—commonly found in the mouth; accounts for 15% of genital infections
     b. Type II (HSV-2)—causes 85% of genital infections
  2. Approximately 50 million people infected; 1 million new cases each year
  3. An estimated 80%–90% of people with HSV-2 infection report no history of signs/symptoms
  4. Asymptomatic shedding of the virus accounts for the majority of transmission
  5. Usually transmitted by skin-to-skin contact; rarely spread by fomite transmission
  6. Approximately 80%–90% chance that a female will develop herpes following sexual contact with an infected male; little data available on female-to-male, male-to-male, female-to-female transmission rates
  7. Risk factors
     a. Previous or present STI
     b. Trauma to skin (portal of entry for virus)
     c. Immunosuppressed individual
     d. Multiple sexual partners
  8. Complications
     a. Herpes encephalitis
     b. Herpes meningitis
     c. Diffuse infection in immunocompromised individuals
     d. Perinatal infection
  9. Genital herpes and pregnancy
     a. Most individuals with infected neonates have no known history of HSV
     b. Infection is transmitted during labor and birth
     c. Risk for transmission to the neonate is highest if the pregnant individual has primary infection near the time of birth—30% to 50%; <1% if has a recurrent episode near the time of birth
- Symptoms—three HSV syndromes (primary infection, nonprimary first-episode infection, and recurrent infection)
  1. Primary infection
     a. Systemic symptoms—two-thirds have systemic symptoms; flu-like symptoms—fever, malaise, headache; symptoms usually begin within 1 week of exposure, peak within 4 days, and subside over the next week
     b. Localized genital pain

c. Course of genital lesions
   (1) Local prodrome; pruritus, erythema about 1–2 days before the appearance of lesions
   (2) Formation of small, painful vesicles over labia majora, minora, mons pubis, vagina; penis; perianal area (4–10 days)
   (3) Vesicles rupture, forming shallow, painful, wet ulcerations lasting 1–2 weeks
   (4) Lesions heal without scarring
d. Tender inguinal lymphadenopathy may be the last symptom to resolve
e. 75% of women have a vaginal discharge
f. 90% of women have cervical involvement characterized by vesiculation and a tendency to bleed easily
2. Nonprimary first-episode infection—initial clinical episode in patients with previously circulating antibodies to HSV-1 or HSV-2
   a. Symptoms same as for primary infection
   b. Few constitutional symptoms
   c. Shorter, milder course
3. Recurrent genital herpes infection
   a. Symptoms same as for primary infection, but usually milder
   b. Usually no constitutional symptoms
   c. Shorter duration of symptoms (resolves in 7–10 days)
      (1) Prodrome—1 to 2 days
      (2) Vesicles—3 to 5 days
      (3) Dry-out days—2 to 3 days
- Physical findings
1. Small, painful vesicles and ulceration at varying stages of progression
2. Exquisite pain at the site of the lesion
3. Inguinal lymphadenopathy
- Diagnostic tests/findings
1. HSV culture collected from the base of the vesicle or ulcer (may have low sensitivity depending on the stage of the lesion)
2. Cervical cytology—low sensitivity, high specificity
3. Nonculture methods—polymerase chain reaction (PCR) assay for HSV DNA; most sensitive test
4. Type-specific serologic tests (TSSTs) are available to identify HSV-1 and HSV-2 antibodies; low sensitivity for HSV-1; HSV-2 sensitivity of 91%–100%, specificity of 92%–98% at 6–12 weeks after initial infection; most useful in identifying HSV-2 antibodies as up to 97% of women have antibodies to HSV-1
5. Serologic testing for syphilis; tests for other STIs; consider HIV testing
- Management/treatment
1. HSV-1 and HSV-2 have no cure; systemic antiviral drugs partially control symptoms; do not eradicate the latent virus or affect the risk, recurrence, frequency, or severity of the symptoms once drug is discontinued; suppressive therapy may reduce viral shedding
2. Medical management
   a. First clinical episode
      (1) Acyclovir 400 mg PO TID for 7 to 10 days
      (2) Famciclovir 250 mg PO TID for 7 to 10 days
      (3) Valacyclovir 1 g PO BID for 7–10 days
         (a) Episodic treatment for recurrent genital herpes initiates within 1 day of lesion onset or during prodrome
      (4) Acyclovir 800 mg PO BID for 5 days
      (5) Acyclovir 800 mg PO TID for 2 days
      (6) Famciclovir 125 mg PO BID for 5 days
      (7) Famciclovir 1,000 mg PO BID for 1 day
      (8) Famciclovir 500 mg once, followed by 250 mg PO BID for 2 days
      (9) Valacyclovir 500 mg PO BID for 3 days
      (10) Valacyclovir 1 g PO once a day for 5 days
         (a) Suppressive treatment of recurrent genital herpes—reduces the frequency of recurrences, decreases the rate of transmission of HSV-2 to sexual partners
      (11) Acyclovir 400 mg PO BID
      (12) Famciclovir 250 mg PO BID
      (13) Valacyclovir 500 mg or 1.0 g PO once a day
      (14) Asymptomatic—counsel; encourage self-examination; encourage use of condoms or dental dams
      (15) Symptomatic—use same treatment regimens
      (16) Prevention of transmission to uninfected pregnant woman when the sexual partner has a known or suspected history of genital herpes
         (a) Advise use of condoms with all genital-to-genital contact
         (b) Advise no genital-to-genital contact when the partner has genital lesions or prodrome
         (c) Consider abstaining from genital-to-genital contact near the estimated time of birth
         (d) Consider suppressive therapy for an infected partner to reduce the risk of transmission
   b. Pregnancy and lactation
      (1) Ask about the history of herpes or genital lesions at the initial visit during pregnancy
      (2) Acyclovir can be safely used in all stages of pregnancy; may be used during lactation
      (3) Famciclovir and valacyclovir—limited data; animal trials suggest low risk in pregnant patients
      (4) Consider a suppressive therapy regimen for pregnant individuals with recurrent genital herpes starting at 36 weeks' gestation
      (5) No data to support the use of antiviral therapy among pregnant individuals without a history of genital herpes but who are HSV-seropositive
      (6) At the onset of labor/admission to the hospital or birth center, inquire about prodromal symptoms for herpes and perform a careful examination for herpetic lesions
      (7) Cesarean section should be offered if the individual has active genital lesions or prodromal symptoms
   c. Special considerations
      (1) Allergy, intolerance, and adverse reaction—rare; desensitization may be necessary

(2) HIV infection
  (a) Episodes may be prolonged or more severe in persons infected with HIV
  (b) Episodic or suppressive therapy is often beneficial for HSV symptoms; does not reduce the risk of HIV transmission
  (c) Acyclovir, famciclovir, and valacyclovir are safe for use in immunocompromised individuals in recommended doses
(3) Severe infection—hospitalize for IV acyclovir therapy
(4) Nonpharmacologic symptom relief
  (a) Cool, topical compresses with Burow's solution as needed; reduces swelling and inflammation
  (b) Local hygiene; topical anesthetics; cool air with a fan or hair dryer

Molluscum Contagiosum

- Definition—a mildly contagious viral epithelium proliferation of the skin
- Etiology/incidence
  1. Caused by the virus *Molluscum contagiosum*, an unassigned pox virus containing double-stranded DNA
  2. Occurs worldwide—more common in tropical and subtropical regions
  3. Most common in children and young adults
  4. Transmitted by skin to skin, fomite, and autoinoculation
  5. Incubation period—2 to 7 weeks
- Symptoms
  1. Flesh-colored, white, or pink, waxy, smooth, firm, spherical papules; umbilicated apex contains central plug; usually fewer than 20 lesions, ranging from pinhead size to 2 to 5 mm in diameter
  2. Presents on trunk and lower extremities in children
  3. Presents on the lower abdominal wall, inner thigh, pubic area, genitalia in adults
  4. Usually asymptomatic; may have pain, pruritus, and inflammation
- Physical findings
  1. Lesions are multiple but usually number fewer than 20
  2. Characteristic light-colored papules with an umbilicated center
  3. Lesions found on face, neck, trunk, lower extremities, abdomen, inner thigh, genital area
- Differential diagnosis
  1. Varicella
  2. Lichen planus
  3. Warts/condyloma
  4. Keratoacanthomas
  5. Subepidermal fibrosis
  6. Epidermal cysts
- Diagnostic tests/findings
  1. Biopsy usually not indicated—cytoplasmic inclusions; molluscum bodies
  2. Test for other STIs in young adults
- Management/treatment
  1. Usually resolve spontaneously without scarring

2. Superficial incision; express contents with comedone extractor
3. Curettage with cautery
4. For multiple lesions, cryotherapy with liquid nitrogen, silver nitrate
5. Treatment may cause scarring

Mycoplasma Genitalium

- Definition—*Mycoplasma genitalium* (or *Mgen*) is a sexually transmitted bacteria that can cause reproductive tract infections of the urethra or cervix. It causes symptomatic and asymptomatic urethritis. It may also play a role in cervicitis (CDC, 2021b), pelvic inflammatory disease, preterm delivery, spontaneous abortion, and infertility
- Etiology/incidence
  1. *Mgen* spreads through vaginal and anal sex without a condom with someone who has the infection. Researchers are still determining whether sex partners can spread *Mgen* through oral sex. People treated for *Mgen* can get reinfected.
  2. The 2017–2018 National Health and Nutrition Examination Survey estimates the overall prevalence of urogenital *Mgen* to be 1.7% among people aged 14–59 years in the United States. The survey reported a similar prevalence among males at 1.8% and females at 1.7%
  3. Etiology of approximately 15%–20% of NGU, 20%–25% of nonchlamydial NGU, and 40% of persistent or recurrent urethritis (*697,909,910*). Infection with *C. trachomatis* is common in selected geographic areas (*911–913*), although *M. genitalium* is often the sole pathogen.
- Symptoms/Physical Findings
  1. *Mgen* causes symptomatic and asymptomatic urethritis among men. When present, the typical symptoms of *Mgen-* urethritis include:
    a. dysuria
    b. urethral pruritus
    c. purulent or mucopurulent urethral discharge
      (1) Among women, *Mgen* may cause cervicitis and PID, though individuals with cervicitis due to *Mgen* often are asymptomatic. When present, symptoms associated with *Mgen* cervicitis include:
        (a) vaginal discharge
        (b) vaginal itching
        (c) dysuria
        (d) pelvic discomfort
- Differential diagnosis
  1. BV
  2. Candida
  3. Trichomonas
  4. PID
  5. Urethritis
- Diagnostic tests/findings
  1. *M. genitalium* is an extremely slow-growing organism. Culture can take up to 6 months, and technical laboratory capacity is limited to research settings. NAAT for *M. genitalium* is FDA cleared for use with urine and urethral, penile meatal, endocervical, and vaginal swab samples

- Management/treatment
  1. Recommended regimens if *M. genitalium* resistance testing is available
     a. If *macrolide sensitive:* Doxycycline 100 mg orally 2 times/day for 7 days, followed by azithromycin 1 g orally initial dose, followed by 500 mg orally once daily for 3 additional days (2.5 g total)
     b. If macrolide resistant: Doxycycline 100 mg orally 2 times/day for 7 days followed by moxifloxacin 400 mg orally once daily for 7 days
  2. Recommended Regimens if *M. genitalium* resistance testing is not available
     a. If *M. genitalium* is detected by an FDA-cleared NAAT: Doxycycline 100 mg orally 2 times/day for 7 days, followed by moxifloxacin 400 mg orally once daily for 7 days

Syphilis

- Definition—a chronic, infectious, sexually transmitted process that progresses predictably through distinct stages
- Etiology/incidence
  1. Caused by *Treponema pallidum*
  2. Organism enters skin through microscopic breaks in the skin during sexual contact
  3. Incubation period—10 to 90 days, average 21 days
  4. Occurs worldwide, primarily involving adults 20 to 35 years of age; has become epidemic in the United States; includes syphilis in pregnancy and congenital syphilis
  5. Increased incidence associated with greater use of illicit drugs and high-risk behavior associated with drug use
  6. Approximately 90,000 cases annually in the United States
- Symptoms
  1. Four stages of syphilis
     a. Primary
        (1) May be asymptomatic
        (2) Primary lesion (chancre) arises at the point of entry—evident 10 to 90 days following contact
        (3) Painless, ulcerated lesion with raised border and indurated base, rolled edges—spontaneously disappears in 3 to 6 weeks
        (4) May appear anywhere the organism enters; genitals, mouth, or anus
        (5) Painless lymphadenopathy may occur
     b. Secondary
        (1) Follows resolution of the primary stage; symptoms become systemic
        (2) Localized or diffuse mucocutaneous lesions (palms, soles, mucous patches, and condylomata lata) with generalized lymphadenopathy along with flulike symptoms (low-grade fever, headache, sore throat, malaise, arthralgias)
        (3) May begin 4 to 6 weeks after the appearance of the primary lesion and resolve in 1 week to 2 months
     c. Latent
        (1) Begins after spontaneous resolution of secondary stage

        (2) No clinical manifestation
        (3) Detected by serologic testing
        (4) If no treatment, the patient goes into the latent phase (asymptomatic)
        (5) Early latent phase—within 1 year of acquiring the disease
        (6) Late latent phase—after 1-year duration
        (7) Late latent phase of unknown duration
        (8) May remain in this stage or progress to the tertiary stage
     d. Tertiary
        (1) Characterized by gummas (nodular lesions) involving skin, mucous membranes, skeletal system, and viscera
        (2) Cardiac symptoms, aortitis, aneurysm, or aortic regurgitation
        (3) Neurosyphilis may present without symptoms or with nerve dysfunction, acute or chronic meningitis, stroke, tabes dorsalis, meningovascular syphilis, general paralysis, insanity, iritis, chorioretinitis, and leukoplakia
        (4) Not infectious
- Physical findings
  1. Chancre on vulva, vagina, cervix, penis, or at site of entry of organism—begins primary stage
  2. Secondary stage manifestations—generalized maculopapular rash, mucocutaneous lesion, adenopathy
  3. Condyloma lata—wartlike lesions on the vulva, penis, perianal region, and upper thighs
  4. Tertiary stage may manifest as multiple organ involvement
  5. Gummas—tertiary manifestation; appear as nodules that enlarge, ulcerate, and become necrotic
- Differential diagnosis
  1. Other genito-ulcerative diseases; herpes, chancroid, lymphogranuloma venereum, granuloma inguinale
  2. Genital carcinoma
  3. Trauma
- Diagnostic tests/findings
  1. Darkfield microscopy of fluid from lesions reveals *Treponema*
  2. Serologic testing
     a. Nontreponemal—Venereal Disease Research Laboratory (VDRL), rapid plasma reagin (RPR); 80%–90% accurate in making a diagnosis; nonspecific
     b. Treponemal—fluorescent treponemal antibody absorption test (FTA-ABS), *T. pallidum* particle agglutination (TP-PA); specific
     c. A positive RPR or VDRL test must be confirmed with an FTA-ABS or TP-PA
     d. Although not common (1%), false positives may occur; more likely with nontreponemal tests; causes may include autoimmune disease, Lyme disease, pregnancy, recent immunization, substance use disorder
     e. Treponemal tests tend to remain positive for a lifetime regardless of treatment for syphilis
     f. Nontreponemal test titers usually correlate with disease activity; results should be reported quantitatively; a fourfold change in titer is equal to two dilutions (e.g., 1:16 to 1:4 or 1:8 to 1:32)

3. Lumbar puncture for testing of cerebrospinal fluid (CSF) to detect neurosyphilis—late latent or tertiary stage
4. Tests for other STIs including HIV
- Management/treatment
  1. Who must be treated
     a. Pregnant individuals
     b. Individuals with positive dark-field examination or positive treponemal antibody test
     c. People treated previously who have a fourfold rise in quantitative nontreponemal test
     d. Patients with uncertain diagnosis
     e. Persons who were exposed within 90 days preceding the diagnosis of primary, secondary, or early latent syphilis in a sexual partner—treated presumptively even if seronegative
     f. Persons who were exposed more than 90 days before the diagnosis of any stage of syphilis in a sexual partner—treat presumptively if test results are not immediately available and the opportunity for follow-up is uncertain
  2. Treatment (CDC, 2015)
     a. Primary, secondary, and early latent syphilis
        (1) Benzathine penicillin G 2.4 million IM in a single dose
     b. Latent syphilis
        (1) Early latent—benzathine penicillin G 50,000 units/kg IM, up to the adult dose of 2.4 million units in a single dose
        (2) Late latent or latent of unknown duration—benzathine penicillin G 7.2 million units total administered as 3 doses of 2.4 million units given IM at 1-week intervals (total 150,000 units/kg up to the adult dose of 7.2 million units)
     c. Tertiary syphilis with normal CSF examination—benzathine penicillin G 7.2 million units total, administered as 3 doses of 2.4 million units IM each at 1-week intervals
     d. Neurosyphilis and ocular syphilis
        (1) Aqueous crystalline penicillin G—18 to 24 million units per day, administered as 3 to 4 million units IV every 4 hours or continuous infusion, for 10–14 days
        (2) If compliance with therapy can be ensured:
            (a) Procaine penicillin G 2.4 million units IM once daily *plus*
            (b) Probenecid 500 mg QID
            (c) Both for 10–14 days
     e. Treatment in pregnancy—treat pregnant individuals with the penicillin regimen appropriate for their stage of infection
     f. HIV-positive individuals
        (1) May have a higher incidence of neurologic involvement and a higher rate of treatment failure—careful follow-up is important
        (2) Serologic test results may be atypical
        (3) When the clinical picture is positive and the serologic test is negative, biopsy, darkfield, or direct fluorescent antibody staining is done

3. Follow-up
   a. Quantitative nontreponemal serologic tests repeated at 6, 12, and 24 months
   b. Titers should decline at least fourfold within 12 to 24 months
   c. A fourfold increase in titer indicates inadequate treatment or a new infection
   d. Pregnant individuals without a fourfold drop in titer in a 3-month period need repeat treatment
   e. Treponemal tests remain positive for a lifetime in most individuals regardless of treatment or disease activity
   f. Report all cases to the proper agency for follow-up of sexual contacts

Chancroid

- Definition—an acute, contagious, ulcerative, bacterial infection that is sexually transmitted
- Etiology/incidence
  1. *Haemophilus ducreyi* is a short, nonmotile, gram-negative rod (anaerobe) that grows in chains known as a school-of-fish pattern
  2. Incubation period—4 to 5 days
  3. Occurs only in a few areas of the United States in discrete outbreaks; associated with drug use, commercial sex, and acquisition of infection outside the United States
  4. Most often seen in tropical and subtropical climates, in regions of Africa and the Caribbean
  5. Increases risk for both acquisition and transmission of HIV
- Symptoms
  1. May be asymptomatic
  2. Papules or painful ulcerations on labia, anogenital skin, vagina, cervix in women; around the prepuce, around the frenulum, on coronal sulcus in men
  3. May have a foul odor
  4. One week after onset, bilateral, tender, suppurant inguinal lymphadenopathy (bubo) develops (30%–60% of cases)
  5. Lesions resolve in 1–2 weeks if treated; 1–3 months if untreated
- Physical findings
  1. Deep ulcerations with irregular, scalloped borders
  2. Bilateral, tender, suppurant inguinal lymphadenopathy
  3. Lesions found on labia, vagina, anogenital skin, penis, and cervix
  4. May have a foul odor
- Differential diagnosis
  1. Genital herpes
  2. Syphilis
  3. Malignancy of the vulva or penis
  4. Trauma
  5. Donovanosis
- Diagnostic tests/findings
  1. Gram stain reveals gram-negative rods or chains
  2. Definitive test is culture to identify *H. ducreyi*—collected from lesion or bubo; difficult to isolate on culture; use specific medium (sensitivity < 80%)

3. Clinical signs are pathognomonic
   a. Genital ulcers with typical characteristics
   b. Regional lymphadenopathy
   c. Negative test for HSV
   d. Suppurant inguinal adenopathy
4. Serologic testing for syphilis and HIV
- Management/treatment
  1. Cured with treatment; may leave scarring in severe cases
  2. CDC (2021a) recommendations
     a. Azithromycin 1 g PO in a single dose
     b. Ceftriaxone 250 mg IM in a single dose
     c. Ciprofloxacin 500 mg PO BID for 3 days
     d. Erythromycin base 500 mg PO BID for 7 days
  3. Treatment in pregnancy and lactation
     a. Ciprofloxacin presents a low risk to the fetus during pregnancy
     b. Ciprofloxacin use during lactation has the potential for toxicity for infant
  4. Follow-up—reexamine in 3 to 7 days; if ulcerations have not improved, reevaluate
  5. Management of sexual partners—if sexual contact occurred during 10 days preceding the onset of the patient's symptoms, evaluate and treat

Lymphogranuloma Venereum (LGV)

- Definition—an ulcerative, bacterial STI
- Etiology/incidence
  1. Caused by serotypes L1, L2, and L3 of *Chlamydia trachomatis*, an obligate, intracellular parasite that infects the columnar epithelium
  2. Occurs infrequently in the United States
  3. Endemic in tropical areas
  4. Incubation period—5 to 21 days or longer
  5. Infects males more than females (5:1)
- Symptoms
  1. May be asymptomatic
  2. Painless ulcerations that heal within a few days (50%)
  3. Tender adenopathy usually occurs 1–4 weeks after the ulcer; may have a fever, malaise, headache, myalgia
  4. Painful bowel movements; blood or pus from the rectum
- Physical findings
  1. Painless genital ulcer at the site of inoculation; disappears in a few days
  2. Tender inguinal and/or femoral lymphadenopathy; most commonly unilateral
  3. Rectal exposure may result in proctocolitis or inflammatory involvement of perirectal or perianal lymphatic tissues, leading to fistulas and strictures
- Differential diagnosis
  1. Chancroid
  2. HSV
  3. Syphilis
  4. Malignancy of the vulva or penis
- Diagnostic tests/findings
  1. Aspiration and culture or NAAT of material from fluctuant lymph nodes—50% of cases show chlamydia
  2. Serologic testing—titer of more than 1:64 shows active disease
  3. CBC shows mild leukocytosis or monocytosis

4. Elevated sedimentation rate
5. Screening for other STIs
6. Encourage HIV screen
- Management/treatment
  1. Treatment recommendations (CDC, 2021a)
     a. Doxycycline 100 mg PO BID for 21 days *Or alternatives*
     b. Azithromycin 1 g orally once weekly for 3 weeks
     c. Erythromycin base 500 mg PO QID for 21 days
  2. Treatment in pregnancy and lactation
     a. Pregnant and lactating individuals should be treated with erythromycin
     b. Doxycycline should be avoided in the second and third trimesters of pregnancy due to the risk of discoloration of fetal teeth and bones; compatible with breastfeeding/chestfeeding
  3. Follow-up—follow clinically until signs and symptoms have resolved
  4. Management of sexual partners
     a. Examine and test those who had sexual contact with the patient during the 60 days before the onset of symptoms and treat with a chlamydia regimen (azithromycin 1 g orally single dose or doxycycline 100 mg orally twice a day for 7 days)
     b. Evaluate for other STIs

Pelvic Inflammatory Disease (PID)

- Definition—comprises a spectrum of inflammatory disorders of the upper female genital tract, including any combination of salpingitis, endometritis, tubo-ovarian abscess, and pelvic peritonitis
- Etiology/incidence
  1. Causative organisms—*Chlamydia trachomatis, Neisseria gonorrhea*, polymicrobial infection (*Escherichia coli, Gardnerella vaginalis, Haemophilus influenzae, Mycoplasma hominis*)
  2. One million cases are diagnosed annually
  3. Approximately 200,000 hospitalizations at a cost of $5 billion
  4. An estimated 25% of cases result in infertility, ectopic pregnancy, or chronic pelvic pain
  5. One-third of individuals with gonorrhea or chlamydia cervicitis progress to PID if not treated
  6. Teenagers account for one-fifth of total cases
  7. Risk factors
     a. Sexually active females younger than 20 years
     b. Multiple sexual partners
     c. Previous episode of PID
     d. Presence of chlamydia, gonorrhea, and/or BV
     e. Vaginal douching
- Symptoms
  1. May be acute or mild
  2. Abdominal pain
  3. Vaginal discharge
  4. Fever
  5. Dysuria
  6. Dyspareunia
  7. Nausea/vomiting
  8. Vaginal spotting or bleeding (30%)

- Physical findings
  1. Minimum criterion for empirical treatment of PID in sexually active young individuals and others at risk for STIs with a complaint of pelvic or lower abdominal pain—the presence of one or more of these three findings on pelvic examination
     a. Cervical motion tenderness
     b. Uterine tenderness
     c. Adnexal tenderness
  2. Additional criteria that enhance the specificity of the minimum criterion and support PID diagnosis
     a. Fever > 101°F (> 38.4°C) orally
     b. Mucopurulent cervical or vaginal discharge
     c. Abundant WBCs on microscopic wet-mount evaluation of vaginal fluid
     d. Elevated erythrocyte sedimentation rate (ESR)
     e. Elevated C-reactive protein level
     f. Laboratory documentation of cervical infection with *N. gonorrhoeae* or *C. trachomatis*
- Differential diagnosis
  1. Ectopic pregnancy
  2. Appendicitis
  3. Ruptured ovarian cyst
  4. Torsion of adnexal mass
  5. Ulcerative colitis
  6. Degenerative leiomyoma
  7. Renal calculus
- Diagnostic tests/findings
  1. Chlamydia and gonorrhea tests
  2. ESR and/or C-reactive protein—elevated
  3. Criteria for definitive diagnosis (in case of unsure diagnosis or poor response to treatment)
     a. Histologic evidence of endometritis on endometrial biopsy
     b. Ultrasound or other radiographic tests revealing tubo-ovarian abscess
     c. Laparoscopy—abnormalities consistent with PID
- Management/treatment
  1. Presumptive treatment for PID should be initiated in sexually active young individuals and others at risk for STDs who report pelvic or lower abdominal pain and no other reason for the illness can be identified *and* one of these clinical criteria is present:
     a. Cervical motion tenderness
     b. Uterine tenderness
     c. Adnexal tenderness
  2. Parenteral treatment
     a. Hospitalization for at least 24 hours to initiate parenteral therapy for patients with tubo-ovarian abscess
     b. Ceftriaxone 1 g IV every 24 hours *plus* doxycycline 100 mg PO or IV every 12 hours plus metronidazole 500 mg orally or by IV every 12 hours
     c. Cefotetan 2 g IV every 12 hours *plus* doxycycline 100 mg PO or IV every 12 hours *or*
     d. Cefoxitin 2 g IV every 6 hours *plus* doxycycline 100 mg PO or IV every 12 hours *or Alternatives*
     e. Clindamycin 900 mg IV every 8 hours *plus* gentamicin loading dose IV or IM (2 mg/kg) followed

by a maintenance dose (1.5 mg/kg) every 8 hours; single daily dosing (3–5 mg/kg) can be substituted
     f. Ampicillin-sulbactam 3gm by IV every 6 hours *plus* doxycycline 100 mg PO or IV every 12 hours
  3. Recommended intramuscular/oral regimens
     a. Ceftriaxone 500 mg IM in a single dose *plus* doxycycline 100 mg PO BID for 14 days *with* metronidazole 500 mg PO BID for 14 days *or*
     b. Cefoxitin 2 g IM in a single dose and probenecid 1 g PO administered concurrently in a single dose *plus* doxycycline 100 mg PO BID for 14 days *with* metronidazole 500 mg PO BID for 14 days
  4. Criteria for hospitalization
     a. Patient is pregnant
     b. Pelvic abscess is suspected
     c. When a surgical emergency cannot be ruled out (ectopic pregnancy, appendicitis)
     d. Severe illness, high fever, nausea, and vomiting
     e. Failure of outpatient therapy
  5. Follow-up—reexamine within 72 hours
     a. If not significantly improved, review diagnosis and treatment; the patient may need hospitalization
     b. Criteria for improvement—abatement of fever, reduction in direct or rebound abdominal tenderness; reduction in adnexal, uterine, and cervical motion tenderness
     c. Counsel on safer sexual practices
  6. Partner treatment—evaluate, test, and treat presumptively for gonorrhea and chlamydia if contact occurred with the patient during the 60 days before the onset of symptoms
  7. Treatment in pregnancy
     a. Pregnant patients with PID have a high risk for perinatal morbidity and preterm delivery
     b. Need hospitalization and parenteral treatment with antibiotics

Vulvar Conditions

Vulvar Dermatoses

- Definition—nonneoplastic disorders of vulvar epithelium producing a number of visible changes as well as pain/pruritis that may be severe; three major vulvar dermatoses: lichen sclerosus, lichen planus, lichen simplex chronicus
- Etiology/incidence
  1. Lichen sclerosus—chronic, progressive inflammatory skin condition primarily affecting the perineal and perianal areas, most common in postmenopausal individuals; multifactorial: genetic, familial disposition, autoimmune
  2. Lichen planus—inflammatory skin condition manifested in the vulva, vagina, and other mucous membranes; typically seen in perimenopausal and postmenopausal individual; flares and remits spontaneously; lasts from several weeks to years; thought to be autoimmune
  3. Lichen simplex chronicus—thickening of skin in response to chronic rubbing or scratching; may be

Table 5-2 Symptoms and Physical Findings of Vulvar Dermatoses

	Lichen Sclerosus	Lichen Planus	Lichen Simplex Chronicus
Symptoms	■ Pruritus ■ Dyspareunia ■ Dysuria	■ Pruritus, burning, raw sensation ■ Vaginal discharge/bleeding ■ Dyspareunia ■ Dysuria	■ Pruritus ■ Chronic itch–scratch cycle ■ Dyspareunia ■ Dysuria
Physical findings	■ Maculopapular lesions, plaques ■ Loss of pigmentation ■ Markedly thin, white epidermis ■ Symmetry of distribution extends around anal region (figure of eight) ■ Loss of vulvar architecture with obliteration of the clitoris ■ Introital stenosis	■ Sharply demarcated, shiny, erythematous papules/patches ■ Gray-white lace strands of hyperkeratosis overlay patches ■ Vaginal erythema, erosions, adhesions ■ Loss of vulvovaginal architecture ■ May involve other mucosal tissues	■ Thickened, leathery plaques on labia majora ■ Excoriations and erosions from scratching ■ May involve other body areas—nape of neck, ankle, forearm, antecubital and popliteal fossae, scalp

atopic reaction; sometimes reaction to chronic inflammation from underlying skin condition

4. Associated autoimmune disorders may be seen with lichen sclerosus and lichen planus—vitiligo, thyroid disorder, alopecia areata, ulcerative colitis, other
- Symptoms and physical findings (**Table 5-2**)
- Differential diagnosis
  1. Vitiligo
  2. Vulvar carcinoma
  3. Seborrheic dermatitis
  4. Psoriasis
  5. Tinea
  6. Vaginitis
  7. STI
  8. Parasitic infection
- Diagnostic tests/findings
  1. Biopsy—confirm diagnosis, may be inconclusive in early-stage disease, imperative if no improvement with treatment
  2. Saline and KOH wet mount to rule out vaginitis
  3. STI testing if indicated
  4. Thyroid function tests—autoimmune connection
- Management/treatment
  1. Remove all contact irritants
  2. Skin emollients—vegetable-based oils
  3. Skin protectants—vitamin A and D ointment, zinc oxide
  4. Baking soda or Domeboro soaks
  5. Treat any underlying infections
  6. High-potency topical corticosteroids, ointment base best for vulva instead of cream; taper as symptoms improve and may continue for maintenance
  7. Oral or injected corticosteroids may be needed with lichen planus
  8. Vaginal dilators if needed to maintain vaginal patency
  9. Referral to dermatologist for severe symptoms, no relief with treatment, or unsure diagnosis
  10. Long-term/chronic conditions; counseling may be beneficial
  11. Increased risk for vulvar squamous cell carcinoma (4%–5%) with lichen sclerosus—yearly vulvar exam with biopsies as needed

Vulvodynia

- Definition—chronic vulvar discomfort, often described as burning pain, occurring in the absence of relevant physical findings or a specific clinically identifiable neurologic disorder; may be generalized or localized to vestibule
- Etiology/incidence
  1. Multifactorial—altered immune-inflammatory process, chronic inflammation, neurologic dysfunction (heightened sensitivity, nerve fiber proliferation)
  2. Incidence—8% to 16% of women in a lifetime, prevalence 3%–8%
  3. Commonly associated conditions are irritable bowel syndrome, interstitial cystitis/painful bladder syndrome, fibromyalgia
- Symptoms
  1. Generalized vulvodynia—severe burning, stinging, irritation, rawness; may involve mons pubis, labia majora, labia minora, perineum; constant
  2. Provoked, localized vulvodynia–involves vestibule and clitoris provoked by any attempt at vaginal penetration or tampon insertion—burning; stinging; tearing; throbbing; razorblades or cut-glass sensation; entry dyspareunia; dysuria
- Physical findings—no visible dermatoses or inflammation
- Differential diagnosis
  1. Vulvovaginal infection
  2. Estrogen deficiency
  3. Urinary tract infection
  4. Allergy/hypersensitivity
  5. Physical trauma to the area
  6. Psychogenic disorder—resulting from a history of sexual abuse, rape, incest
- Diagnostic tests/findings
  1. Cotton swab test for localized, provoked vulvodynia—light touch applied to inner thighs, labia majora, vestibular duct openings, clitoris/hood, and perineum to localize areas of altered sensation
  2. Tests for vulvovaginal infections or UTIs
  3. Colposcopy of vulva/with biopsy of suspicious findings to rule out dermatoses, pathology

- Management/treatment—largely empirical, with limited data to support any one therapy
  1. Treat infections as appropriate
  2. Topical ointments—lidocaine, capsaicin, gabapentin, nitroglycerine, amitriptyline with baclofen
  3. Oral neuropathic pain medications—amitriptyline, desipramine, gabapentin
  4. Injections—interferon, steroids, botulinum toxin type A
  5. Physical therapy with pelvic floor muscle specialist
  6. Surgery (laser) or excision may be useful if intractable symptoms persist after all other treatments
  7. Counseling or psychological support for chronic pain
  8. Expect long-term chronic therapy—may not have complete resolution of symptoms

Bartholin Gland Cyst/Abscess

- Definition—cystic growth in the duct of the greater vestibular gland (also known as Bartholin gland)
- Etiology/incidence
  1. Ductal obstruction due to infection or thickened mucus leads to cyst formation
  2. Most common cystic growth in the vulva, primarily in younger reproductive-age individuals
- Symptoms
  1. Usually nontender, unless abscess
  2. May cause discomfort during sexual intercourse, walking, or sitting
- Physical findings
  1. Medially protruding cystic structure at the inferior aspect of labia (4 and 8 o'clock positions)
  2. Most are 1–3 cm in size
  3. Usually unilateral
  4. Nontender, unless abscess
- Differential diagnosis
  1. Epidermal inclusion cyst
  2. Vulvar lipoma
  3. Vulvar hematoma
  4. Adenocarcinoma of the greater vestibular gland (very rare)
- Diagnostic tests/findings
  1. Usually none needed—diagnosis based on clinical presentation
  2. Culture of abscess—if positive usually polymicrobial
  3. NAAT for chlamydia and gonorrhea if indicated
  4. Biopsy of the greater vestibular glands if older than 40 years of age to rule out carcinoma
- Management/treatment
  1. Dependent on symptoms, size of cyst, whether recurrent or infected
  2. Needle aspiration
  3. Incision and drainage with or without placement of Word catheter
  4. Word catheter allows for the formation of the epithelialized tract and continued drainage of the gland, reducing recurrences
     a. Make a small incision proximal to the hymenal ring; insert and inflate the catheter; tuck the end of the catheter into the vagina

b. Leave in place for 4 to 6 weeks until the fistulous tract forms
     c. Complications—pain during and after placement, difficulty maintaining the catheter in place
  5. Duct marsupialization or gland excision
     a. Incision of cyst or abscess and suturing of edges of the cavity to the skin just distal to the hymenal ring within the introitus into region of normal duct
     b. May be done in office with local anesthesia or pudendal block
     c. Complications—pain, hematoma formation, prolonged healing, dyspareunia due to scarring
  6. Broad-spectrum antibiotic coverage tailored to culture results if cellulitis is present

Cervical Cancer Screening Abnormalities

- Definition—findings on microscopic evaluation of epithelial cells of the cervix and endocervix suggestive of future or current cervical cancer; results may range in degree from atypia to mild, moderate, and severe abnormalities, to invasive cancer
- The 2014 Bethesda System for interpreting results of cervical cytology includes the following:
  1. Specimen type—conventional Pap slide test or liquid-based preparation
  2. Specimen adequacy
     a. Satisfactory for evaluation; will note presence/absence of endocervical/transformation zone component
     b. Unsatisfactory for evaluation—specimen obscured by blood or inflammation, inadequate number of squamous cells, air-dried slide, not processed because unlabeled
  3. General categorization (optional)
     a. Negative for intraepithelial lesion or malignancy
     b. Epithelial cell abnormality—specifies whether squamous or glandular cells
     c. Other—for example, endometrial cells in individuals aged 45 or older
  4. Interpretation/result
     a. Nonneoplastic cellular changes (optional to report)
        (1) Nonneoplastic variations—for example, squamous metaplasia, atrophy, pregnancy-associated changes
        (2) Reactive cellular changes associated with inflammation, radiation, IUD
        (3) Glandular status after a hysterectomy
     b. Organisms
        (1) *Trichomonas*
        (2) Fungal organisms consistent morphologically with *Candida* species
        (3) Shift in vaginal flora suggestive of BV
        (4) Bacteria morphologically consistent with *Actinomyces* species
        (5) Cellular changes consistent with HSV
        (6) Cellular changes consistent with cytomegalovirus

c. Other—for example, endometrial cells in individuals aged 45 or older

5. Epithelial cell abnormalities
   a. Squamous cell abnormalities
      (1) Atypical squamous cells of undetermined significance (ASC-US)—squamous cells do not appear completely normal but not able to determine the cause of abnormal cells
      (2) Atypical squamous cells—cannot exclude high-grade squamous intraepithelial lesion (ASC-H)
      (3) Low-grade squamous intraepithelial lesion (LSIL)—encompasses transient HPV infection/mild dysplasia/cervical intraepithelial neoplasia 1 (CIN 1)
      (4) High-grade squamous intraepithelial lesion (HSIL)—encompasses persistent HPV infection/moderate dysplasia (CIN 2)/severe dysplasia or carcinoma in situ (CIN 3); includes identification of features consistent with invasion
      (5) Squamous cell carcinoma
   b. Glandular cell abnormalities
      (1) Atypical specified as endocervical, endometrial, glandular cells, or not otherwise specified (NOS)
      (2) Atypical specified as endocervical or glandular cells favoring neoplastic disease
      (3) Endocervical adenocarcinoma in situ (AIS)
      (4) Adenocarcinoma identified as endocervical, endometrial, extrauterine, or NOS
   c. Other—endometrial cells in women 45 years of age or older

- Management/treatment
  1. Specimen adequacy
     a. Satisfactory for evaluation—no action needed
     b. Unsatisfactory for evaluation—HPV unknown (any age) or HPV negative (age $\geq$ 30), repeat cervical cytology test in 2 to 4 months; HPV positive (age $\geq$ 30), colposcopy or repeat cervical cytology in 2 to 4 months; if two consecutive unsatisfactory results, perform colposcopy
  2. Organisms
     a. *Trichomonas vaginalis*—highly predictive but not 100%; treat if indicated
     b. *Candida* species—most are asymptomatic colonization and require no treatment; if symptomatic, treat
     c. Shift in flora suggestive of BV—insensitive and nonspecific indicator of BV; do not use for diagnosis
     d. *Actinomyces*—evaluate for signs/symptoms of pelvic infection if intrauterine contraceptive (IUC) present; if the patient has a pelvic infection, remove IUC and treat with antibiotics; otherwise, no treatment or IUC removal needed
     e. HSV—high predictive value; counsel patient; may consider type-specific serology to confirm prior infection and whether HSV-1 or HSV-2
     f. Cytomegalovirus—not likely to have clinical significance in asymptomatic, nonimmunocompromised women
  3. Reactive changes associated with inflammation
     a. Examine—microscopy; STI tests as indicated
     b. Treat any identified cause
  4. Endometrial cells in premenopausal women with normal menstrual pattern—insignificant; must be evaluated with endometrial biopsy in postmenopausal women or in premenopausal individuals with abnormal bleeding
  5. Atrophy—treat if symptomatic
  6. Epithelial cell abnormalities **Table 5-3**
     a. Risk-based management consensus guidelines developed by ASCCP (2019)
     b. Framework for managing abnormal cervical cancer screening (CCS) results based on the risk of currently having or developing high-grade precancer, defined as CIN3 or higher (CIN3+)

Table 5-3 Epithelial Cell Abnormalities

Squamous Cell Abnormalities	Glandular Cell Abnormalities
Atypical squamous cells of undetermined significance (ASC-US)	Atypical endocervical cells (not otherwise specified [NOS] or specify in comments)
Atypical squamous cells cannot exclude HSIL (ASC-H)	Atypical endometrial cells (NOS or specify in comments)
Low-grade squamous intraepithelial lesion (LSIL) encompassing HPV/mild dysplasia/cervical intraepithelial 1 (CIN1)	Atypical glandular cells (NOS or specify in comments)
High-grade squamous intraepithelial lesion (HSIL) encompassing moderate and severe dysplasia, CIN 2, CIN 3	Atypical endocervical cells, favor neoplasia
Squamous cell carcinoma	Atypical glandular cells, favor neoplasia
	Endocervical adenocarcinoma in situ
	Adenocarcinoma

Data from Perkins, R. B., Guido, R. S., Castle, P. E. et al. (2020). 2019 ASCCP risk-based management consensus guidelines for abnormal cervical cancer screening tests and cancer precursors. *Journal of Lower Genital Tract Disease, 24*(2),102–131.

c. All positive primary HPV screening results should have reflex testing to include both genotyping if not already done and cytology from the same specimen to inform decision-making

d. Estimation of risk of CIN3+ is based on a combination of current CCS results and past results

e. If immediate CIN3+ risk is 4% or higher, clinical actions fall into categories of colposcopy or expedited treatment depending on how high the immediate risk is estimated to be

f. If immediate CIN+3 risk is less than 4% this is below the threshold for colposcopy; surveillance with repeat HPV testing or co-testing at 1, 3, or 5 years is recommended with intervals determined by estimated 5-year CIN3+ risk

g. Observation is preferred for CIN1 to avoid unnecessary procedures in low-risk patients, but treatment is acceptable with persistent CIN1 for 2 years or more

h. Management for all categories of atypical glandular cells and adenocarcinoma in situ, except when atypical endometrial cells are specified, is colposcopy with endocervical sampling except in pregnancy

i. ASCCP provides an app and web application system for decision-making http://www.asccp.org/management-guidelines

Diethylstilbestrol (DES) in Utero

- Definition—a synthetic nonsteroidal estrogen approved by the FDA for use from 1940 to 1971 to prevent miscarriage and premature labor; prenatal DES exposure increased risk for reproductive abnormalities, infertility, clear cell adenocarcinoma of the cervix and vagina
- Etiology/incidence
  1. Vagina is originally lined with columnar epithelium, which is eventually replaced with squamous epithelium; if DES is introduced, that transformation is not completed; one-third of exposed individuals have columnar epithelium in the vagina (adenosis)
  2. Structural changes of the cervix and vagina occurred in 25% of females exposed in utero to DES; transverse vaginal septum, cervical collar, uterine constriction band
  3. Occurrence of these abnormalities was related to the dose of medication and the first time exposure; risk is significant if the administration was begun after the 18th week of gestation
  4. Increased incidence of preterm delivery, spontaneous abortion, and ectopic pregnancy
  5. Clear cell carcinoma of the vagina occurs rarely—a 1/1000 risk; highest risk for DES-exposed individuals in their early 20s
  6. Columnar epithelium of the vagina is especially susceptible to HPV
  7. Approximately 25% of male offspring affected with cryptorchidism, small testes, epididymal cysts

  8. Most individuals exposed to DES in utero are now 51 years of age or older
  9. Few data thus far support that reproductive tract effects may be passed on to DES granddaughters and grandsons, but studies are ongoing
- Symptoms
  1. Asymptomatic unless has complications related to exposure
  2. May have discharge, postcoital bleeding with cervical or vaginal cancer
  3. May report infertility; poor pregnancy outcomes
- Physical findings
  1. Vaginal adenosis (most common)—glandular tissue extends from the endocervix into the vagina with a red, granular appearance
  2. Nodularity of cervix or vagina
  3. Visible cervical abnormalities (e.g., ridges, cockscomb, collar, hood on anterior cervix, pseudopolyps, hypoplasia)
  4. Transverse or longitudinal vaginal septum
  5. Uterine abnormalities—T-shaped uterus, bicornate or didelphis uterus, septate uterus
- Differential diagnosis
  1. Congenital anomalies
  2. Genetic disorders
- Diagnostic tests/findings
  1. Cervical cancer screening of cervix and all four vaginal walls to rule out malignancy
  2. Colposcopy and biopsy of suspicious areas
  3. Hysterosalpingogram or ultrasonography to evaluate structural anomalies
- Management/treatment
  1. Follow annually with a cervical cancer screening test, with separate specimens from the cervix and all four vaginal walls
  2. Thorough palpation of the cervix and vaginal walls for masses
  3. Colposcopy and/or iodine staining to enhance vaginal wall inspection for adenosis may be considered
  4. Refer if abnormality suspected

Chronic Pelvic Pain

- Definition—noncyclic pain that lasts longer than 6 months, localized to pelvic/lower abdominal/lumbosacral region, and of sufficient severity to cause functional disability and/or lead individual to seek medical care
- Etiology/incidence
  1. Gynecologic, musculoskeletal, GI, urologic, neurologic, and psychosomatic origin
  2. Relationship between pelvic pain and the underlying gynecologic pathology is often inexplicable
  3. Gynecologic causes
     a. Endometriosis
     b. Post-PID chronic pain
     c. Adhesions
     d. Pelvic varicosity pain syndrome/pelvic congestion syndrome
     e. Ovarian mass

f. Uterine fibroids

g. Adenomyosis

h. Vulvodynia

i. Gynecologic malignancies (especially late stage)

4. Nongynecologic causes

a. Painful bladder syndrome/interstitial cystitis

b. Myofascial pain syndrome—may result from repeated microtrauma, acute trauma, or postural misalignment

c. Irritable bowel syndrome

d. GI or urologic malignancies

5. Affects 15%–20% of women aged 18–50 years in the United States

6. Often associated with negative cognitive, behavioral, sexual, and emotional consequences

7. Psychological factors, such as a history of/current physical, sexual, or emotional abuse; depression; and anxiety, are associated with greater pain-related disability

8. Diagnosis is difficult, and patients are often referred to many specialists while becoming frustrated, angry, and/or defensive

- Symptoms

1. Paroxysms of sharp, stabbing, sometimes crampy, or dull continuous pain, usually severe

2. Dysmenorrhea, dyspareunia, dysuria, vulvar or vaginal pain

3. Pain may or may not be reproducible during abdominal and pelvic examination

4. Feeling of pelvic pressure or heaviness

5. Pain history is important—*Onset*, *Location*, *Duration*, *Characteristics*, *Alleviating/aggravating* factors and associated symptoms, *Radiation*, *Temporal*, *Severity* (OLDCARTS)

6. Pelvic pain assessment forms are helpful

- Physical findings

1. Physical and gynecologic examination may be normal

2. Findings consistent with specific gynecologic, urologic, musculoskeletal, neurologic, GI disorder

3. Pain mapping may help to locate painful areas more specifically

- Differential diagnosis—see Etiology/Incidence section

- Diagnostic tests/findings

1. Laboratory studies are often of little value in the diagnosis of chronic pelvic pain

2. Pregnancy test, CBC, ESR, urinalysis, tests for vaginal infections and STIs; stool for occult blood test

3. Pelvic ultrasonography, hysteroscopy

4. If bowel or urinary symptoms—barium enema, upper GI series, IV pyelogram

5. If musculoskeletal disease suspected—lumbosacral radiography and orthopedic consultation

6. Diagnostic laparoscopy

- Management/treatment

1. Treatment of organic pathology if identified (e.g., endometriosis, uterine fibroids, painful bladder syndrome, irritable bowel syndrome, myofascial pain syndrome)

2. Referral for mental health counseling as needed; counseling for prior abuse or trauma

3. May need both medical and psychological management

4. Supplemental therapies may include biofeedback and relaxation techniques, acupuncture, transcutaneous electrical nerve stimulation (TENS), cognitive behavioral therapy

Pelvic Relaxation Disorders

- Definition—nonspecific term denoting a condition occurring chiefly as a result of weakness or defect in supportive muscles and ligaments of the pelvis

1. Cystocele—bulging of the posterior bladder and overlying anterior vaginal wall into the vaginal canal

2. Urethrocele—bulging of the urethra into the anterior wall of the vagina

3. Rectocele—bulging of the anterior rectal wall and posterior vaginal wall into the vaginal canal

4. Enterocele—bulging of a portion of the small intestine into the rectovaginal space between the rectum and posterior vaginal wall

5. Uterine prolapse—descent of the uterus and cervix into the vaginal canal

- Etiology/incidence

1. Weakness in supporting structures including the pelvic diaphragm, ligaments, and fascia—commonly related to neuromuscular injury during vaginal childbirth, which results in denervation injury of the muscular floor; increased incidence with advancing age

2. Other conditions that cause a chronic increase in abdominal pressure—obesity, straining, chronic lung disease (coughing); nerve function altered by diabetes, pelvic surgery, neurologic disorders; hypoestrogenism

- Symptoms

1. May be asymptomatic and discovered during routine examination

2. Pelvic, vaginal, and low back pain and pressure

3. Bulging or mass in the vagina; may make walking uncomfortable; the sensation that things are falling out

4. Urinary incontinence; incomplete bladder emptying; fecal incontinence; difficulty in evacuation of feces

5. Dyspareunia

6. Exposed vagina may become dry and ulcerated; purulent discharge

- Physical findings

1. Bulging of the anterior or posterior vaginal walls; various degrees of descent of the cervix into the vagina indicating uterine prolapse; may need patient to do Valsalva straining maneuvers to assess the full extent of prolapse

2. Poor muscle strength in pubococcygeal muscles

3. Complete prolapse of the uterus (prodentia); ulceration, purulent discharge, bleeding

- Differential diagnosis

1. Tumors of the pelvis or abdomen involving any abdominal structure

2. Diverticulum of urethra

- Diagnostic tests/findings—rule out tumors with appropriate evaluation as indicated
- Management/treatment
    1. Pelvic floor muscle strengthening exercises—Kegel's
    2. Physical therapy with a pelvic floor muscle specialist—may include biofeedback and other modalities to improve the quality of pelvic floor muscle exercises
    3. Local estrogen therapy for postmenopausal individuals
    4. Pessary—alternative to surgery, temporary relief before surgery, requires fitting and patient instruction on insertion/removal and care
    5. Surgical repair for severe prolapses

Toxic Shock Syndrome (TSS)

- Definition—rare, potentially fatal, febrile condition affecting multiple systems
- Etiology/incidence
    1. Associated with toxins produced by strains of *Staphylococcus aureus*
    2. Occurs most often in White individuals younger than 30 years of age using highly absorbent tampons during menstruation; rarely associated with other articles placed in the vagina, such as diaphragms, sponges, and cervical caps
    3. Incidence is 1 to 2 per 100,000 per year in individuals using tampons
    4. Approximately 10% of the population lacks sufficient antitoxin antibodies to *S. aureus*
    5. Nonmenstruation-associated cases (55%)—caused by puerperal sepsis, post-cesarean endometritis, mastitis, PID, wound infection, insects
- Symptoms
    1. Sudden-onset fever, 101°F or greater
    2. Diffuse macular sunburn-like rash over face, trunk, and extremities that desquamates 1–2 weeks after onset
    3. Hyperemia of conjunctiva, oropharynx, tongue, vagina
    4. GI symptoms—nausea, vomiting, diarrhea, abdominal tenderness, dysphagia
    5. Genitourinary symptoms—vaginal discharge, adnexal tenderness
    6. Flulike symptoms—headache, sore throat, myalgia, rigors, photophobia, arthralgia
    7. Cardiorespiratory symptoms—symptoms of pulmonary edema, disseminated intravascular coagulation (DIC), endocarditis, acute respiratory distress syndrome (ARDS)
    8. Organ failure symptoms—renal, hepatic
- Physical findings
    1. Fever
    2. Diffuse macular erythematous rash and desquamation
    3. Hyperemia of conjunctiva, oropharynx, tongue, vagina
    4. Orthostatic hypotension
    5. Abdominal tenderness
    6. Vaginal discharge, adnexal tenderness
    7. Physical signs of pulmonary edema, DIC, endocarditis, ARDS
    8. Altered sensorium
- Differential diagnosis
    1. Septic shock
    2. Rocky Mountain spotted fever
    3. Scarlet fever
    4. Staphylococcal food poisoning
    5. Meningococcemia (meningitis)
    6. Legionnaires' disease
    7. PID
- Diagnostic tests/findings
    1. Cultures to determine the source of infection (e.g., throat, vagina, cervix, blood)
    2. Serologic tests to rule out Rocky Mountain spotted fever, syphilis, rubeola
    3. Urinalysis
    4. Evaluation for the presence of multiple-organ involvement—serum multichemical analysis, clotting profile, blood gases, CBC with differential (platelets numbering 100,000/mm^3)
    5. Diagnostic criteria—involvement of three or more organs or systems that include cardiopulmonary, CNS, hematologic, liver, renal, mucous membranes, musculoskeletal, GI
- Management/treatment
    1. Refer immediately to the hospital for emergency treatment in an intensive care setting
    2. Prevention
        a. Avoidance of tampons, in particular super-absorbent tampons, or leave in place no longer than 4 hours; alternate with pads
        b. Educate regarding signs and symptoms if using a cervical cap, diaphragm, sponge and need for removal as soon as possible if symptoms present and the need for prompt treatment
        c. History of TSS—avoid tampons, cervical caps, diaphragms, sponges

Sexual Dysfunction

- Definition—heterogeneous group of disorders typically characterized by an individual's lowered sexual drive or response, including decreased or absent sexual pleasure when sexual arousal and/or pleasure is desired by the individual; *DSM-5* criteria include experiencing the disorder at least 75% of the time for at least 6 months and causing significant distress for the individual
    1. Female
        a. Hypoactive sexual desire disorder (HSDD)—persistent or recurrent deficient or absent sexual fantasies and desire for sexual activity
        b. Sexual interest/arousal disorder—complete lack of or significant reduction in sexual interest or sexual arousal
        c. Orgasmic disorder—marked delay in, marked infrequency of, or absence of orgasm or reduction of intensity in all or almost all occasions of sexual activity

d. Genito-pelvic pain/penetration disorder—persistent or recurrent difficulties in relation to vaginal penetration
    (1) Dyspareunia—marked vulvovaginal or pelvic pain during sexual intercourse or penetration attempts
    (2) Vaginismus—recurrent or persistent involuntary spasm of the musculature of the outer third of the vagina
    (3) Noncoital pain—for example, vulvodynia, endometriosis, bladder pain syndrome
    (4) Marked fear or anxiety about vulvovaginal or pelvic pain; marked voluntary tensing or tightening of pelvic floor muscles during attempted vaginal penetration
2. Male
    a. Delayed ejaculation—unable to ejaculate during sexual activity, specifically after 25 to 30 minutes of continuous sexual stimulation
    b. Premature ejaculation—early ejaculation during vaginal intercourse; individual feels unable to control orgasm, climaxes in less than 1 minute after vaginal penetration; no duration for oral or manual stimulation established
    c. Erectile disorder (ED)—recurrent inability to achieve or maintain an adequate erection during partnered sexual activities
- Etiology/incidence
1. Prevalence of Female Sexual Problems Associated with Distress and Determinants of Treatment Seeking (PRESIDE) Survey—more than 30,000 participants; 43% reported at least one problem with sexual desire, arousal, or orgasm with or without personal distress; 22% of those reporting a problem indicated personal distress
2. Causes
    a. Relationship factors; other life stressors; medical conditions; medications; substance misuse/disorder; current or past physical, emotional, or sexual abuse; history of sexual assault
    b. Medical conditions—depression; diabetes; thyroid disease; cardiovascular disease; neurologic diseases; chronic pain syndromes; urinary incontinence; androgen insufficiency; estrogen deficiency
    c. Medications—some antidepressants, antihypertensives, lipid-lowering agents, digoxin, combined hormonal contraceptives, histamine H2-receptor blockers, opioids, amphetamines, anticonvulsants
- Symptoms—see definitions for specific sexual dysfunctions; may be lifelong, acquired, or situational
- Physical findings
1. Related to contributing medical conditions
2. Female—genital/pelvic tenderness, lesions, tissue atrophy, masses, muscle spasms related to the underlying cause for genito-pelvic pain/penetration disorder
3. Male—testicular atrophy, abnormal genital reflexes, penile abnormalities related to underlying causes for HSDD or ED
- Differential diagnosis—focused on determining causative factors

- Diagnostic tests/findings—only if indicated by history and physical exam findings; androgen levels and estrogen levels are not recommended
- Management/treatment—dependent on specific dysfunction and causative factors
1. PLISSIT model
    a. *Permission*—validate concerns, express that sexual problems are real and prevalent
    b. *Limited Information*—provide basic education about the sexual response cycle, components of desire, identified causes of problem
    c. *Specific Suggestions*—lubricants, erotica, enhancing clitoral stimulation, positioning for comfort
    d. *Intensive Therapy*—referral to a sex specialist for cognitive-behavioral psychotherapy focused on sexual concerns and solutions
2. Treat underlying medical conditions and consider change in causative medications when appropriate
3. Treat specific causes of genito-pelvic pain if identified
4. Low-dose localized estrogen for postmenopausal vulvovaginal atrophy
5. Flibanserin (Addyi)—FDA approved with indication for treatment of HSDD in premenopausal individuals; oral tablet taken once daily at bedtime
6. Bremelanotide (Vyleesi)—FDA approved with indication for treatment of acquired, generalized HSDD in premenopausal individuals; self-administered subcutaneously into the abdomen or thigh at least 45 minutes before anticipated sexual activity
7. Sildenafil (Viagra), vardenafil, tadalafil—FDA approved with indication for treatment of ED; not FDA approved for use in women
8. Prasterone (Intrarosa)—FDA approved for treatment of postmenopausal individuals experiencing moderate to severe dyspareunia; dehydroepiandrosterone preparation converted into active androgens and estrogens; intravaginal insert used once daily at bedtime
9. Referral to a therapist specializing in sexual dysfunction, mental health specialist, physical therapist specializing in pelvic floor dysfunction, urologist for individuals with ED

Infertility

- Definition—no conception after 1 year of unprotected coitus if younger than age 35; after 6 months if age 35 years or older; inability to carry a pregnancy to live birth
- Etiology/incidence
1. Estimated infertility in the United States is 15% of couples
2. Female factors (25%–50%)
    a. Age-related
    b. Altered menstrual pattern/ovulatory dysfunction—anovulation, luteal-phase insufficiency, inadequate cervical mucus
    c. Pelvic pathology—uterine anomaly, adhesions from surgery or peritonitis, tubal occlusion, endometriosis, leiomyomas
    d. High adverse childhood experiences (ACE) scores

e. History of STIs

f. Genetic or chromosomal differences

g. Endocrine disorders (PCOS, thyroid dysfunction, hyperprolactinemia)

h. Premature ovarian insufficiency

i. Disordered eating, current or history

j. Autoimmune conditions

k. Tubal ligation, known or unknown

3. Sperm-related factors (25%–50%)

   a. Low sperm production—low testosterone (hypogonadism), varicocele, toxin exposure (radiation, chemicals, drugs), chronic overheating of testicles, mumps orchitis (testicular inflammation)

   b. Adhesions in vas deferens—epididymitis, genital tract surgery

   c. Structural/Anatomic abnormalities

     (1) Varicocele—abnormal dilation of peritesticular veins resulting in varicose veins in the spermatic cord

     (2) Hypospadias—a congenital anomaly in which the urethral meatus is located on the ventral surface of the glans, penile shaft, or perineal area

     (3) Phimosis—tight foreskin that cannot be retracted, may be congenital or the result of recurrent infections of the glans penis and prepuce

     (4) Retrograde ejaculation (obstruction)

     (5) History of pelvic/groin surgery, scarring

     (6) Testicular injury or trauma

   d. Erectile dysfunction, anxiety

   e. History of viral infection

   f. Known endocrine disorders

   g. Medications that lowered sperm count

   h. Chemical/Environmental exposure

   i. Age

   j. Chromosomal differences

   k. Genetic disorders

   l. Prior vasectomy, disclosed or undisclosed

   m. History of STIs

4. Combined male and female factors (30%)

5. Unexplained cause (10%–25%)

- Assessment

1. Focused history—both partners

   a. Prior pregnancies, duration of infertility, any previous evaluation and treatment, frequency of intercourse, sexual dysfunction

   b. History of STIs, other genitourinary infections, pelvic or abdominal surgeries

   c. Symptoms of or known diagnosis of endocrine disorders

   d. Prior chemotherapy or treatments for cancer

   e. Current medications (prescription and over the counter)

   f. Smoking, marijuana use, alcohol use, illicit drugs

   g. Exposure to toxic environmental or chemical substances

   h. Family history of congenital anomaly or infertility

2. Additional female medical history—menstrual history, dyspareunia, abnormal cervical cancer screening and treatment

3. Additional male medical history—history of mumps, testicular torsion, regular exposure to high levels of heat, use of anabolic steroids

4. Physical examination—female

   a. Vital signs and BMI

   b. Signs of potential genetic or hormonal abnormalities—short stature, acne, alopecia, hirsutism, galactorrhea, thyroid enlargement, or nodules

   c. Pelvic examination—signs of anatomic abnormalities, masses, infections, hormonal status

5. Physical examination—male

   a. Vital signs and BMI

   b. Breast examination—gynecomastia

   c. Thyroid examination—enlargement, masses

   d. Signs of androgen deficiency

   e. Genital examination—varicocele, infections, hypospadias, phimosis

- Differential diagnosis—related to determining specific cause or causes

- Diagnostic tests/findings

1. Pelvic ultrasound—antral follicle count; uterine anomalies; ovarian volume or mass; persistent ovarian cysts

2. Hysterosalpingogram—tubal patency

3. Basal body temperatures for ovulation detection

4. Ovulation prediction tests—home urine tests to detect LH surge; predicts ovulation within 24 to 36 hours

5. Anti-Müllerian hormone (AMH) level and antral follicle count to determine ovarian reserve

6. FSH, LH, estradiol (E_2), progesterone levels at baseline during cycle days 2–5

7. Progesterone level in the luteal phase, typically day 21 in a 28-day cycle

8. Thyroid panel

9. STI screening if indicated

10. Semen analysis—semen volume; sperm number; sperm concentration, motility, vitality, morphology, pH

- Management/treatment

1. Ovulatory dysfunction—ovulation induction therapy with clomiphene citrate, letrozole

2. Luteal-phase insufficiency—vaginal suppositories, though research indicates minimal to no benefit

3. Infections/endometriosis—appropriate therapy

4. Tubal occlusion/obstruction—consider IVF as the next step vs surgical intervention to attempt clearing blockage

5. Varicocele—surgical repair

6. Intrauterine insemination—if the partner has oligospermia and the gestational partner has normal evaluation, washed sperm (separate motile from nonmotile sperm and other seminal material that may have detrimental effects on fertilization) may be placed in fundus using a catheter; may combine with ovulation induction medications; may be used by a fertile individual who desires pregnancy but does not have a sperm-producing sexual partner (e.g., lesbian, single, transgender male)

7. Assisted reproductive technology (ART)—all the techniques used to achieve pregnancy that involve direct retrieval of oocytes from the ovary

a. In vitro fertilization (IVF)—stimulate multiple eggs to maturation w/FSH/LH containing injectable medications. Oocytes are extracted via ultrasound-guided transvaginal egg retrieval (surgical/under anesthesia) fertilized in the laboratory and monitored for 3–5 days, then transferred via embryo transfer with a small catheter through the cervix into the uterus (success rate dependent on age, up to 70% if genetically tested and found to be euploid
   (1) Recommend single embryo transfer
   (2) Reciprocal IVF with 2 uterus-having partners→ One set of DNA, one carrying partner
b. Intracytoplasmic sperm injection (ICSI)—oocyte directly injected with one sperm; used when the male has a low sperm count; combined with IVF
c. Preimplantation genetic testing–aneuploid (PGT-A) or preimplantation genetic testing–monogenic or single gene disorder (PGT-M) recommended for individuals who are at an increased risk of having a child with a specific genetic disorder
d. Donor egg, donor sperm, donor embryo
8. Sensitive counseling; infertility support groups

Congenital and Chromosomal Abnormalities

Müllerian Abnormalities

- Definition—congenital anomalies involving the uterus, uterine (also called fallopian) tubes, and upper vagina resulting from defects in development of the Müllerian ducts
- Etiology/incidence
  1. Possible causes—teratogenesis, genetic inheritance, and multifactorial expression
  2. As many as 15% of women with recurrent spontaneous abortion and 5%–19% of infertile women have Müllerian abnormality
- Symptoms
  1. History of pregnancy loss or infertility
  2. Amenorrhea, dysmenorrhea
  3. Dyspareunia
- Physical findings
  1. Many variations may occur
     a. Lack of development (agenesis)—no vagina, uterus, tubes, uterine cavity
     b. Incomplete development (hypoplasia)—partial vagina, bicornate uterus, partial uterine cavity
     c. Incomplete canalization (atresia)—imperforate hymen, cervical atresia
     d. One-third have urinary tract abnormalities (e.g., ectopic kidney, renal agenesis, horseshoe-shaped kidney, abnormal collecting ducts)
  2. Ovaries may be developed, resulting in well-developed secondary sexual characteristics

- Differential diagnosis
  1. Various congenital anomalies
  2. Anomalies of the urinary tract
  3. Primary amenorrhea
- Diagnostic tests/findings
  1. Structural abnormalities detected by ultrasonography, MRI, hysterosalpingogram, laparoscopy
  2. Chromosomal abnormalities ruled out with karyotyping (46XX)
- Management/treatment
  1. Referral to reproductive endocrinologist
  2. Surgical intervention

Androgen Insensitivity/Resistance Syndrome

- Definition—genetically transmitted androgen receptor defect; the individual is genotypic male (46XY) but phenotypic female or has both female and male characteristics; the individual has testes that may be partially descended or intra-abdominal
- Etiology/incidence
  1. Transmitted by maternal X-linked recessive gene; a defect in androgen receptors; 25% risk of affected child; 25% risk of carrier
  2. Third most common cause of primary amenorrhea; represents 10% of all cases
  3. Risk of malignant transformation of gonads (5%); incidence of malignancy is rare before puberty
- Symptoms
  1. Often not detected until puberty
  2. Primary amenorrhea
  3. Infertility
- Physical findings
  1. Uterus and ovaries are absent, and a blind pouch vagina is present; labia underdeveloped; absent or scant pubic hair
  2. Normally developed breast with small nipples and pale areola
  3. Inguinal hernias (50%) or labial masses in infant children due to partially descended testes; testes may be intra-abdominal
  4. Scant body hair
  5. Growth and development are normal; overall height usually greater than the female average
  6. May have horseshoe kidneys
- Differential diagnosis
  1. Müllerian anomalies (agenesis)
  2. Incomplete androgen insensitivity
- Diagnostic tests/findings
  1. Karyotype reveals 46XY; phenotypically female or has both female and male characteristics
  2. Testosterone greater than 3 ng/mL and LH levels normal to slightly elevated
- Management/treatment
  1. Once full development is attained (after puberty), gonads should be removed at about age 16 to 18 years
  2. Estrogen replacement therapy after gonads removed
  3. Evaluate other family members; sensitive counseling

Turner Syndrome

- Definition—gonadal dysgenesis; an abnormality in or an absence of one of the X chromosomes; phenotypically female
- Etiology/incidence
  1. Usually a deficiency of paternal contribution of sex chromosomes, reflecting paternal nondisjunction
  2. Occurs in 1 out of 2,500 to 5,000 live-born girls
  3. Most common chromosomal abnormality found on spontaneous abortuses (45X)
  4. Approximately 60% of individuals with Turner syndrome have a total loss of one X chromosome; 40% are mosaics or have structural aberrations in the X or Y chromosome
- Symptoms
  1. Amenorrhea
  2. Lack of sexual development
  3. Infertility
  4. May have autoimmune disorders; Hashimoto's thyroiditis (hypothyroidism [10%] with goiter formation), Addison's disease (adrenal insufficiency), alopecia, and vitiligo
  5. Hearing loss
  6. Normal intelligence; may have difficulty with mathematical ability, visual–motor coordination, and spatial–temporal processing
- Physical findings
  1. No secondary sex characteristics
  2. Uterus and vagina present; absent or streak ovaries; infertile
  3. Short stature, webbed neck, shield chest with widely spaced nipples, increased carrying angle of elbow, arched palate, low neck hairline, short fourth metacarpal bones, disproportionately short legs, swollen hands and feet, lack of breast development, scant pubic hair
  4. Renal (horseshoe kidney) and cardiac anomalies (coarctation of aorta, bicuspid aortic valves, mitral valve prolapse, aortic aneurysm)
  5. Hearing loss
  6. Signs of hypothyroidism, adrenal insufficiency
  7. Alopecia, vitiligo
- Differential diagnosis—other forms of gonadal dysgenesis
- Diagnostic tests/findings
  1. Genetic karyotyping
  2. Ultrasonography or MRI scan
  3. Renal ultrasonography, cardiology consultation
- Management/treatment
  1. Refer to endocrinologist; may need multiple medical specialists to manage multisystem involvement
  2. Estrogen and progesterone replacement
  3. Human growth hormone
  4. Genetic support group

Breast Disorders

Fibrocystic Breast Changes

- Definition—"nondisease" that includes nonproliferative microcysts, macrocysts, and fibrosis, as well as proliferative changes, such as hyperplasia and adenosis;

hyperplasia with atypia is associated with a moderate risk for breast cancer
  1. Cystic changes—refers to dilation of ducts; may regress with menses, may persist, or may disappear and reappear
  2. Fibrous change—mass develops following an inflammatory response to ductal irritation
  3. Hyperplasia—a layering of cells; has malignant potential if atypical
  4. Adenosis—related to changes in the acini in the distal mammary lobule; ducts become surrounded by a firm, hard, plaque-like material
- Etiology/incidence
  1. Etiology not understood; occurs in response to endogenous hormone stimulation, primarily estrogen
  2. Conflicting studies on association with ingestion of foods or beverages containing methylxanthines
  3. Most common benign breast condition in women
  4. Palpable nodular changes observed in more than half of adult women 20 to 50 years of age; most common ages 35 to 50 years
  5. Detectable on radiography in 90% of women age 40 or older
  6. Usually a regression of the signs after menopause
- Symptoms
  1. Breast pain and nodularity; usually bilateral
  2. Frequently occurs or increases 1–2 weeks before menses
  3. May have spontaneous, clear, or white nipple discharge
- Physical findings
  1. Multiple, usually cystic masses that are well defined, mobile, and often tender
  2. Absence of breast skin changes
  3. Most common sites—upper outer quadrant and axillary tail
  4. May have clear to white multi-duct nipple discharge—bilateral or unilateral
- Differential diagnosis
  1. Carcinoma
  2. Galactorrhea
  3. Mastitis
  4. Costochondritis
- Diagnostic tests/findings
  1. Usually none needed
  2. Mammography to identify and characterize masses if age 40 or older
  3. Ultrasound to determine whether the mass is cystic or solid
  4. Fine-needle aspiration (FNA) if dominant mass; cytologic evaluation
  5. Biopsy or excision if dominant mass or the following findings are present:
     a. Bloody fluid on aspiration
     b. Failure of mass to disappear after aspiration
     c. Recurrence of a cyst after two aspirations
     d. Solid mass not diagnosed as fibroma
- Management/treatment
  1. Treatment not necessary
  2. Aspiration of palpable cysts may be curative

3. Patients with symptomatic nodularity or with mastalgia may be treated with nonpharmacologic or pharmacologic therapies
   a. Reassurance; supportive bra
   b. NSAIDs—oral or topical
   c. Reduction in methylxanthines (caffeine, tea, cola, chocolate) has shown limited effectiveness
   d. Hormonal contraception may decrease or increase mastalgia
   e. Danazol, tamoxifen, bromocriptine have all been used to treat severe mastalgia; each has major side effects that limit utility; mastalgia typically returns when discontinuing use

Fibroadenoma

- Definition—benign breast mass derived from fibrous and glandular tissue
- Etiology/incidence
  1. Etiology unknown—development soon after menarche; appears to be hormone related
  2. Most common benign, dominant mass in younger women
  3. Occurs most often in women 15 to 25 years of age
  4. Pregnancy may stimulate growth; may regress with menopause
- Symptoms
  1. Painless, usually single mass
  2. No nipple discharge
  3. Does not change with menstrual cycle
- Physical findings
  1. Firm, well-delineated, freely movable, smooth, rubbery, round, typically 2 to 4 cm marble-sized, nontender mass; usually unilateral; may grow up to 15 cm
  2. No nipple discharge
  3. No breast skin changes
- Differential diagnosis
  1. Carcinoma of the breast
  2. Cystosarcoma phyllodes
  3. Benign cyst
- Diagnostic tests/findings
  1. FNA to determine whether cystic or solid
  2. Excisional biopsy
  3. Ultrasonography and/or mammography will help distinguish singular from multiple nonpalpable masses (ultrasound is the best choice for young women)
- Management/treatment
  1. Observation, if the diagnosis is confirmed and the patient is younger than 25 years
  2. May be removed to alleviate patient anxiety or if the diagnosis is uncertain
  3. Follow up with regular clinical breast examination; screening mammograms per current professional organization recommendations
  4. Key points
     a. No mass is obviously benign—each should be carefully evaluated to rule out carcinoma
     b. Nipple discharge is seldom associated with carcinoma of the breast; when there is spontaneous clear, serous, or bloody discharge or postmenopausal discharge present, cancer should be ruled out with a thorough evaluation
     c. Breast discomfort is usually associated with fibrocystic changes

Intraductal Papilloma

- Definition—benign lesion of the lactiferous duct; most common in the perimenopausal age group, 35–50 years old
- Etiology/incidence
  1. Proliferation and overgrowth of epithelial tissue of the subareolar collection duct
  2. Most common cause of pathologic nipple discharge
- Symptoms
  1. Bloody, serous, or turbid discharge (not milk), which may occur spontaneously
  2. Mass not usually palpable
  3. Feeling of fullness or pain beneath the areola (possible)
- Physical findings
  1. Expression of serosanguinous nipple discharge from a single duct when pressure applied to the affected duct
  2. Poorly delineated, soft mass may be palpated
  3. Usually singular papilloma
  4. No breast skin changes
- Differential diagnosis
  1. Intraductal carcinoma
  2. Multiple papillomatosis
- Diagnostic tests/findings
  1. Excisional biopsy of the duct allows for definitive evaluation
  2. Cytology of fluid—false-negative rates of 20% for cancer
  3. Mammography and/or ultrasound depending on age
  4. Radiologic ductogram—use is controversial, low sensitivity
- Management
  1. Refer for surgical excision
  2. Excisional biopsy is curative

Nonpuerperal/Periductal Mastitis

- Definition—periareolar inflammation with mass or abscess in an individual who is not lactating; most common in reproductive-age group
- Etiology/incidence
  1. May be associated with breast cysts and cyst rupture
  2. Commonly related to *Staphylococcus aureus*
  3. Risk factors—smoking, nipple piercing
- Symptoms
  1. Reddened, painful nipple or breast
  2. May or may not have mass
  3. May or may not have spontaneous purulent nipple discharge
- Physical findings
  1. Subareolar warmth, tenderness, erythema
  2. Fluctuant or indurated mass
  3. Dimpling, nipple retraction
  4. Purulent nipple discharge
  5. Mammary duct fistula at the areolar margin

- Differential diagnosis
  1. Inflammatory breast cancer
  2. Paget's disease of the breast
- Diagnostic tests/findings
  1. Breast ultrasound to assess for abscess and fistula
  2. Biopsy if mass or inflammation persists after treatment
- Management
  1. Oral antibiotic for 10 days with an agent that covers gram-positive organisms—amoxicillin-clavulanate, dicloxacillin, cephalexin
  2. If poor response to the initial antibiotic, culture for methicillin-resistant *Staphylococcus aureus* (MRSA), if positive treat with doxycycline or sulfamethoxazole/trimethoprim
  3. Aspiration or incision and drainage of abscess
  4. Removal of foreign objects (e.g., nipple ring, nipple bar)
  5. Warm packs and NSAIDs for pain relief
  6. Smoking cessation

Mammary Duct Ectasia

- Definition—dilation of ducts with surrounding inflammation and fibrosis
- Etiology/incidence
  1. Most common age 50 and older; increased incidence in smokers
  2. Widening of ducts and thickening of duct walls—ducts fill with desquamated ductal epithelium and secretory proteinaceous contents
  3. Skin bacteria collecting in ducts may cause inflammation and pain
- Symptoms
  1. Green, brown, or black discharge; spontaneous; often bilateral
  2. May have burning, itching, sensation of pulling in the nipple area
- Physical findings
  1. Multicolor, sticky, bilateral, multiductal discharge
  2. May have palpable mass behind the nipple
  3. No breast skin changes
- Differential diagnoses
  1. Intraductal carcinoma
  2. Breast cancer
- Diagnostic tests/findings
  1. Mammography
  2. Ductography
  3. Biopsy if mass is present
- Management
  1. Anti-inflammatory drugs
  2. Antibiotics
  3. Smoking cessation

Breast Carcinoma

- Definition—malignant neoplasm of the breast
- Etiology/incidence
  1. Possible interaction of ovarian estrogen and nonovarian estrogen; estrogen of exogenous origin with susceptible breast tissue
  2. Most common female malignancy—second to lung cancer as the leading cause of cancer-related death
  3. Approximately 287,850 new cases of breast cancer diagnosed and 43,250 deaths from breast cancer in 2022
  4. Incidence increases with age (75% of patients are older than age 40 years)
  5. Cumulative lifetime risk is 12.3%, or 1 in 8
  6. Risk factors
     a. Advancing age
     b. Family history of breast cancer in one or more first-degree relative especially at early age or if male relative
     c. Inherited pathogenic gene variants (previously called mutations) are responsible for approximately 5%–10% of breast cancers; most common in *BRCA1* or *BRCA2* genes
        (1) An estimated 1 in 300–500 individuals in the general population carry a pathogenic variant in *BRCA1* or *BRCA2* genes inherited from a parent—hereditary breast and ovarian cancer (HBOC) syndrome
        (2) An estimated 1 in 40 individuals of Ashkenazi Jewish ancestry carry the pathogenic variant
        (3) Lifetime risk of breast cancer with a *BRCA1* pathogenic variant on average is 57% but may be as high as 85%; the lifetime risk with a *BRCA2* pathogenic variant is approximately 47%; the lifetime risk without a pathogenic variant is 13%
        (4) Approximately 6% of males with a *BRCA2* pathogenic variant eventually develop breast cancer
        (5) Personal and family history is key to determining if an individual is a candidate for genetic counseling and possibly genetic testing; include at minimum first- and second-degree relatives on both sides of the family; specific types of cancer, primary cancer sites, age at diagnosis; update regularly
            (a) Personal history of breast cancer at age ≤ 50 years; triple-negative breast cancer at age ≤ 60 years; breast cancer at any age if Ashkenazi Jewish inheritance; ovarian, fallopian tube, pancreatic, or primary peritoneal cancer; multiple primary cancers
            (b) Family history of known pathogenic gene variant carrier; breast cancer age ≤ 50 years; male breast cancer; ovarian, fallopian tube, primary peritoneal, pancreatic, or metastatic prostate cancer; multiple primary cancers on same side of family
        (6) Goal of risk assessment—identify individuals who may benefit from genetic counseling, genetic testing, enhanced surveillance, other risk management strategies
        (7) Consider genetic counseling and genetic testing for the following:
            (a) Individuals with breast cancer diagnosis who have risk factors for HBOC syndrome

(b) Family members if the individual with breast cancer diagnosis has a positive test for a *BRCA1/BRCA2* pathogenic variant

(c) Individuals assessed to be at high risk for HBOC syndrome because of specific personal or family cancer history characteristics or known *BRCA1/BRCA2* pathogenic variant in family member; results may guide discussion regarding additional or more frequent screening and risk-reducing surgeries

(d) All men with breast cancer diagnosis

d. Other hereditary cancer syndromes associated with breast cancer—Li-Fraumeni, Cowden, and Peutz-Jeghers; pathogenic gene variations in these syndromes often result in cancers that affect multiple organs

e. Personal history of breast, endometrial, or colon cancer

f. Biopsy-confirmed atypical hyperplasia

g. High-dose radiation to the chest

h. High bone density (postmenopausal)

i. Menarche before age 12; menopause after age 55

j. Nulliparity, first full-term pregnancy after 30

k. Obesity (postmenopausal)

l. Heavy alcohol use

m. Dense breasts

(1) Breast density is a measure used to describe the proportion of fibroglandular tissue to fat seen on a mammogram; the greater the amount of fibroglandular tissue, the greater the density

(2) Increased breast density can mask cancers that present as masses on mammography

(3) Increased breast density is an independent risk factor for breast cancer

(4) FDA federal regulations require all mammography facilities to notify patients about the density of their breasts, explain that breast density can influence the accuracy of a mammogram, and recommend they talk to their health care provider about risks for breast cancer and their individual situation No current evidence base for recommendation of alternative or adjunctive tests to screening mammography for individuals with dense breasts who are asymptomatic and have no other risk factors

(5) Individuals with increased breast density and other factors that place them in a high-risk category (e.g., personal or family-known pathogenic variant in a cancer susceptibility gene, strong family history, history of chest radiation therapy) may consider annual screening mammogram and breast MRI (can alternate every 6 months)

- Symptoms
  1. Breast mass—most often upper-outer quadrant
  2. May have spontaneous clear, serous, or bloody nipple discharge
  3. May have retraction, dimpling, skin edema, erythema, irritation
- Physical findings
  1. Mass fixed, poorly defined, irregular, usually nontender
  2. May have nipple discharge, retraction
  3. May have breast skin changes—dimpling, edema, color changes
  4. Enlarged lymph nodes—axillary, supraclavicular, infraclavicular
- Differential diagnosis
  1. Fibroadenoma
  2. Fibrocystic breast changes
  3. Trauma
  4. Mastitis
- Diagnostic tests/findings
  1. Mammogram detects 30%–50% of cancers
  2. Ultrasound to distinguish solid from cystic mass
  3. Histology for definitive diagnosis—specimen obtained through open biopsy, needle biopsy, FNA, or stereotactic core-needle biopsy
  4. MRI—may be useful in identification of multifocal, multicentric, or contralateral tumors
  5. CT scan of liver, lungs, bones to rule out metastasis
  6. Presence of estrogen receptors determined by assay
  7. Sentinel node biopsy
  8. Negative mammogram and negative aspiration cytology do not exclude malignancy
- Management/treatment
  1. Referral to oncologist if malignancy is suspected; staging determines appropriate treatment options
  2. Early breast cancer—surgery or surgery plus radiation; 60%–70% choose lumpectomy, axillary node dissection, and breast radiation
  3. Medical therapy for hormone receptor–positive tumors—tamoxifen, aromatase inhibitors
  4. Radiotherapy and cytotoxic chemotherapy are adjuvant therapy in late disease

Questions

Select the best answer.

1. PMS is suspected when an individual experiences symptoms only during:
   a. ovulation
   b. the luteal phase
   c. the LH surge
   d. the follicular phase

2. Primary dysmenorrhea can best be treated with:
   a. dopamine agonists
   b. GnRH agonists
   c. prostaglandin inhibitors
   d. tricyclic antidepressants

3. The most common cause of chronic pelvic pain in reproductive-age women is:
   a. adenomyosis
   b. endometriosis
   c. pelvic inflammatory infection
   d. uterine fibroids

4. Which of the following contraceptive methods has also been FDA approved for the treatment of endometriosis?
   a. Combination oral contraceptive pills
   b. Levonorgestrel IUS
   c. Progestin-only contraceptive pills
   d. Subcutaneous 104 DMPA

5. A complication of PID is:
   a. adenomyosis
   b. endometriosis
   c. infertility
   d. irritable bowel syndrome

6. The ovulation prediction urine test:
   a. detects the LH surge
   b. detects an increase in progesterone
   c. predicts fertility level
   d. predicts ovulation within 12 hours

7. During a vaginal examination, you observe bulging of the anterior wall when you ask the patient to bear down. This is most likely a:
   a. congenital abnormality
   b. cystocele
   c. rectocele
   d. uterine prolapse

8. The definitive diagnosis of endometriosis is made with:
   a. CT scan
   b. laparoscopy
   c. serum CA-125
   d. transvaginal ultrasound

9. Adenomyosis can be suspected when which of the following is found on physical exam?
   a. boggy, tender uterus
   b. enlarged, irregularly shaped uterus
   c. fixed, retroverted uterus
   d. prolapsed uterus

10. The most common benign neoplasm of the cervix is:
    a. greater vestibular (Bartholin) gland cyst
    b. squamous papilloma
    c. pedunculated myoma
    d. polyp

11. A 22-year-old individual presents with a complaint of clumpy white vaginal discharge and vulvar itching. On examination, a white, thick nonodorous vaginal discharge is noted, along with vulvar and vaginal erythema. pH was performed and was 4.5. The most likely findings on a wet-mount examination will be:
    a. clue cells
    b. lactobacilli
    c. pseudohyphae
    d. trichomonads

12. Characteristics of Turner's syndrome include:
    a. uterus absent, ovaries absent
    b. uterus absent, ovaries present

c. uterus present, ovaries absent
d. uterus present, ovaries present

13. A 58-year-old individual complains of severe vulvar pruritus. On examination of the patient's vulva, you note thinning of the epidermis and loss of pigmentation, as well as maculopapular lesions. You suspect the diagnosis may be:
    a. lichen sclerosus
    b. local allergic reaction
    c. lichen simplex chronicus
    d. vulvodynia

14. Treatment of molluscum contagiosum includes:
    a. azithromycin 1 g orally in a single dose
    b. erythromycin base 500 mg orally four times a day for 21 days
    c. trichloroacetic or bichloroacetic acid (80%–90% solution)
    d. cryotherapy with liquid nitrogen

15. Which of the following best describes the mechanism of action of tranexamic acid in the treatment of heavy menstrual bleeding?
    a. Acts as an antifibrinolytic to block lysis of fibrin clots
    b. Causes rapid growth of the endometrium to control an acute, heavy bleeding episode
    c. Increases the ratio of vasoconstricting prostaglandins to vasodilating prostaglandins
    d. Suppresses endometrial proliferation to manage chronic heavy menstrual bleeding

16. Hirsutism is most commonly seen with:
    a. androgen insensitivity syndrome
    b. Asherman's syndrome
    c. PCOS
    d. Turner's syndrome

17. A 22-year-old patient experiences 6 months of amenorrhea. Laboratory test results include normal prolactin and TSH and a negative pregnancy test. The next action will be to:
    a. administer a progestin challenge test
    b. measure testosterone
    c. order a hysterosalpingogram
    d. order an MRI or CT scan of the pituitary gland

18. A 24-year-old patient presents for a routine wellness visit without any concerns. On physical examination, you note a 2-cm, nontender, fluctuant mass at the inferior aspect of the left labia. The most likely diagnosis is:
    a. greater vestibular (Bartholin) gland cyst
    b. epidermal inclusion cyst
    c. vestibulitis
    d. vulvar carcinoma

19. The pain of primary dysmenorrhea is:
    a. always associated with pathology such as endometriosis
    b. colicky, spasmodic, and sometimes radiating up the back to the shoulders
    c. colicky, spasmodic, and sometimes radiating to the thighs and low back
    d. a dull ache associated with underlying pathology

20. A 16-year-old patient has not yet begun menstruating but does have pubic hair. The patient is best described as having:
    a. Asherman's syndrome
    b. oligomenorrhea
    c. primary amenorrhea
    d. secondary amenorrhea

21. Which of the following is the most accurate method to predict the occurrence of ovulation in an individual with regular 28-day cycles?
    a. Counting cycle length
    b. Evaluation of cervical mucus
    c. LH surge test
    d. Basal body temperature

22. TSS should be suspected in a patient presenting with sudden-onset fever, flulike symptoms, recent tampon use, and:
    a. dysuria
    b. heavy vaginal bleeding
    c. pale conjunctiva and vaginal walls
    d. macular rash on the face and trunk

23. Which of the following components of the PLISSIT model would best describe instructing a couple on the use of water-soluble lubrication for dyspareunia caused by vaginal dryness?
    a. Permission giving
    b. Limited information
    c. Specific suggestions
    d. Intensive therapy

24. PCOS predisposes individuals to an increased incidence of:
    a. adrenal tumors
    b. endometriosis
    c. endometrial cancer
    d. ovarian cancer

25. With which of the following conditions would you expect to see a positive progestin challenge test?
    a. Androgen insensitivity syndrome
    b. Asherman's syndrome
    c. PCOS
    d. Turner's syndrome

26. The most common presenting symptom of vulvar cancer is:
    a. bleeding
    b. pruritus
    c. vaginal discharge
    d. vaginal odor

27. Which treatment for chlamydia should not be used in pregnancy because it may lead to the discoloration of teeth in children?
    a. Ciprofloxacin
    b. Doxycycline
    c. Penicillin
    d. Trimethoprim

28. The ASCCP recommendation for the management of a positive primary HPV screening result is:
    a. colposcopy
    b. reflex testing with genotyping and cytology on specimen
    c. HPV screening with cytology (co-testing) in 1 year
    d. repeat HPV screening in 6 months

29. A 24-year-old nulliparous patient with occasional spontaneous, bilateral milky nipple discharge has no other significant breast findings. The patient has regular menses, a negative pregnancy test, no medications, and reports no use of illicit drugs. Prolactin and TSH levels are normal. An appropriate next step in management for this patient would be:
    a. advise a repeat prolactin level in 1 year
    b. order a breast ultrasound
    c. order an MRI or CT scan of the pituitary gland
    d. start her on a low-dose dopamine agonist

30. A 24-year-old patient presents with a concern regarding a nontender mass in the left breast that does not change during the menstrual cycle. On examination, you note a freely movable, 0.5 cm × 1 cm, firm, rubbery nontender mass. The most likely diagnosis is:
    a. fibroadenoma
    b. fibrocystic breast changes
    c. intraductal papilloma
    d. cystosarcoma phyllodes

31. The ASCCP recommendation for the management of CIN1 is based on:
    a. age
    b. family history of cervical cancer
    c. HPV test results
    d. Previous history of CIN1

32. Which of the following is a potential cause of galactorrhea?
    a. Hyperthyroidism
    b. NSAID use
    c. X-linked genetic conditions
    d. Herpes simplex virus

33. Leiomyomas occurring within the uterine wall are described as:
    a. intramural
    b. pedunculated
    c. subserosal
    d. submucosal

34. The most common presenting symptom of leiomyoma (fibroids) is:
    a. heavy or prolonged menses
    b. GI symptoms
    c. infertility
    d. urinary frequency

35. Another name for a dermoid cyst is:
    a. benign cystic teratoma
    b. follicular cyst
    c. hyperplastic endometrioma
    d. Müllerian cyst

36. Your examination of a 23-year-old patient reveals a diagnosis of external genital warts. You will want to explain to the patient that:
    a. Any sexual partners should have a blood test to see if they have a subclinical infection.
    b. The patient should have cervical cancer screening performed every 6 months.
    c. There is no therapy that will eliminate the HPV virus.
    d. You can prescribe a topical medication today that will eliminate the HPV virus.

37. A 36-year-old patient is seen in your office for her routine annual examination. She has no concerns and is on day 19 of her cycle, which is normally 28 days in length. The pelvic examination reveals a 9-cm firm pelvic mass anterior to the uterus. The most likely diagnosis is:
    a. benign cystic teratoma
    b. ectopic pregnancy
    c. endometrioma
    d. follicular cyst

38. The term for the anatomic abnormality in which an individual has a tight foreskin that cannot be retracted is:
    a. hypospadias
    b. Peyronie's disease
    c. phimosis
    d. varicocele

39. Identify risk factors for cancer of the vulva.
    a. Alcohol intake
    b. Low-risk type HPV infection
    c. Lichen sclerosus
    d. Multiparity

40. The most common presenting symptom of cervical cancer is:
    a. dyspareunia
    b. lower abdominal pain
    c. irregular bleeding
    d. yellow vaginal discharge

41. The ASCCP risk-based management consensus guidelines for cervical cancer screening (CCS) are based on:
    a. current CCS results and past results
    b. the age of the patient
    c. Use of HPV and cytology co-testing
    d. Use of primary HPV screening

42. Persistent vague abdominal pain or discomfort in a 65-year-old woman may be an early sign of:
    a. choriocarcinoma
    b. benign cystic teratoma
    c. endometrial cancer
    d. ovarian cancer

43. A risk factor for endometrial cancer is:
    a. type 1 diabetes
    b. late menopause
    c. low BMI
    d. multiparity

44. The most lethal gynecologic malignancy is:
    a. cervical carcinoma
    b. choriocarcinoma
    c. endometrial carcinoma
    d. ovarian carcinoma

45. A positive "whiff" or amine test is suggestive of:
    a. atrophic vaginitis
    b. bacterial vaginosis
    c. chronic lichen sclerosus
    d. recurrent candidiasis

46. An indicator of loss of lactobacilli in the vagina is:
    a. elevated pH
    b. increased WBCs on wet mount
    c. malodorous vaginal discharge
    d. vaginal itching

47. Trichomoniasis is best treated with:
    a. oral fluconazole
    b. oral metronidazole
    c. topical clindamycin cream
    d. topical metronidazole cream

48. Which of the following treatments for genital warts may be used during pregnancy?
    a. Imiquimod cream
    b. Podophyllin resin
    c. Podofilox gel
    d. Trichloroacetic acid

49. A sexually active 18-year-old patient presents with postcoital spotting, dysuria, and a yellow discharge. On examination, you find the cervix is erythematous and bleeds with contact. The most likely diagnosis is:
    a. cervical cancer
    b. chlamydia
    c. primary syphilis
    d. tampon injury

50. Risk factors for ovarian cancer include:
    a. diabetes
    b. late menopause
    c. history of HPV
    d. oral contraceptive pill use for more than 5 years

51. Recommendations for repeat testing after treatment for chlamydia with doxycycline include:
    a. test of cure 1–2 weeks after treatment if nonadherence is suspected
    b. test of cure 3–4 weeks after treatment for all patients
    c. test for possible reinfection 1 month after treatment
    d. test for possible reinfection 3 months after treatment

52. An effective treatment for the symptomatic relief of herpes genitalis is:
    a. ceftriaxone
    b. famciclovir
    c. silver nitrate
    d. tetracycline

53. A lesion associated with secondary syphilis is:
    a. condyloma acuminata
    b. condyloma lata
    c. molluscum contagiosum
    d. inguinal bubo

54. Primary syphilis may be suspected when the patient presents with:
    a. a maculopapular rash
    b. an indurated, painless ulcer on the cervix
    c. enlarged, tender inguinal lymph nodes
    d. tender vesicles and papules on the vulva

55. Which of the following is considered to be a risk factor for nonpuerperal mastitis?
    a. Cigarette smoking
    b. Dense breast tissue
    c. Fibrocystic breast condition
    d. Heavy alcohol use

56. A 66-year-old patient with a history of pruritus presents with an ulceration of the vulva. The most likely diagnosis is:
   a. chancroid
   b. secondary trauma
   c. syphilis
   d. vulvar carcinoma

57. A 26-year-old patient presents with multiple, painless, umbilicated papules on the mons pubis. The most likely diagnosis is:
   a. condyloma acuminata
   b. condyloma lata
   c. lymphogranuloma venereum
   d. molluscum contagiosum

58. Recurrent Herpes Genitalium usually presents with
   a. a white, curdy, nonodorous discharge
   b. systemic symptoms, such as fever and malaise.
   c. no symptoms at all
   d. prodromal symptoms and localized pain.

59. A menopausal individual with obesity and a history of complicated vaginal childbirth is at increased risk for:
   a. chronic pelvic pain
   b. pelvic relaxation disorders
   c. recurrent UTIs
   d. vulvodynia

60. A 58-year-old patient reports the feeling of "sitting on a ball." The patient has significant constipation and rectal pressure. On examination, you will most likely find a:
   a. cystocele
   b. hemorrhoid
   c. rectocele
   d. urethrocele

61. Vaginal cancer is most commonly found in which part of the vagina?
   a. The hymenal ring
   b. Midway of the vagina
   c. The posterior fourchette
   d. The upper one-third of the vagina

62. Female infants exposed to diethylstilbestrol (DES) in utero are at increased risk for:
   a. breast cancer
   b. ovarian cancer
   c. vaginal cancer
   d. vulvar cancer

63. Initial management for a 30-year-old woman whose brother had breast cancer should be to:
   a. discuss having a risk-reducing bilateral mastectomy
   b. discuss starting her on a selective estrogen receptor modulator
   c. encourage her to have her son tested for *BRCA1/BRCA2* pathogenic variants
   d. refer her for genetic counseling and possible genetic testing

64. The test/procedure used in an infertility workup to help determine ovarian reserve is:
   a. an AMH level
   b. basal body temperature charting
   c. LH levels
   d. hysterosalpinogram

65. The most common cause of pathologic nipple discharge in perimenopausal individuals is:
   a. breast cancer
   b. fibroadenoma
   c. intraductal papilloma
   d. prolactin-secreting pituitary adenoma

66. Pathologic variants (formerly called mutations) in *BRCA1* and/or *BRCA2* genes are responsible for approximately what percentage of female breast cancers?
   a. Less than 5%
   b. 5%–10%
   c. 15%–20%
   d. More than 20%

67. An examination finding that is considered a minimum criterion for empirical treatment of PID in a sexually active patient presenting with lower abdominal or pelvic pain is:
   a. adnexal mass
   b. cervical motion tenderness
   c. fever > 101°F (38.4°C)
   d. vaginal discharge

68. A 16-year-old patient comes to the office because the patient has never had a menstrual period. The patient has normal breast development, scant pubic hair, a vaginal pouch without a cervix, and no palpable uterus or ovaries. The most likely diagnosis is:
   a. androgen insensitivity/resistance syndrome
   b. Müllerian agenesis
   c. Sheehan's syndrome
   d. Turner syndrome

69. The gonads should be removed after puberty in a person with androgen insensitivity/resistance syndrome to prevent:
   a. endometrial hyperplasia
   b. gonadal malignancies
   c. increased risk for breast cancer
   d. psychological trauma

70. The most commonly used method of ART is:
   a. laparoscopy
   b. intracytoplasmic sperm injection (ICSI)
   c. in-vitro fertilization (IVF)
   d. preimplantation genetic testing for monogenic disorders (PGT-M)

71. Turner syndrome can be suspected when the patient has primary amenorrhea and:
   a. a vaginal pouch with an imperforate hymen
   b. cognitive impairments and visual disturbances
   c. normal breast development but lack of pubic and axillary hair growth
   d. short stature and a webbed neck

72. The most common chromosomal abnormality found in pregnancy tissue analyzed after a spontaneous abortion is:
   a. Fitz-Hugh-Curtis syndrome
   b. fragile X syndrome
   c. Müllerian duct abnormalities
   d. Turner syndrome

73. Which of the following statements concerning ovarian cancer is *true*?
    a. *BRCA1* pathogenic variants (previously called mutations) increase risk, but *BRCA2* pathogenic variants do not.
    b. The lifetime risk of ovarian cancer in the general population is 1%–2%.
    c. Ovarian cancer rates are highest among individuals aged 30–45 years.
    d. Use of oral contraceptives for more than 5 years increases the risk of developing ovarian cancer.

74. A patient with latent syphilis may present with:
    a. a maculopapular rash
    b. an indurated painless ulcer
    c. condyloma lata
    d. no signs of infection

75. The CDC recommendation for follow-up of a patient treated for PID with a recommended outpatient regimen is:
    a. Advise the patient to return if pain and/or fever persists more than 5 days.
    b. Reexamine the patient within 72 hours after initiation of treatment.
    c. Retest for chlamydia and gonorrhea in 2 weeks.
    d. See the patient in 1 week to administer a second dose of ceftriaxone IM.

76. Which of the following medications is most likely to cause a metallic taste?
    a. Acyclovir
    b. Azithromycin
    c. Fluconazole
    d. Metronidazole

77. A patient-applied treatment for genital warts is:
    a. bichloroacetic acid
    b. clindamycin cream
    c. imiquimod
    d. podophyllin resin

78. A patient reports a noticeable reduction in sexual interest and arousal. Which of the following criteria must be met for these symptoms to meet the *DSM-5* criteria for sexual dysfunction?
    a. The patient must experience the symptoms 100% of the time.
    b. The symptoms must have been present for at least 1 year.
    c. The patient must also have a decrease in orgasms and/or pain with sex.
    d. The symptoms must cause the patient significant distress.

79. Characteristic "strawberry spots" on the cervix may be seen with:
    a. bacterial vaginosis
    b. chlamydia
    c. herpes genitalis
    d. trichomoniasis

80. Characteristics of vulvodynia include:
    a. diagnosis of a specific cause is needed to guide treatment.
    b. pain is rarely chronic often resolving on its own over time.
    c. pain may be generalized or localized to the vestibule.
    d. dermatoses or inflammation is visible on physical examination.

81. A word "catheter" is used in the treatment of a greater vestibular (also called Bartholin) gland cyst to:
    a. instill local antibiotics to treat or prevent infection
    b. form a fistulous tract to prevent cyst recurrence
    c. provide a permanent structure for drainage of the gland
    d. allow for injection of local anesthesia for pain management

82. A 20-year-old patient presents frequent lower abdominal pain that the patient describes as cramping and sometimes sharp for the past 8 months. The patient has never had sexual intercourse and has mild dysmenorrhea relieved by over-the-counter medications. The lower abdominal pain is severe enough to interfere with normal activities. The most appropriate next question would be:
    a. Is there anything that makes the pain better or worse?
    b. Do you have plans for future pregnancies?
    c. Do you think you might have a sexually transmitted infection?
    d. Do you have any problems with breathing or shortness of breath?

83. A characteristic of lichen simplex chronicus that differentiates it from lichen planus is:
    a. dyspareunia
    b. involvement of other mucosal tissues
    c. thickened, leathery plaques on the labia majora
    d. vaginal discharge/bleeding

84. A routine screening mammogram for a 45-year-old patient indicates dense breast tissue. The patient has no other known risk factors for breast cancer. You would inform the patient that:
    a. annual screening mammograms and breast MRIs are indicated.
    b. testing for BRCA1/2 pathogenic variants is indicated.
    c. there is no increased risk of breast cancer associated with increased breast density.
    d. there may be moderately reduced sensitivity of a mammogram in identifying masses.

85. The recommended treatment regimen for an unpregnant adult weighing 110 kilograms who tested positive for gonococcal infection without concurrent chlamydia on a swab of the pharynx?
    a. Ceftriaxone 500 mg IM in a single dose
    b. Gentamycin 250 mg IM in two divided doses
    c. Doxycycline 100 mg orally 2 times/day for 7 days
    d. Metronidazole 500 mg orally 2 times/day for 7 days

86. Which of the following is recommended during parenteral treatment of pelvic inflammatory disease?
    a. In-patient monitoring for 12 hours
    b. Transition to oral therapy after 24 hours
    c. Oral doxycycline to limit pain on infusion
    d. Concurrent administration of IV glucose

Answers with Rationales

1. **b.** the luteal phase
   PMS is the cyclic occurrence of a group of distressing physical and psychological symptoms in the luteal phase that begins about 5 to 7 days before menses and resolves within about 4 days after the onset of menses.

2. **c.** prostaglandin inhibitors
   Prostaglandin synthetase inhibitors, which are NSAIDs, are the treatment of choice for primary dysmenorrhea. They work best if they are begun at the onset of menses and are continued for 48 to 72 hours. Agents shown to be effective include mefenamic acid, naproxen sodium, ibuprofen, and indomethacin.

3. **b.** endometriosis
   Approximately 7%–10% of premenopausal women are affected by endometriosis; it is the most common cause of chronic pelvic pain.

4. **d.** Subcutaneous 104 DMPA
   Subcutaneous 104 DMPA is an FDA-approved medication for the treatment of endometriosis. Other medical management includes analgesics (NSAIDs) are the first choice), GnRH agonists, and danazol to induce regression of endometrial implants; IM DMPA has also been found to be effective.

5. **c.** infertility
   Approximately 25% of cases of PID result in infertility, ectopic pregnancy, or chronic pelvic pain.

6. **a.** detects the LH surge
   The ovulation prediction urine test detects the LH surge and predicts ovulation within 24 to 36 hours.

7. **b.** cystocele
   A cystocele involves bulging or herniation of the bladder into the vaginal lumen.

8. **b.** laparoscopy
   Direct visualization with laparoscopy or laparotomy reveals classic implants with endometriosis, classified as Stage I—minimal, Stage II—mild, Stage III—moderate, and Stage IV—severe.

9. **a.** boggy, tender uterus
   Physical findings with adenomyosis include a boggy, tender uterus and diffuse globular enlargement (may be 8 to 10 weeks' gestation size) and potentially evidence of anemia.

10. **d.** polyp
    Polyps are the most common benign neoplasm of the cervix. They are seen most often in perimenopausal and multigravida women between the ages of 30 and 50 years.

11. **C.** pseudohyphae
    Symptoms of candidiasis include a curdy white vaginal discharge; vulvar irritation; pruritus; and occasionally dysuria, urgency, frequency of urination, and dyspareunia. The onset of symptoms often occurs after menses or after antibiotic use. In addition to vaginal discharge, physical examination findings may include erythema of the vulva secondary to itching and a white, thick vaginal discharge that can adhere to the vaginal side walls.

12. **c.** uterus present, ovaries absent
    Physical characteristics found in persons with Turner syndrome include lack of breast development, scant pubic hair, normal uterus and vagina, absent or streak ovaries, short stature, webbed neck, and shield chest with widely spaced nipples. Cardiac and renal anomalies may also be present.

13. **a.** lichen sclerosus
    Lichen sclerosus is a chronic, progressive inflammatory skin condition primarily affecting the perineal and perianal areas. Symptoms include pruritus, dysuria, and dyspareunia. Physical examination findings include maculopapular lesions and plaques; loss of pigmentation; markedly thin, white epidermis; loss of vulvar architecture with obliteration of the clitoris; and introital stenosis. There is symmetry in the distribution of skin changes extending around the anal region (figure of eight).

14. **d.** cryotherapy with liquid nitrogen
    Molluscum contagiosum usually resolves spontaneously without scarring. Treatment options include superficial incision, expressing contents with a comedone extractor, curettage with cautery, and cryotherapy with liquid nitrogen (most often used if the patient has multiple lesions).

15. **a.** Acts as an antifibrinolytic to block lysis of fibrin clots
    Tranexamic acid is effective in blocking lysis of fibrin clots and, when taken up to the first 5 days of menses, reduces heavy menstrual bleeding in women who have increased endometrial plasminogen activity.

16. **c.** PCOS
    Physical findings related to androgen excess with PCOS may include acne, hirsutism, male pattern baldness, deepening of the voice, and enlargement of the clitoris.

17. **a.** administer a progestin challenge test
    To evaluate an amenorrheic patient, obtain a pregnancy test, serum prolactin level, and TSH test. If all these tests are negative or normal, evaluate the availability of estrogen with a progestin challenge test. Provide oral progestin each day for 10 to 14 days, and then wait for bleeding, which should occur within 7 to 14 days. A positive progestin challenge test indicates adequate estrogen production and stimulation as well as no problem with outflow tract.

18. **a.** Greater vestibular (also called Bartholin) gland cyst
    The greater vestibular glands are located at the inferior aspects of the labia (4 o'clock and 8 o'clock). Cysts within these glands are generally unilateral, 1 to 3 cm in size, nontender (unless there is an abscess), and fluctuant.

19. **c.** colicky, spasmodic, and sometimes radiating to the thighs and low back
    Primary dysmenorrhea is characterized by pain that begins shortly before the onset of menses and usually lasts no longer than 2 days. The pain is described as colicky, crampy, and spasmodic in the lower abdomen, but sometimes radiates to the lower back and thighs. There is no associated underlying pathology.

20. **c.** primary amenorrhea
    Primary amenorrhea is characterized by no menstruation by age 14 in the absence of secondary sex characteristics or by age 16, regardless of the development of secondary sex characteristics.

21. **c.** LH surge test
    Ovulation prediction tests detect LH in the urine. A surge of LH precedes ovulation. LH can be detected in the urine a few hours after the surge and within 24 to 26 hours of ovulation.

22. **d.** macular rash on the face and trunk
    TSS is characterized by sudden-onset fever of 102°F or greater and a diffuse macular sunburn-like rash over the face, trunk, and extremities that desquamates 1 to 2 weeks after onset.

23. **c.** Specific suggestions
    The PLISSIT model (P = permission giving, LI = limited information, SS = specific suggestions, IT = intensive therapy) may be used by clinicians who are not sex therapists when counseling patients with sexual dysfunction. Instructing a couple on the use of water-soluble lubrication for dyspareunia caused by vaginal dryness constitutes a specific suggestion.

24. **c.** endometrial cancer
    Individuals with PCOS are at risk for future development of endometrial cancer related to chronic anovulation and unopposed estrogen.

25. **c.** PCOS
    A positive progestin challenge test indicates the individual who is not having menses has adequate production of estrogen, is able to develop a proliferative endometrium, and has an unobstructed outflow tract.

26. **b.** pruritus.
    Symptoms associated with vulvar cancer include vulvar pruritus (most common), pain, burning, bleeding, odorous discharge that may be tinged with blood, and lesions.

27. **b.** Doxycycline
    Doxycycline should not be used in pregnancy because it may cause discoloration of teeth in children.

28. **b.** reflex testing with genotyping and cytology on specimen.
    ASCCP recommendation is that all positive primary HPV screening results should have reflex testing to include both genotyping if not already done and cytology from the same specimen, if possible, to inform decision making

29. **a.** advise a repeat prolactin level in 1 year
    The patient with galactorrhea who has regular menses and normal prolactin and TSH levels may be followed with yearly prolactin levels.

30. **a.** fibroadenoma
    Fibroadenomas are firm, well-delineated, freely movable, smooth, rubbery, round, typically marble-sized, nontender masses. They usually occur on a unilateral basis.

31. **d.** previous history of CIN1
    The ASCCP preferred recommendation for management of CIN1 is observation to avoid unnecessary procedures in low-risk patients, but treatment is acceptable with persistent CIN1 for 2 years or more.

32. **a.** Hyperthyroidism
    Potential causes of galactorrhea include hypothyroidism/hyperthyroidism, use of some medications, use of opiates or cannabis, excessive breast stimulation, and pituitary adenoma.

33. **a.** intramural
    Leiomyomata can be found in different areas within and around the uterine cavity and surrounding ligaments. Submucosal myomas protrude into the uterine cavity. Subserosal myomas bulge through the outer uterine wall. Intraligamentous myomas are found within the broad ligament. Intramural myomas stay within the uterine wall; they are the most common form of myoma. Pedunculated myomas are found on a thin pedicle or stalk attached to the uterus.

34. **a.** heavy or prolonged menses
    Patients with leiomyomata uteri (fibroids) are usually asymptomatic. If they do have symptoms, heavy or prolonged menstrual bleeding is the most common presentation.

35. **a.** benign cystic teratoma
    A dermoid cyst is also known as a benign cystic teratoma. It is the most common ovarian germ cell tumor.

36. **c.** There is no therapy that will eliminate the HPV virus.
    The goal of treatment for genital warts is to eliminate visible lesions; however, no therapy can completely eliminate the HPV virus.

37. **a.** benign cystic teratoma
    Benign cystic teratomas usually measure between 5 and 10 cm in diameter and are composed of well-differentiated tissue from all three germ layers. They are often located anterior to the uterus. Patients are usually asymptomatic but may experience acute pain if the teratoma twists or ruptures.

38. **c.** phimosis
    The term for the anatomic abnormality in which an individual has a tight foreskin that cannot be retracted is phimosis. Phimosis may be congenital or the result of recurrent infections of the glans penis and prepuce and may contribute to infertility.

39. **c.** Lichen sclerosus
    Risk factors for vulvar cancer includes high-risk type HPV infection, lichen sclerosus, and cigarette smoking.

40. **c.** irregular bleeding
    Early in the disease process, individuals with cervical carcinoma may be asymptomatic. The most common presenting symptom of advanced cervical cancer is irregular, painless bleeding or odorous, bloody, or purulent discharge. Late symptoms include pelvic or epigastric pain and urinary or rectal symptoms.

41. **a.** current CCS results and past results
    The ASCCP recommendations for management of CCS results are based on an estimation of risk of CIN3+ based on combination of current CCS results and past results.

42. **d.** ovarian cancer
    Early signs of ovarian carcinoma include abdominal discomfort or pain, pressure sensation on the bladder or rectum, pelvic fullness or bloating, and vague GI symptoms.

43. **b.** late menopause
    Risk factors for endometrial carcinoma include type 2 diabetes, BMI greater than 25, hypertension, family history, early menarche, late menopause, unopposed estrogen therapy, oligo-ovulation, anovulation, and estrogen-secreting tumors (granulosa cell).

44. **d.** ovarian carcinoma
    The mortality rate for ovarian carcinoma exceeds that of all other genital tract malignancies.

45. **b.** bacterial vaginosis
    A positive "whiff" test is the fishy odor that may be found when 10% KOH is added to a vaginal discharge sample of a patient with bacterial vaginosis. The whiff test is part of Amsel's criteria for diagnosing bacterial vaginosis, along with vaginal pH ≥ 4.5, clue cells on saline wet mount, and homogeneous white discharge coating the vaginal wall.

46. **a.** elevated pH
    Loss of lactobacilli (hydrogen peroxide–producing strains) in the vagina results in an elevated pH. An elevated pH may predispose an individual to bacterial vaginosis.

47. **b.** oral metronidazole
    For the treatment of trichomoniasis, the CDC recommends metronidazole 2 g orally in a single dose.

48. **d.** Trichloroacetic acid
    For the treatment of genital warts in pregnancy, the CDC recommends trichloroacetic or bichloroacetic acid (80%–90% solution). Imiquimod cream, podophyllin resin, and podofilox gel should not be used during pregnancy.

49. **b.** chlamydia
    Symptoms of chlamydia may include postcoital bleeding; intermenstrual bleeding or spotting; symptoms of urinary tract infection—dysuria, frequency; vaginal discharge; and abdominal pain. Physical findings may include mucopurulent endocervical discharge; an edematous, tender cervix with easily induced bleeding; and slight tenderness upon palpation of the suprapubic area.

50. **b.** late menopause
    Risk factors for ovarian carcinoma include low parity; early menarche; late menopause; and history of breast, colon, or endometrial cancer.

51. **d.** test for possible reinfection 3 months after treatment.
    A test of cure is not recommended for nonpregnant individuals after treatment for chlamydia with a CDC-recommended regimen. A majority of posttreatment infections are reinfections. The CDC recommends retesting the patient 3 months after treatment ends.

52. **b.** famciclovir
    Acyclovir, famciclovir, and valacyclovir are systemic antiviral drugs that partially control the symptoms of herpes genitalis. These medications do not eradicate latent virus or affect the risk, recurrence, frequency, or severity of symptoms once the drug is discontinued; suppressive therapy may reduce viral shedding.

53. **b.** condyloma lata
    Patients with secondary syphilis may present with localized or diffuse mucocutaneous lesions on the palms and soles, mucous patches, and condyloma lata. They may also have generalized lymphadenopathy along with flu-like symptoms (low-grade fever, headache, sore throat, malaise, arthralgias).

54. **b.** an indurated, painless ulcer on the cervix
    Primary syphilis should be suspected if a person presents with a painless, ulcerated lesion with raised border; indurated base; and rolled edges on the vulva, vagina, cervix, penis, or other site of potential entry of the syphilis organism. The primary syphilis lesion spontaneously disappears in 1 to 6 weeks.

55. **a.** Cigarette smoking
    Cigarette smoking and nipple piercing are considered to be risk factors for nonpuerperal mastitis.

56. **d.** vulvar carcinoma
    The most common signs and symptoms of vulvar carcinoma include pruritus (most common); pain; burning; bleeding lesions that may be darkly or irregularly pigmented, white or red, multifocal or singular, and flat, wartlike, or scaly; erythematous irritated ulceration; and odorous discharge that may be tinged with blood.

57. **d.** molluscum contagiosum
    Molluscum contagiosum presents with characteristic light-colored papules with umbilicated centers on the trunk, lower extremities, abdomen, inner thigh, or genital area.

58. **d.** prodromal symptoms and localized pain
    A recurrent genital herpes infection usually is associated with prodromal symptoms followed by localized pain or tingling sensation. A primary outbreak typically presents with systemic symptoms such as fever, malaise, and headache.

59. **b.** pelvic relaxation disorders
    Pelvic relaxation disorders result from weakness in supporting structures, including the pelvic diaphragm, ligaments, and fascia. Causes include neuromuscular injury at childbirth, which results in denervation injury of the muscular floor, as well as conditions that cause a chronic increase in abdominal pressure—obesity, straining, chronic lung disease (coughing); nerve function altered by diabetes, pelvic surgery, neurologic disorders; and hypoestrogenism.

60. **c.** rectocele
    A rectocele typically presents as a bulging or herniation of the anterior rectal wall and posterior vaginal wall into the opening of the vagina. Constipation, rectal pressure, and a sensation of "sitting on a ball" are symptoms that may occur with a significant rectocele.

61. **d.** The upper one-third of the vagina
    The most common site of vaginal carcinoma is the upper one-third of the vagina.

62. **c.** vaginal cancer
    Females exposed to DES in utero are at increased risk for clear cell carcinoma of the vagina (although rarely; the risk is 1 in 1,000).

63. **d.** refer her for genetic counseling and possible genetic testing

    Having a brother with breast cancer places a woman at high risk for hereditary breast and ovarian cancer syndrome. Genetic counseling and genetic testing may guide the discussion regarding additional or more frequent screening and risk-reducing surgeries.

64. **a.** an AMH level

    The test commonly used in an infertility workup to determine an individual's ovarian reserve is an AMH level.

65. **c.** intraductal papilloma

    An intraductal papilloma is a benign lesion of the lactiferous duct found most commonly in the perimenopausal age group, 35–50 years old. It is the most common cause of pathologic nipple discharge.

66. **b.** 5%–10%

    Pathogenic variants in *BRCA1* and/or *BRCA2* genes are responsible for approximately 5%–10% of female breast cancers.

67. **b.** cervical motion tenderness

    The minimum criterion for empirical treatment of PID in sexually active young individuals and others at risk for STIs with a complaint of pelvic or lower abdominal pain includes the presence of one or more of these three findings on pelvic examination: uterine tenderness, adnexa tenderness, cervical motion tenderness.

68. **a.** androgen insensitivity/resistance syndrome

    Androgen insensitivity/resistance syndrome is a genetically transmitted androgen receptor defect. The individual is a genotypic male (46XY) but a phenotypic female or has both female and male characteristics. The individual has normally developed breasts with small nipples and areola, scanty or absent pubic hair, a blind vaginal pouch, and no uterus or ovaries. Testes are present and may be partially descended or intra-abdominal.

69. **b.** gonadal malignancies

    Once full development is attained (after puberty) in a person with androgen insensitivity syndrome, gonads should be removed at about age 16–18 years to reduce the risk of malignant transformation of the gonads (5%). Incidence of malignancy is rare before puberty.

70. **c.** in-vitro fertilization (IVF)

    IVF is the most commonly used ART, with a success rate of 15%–20%. IVF comprises a series of complex procedures wherein the oocytes are extracted, fertilized in the laboratory, and then transferred through the cervix into the uterus.

71. **d.** short stature and a webbed neck.

    Individuals with Turner syndrome phenotypically present with short stature, a webbed neck, a shield chest with widely spaced nipples, increased carrying angle of the elbow, an arched palate, a low-neck hairline, short fourth metacarpal bones, disproportionately short legs, swollen hands and feet, lack of breast development, and scant pubic hair.

72. **d.** Turner syndrome

    Turner syndrome (45X) is the most common chromosomal abnormality found in spontaneous abortuses.

73. **b.** The lifetime risk of ovarian cancer in the general population is 1%–2%

    The lifetime risk for ovarian cancer in the general population is 1%–2%. The presence of *BRCA1* or *BRCA2* pathogenic gene variants (formerly called mutations) increases this risk. The use of oral CHCs for more than 5 years decreases the risk.

74. **d.** no signs of infection

    Patients with latent syphilis show no signs of infection; detection is through serologic testing.

75. **b.** Reexamine the patient within 72 hours after initiation of treatment.

    After treatment for PID, follow-up and reexamination within 72 hours posttreatment are recommended. If the patient has not significantly improved, review the diagnosis and treatment; the patient may need hospitalization.

76. **d.** Metronidazole

    Side effects of metronidazole include metallic taste, nausea, headache, dry mouth, and dark-colored urine.

77. **c.** imiquimod

    Patient-applied treatments for genital warts include imiquimod cream, podofilox gel or solution, and sinecatechins ointment.

78. **d.** The symptoms must cause the patient significant distress.

    The *DSM-5* criteria for the diagnosis of sexual dysfunction include sex-related symptoms that occur at least 75% of the time for at least 6 months and cause significant distress for the individual.

79. **d.** trichomoniasis

    A classic (although not always present) examination finding with trichomoniasis is punctate red lesions on the cervix often called "strawberry spots."

80. **c.** pain may be generalized or localized to the vestibule.

    Generalized vulvodynia may involve the mons pubis, labia majora, labia minora, and perineum. Provoked, localized vulvodynia involves the vestibule and clitoris and is provoked by any attempt at vaginal penetration or tampon insertion. By definition, vulvodynia occurs in the absence of relevant physical findings or a specifically clinically identifiable neurologic disorder. Long-term chronic therapy is often needed.

81. **b.** form a fistulous tract to prevent cyst recurrence

    A Word catheter can be placed near the incision and drainage of a greater vestibular (also called Bartholin) gland cyst for 4–6 weeks until a fistulous tract forms for continuous drainage and prevention of recurrence.

82. **c.** Do you think you might have a sexually transmitted infection?

    The patient reported never having sexual intercourse. Chronic pelvic pain can have gynecologic or nongynecologic causes. Questions concerning symptoms (e.g., gastrointestinal, urologic) of potential nongynecologic causes should be included in the history. Asking if anything makes the pain better or worse is a component of any assessment regarding pain.

83. **c.** thickened, leathery plaques on the labia majora
Lichen simplex chronicus is a thickening of the skin in response to chronic rubbing or scratching. It may be an atopic reaction or a reaction to a chronic underlying skin condition. Excoriations and erosions from scratching may be seen. Symptoms include a chronic itch-scratch cycle.

84. **d.** there may be moderately reduced sensitivity of a mammogram in identifying masses.
Increased breast density can mask cancers that present as masses on mammography. Increased breast density is an independent risk factor for breast cancer. There is no current evidence for recommending alternative or adjunctive tests if the individual is asymptomatic and has no other risk factors.

85. **a.** Ceftriaxone 500 mg IM in a single dose
Per the CDC guidelines (2021), a single 500 mg dose of IM ceftriaxone. If chlamydial infection has not been excluded, concurrent treatment for chlamydia with doxycycline 100 mg orally 2 times/day for 7 days is warranted. For persons weighing ≥150 kg, 1 g ceftriaxone should be administered.

86. **c.** Oral doxycycline to limit pain on infusion
Doxycycline can be associated with pain on IV infusion, thus oral administration should be offered where possible. There is no difference in bioavailability between oral and parenteral administration.

Bibliography

American Cancer Society. (2022a). *Breast cancer*. https://www.cancer.org/cancer/breast-cancer.html

American Cancer Society. (2022b). *Breast cancer in men*. https://www.cancer.org/cancer/breast-cancer-in-men.html

American Cancer Society. (2022c). *Cancer facts & figures*. https://www.cancer.org/research/cancer-facts-statistics/all-cancer-facts-figures/cancer-facts-figures-2022

American College of Obstetrics and Gynecologists. (2012, reaffirmed 2016). Practice bulletin 128: Diagnosis of abnormal uterine bleeding in reproductive-aged women. *Obstetrics and Gynecology*, 120(1), 197–206.

American College of Obstetricians and Gynecologists. (2013a, reaffirmed 2019). Committee opinion 557: Management of acute abnormal uterine bleeding in nonpregnant reproductive-aged women. *Obstetrics and Gynecology*, 121(4), 891–896.

American College of Obstetricians and Gynecologists. (2017a, reaffirmed 2019). Practice bulletin 179: Breast cancer risk assessment and screening in average-risk women. *Obstetrics & Gynecology*, 130:e-1–16. https://doi.org/10.1097/AOG.0000000000002158.

American College of Obstetricians and Gynecologists. (2017b, reaffirmed 2019). Practice bulletin 182: Hereditary breast and ovarian cancer syndrome. *Obstetrics and Gynecology*, 130(3), e110–e126.

American College of Obstetricians and Gynecologists. (2019a). Committee opinion 781: Infertility workup for the women's health specialist. *Obstetrics and Gynecology*, 133(6), e377–e384.

American College of Obstetricians and Gynecologists. (2019b). Practice Bulletin 213: Female sexual dysfunction. *Obstetrics and Gynecology*, 134(1), e1–e13.

American College of Obstetricians and Gynecologists. (2019c). Practice bulletin 214: Pelvic organ prolapse. *Obstetrics and Gynecology, 134*(5), e126–140.

American College of Obstetricians and Gynecologists. (2020). Practice bulletin 218: Chronic pelvic pain. *Obstetrics and Gynecology, 135*(3), e98–108.

American Psychiatric Association. (2022). *Diagnostic and statistical manual of mental disorders* (5th ed. with text revision [DSM-5-TR]). American Psychiatric Association.

Ball, J., Dains, J., Flynn, J., Solomon, B., & Stewart, R. (2019). *Seidel's guide to physical examination* (9th ed.). Mosby.

Barnabei, V. M. (2020). Vulvodynia. *Clinical Obstetrics and Gynecology, 63*(4), 752–769.

Centers for Disease Control and Prevention. (2021a). Sexually transmitted diseases treatment guidelines, 2021. *Morbidity and Mortality Weekly Report, 70*(4);1–187.

Centers for Disease Control and Prevention. (2021b). *Diseases characterized by urethritis and cervicitis*. Sexually transmitted diseases treatment guidelines, 2021. https://www.cdc.gov/std/treatment-guidelines/urethritis-and-cervicitis.htm

Egger, M., & Lam, D. (2018). Dense breasts: Cancer risk and supplemental imaging modalities. *Women's Healthcare: A Clinical Journal for NPs, 6*(1), 10–14.

Gershenson, G., Lentz, G., Valea, F., & Lobo, R. (2021). *Comprehensive gynecology* (8th ed.). Elsevier.

Holland, A., & Choma, K. (2021). Cervical cancer prevention: review of the past, present, and future. *Women's Healthcare: A Clinical Journal for NPs, 9*(1), 16–20, 29.

International Pelvic Pain Society. (2009). *Pelvic pain assessment form*. https://www.pelvicpain.org

Marnach, M. L., & Laughlin-Tommaso, S. K. (2019). Evaluation and management of abnormal uterine bleeding. *Mayo Clinic Proceedings, 94*(2), 326–335.

Mahshid, T., Azam, B., Abbas, R. F., Nikmanesh, B., & Modarres, M. (2015). Treatment of vitamin D deficiency is an effective method in the elimination of asymptomatic bacterial vaginosis: A placebo-controlled randomized clinical trial. *Indian Journal of Medical Research, 141*(6): 799–806.

McCabe, M. P., Sharlip, I. D., Lewis, R., et al. (2016). Incidence and prevalence of sexual dysfunction in women and men: A consensus statement from the Fourth International Consultation on Sexual Medicine 2015. *Journal of Sexual Medicine,13*(2), 144–152.

McCance, K., & Huether, S. (2017). *Pathophysiology: The biologic basis for disease in adults and children* (8th ed.). St. Louis, MO: Mosby.

Munro, M. G., Critchley, H. O., Broder, M. S., & Fraser, I. S. (2011). FIGO classification system (PALM-COEIN) for causes of abnormal uterine bleeding in nongravid women of reproductive age. FIGO Working Group on Menstrual Disorders. *International Journal Gynaecology and Obstetrics, 113*, 3–13.

National Association of Nurse Practitioners in Women's Health. (2022). *NPWH Position Statement: Hereditary Breast and Ovarian Cancer Risk Assessment*. National Association of Nurse Practitioners in Women's Health.

National Cancer Institute (NCI). (2019b). *Cancer stat facts: Ovarian cancer*. https://seer.cancer.gov/statfacts/html/ovary.html

National Cancer Institute (NCI). (2022). *Cancer stat facts: Female breast cancer*. https://seer.cancer.gov/statfacts/html/breast.html

National Comprehensive Cancer Network (NCCN). (2022). *NCCN clinical practice guidelines in oncology*. https://www.nccn.org/professionals/physician_gls/default.aspx

Perkins, R. B., Guido, R. S., Castle, P. E. et al. (2020). 2019 ASCCP risk-based management consensus guidelines for abnormal cervical cancer screening tests and cancer precursors. *Journal of Lower Genital Tract Disease, 24*(2),102–131.

Phillippi, J. & Kantrowitz-Gordon, I. (Eds.). (2025). *Varney's midwifery* (7th ed.). Jones & Bartlett Learning.

Schadewald, D., Pritham, U., Youngkin, E., Davis, M., & Juve, C. (2020). *Women's health: A primary care clinical guide* (5th ed.). Pearson Education.

Schuiling, K. D., & Likis, F. E. (2022). *Gynecologic health care* (4th ed.). Jones & Bartlett Learning.

Shifren, J., Monz, B., Russo, P., Segreti, A., & Johannes, C. (2008). Sexual problems and distress in United States women: Prevalence and correlates. *Obstetrics and Gynecology*, 112, 970–978.

Taylor, H. S., Pal, L., & Seli, E. (2019). *Speroff's clinical gynecology, endocrinology, and infertility* (9th ed.). Lippincott Williams & Wilkins.

Tharpe, N. L., Farley C. L., & Jordan, R. G. (2022). *Clinical practice guidelines for midwifery and women's health* (6th ed.). Jones & Bartlett Learning.

United States Prevention Services Task Force. (2019). *BRCA-related cancer: Risk assessment, genetic counseling, and genetic testing.* https://www.uspreventiveservicestaskforce.org/uspstf/recommendation/brca-related-cancer-risk-assessment-genetic-counseling-and-genetic-testing

Wellette, J. N., Rivas, S. J., & Davis, M. G. (2023). Clinical presentation, diagnosis, and management of mycoplasma genitalium. *Women's Healthcare: A Clinical Journal for NPs, 11*(1), 33–35.

Yudasz, S. (2020). Assessment and management of benign breast lesions: Role of the WHNP. *Women's Healthcare: A Clinical Journal for NPs, 8*(6), 32–36.

CHAPTER 6

Prenatal Care and Assessment of Fetal Well-Being

Jamille Nagtalon-Ramos
Melicia Escobar

Human Reproduction and Fertilization

- Process of gametogenesis
  1. Definition—development of gametes; oogenesis or spermatogenesis
  2. Essential concepts
     a. Oogenesis—developmental process by which the mature human ovum is formed; haploid number of chromosomes
     b. Spermatogenesis—formation of mature functional spermatozoa; haploid number of chromosomes
     c. Meiosis—a process of two successive cell divisions, producing cells, egg, or sperm that contain half the number of chromosomes found in somatic cells
     d. Mitosis—type of cell division of somatic cells in which each daughter cell contains the same number of chromosomes as the parent cell
     e. Haploid number of chromosomes 23—possessing half the diploid or normal number of chromosomes (i.e., 46) as found in somatic or body cells
- Process of fertilization
  1. Definition—the union of ovum and spermatozoon; usually occurs in a fallopian tube within minutes or no more than a few hours of ovulation; most pregnancies occur when intercourse or insemination occurs within 2 days of ovulation
  2. Stages of development

     a. Zygote—a diploid cell with 46 chromosomes that results from the fertilization of the ovum by a spermatozoon
     b. Blastomeres—mitotic division of the zygote (cleavage) yields daughter cells called blastomeres
     c. Morula—the solid ball of cells formed by 16 or so blastomeres; a mulberry-like ball of cells that enters the uterine cavity 3 days after fertilization
     d. Blastocyst—after the morula reaches the uterus, fluid accumulates between blastomeres, converting the morula to a blastocyst; the inner cell mass at one pole becomes the embryo, the outer cell mass becomes a trophoblast
     e. Embryo—stage in prenatal development between the fertilized ovum and the fetus (i.e., between 2nd and 8th weeks inclusive)
     f. Fetus—the developing conceptus after the embryonic stage
     g. Conceptus—all tissue products of conception: embryo or fetus, fetal membranes, and placenta
- Physiology of implantation of the blastocyst
  1. Definition—blastocyst adheres to the endometrial epithelium by gently eroding between the epithelial cells of the surface endometrium; invading trophoblasts burrow into the endometrium; the blastocyst becomes encased and covered over by the endometrium
  2. Implantation occurs 6–7 days after fertilization and usually in the upper, posterior wall of the uterus
  3. Provides physiologic exchange between the maternal and embryonic environment prior to full placental function

Development of the Placenta, Membranes, and Amniotic Fluid

- Essential concepts
  1. Chorion—an extra-embryonic membrane that, in early development, forms the outer wall of the blastocyst; from it develops the chorionic villi, which establish an intimate connection with the endometrium, giving rise to the placenta
  2. Chorion frondosum—the outer surface of the chorion whose villi contact the decidua basalis; the placental portion of the chorion
  3. Chorion laeve—smooth, nonvillous portion of the chorion
  4. Syncytiotrophoblast—the outer layer of cells covering the chorionic villi of the placenta that are in contact with the maternal blood or decidua
  5. Cytotrophoblast—the thin inner layer of the trophoblast composed of cuboidal cells
  6. Decidua capsularias—the part of the decidua that surrounds the chorionic sac
  7. Decidua basalis—the part of the uterine decidua that unites with the chorion to form the placenta
  8. Decidua parientalis (vera)—the endometrium during pregnancy, except at the site of the implanted blastocyst
  9. Amnion—the innermost fetal membrane; a thin, transparent sac that holds the fetus suspended in the amniotic fluid; it grows rapidly at the expense of the extra-embryonic coelom; by the end of the 3rd month, it fuses with the chorion, forming the amniochorionic sac, commonly called the "bag of waters"
- Placenta
  1. Function—serves as fetal lungs, liver, and kidneys until birth, while growing and maintaining the conceptus in a balanced, healthy environment
  2. Anatomy
     a. Trophoblasts
     b. Chorionic villi
     c. Intervillous spaces
     d. Chorion
     e. Amnion
     f. Decidual plate
  3. Steroid and protein hormones—human trophoblasts produce more diverse steroid and protein hormones in greater amounts than any endocrine tissue in all of mammalian physiology
     a. Steroid hormones
        (1) Estradiol-17B—responsible for the growth of the uterus, fallopian tubes, vagina, and mammary development
        (2) Estriol—estrogen metabolite excreted by the placenta during pregnancy; found in the urine of pregnant people
        (3) Progesterone—secreted by the corpus luteum; essential in preparing the uterus for implantation of the fertilized ovum and maintaining the pregnancy
        (4) Aldosterone—responsible for the regulation of the body's salt and water balance
        (5) Cortisol—plays a role in the metabolism of fats, glucose, and proteins
     b. Protein and peptide hormones
        (1) Human placental lactogen (hPL)—a placental hormone that inhibits maternal insulin activity during pregnancy; decreases to undetectable levels soon after delivery of the placenta
        (2) Human chorionic gonadotropin (hCG)—a hormone secreted by the placenta to help maintain corpus luteum function and production of progesterone; found in serum and urine assays of pregnant persons as early as a week after conception
        (3) Placental adrenocorticotropin hormone (ACTH)—plays a role in the regulation of the secretion of glucocorticoids
        (4) Pro-opiomelanocortin—a precursor polypeptide
        (5) Chorionic thyrotropin—a type of hormone similar to thyroid-stimulating hormone (TSH) that can increase metabolism
        (6) Growth hormone variant—a hormone that plays a vital role in growth control
        (7) Parathyroid hormone-related protein (PTH-rP)—essential for bone differentiation and formation and development of mammary gland
        (8) Calcitonin—the hormone responsible for calcium balance
        (9) Relaxin—produced in the placenta and corpus luteum; believed to help with relaxing the uterine myometrium during pregnancy
     c. Hypothalamic-like releasing and inhibiting hormones
        (1) Thyrotropin-releasing hormone (TRH)—responsible for the regulation of TSH
        (2) Gonadotropin-releasing hormone (GnRH)—essential in controlling the secretion of luteinizing hormone (LH) and follicle-stimulating hormone (FSH)
        (3) Corticotropin-releasing hormone (CRH)—works with vasopressin hormone to regulate the release of ACTH
        (4) Somatostatin—responsible for inhibiting the release of growth hormone, prolactin, and thyrotropin
     d. Regulation of blood flow in the placenta—maternal blood traverses the placenta randomly without preformed channels and enters the intervillous spaces in spurts, propelled by the maternal arterial pressure
     e. Placental "barrier"—the placenta does not maintain absolute integrity between maternal and fetal circulations, as indicated by the presence of fetal blood cells in maternal circulation and the development of erythroblastosis fetalis
     f. Oxygen and glucose are transported across the placenta via facilitated diffusion

- Umbilical cord
  1. Anatomy
     a. Vessels—two arteries carry fetal deoxygenated blood to the placenta, smaller in diameter than the vein; one vein carries oxygenated blood from the placenta to the fetus, characterized by twisting or spiraling to minimize snarling
     b. Measurements—0.8–2 cm in diameter; average length of 55 cm, with range of 30–100 cm
     c. Wharton's jelly—extracellular matrix consisting of specialized connective tissue that serves as protection for the umbilical cord
  2. Abnormalities of length—positively influenced by amniotic fluid volume (AFV) and fetal mobility
     a. Extremely short cord—associated with abruptio placentae or uterine inversion; the latter is rare
     b. Abnormally long cord—associated with vascular occlusion by thrombi and true knots
- Amniotic fluid
  1. Production—produced by amniotic epithelium; water transfers across amnion and through fetal skin; in the second trimester, the fetus starts to swallow, urinate, and inspire amniotic fluid
  2. Volume maintenance—fetal swallowing seems to be a critical mechanism affecting fluid volume; polyhydramnios is consistently present when fetal swallowing is inhibited; other factors, such as tracheoesophageal atresia, also contribute to volume balance
  3. Polyhydramnios (hydramnios)—in a singleton pregnancy, an excess of amniotic fluid; amniotic fluid index (AFI) ≥24 cm or a maximum deepest vertical pocket ≥8 cm
     a. Incidence—approximately 1% of all pregnancies
     b. Etiology—50% to 60% are idiopathic; also associated with fetal anomalies, fetal infection, twin-to-twin transfusion syndrome, alloimmunization, or multiple gestation
     c. Signs and symptoms—uterine size larger than expected for gestational age (GA), difficulty auscultating fetal heart rate (FHR) and palpating fetal parts, mechanical pressure exerted by the large uterus (i.e., dyspnea, edema, heartburn, nausea)
     d. Diagnosis
        (1) Physical findings—a fundal height measurement that is 3–4 cm greater than the normal height warrants an ultrasound to determine the reason for the enlarged uterus; palpation of fetal parts and auscultation of fetal heartbeat may be difficult
        (2) Ultrasonography (US)—AFI >24 cm or a single deepest vertical pocket ≥8 cm confirms polyhydramnios diagnosis; US may also identify an associated fetal anomaly
     e. Pregnancy outcome—hydramnios has been linked to fetal macrosomia; the greater the polyhydramnios, the higher the perinatal mortality; preterm labor increases; risk for postpartum hemorrhage (PPH) is higher given that the uterus is enlarged; increased risk for cord prolapse with rupture of membranes; also associated with erythroblastosis

     f. Management—treat only if symptomatic and if benefits outweigh risks; antenatal monitor is not required for mild idiopathic polyhydramnios alone; however, serial antenatal testing may be indicated in the setting of additional perinatal or fetal complications contributing to the polyhydramnios.
        (1) Amnioreduction via amniocentesis—to reduce fluid volume if polyhydramnios is severe (AFI >35 cm), severe maternal discomfort, and/or dyspnea; amniotic fluid can be tested for fetal lung maturity and also sent for chromosomal studies
        (2) Indomethacin—SHOULD NOT be used to decrease amniotic fluid due to findings of neonatal complications and absence of data to support improved perinatal or neonatal outcomes
        (3) Birth at a tertiary center is recommended for birthing people with severe polyhydramnios given the high probability of fetal anomalies
  4. Oligohydramnios—decreased AFV, defined as AFI of 5 cm or a maximum deepest vertical pocket of fluid <2 cm
     a. Conditions associated with oligohydramnios
        (1) Fetal—almost always present with fetal urinary tract obstruction or renal agenesis
           (a) Chromosomal abnormalities
           (b) Congenital anomalies
           (c) Growth restriction
           (d) Demise
           (e) Postterm pregnancy
           (f) Ruptured membranes; premature rupture of membranes (PROM)
        (2) Placental
           (a) Abruption
           (b) Twin-to-twin transfusion syndrome
        (3) Perinatal
           (a) Uteroplacental insufficiency
           (b) Hypertensive disorders (chronic, gestational, superimposed)
           (c) Diabetes
        (4) Drugs
           (a) Prostaglandin synthesis inhibitors
           (b) Angiotensin-converting enzyme inhibitors
        (5) Idiopathic
     b. Prognosis
        (1) Early-onset diabetes has poor outcomes, and the risk of pulmonary hypoplasia is greatly increased; if due to early PROM, the risk of stillbirth increased
        (2) Late pregnancy onset leads to more cesarean sections for fetal distress
     c. Management
        (1) Ultrasonographic evaluation for fetal anomalies and growth restriction
        (2) Amnioinfusion in the intrapartum period for the treatment of repetitive variable decelerations

Embryonic and Fetal Development

- Embryonic development
  1. Period of organogenesis; begins in the 3rd week after fertilization and spans 8 weeks; serum and urine assays can detect hCG as early as a week after conception
  2. 4th week—partitioning of the heart begins; arm and leg buds form; amnion begins to unsheathe the body stalk that becomes the umbilical cord
  3. 6th week—head is much larger than the body; the heart is completely formed; fingers and toes present
  4. All major organ systems are formed except for the lungs
- Fetal development
  1. Begins 8 weeks after fertilization; 10 weeks after onset of last menstrual period (LMP)
  2. At 12 weeks—uterus palpable at the symphysis; the fetus begins to make spontaneous movements
  3. At 16 weeks—experienced observers can determine sex on ultrasound
  4. At 20 weeks—fetus weighs 300 g; weight now begins to increase in a linear manner
  5. At 24 weeks—fetus weighs 630 g; fat deposition begins; terminal sacs in the lungs still not completely formed
  6. At 28 weeks—the fetus weighs 1,100 g; the papillary membrane has just disappeared from the eyes; has a 90% chance of survival if otherwise normal
  7. At 32 to 36 weeks—the fetus continues to increase in weight as more subcutaneous fat accumulates

Diagnosis and Dating of Pregnancy

- Diagnosis
  1. Signs of pregnancy
     a. Presumptive—subjective (what the pregnant person reports)
        (1) Amenorrhea
        (2) Nausea and/or vomiting
        (3) Urinary frequency; nocturia
        (4) Fatigue
        (5) Breast tenderness, tingling, enlargement, and changes in color
        (6) Vasomotor symptoms
        (7) Skin changes
        (8) Congestion of vaginal mucus
        (9) The pregnant person's belief that they are pregnant
     b. Presumptive—objective (physical examination)
        (1) Continuation of elevated basal body temperature
        (2) Bluish discoloration of the cervix, vagina, and vulva (observable as early as 6–8 weeks after conception)
        (3) Appearance of sebaceous glands on the surface of the dark area of the nipple
        (4) Expression of colostrum
        (5) Mammary tissue changes
     c. Probable
        (1) Enlargement of the abdomen
        (2) Enlargement of the uterus
        (3) Palpation of the fetal outline
        (4) Ballottement
        (5) Change in the shape of the uterus
        (6) A palpable lateral bulge or soft prominence where the zygote has implanted
        (7) Softening of the uterine isthmus
        (8) Softening of the cervix
        (9) Palpation of Braxton Hicks contractions
        (10) Positive pregnancy test
     d. Positive
        (1) Fetal heart tones (FHTs)—heard with a fetoscope at approximately 18–20 weeks and/or by Doppler ultrasound as early as 10 weeks' gestation
        (2) Ultrasonographic evidence of pregnancy
        (3) Palpation of fetal movement
  2. Differential diagnosis
     a. Pregnancy
     b. Leiomyoma
     c. Ovarian cyst
     d. Pseudocyesis
- Dating of pregnancy
  1. Determining estimated date of delivery (EDD), estimated date of confinement (EDC), or estimated date of birth (EDB)
  2. Average duration of human pregnancy—280 days, 10 lunar months, 9 calendar months
  3. Methods for determining EDD, EDC, and EDB
     a. Naegele's rule—subtract 3 months, add 7 days to the first day of the LMP, then add 1 year *or* add 9 months and 7 days to the first day of the LMP
     b. Additional information needed to determine EDD more precisely
        (1) Complete menstrual history
        (2) Contraceptive history
        (3) Sexual history
        (4) Physical examination for signs and symptoms of pregnancy
        (5) Quickening—maternal perception of fetal movement, which usually occurs between 18 and 20 weeks for primiparas; earlier for multiparas, at about 14–18 weeks
  4. USG for GA determination
     a. A combination of measurements is more accurate than any one of the following measurements
        (1) Crown–rump length (CRL)
        (2) Biparietal diameter (BPD)
        (3) Head circumference (HC)
        (4) Abdominal circumference (AC)
        (5) Femur length (FL)
     b. Accuracy by trimester
        (1) First trimester—CRL is accurate to 3–5 days

(2) Second trimester—BPD and FL are most accurate to within 7–10 days

(3) Third trimester—after 26 weeks, all measurements are less accurate; variation in BPD and FL is 14–21 days

Maternal Physiologic Adaptations to Pregnancy

- Effects of pregnancy on the organs of reproduction and implications for clinical practice
  1. Uterus
     a. Nonpregnant uterus is about 70 g with a 10-mL cavity
     b. First trimester—at 6 weeks, the uterus is soft, globular, and asymmetric; at 12 weeks, it is 8–10 cm and is rising out of the pelvis
     c. Early second trimester—at 14 weeks, the uterus is one-fourth of the way to the umbilicus; at 16 weeks, it is halfway to the umbilicus; at 20 weeks, the fundus is approximately at the umbilicus
     d. After 20 weeks, the number of centimeters with tape measure equals the number of weeks of gestation within 2 cm
     e. By term, the uterus weighs about 1,100 g with a 5-L volume
  2. Cervix
     a. Develops increased vascularity
     b. Softening of the isthmus
     c. Bluish color of the cervix
     d. Softening of the cervix
     e. Thick mucus plug forms secondary to glandular proliferation
  3. Ovaries—corpus luteum
     a. Anovulation secondary to hormonal interruption of the feedback loop
     b. Corpus luteum persists under the influence of the hormone hCG until about 12 weeks
     c. Corpus luteum is responsible for the secretion of progesterone to maintain the endometrium and pregnancy until the placenta takes over production
     d. Ovaries also thought responsible for producing relaxin
  4. Vagina
     a. Bluish color
     b. Thickening of vaginal mucosa
     c. Increase in vaginal secretions
     d. Some loosening of connective tissue in preparation for birth
  5. Breasts
     a. Increase in size secondary to mammary hyperplasia
     b. Areola becomes more deeply pigmented and increases in size
     c. Colostrum may be expressed after the first several months of pregnancy
     d. Appearance of sebaceous glands on the surface of the dark area of the nipple
     e. Vascularity increases
  6. Pelvis—responsible for load transfer of body weight and gravity, which increases in pregnancy; changes in pelvic alignment occur in pregnancy
     a. Progressive anterior tilt throughout the pregnancy
     b. Elasticity in the joints can lead to distortion and asymmetry
     c. Weakening of the pubic symphysis
- Effects of pregnancy on major body systems, with related clinical implications and patient education needs
  1. Gastrointestinal (GI)
     a. Mouth and pharynx
        (1) Gingivitis is common and may result in bleeding of the gums
        (2) Increased salivation
        (3) Epulis (focal swelling of gums) may develop and resolves after the birth
        (4) Pregnancy does not increase tooth decay
     b. Esophagus
        (1) Decreased lower esophageal sphincter pressure and tone
        (2) Widening of hiatus with decreased tone
        (3) Heartburn is common
     c. Stomach
        (1) Decreased gastric emptying time
        (2) Decreased gastric acidity and histamine output
     d. Large and small intestines
        (1) Decreased tone and motility
        (2) Altered enzymatic transport across villi, resulting in increased absorption of vitamins
        (3) Displacement of intestines, cecum, and appendix by the enlarging uterus
     e. Gallbladder
        (1) Decreased tone
        (2) Decreased motility
     f. Liver
        (1) Altered production of liver enzymes
        (2) Altered production of plasma proteins and serum lipids
  2. Genitourinary/renal
     a. Dilation of renal calyces, pelvis, and ureters, resulting in increased risk of urinary tract infection (UTI)
     b. Decreased bladder tone
     c. Renal blood flow increases 35%–60%
     d. Decreased renal threshold for glucose, protein, water-soluble vitamins, calcium, and hydrogen ions
     e. Glomerular filtration rate increases from 40% to 50%
     f. All components of the renin–angiotensin–aldosterone system increase, resulting in retention of sodium and water, resistance to the pressor effect of angiotensin II, and maintenance of normal blood pressure
  3. Musculoskeletal
     a. Relaxin and progesterone affect cartilage and connective tissue
        (1) Results in loosening of sacroiliac joint and symphysis pubis

      (2) Encourages development of the characteristic gait of pregnancy

   b. Lordosis

4. Respiratory
   a. Level of the diaphragm rises about 4 cm because of the increase in uterine size
   b. Thoracic circumference increases by 5–6 cm and residual volume is decreased
   c. A mild respiratory alkalosis occurs because of decreased P_{CO_2}
   d. Congestion of nasal tissues occurs
   e. Respiratory rate changes very little, but the tidal volume, minute ventilatory, and minute oxygen uptake all increase appreciably
   f. Possible experience of physiologic dyspnea due to the increased tidal volume and lower P_{CO_2}

5. Hematologic changes
   a. Blood volume increases from 30% to 50% from nonpregnant levels
   b. Plasma volume expands, resulting in physiologic anemia
   c. Hemoglobin averages 12.5 g/dL
   d. Potential need for iron supplementation during pregnancy
   e. Pregnancy can be considered a hypercoagulable state because fibrinogen (factor I) and factors VII–X increase during pregnancy

6. Cardiovascular system
   a. Cardiac volume increases by approximately 10% and peaks at about 20 weeks
   b. Resting pulse increases by 10–15 beats per minute, with the peak at 28 weeks
   c. Slight cardiac shift (up and to the left) due to the enlarging uterus
   d. Approximately 90% of pregnant individuals develop a physiologic systolic heart murmur
   e. May have exaggerated splitting of S_1, audible third sound, or soft transient diastolic murmur
   f. Cardiac output is increased
   g. Diastolic blood pressure is lower in the first two trimesters because of the development of new vascular beds and relaxation of peripheral tone by progesterone, which results in decreased flow resistance

7. Integumentary system
   a. Vascular changes
      (1) Palmar erythema
      (2) Spider angiomas
      (3) Varicose veins and hemorrhoids
      (4) Hyperpigmentation—believed to be related to estrogens and progesterone, which have a melanocyte-stimulating effect
      (5) Chloasma, freckles, nevi, and recent scars may darken
      (6) Linea nigra
      (7) Increased sweat/sebaceous activity
      (8) Change in connective tissues resulting in striae gravidarum

   b. Hair growth
   (1) Estrogen increases the length of the anagen (growth) phase of the hair follicles
   (2) Mild hirsutism may develop in early pregnancy

8. Endocrine
   a. Pituitary
      (1) Prolactin levels are 10 times higher at term than in the nonpregnant state
      (2) Enlarges by more than 100%
   b. Thyroid
      (1) Increases in size (approximately 13%)
      (2) Normal pregnant individual is euthyroid because of estrogen-induced increase in thyroxin-binding globulin (TBG)
      (3) TSH does not cross the placenta
      (4) Thyroid-stimulating immunoglobulins and TRH cross the placenta
   c. Adrenal glands
      (1) Remain the same size, but an increase in the zona fasciculata that produces glucocorticoid
      (2) Two-fold increase in serum cortisol
   d. Pancreas
      (1) Hypertrophy and hyperplasia of the B cells
      (2) Insulin resistance as a result of the placental hormones, especially hPL

9. Metabolism
   a. Weight gain during pregnancy
      (1) Average weight gain is 28 lb—1.5 lb for placenta, 2 lb for amniotic fluid, 2.5 lb for uterine growth, 3 lb for increased blood volume, 1 lb for increased breast tissue, 7.5 lb for the fetus, and the remainder for maternal fat deposits
      (2) Recommended weight gain in second and third trimesters as per the 2009 Institute of Medicine/National Research Council guided prepregnancy weight and by the weight of the products of conception listed above:
         (a) Prepregnancy BMI less than 18.5: gain 28–40 lb total, at a rate of 1 lb/week
         (b) Prepregnancy BMI 18.5–24.9: gain 25–35 lb total, at a rate of 1 lb/week
         (c) Prepregnancy BMI 25–29.9: gain 15–25 lb total, at a rate of 0.6 lb/week
         (d) Prepregnancy BMI 30 or greater: gain 11–20 lb total, at a rate of 0.5 lb/week
         (e) Note that gestational weight gain is complex. The use of the above guidelines should recognize existing gaps (i.e., lack of data for BMI >35, outcomes stratified by BMIs >30, the generalizability of data, accounting for structural and social determinants of health) and work to mitigate weight stigma and bias
   b. Protein metabolism is increased
   c. Fat deposit and storage are increased to prepare for breastfeeding
   d. Carbohydrate metabolism is altered; blood glucose levels are 10%–20% lower than prepregnant states

Perinatal Psychological/ Social Changes in Pregnancy

- Pregnancy is a time of many transitions that is marked by vulnerability; moods may be labile in the perinatal period
- First trimester (1–13 weeks)—focus on physical changes and feelings
  1. Psychological responses
     a. Ambivalence
     b. Adjustment
  2. Prenatal anticipatory guidance
     a. Review normal changes in pregnancy
        (1) Increased pigmentation
        (2) Linea nigra
        (3) Striae gravidarum
        (4) Breast fullness
        (5) Urinary frequency
        (6) Nausea/vomiting
        (7) Fatigue
     b. Calculate and explain EDD and compare it with uterine size
     c. Develop a shared expectation for prenatal visits
     d. Discuss the importance of ongoing care in pregnancy to promote well-being and prevent and recognize problems
     e. Provide a rationale for nutrition and vitamin/mineral supplementation
     f. Share resources available for education, emergency care, etc.
     g. Discuss/review danger signs and symptoms (e.g., vaginal bleeding) and how to report them
- Second trimester (14–26 weeks)—more aware of fetal movements
  1. Psychological responses
     a. Acceptance
  2. Prenatal anticipatory guidance
     a. Avoid exposure to teratogenic agents
        (1) CMV, HSV, rubella, syphilis, varicella, toxoplasma
        (2) Hyperthermia
        (3) Environmental chemicals, such as herbicides and polychlorinated biphenyl (PCB)
        (4) Substance use/misuse
        (5) If medication required in pregnancy (over-the-counter, herbal, or prescription), the lowest possible dose should be considered, and minimizing first-trimester exposure
     b. Monitor fetal growth, movement, and FHTs
     c. Review personal hygiene, brassieres, vaginal discharge
     d. Learn about infant feeding preferences—breastfeeding, chestfeeding, and/or formula feeding
     e. Educate on avoidance and alleviation of backache, constipation, hemorrhoids, leg aches, varicosities, edema, and round ligament pain
     f. Discuss nutritional needs, diet, and weight gain
     g. Discuss/review danger signs and symptoms (e.g., preterm labor)
- Third trimester
  3. First part (27–36 weeks)—concerned with the fetus' needs; second part (36 weeks–birth)—concerned with birth and postpartum transition
     a. Psychological responses
        (1) Period of watchful waiting
        (2) Nesting
     b. Prenatal anticipatory guidance
        (1) Monitor fetal growth and well-being
        (2) Review hygiene, clothing, body mechanics and posture, positions of comfort
        (3) Affirm physical and emotional changes
        (4) Affirm sexual needs/intercourse
        (5) Educate on the alleviation of backache, Braxton Hicks contractions, dyspnea, round ligament pain, leg aches, or edema
        (6) Confirm infant feeding plans and discuss preparation for the desired method
        (7) Discuss preparation for baby supplies and support at home
        (8) Recommend prenatal classes and/or discuss approaches that may best suit
        (9) Involvement of significant other
        (10) Review danger signs at each visit (e.g., signs/symptoms of preeclampsia)
        (11) Provide contraceptive counseling if the patient desires.
        (12) If planning tubal ligation, prepare papers if required
     c. Anticipation of birth and infant care
        (1) Discuss fetal movement
        (2) Review personal hygiene needs/concerns, alleviation of discomforts of pregnancy
        (3) Discuss recognition of Braxton Hicks and prodromal contractions and differentiation from true labor
        (4) Discuss labor, contractions, and labor progress and expectations of labor
        (5) Review breathing and relaxation techniques; labor support options
        (6) Discuss provisions needed for other children, sibling issues, and care of children during hospital stay
        (7) Review signs of labor
        (8) Continue discussion of relaxation and breathing techniques; latent labor coping skills
        (9) Finalize home preparations
        (10) Discuss procedures particular to the birth setting (i.e., home, birthing center, hospital)—analgesia, IVs, examinations, labor care, birthing plans, postpartum care, and supplies needed
        (11) Confirm plans for transport to the hospital, who to call, and where to go; hospitalization and process of admission

(12) Consider reproductive life plan and contraceptive needs

(13) Discuss emergency arrangements in the event of danger signs, PROM, bleeding, severe headache, pain

- Threats to psychological well-being
  1. Limited support network
  2. High levels of chronic or acute stress
  3. Experiences of racism, discrimination, or marginalization
  4. Psychological and mental health issues
  5. Pregnancies complicated by medical issues
  6. Intimate partner violence

Overview of Antepartum Care

- Purpose and objectives of antepartum care—to differentiate normal and pathologic maternal–fetal alterations throughout pregnancy by employing maternal–fetal assessment methods, techniques, and parameters appropriate to the antepartum period, specifically
  1. Application of the management process, including components of history and physical examination at initial and interval visits
  2. Critical evaluation of indications and techniques for the application of therapeutics during the antepartum period
  3. Incorporation of current evidence and research in the care of childbearing individuals and families during the antepartum period
- Definition of the essential concepts
  1. Fertility rate—number of live births/1,000 females 15–44 years of age
  2. Birth rate—number of births divided by total population in the given year(s)
  3. Live birth—birth of an infant, no matter the age of gestation, showing any signs of life (e.g., spontaneous breathing, beating of the heart, pulsation of the cord, movement of voluntary muscles)
  4. Neonatal period—28 completed days after birth
  5. Perinatal period—from the end of 22 weeks (154 days) GA up to 7 days after birth; also defined as births weighing 500 g or more and ending at 28 completed days after birth
  6. Fetal death—spontaneous intrauterine death of a fetus at any time during the pregnancy; also referred to as stillbirth if it occurs after 20 weeks or more
  7. Stillbirth rate (fetal death rate)—the ratio of fetal deaths divided by the sum of births (including live births and fetal deaths) in any given year
  8. Neonatal death—early neonatal death is death during the first 7 days after birth; late neonatal death is death between 7 and 28 days
  9. Neonatal mortality rate—the number of neonates dying before reaching 28 days of age per 1,000 live births in a given year
  10. Perinatal mortality—the number of stillbirths and deaths in the first week of life
  11. Perinatal mortality rate—the number of stillbirths and perinatal deaths (in the first week of life) per 1,000 total births
  12. Infant mortality—death of an infant in the first 12 months of life
  13. Infant mortality rate—number of infant deaths (in the first 12 months of life) per 1,000 live births
  14. Maternal morbidity—illness or disease associated with childbearing
  15. Maternal mortality ratio—number of maternal deaths that result from the reproductive process/100,000 live births
  16. Abortus—fetus or embryo removed or expelled from the uterus during the first half of gestation (20 weeks or less), weighing less than 500 g
  17. Late preterm infant (34 0/7–36 6/7 weeks of gestation)
  18. Early term infant (37 0/7–38 6/7 weeks of gestation)
  19. Term infant—infant born after 37 completed weeks of gestation up until 42 completed weeks of gestation (260–294 days)
  20. Postterm infant—infant born any time after completion of the 42nd week beginning with day 295
  21. Direct obstetric death—death resulting from obstetric complications of pregnancy, labor, or the puerperium; and from interventions, omissions, incorrect treatment, or a chain of events resulting from any of these factors

Antepartum Visit

- Terminology that describes pregnant individuals and their pregnancies
  1. Gravida—the number of times a person has been pregnant regardless of the result of the pregnancy
  2. Para—the number of pregnancies carried to the 20th week of gestation or the delivery of an infant weighing more than 500 g, regardless of the outcome
  3. Nulligravida—a person who has never been pregnant
  4. Nullipara—a person who has not carried a baby to 500 g or 20 weeks
  5. Primigravida—a person who is pregnant for the first time
  6. Primipara—a person who has carried a pregnancy past the 20th week of gestation or who is currently pregnant for the first time and is carrying past the 20th week
  7. Multigravida—an individual who has been pregnant two or more times
  8. Multipara—a person who has carried two or more pregnancies past the 20th week of gestation or who has birthed an infant weighing more than 500 g more than once
  9. Grand multipara—a person who has given birth seven times or more
  10. TPAL numerical description of parity—a four-digit system that counts all fetuses/babies born rather than pregnancies carried to viability
      a. T = term infants (≥37 weeks or 2,500 g)
      b. P = premature infants (20–36 weeks and 6 days; 500–2,499 g)

c. A = abortions (any fetus born <20 weeks and 500 g)
d. L = current living children

- Components of the antepartum visit (initial and return)
  1. The Pregnant Patient's Bill of Rights
  2. Complete history
     a. Menstrual history
     b. Contraceptive history
     c. Obstetric history, including quickening
     d. Medical–surgical history
     e. Sexual history
     f. History or current physical, sexual, emotional abuse
     g. Medicines and/or complementary alternative medicines and therapies
     h. Family history
     i. Genetic risk
     j. Health habits
     k. Environmental exposures
     l. Social history
     m. Exercise and nutrition history
     n. Immunizations
  3. Physical examination
     a. Height, weight, and vital signs
     b. Complete physical examination
     c. Abdominal examination
        (1) Fundal height—measured in centimeters, from the pubic symphysis to the fundus of the uterus
        (2) Leopold's maneuvers—four abdominal palpation maneuvers used to determine fetal characteristics
           (a) Lie
           (b) Presentation
           (c) Position
           (d) Attitude
           (e) Variety
           (f) Estimated fetal weight
        (3) FHTs—auscultation of presence and pattern of FHR
  4. Laboratory studies used in the provision of antepartum care
     a. Initial visit
        (1) Blood type, Rh factor, antibody screen, complete blood count (CBC), rapid plasma reagin (RPR) or Venereal Disease Research Laboratory (VDRL), rubella titer, hepatitis B surface antigen (HB$_s$Ag), urine culture/screen
        (2) HIV testing should be recommended to all pregnant individuals with the option to decline testing
        (3) Gonorrhea (GC), chlamydia (CT), and wet-mount tests (i.e., vaginal smear, wet prep), TSH, hemoglobin A$_{1c}$ (HbA$_{1c}$), as indicated by history and physical examination findings
        (4) Pap test per routine recommendations
        (5) Positive purified protein derivative (PPD) skin test, hemoglobin (Hgb) electrophoresis, genetic screening tests as indicated by history and risk factors

  b. Prenatal genetic screening tests
     (1) Two main types of prenatal genetic tests
        (a) Prenatal screening tests—tests that provide the risk for certain genetic disorders, such as aneuploidy (a condition in which the infant has either a missing chromosome or an extra chromosome)
        (b) Prenatal diagnostic tests—confirmatory tests using cells from the fetus or placenta
     (2) Different types of prenatal screening tests (**Table 6-1**)
        (a) Carrier screening—serologic or tissue testing performed before or during the pregnancy to determine if the patient carries specific genetic illnesses
        (b) Prenatal genetic screening—serologic testing combined with USG performed during pregnancy to screen for aneuploidy and spine and brain defects
     (3) Common Screening Tests for Chromosomal Abnormalities (Rose et al., 2020)
        (a) Cell-free DNA testing—serologic screening test on mother analyzes the small amount of DNA that is released from the placenta into the bloodstream of the mother; screens for aneuploidy (trisomies 13, 18, 21) and problems with sex chromosomes; this screening test can be performed as early as 10 weeks, and results may take up to 1 week; positive cell-free DNA results need to be followed by a diagnostic test (CVS or amniocentesis)
        (b) First-trimester screening (FTS)—performed between 10 and 13 weeks; serologic testing for pregnancy-associated plasma protein (PAPP-A) and hCG, an ultrasound exam to measure nuchal translucency, and the mother's age are combined to calculate risk for trisomies 18 and 21
        (c) Quadruple marker screen (aka Quad screen)—serologic blood test performed between 15 and 22 weeks to detect neural tube defects and trisomies 18 and 21; serologic testing measuring maternal serum alpha-fetoprotein (MSAFP), estriol, inhibin A, and hCG;
        (d) Integrated Screen—need two serologic samples, one from 10 to 13 weeks and a second between 15 and 22 weeks of gestation, to detect trisomy 18 and 21. This is a combination of NT ultrasound results, PAPP-A, and the quad screen. Of note, the first trimester results are not given. The result is a combination of first and second screenings into one screening result.
        (e) Serum integrated screen—requires two serologic samples, one from 10 to 13 weeks and a second between 15 and 22 weeks of gestation to detect trisomy 18 and 21. Does not include NT ultrasound results. This

Table 6-1 Prenatal Genetic Testing Chart

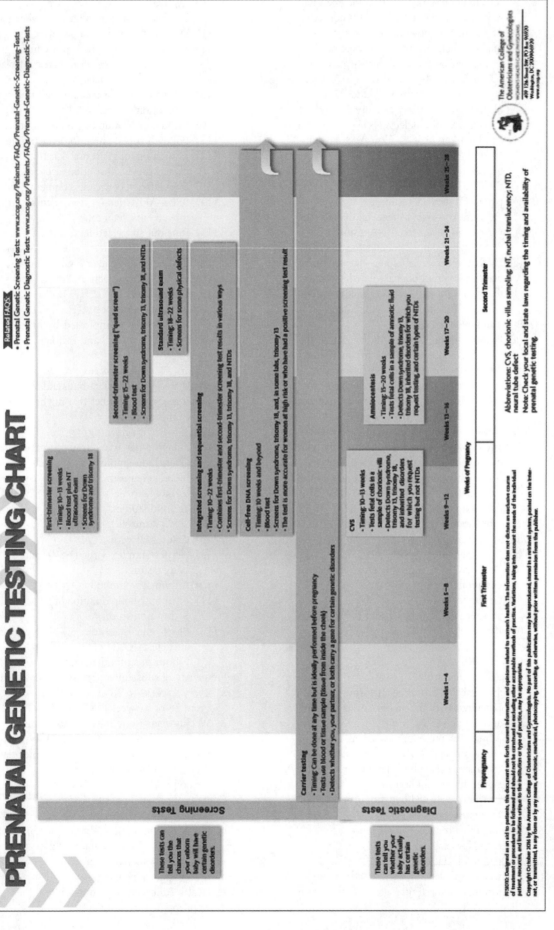

PRENATAL GENETIC TESTING CHART

Related FAQS
- Prenatal Genetic Screening Tests: www.acog.org/Patients/FAQs/Prenatal-Genetic-Screening-Tests
- Prenatal Genetic Diagnostic Tests: www.acog.org/Patients/FAQs/Prenatal-Genetic-Diagnostic-Tests

Screening Tests

These tests can tell you the chances that your unborn baby will have certain genetic disorders.

First-trimester screening
- Timing: 10–13 weeks
- Blood test plus NT ultrasound exam
- Screens for Down syndrome and trisomy 18

Second-trimester screening ("quad screen")
- Timing: 15–22 weeks
- Blood test
- Screens for Down syndrome, trisomy 13, trisomy 18, and NTDs

Standard ultrasound exam
- Timing: 18–22 weeks
- Screens for some physical defects

Integrated screening and sequential screening
- Timing: 10–22 weeks
- Combines first-trimester and second-trimester screening test results in various ways
- Screens for Down syndrome, trisomy 13, trisomy 18, and NTDs

Cell-free DNA screening
- Timing: 10 weeks and beyond
- Blood test
- Screens for Down syndrome, trisomy 18, and, in some labs, trisomy 13
- The test is more accurate for women at high risk or who have had a positive screening test result

Carrier testing
- Timing: Can be done at any time but is ideally performed before pregnancy
- Tests use blood or tissue sample (tissue from inside the cheek)
- Detects whether you, your partner, or both carry a gene for certain genetic disorders

Diagnostic Tests

These tests can tell you whether your baby actually has certain genetic disorders.

CVS
- Timing: 10–13 weeks
- Tests fetal cells in a sample of chorionic villi
- Detects Down syndrome, trisomy 13, trisomy 18, and inherited disorders for which you request testing but not NTDs

Amniocentesis
- Timing: 15–20 weeks
- Tests fetal cells in a sample of amniotic fluid
- Detects Down syndrome, trisomy 13, trisomy 18, inherited disorders for which you request testing, and certain types of NTDs

Pregnancy	First Trimester			Second Trimester			
	Weeks 1–4	Weeks 5–8	Weeks 9–12	Weeks 13–16	Weeks 17–20	Weeks 21–24	Weeks 25–28

Weeks of Pregnancy

Abbreviations: CVS, chorionic villus sampling; NT, nuchal translucency; NTD, neural tube defect

Note: Check your local and state laws regarding the timing and availability of prenatal genetic testing.

The American College of
Obstetricians and Gynecologists
WOMEN'S HEALTH CARE PHYSICIANS
409 12th Street SW, PO Box 96920
Washington, DC 20090-6920
www.acog.org

Reprinted with permission from American College of Obstetricians and Gynecologists. (2019). Prenatal genetic testing chart (infographic). ACOG Patient Education Infographics. Washington, DC: Author.

screening only uses PAPP-A and the quad screen. Of note, the FTS result is not given. The result is a combination of first and second screenings into one screening result.

(f) Sequential stepwise screen—Needs two serologic samples from 10 to 13 weeks and a second between 15 and 22 weeks of gestation to detect trisomy 18 and 21 and neural tube defects (NTD). This is a combination of NT ultrasound results, PAPP-A, beta hCG, and AFP then the quad screen. Unlike the integrated screen, the first-trimester result is provided to the patient. If the FTS results are

   i. Positive—the patient is offered the option of cell-free DNA testing
   ii. Negative—no further testing necessary

(g) Nuchal translucency alone—measurement via ultrasound of nuchal fold (the tissue at the back of a fetus' neck) thickness done between 10 and 13 weeks of gestation

(4) Prenatal screen test results

(a) Positive screening test—indicates that the fetus has an increased risk for aneuploidy relative to the general population; this is only a screening and is not diagnostic; the positive result does not mean that the fetus definitely has the disorder

(b) Negative screening test—indicates that the fetus has a lower risk for aneuploidy relative to the general population; however, this is only a screening, so the possibility that the fetus definitely has the disorder is not completely ruled out

c. Obstetric ultrasound

(1) First-trimester examination

(a) Presence of intrauterine pregnancy

(b) Presence, size, location, and number of gestational sac(s)

(c) Gestational sac is examined for the presence of the yolk sac and embryo/fetus

(d) If embryo/fetus present, measure:
   i. Fetal number
   ii. CRL
   iii. Cardiac activity
   iv. Embryonic or fetal anatomy

(e) Examination of the uterus, cervix, adnexa, and cul-de-sac

(f) Adjunct to procedures, such as chorionic villus sampling (CVS), embryo transfer, localization, and removal of intrauterine device

(g) Screen for aneuploidy

(h) Evaluate suspected hydatidiform mole

(i) Evaluate vaginal bleeding

d. Second- and third-trimester ultrasound

(1) Screening for fetal anomalies

(2) Evaluation of fetal anomaly

(3) Evaluation of fetal growth and dating—macrosomia, intrauterine growth restriction (IUGR), AFI

(4) Evaluation of vaginal bleeding

(5) Evaluation of abdominal and pelvic pain

(6) Determination of fetal presentation

(7) Adjunct to obstetric procedures, such as amniocentesis, cervical cerclage placement, and external cephalic version

(8) Estimated GA for patients with uncertain LMP

(9) Evaluation of fetal well-being

(10) Evaluation of amniotic fluid abnormalities

(11) Follow-up evaluation for fetal anomaly

(12) Evaluation of placental location, grade, suspected previa, abruption, accrete

(13) Evaluation of pelvic mass or uterine abnormality

(14) BPP—AFI, fetal movements, respiratory movements, fetal tone

(15) Rule out suspected fetal demise

e. Gestational diabetes screening at 24–28 weeks (see the diabetes section in Chapter 7, *Complex Pregnancy Care*)

f. Repeat antibody screen at 26–28 weeks for Rh-negative mother

g. Repeat CBC/hematocrit (Hct), VDRL/RPR, CT, GC, HIV, HB_sAg as indicated by history, physical examination findings, and risk factors in the third trimester

h. Group B *Streptococcus* (GBS) screening at 35–37 weeks—vaginal introitus and rectal specimens

i. Other laboratory studies that might be indicated

(1) Amniocentesis or CVS

(2) Tay–Sachs screening

(3) Maternal/paternal chromosomal studies

(4) Chest radiographs

(5) Blood chemistry (basic or comprehensive metabolic panel)

(6) Thyroid studies

(7) Toxoplasmosis testing

(8) Cytomegalovirus (CMV)

(9) Herpes simplex virus (HSV) cultures or antibody testing

(10) Antinuclear antibody (ANA)

(11) Antiphospholipid antibodies

(12) Serum iron studies

(13) Blood glucose studies (3-hour glucose tolerance test [GTT], fasting blood sugar [FBS], 2-hour postprandial, and HbA_{1c})

5. Frequency of subsequent (interval) prenatal visits

a. Every 4 weeks to 28 or 32 weeks

b. From 28 or 32 weeks to 36 weeks, every 2 weeks

c. Weekly visits from 36 weeks to 41 weeks

d. Some prefer biweekly visits from 41 weeks to delivery

e. Schedule more frequent visits as appropriate; some providers recommend fewer prenatal visits if there are no problems

6. Content of prenatal revisits

a. History

b. Physical examination—blood pressure, urine dipstick, weight, FHT, fundal height

c. Anticipatory management

d. Anticipatory guidance

e. Health education and counseling

f. Appropriate screening

- Prenatal risk factors
  1. History
     a. Genetic factors
        (1) Parental age at or older than 35 years
        (2) Previous child with a chromosome abnormality
        (3) Family history of birth defects or mental retardation
        (4) Ethnic/racial origins
            (a) African—sickle cell disease
            (b) Mediterranean or East Asian—B thalassemia
            (c) Jewish—Tay-Sachs disease
     b. Multiple pregnancy losses/previous stillbirths
     c. Psychological/mental health disorders
     d. History of IUGR
     e. Preterm birth(s)
  2. Current pregnancy
     a. Abnormal multiple marker screening
     b. Exposure to possible teratogens
        (1) Radiation
        (2) Alcohol/medications/other substances
        (3) Occupational exposures
        (4) Infections (see section on infection in Chapter 7, *Complex Pregnancy Care*)
            (a) Toxoplasmosis
            (b) Rubella
            (c) CMV
            (d) Herpes
            (e) HIV
            (f) Syphilis
            (g) Zika
     c. IUGR
     d. Oligohydramnios/polyhydramnios
     e. Diabetes
        (1) Pregestational
        (2) Gestational
            (a) Diet-controlled
            (b) Medication-controlled (by insulin or oral medications)
     f. Hypertension (see hypertension section in Chapter 7, *Complex Pregnancy Care*)
        (1) Chronic
        (2) Gestational
        (3) Preeclampsia/eclampsia
     g. Multiple gestation
     h. PROM
     i. Postterm (postdates pregnancy)
     j. Decreased fetal movement
     k. Rh isoimmunization

Common Discomforts of Pregnancy and Comfort Measures

- Nausea and vomiting of pregnancy (NVP)—most common in first trimester
  1. Nausea and vomiting—50% of pregnant individuals; nausea only, 25%; unaffected, 25%
  2. NVP is different from hyperemesis gravidarum (HG)
     a. HG happens much less frequently, in approximately 0.3%–3% of pregnancies
     b. HG is a diagnosis of exclusion when other causes of nausea and vomiting have been explored (see HG discussion in Chapter 7, *Complex Pregnancy Care*)
  3. Nonpharmacologic therapies for NVP
     a. Prevention—pregnant individuals who were taking multivitamins at the time of conception are less likely in need of treatment for vomiting; recommend that childbearing individuals of reproductive age take prenatal vitamins 3 months prior to conceiving to reduce the likelihood and intensity of NVP
     b. Avoid triggers, such as odors, that provoke symptoms
     c. Small, frequent meals every 1–2 hours
     d. Avoid spicy or fatty foods; eat foods that are high in protein
     e. Eat bland or dry foods, such as crackers or toast, before getting up and out of bed
     f. Discontinue prenatal vitamins with iron until nausea and vomiting have resolved, but continue folic acid
     g. Acupressure, acupuncture, or acustimulation at the P6 (Neiguan)—conflicting evidence for this therapy
- Breast tenderness
  1. Good support brassiere
  2. Careful intercourse
  3. Reassurance that it will soon pass
- Backache
  1. Consider other differential diagnoses for musculoskeletal strain, sciatica, sacroiliac joint problem, preterm labor, UTI
  2. Nonpathologic—related to normal changes in pregnancy
     a. Massage
     b. Application of ice or heat
     c. Hydrotherapy
     d. Pelvic rock
     e. Good body mechanics
     f. Pillow in lumbar area when sitting or between legs when lying on side
     g. Pregnancy support harness or girdle
     h. Good support brassiere
     i. Supportive low-heeled shoes
  3. Sacroiliac joint problems
     a. Teach appropriate exercises
     b. Nonelastic sacroiliac belt
     c. Trochanteric belt worn below the abdomen at the femoral heads to increase joint stability
- Fatigue
  1. Reassurance that this is a normal first-trimester problem and will pass
  2. Mild exercise and good nutrition
  3. Decrease activities and plan rest periods
  4. Decrease fluid intake in evening to decrease nocturia
- Heartburn
  1. Small, frequent meals
  2. Decrease amount of fluids taken with meals; drink fluids between meals

3. Papaya (may recommend fresh, dried, juice, or enzymes)
4. Elevate head of bed 10–30 degrees
5. Slippery elm bark throat lozenges
6. Antacids
7. Proton pump inhibitors and H_2 blockers

- Constipation
  1. Increased fluids, fiber
  2. Prune juice or warm beverage in the morning
  3. Encourage exercise
  4. Stool softeners
- Hemorrhoids
  1. Avoid constipation or straining with a bowel movement
  2. Elevate hips with pillow or knee–chest position
  3. Sitz baths
  4. Witch hazel or Epsom salt compresses
  5. Reinsert hemorrhoid with lubricated finger
  6. Kegel exercises
  7. Topical anesthetics; use with caution if combined with steroid
- Varicosities
  1. Support stockings; apply before getting out of bed
  2. Avoid wearing restrictive clothing
  3. Perineal pad if vaginal and vulvar varicosities
  4. Rest periods with legs elevated; avoid crossing legs
- Leg cramps
  1. Decrease phosphate in diet; no more than two glasses of milk per day
  2. Massage affected leg
  3. Do not point toes; flex ankle to stretch calf
  4. Keep legs warm
  5. Walk, exercise
  6. Calcium tablets
  7. Magnesium tablets
- Presyncopal episodes
  1. Change positions slowly
  2. Push fluids; regular caloric/glucose intake
  3. Avoid lying flat on back; avoid prolonged standing or sitting
- Headaches
  1. Rule out migraines and other pathologic causes of headache
  2. Head, shoulder, and/or neck massage
  3. Acupressure
  4. Hot or cold compresses
  5. Rest
  6. Follow a regular sleep schedule
  7. Warm baths
  8. Meditation and biofeedback
  9. Aromatherapy
  10. Eat smaller, more frequent meals
  11. Mild analgesic—such as acetaminophen 325 mg one to three tablets every 4 hours as needed
- Leukorrhea
  1. Rule out vaginitis and sexually transmitted infection (STI)
  2. Good perineal hygiene
  3. Wear cotton underwear and change as often as necessary
  4. Unscented panty liners

5. Instructions to avoid douching and use of feminine sprays
- Urinary frequency
  1. Decrease fluids in evening to avoid nocturia
  2. Avoid caffeine
  3. Rule out UTI
- Insomnia
  1. Warm bath
  2. Hot drink—warm milk, chamomile tea
  3. Quiet, relaxing, minimally stimulating activities
  4. Avoid daytime napping
- Round ligament pain
  1. Rule out other causes of abdominal pain, such as appendicitis, ovarian cyst, placental separation, inguinal hernia
  2. Warm compresses, ice compresses
  3. Hydrotherapy
  4. Avoid sudden movement or twisting movements
  5. Flex knees to abdomen, pelvic tilt
  6. Support uterus with a pillow when lying down
  7. Pregnancy abdominal support or girdle
- Skin rash
  1. Ice
  2. Oatmeal bath
  3. Diphenhydramine—25 mg orally every 4 hours as needed for itching
  4. Dermatology referral, as needed
- Carpal tunnel syndrome (tingling and numbness of fingers)
  1. Good posture
  2. Lying down
  3. Rest and elevate affected hands
  4. Ice, wrist splints
  5. Mild analgesic—such as acetaminophen 325 mg one to three tabs every 4 hours as needed

Nutrition During Pregnancy

- Recommended daily allowances
  1. Calories—2,500 kcal
  2. Protein—average of 60 g/day throughout pregnancy
- Weight gain in pregnancy
  1. Body mass index (BMI; weight/height^2)—only anthropometric measurement with documented clinical value for assessment of gestational weight gain
  2. Weight-for-height categories
     a. Underweight—BMI <18.5
     b. Normal weight—BMI 18.5–24.9
     c. Overweight—BMI 25.0–29.9
     d. Obese—BMI ≥30.0
  3. Determinants of gestational weight gain
     a. Prepregnant weight—if overweight at conception, more likely to gain less weight than normal-weight individual
     b. Low gestational weight gain associated with several factors
        (1) Low family income

(2) Black race
(3) Young age
(4) Unmarried status
(5) Low educational level
  c. Multiple gestation
  d. Developing pathology
4. Consequences of gestational weight gain
  a. Low gestational weight gain is associated with:
    (1) Growth-restricted infants
    (2) Fetal and infant mortality
  b. High gestational weight gain is associated with:
    (1) Greater rate of large infant weight; may increase the risk for several conditions
      (a) Fetopelvic disproportion
      (b) Operative delivery (forceps, vacuum, or cesarean)
      (c) Birth trauma
      (d) Asphyxia
      (e) PPH
      (f) Mortality
    (2) The above associations are more pronounced in short individuals (<157 cm or 62 in)
5. Recommended patterns and quantity of weight gain
  a. Normal prepregnant weight—0.8 to 1.0 lb per week during second and third trimesters, for a total of 25–35 lb for singleton; 50–62 lb if pregnant with twins
  b. Underweight before pregnancy—1.0 to 1.3 lb per week in second and third trimesters, for a total of 28–40 lb for singleton; 37–54 lb if pregnant with twins
  c. Overweight before pregnancy—0.5 to 0.7 lb per week in second and third trimesters, for a total of 15–25 lb for singleton; 31–50 lb if pregnant with twins
  d. Obese before pregnancy—0.4 to 0.6 lb per week in second and third trimesters, for a total of 11–20 lb if singleton; 25–42 lb if pregnant with twins

- Diet history—the recall of fluid and solid food intake in the last 24 hours with the purpose of evaluating the adequacy of nutrition and formulating a plan for nutrition counseling
1. Components of diet history
  a. Qualitative components of the intake
  b. Quantitative components, but only if weight is an issue
  c. Ascertain how typical the last 24-hour intake was relative to the usual intake
2. Components of diet counseling
  a. Diet assessment
  b. Set a weight gain goal with the patient for the pregnancy
  c. Discuss food preferences and their relationship to the goal
  d. Review generally or specifically at each visit, depending on the results
  e. Include fetal growth as part of the parameters
3. Cultural and personal beliefs about nutrition that may modify a diet plan
  a. Pica—ingestion of nonfood substances (i.e., starch, clay)

  b. Vegetarianism
  c. Hot and cold foods and when they can be eaten
  d. Discern eating patterns and beliefs pertinent to pregnancy in the individual's culture

The Childbearing People and Their Families, and Their Families' Role in Pregnancy

- Family
1. Assessment of family size, structure, and relationships
2. Significant individuals involved in pregnancy
3. Family roles and their relationship to family function
  a. Occupations
  b. Income levels
  c. Education levels
  d. Nationality and ethnic background
  e. Relationship status and intensity
4. Feelings and thoughts about this pregnancy and any past pregnancies and births

- Pregnancy as essential, permanent family and life change
1. The significance of change in relation to pregnancy
2. Role adaptation needed to cope successfully with pregnancy
3. Family resources to be mobilized to enable the family to cope
  a. Clear and continuous communication of information
  b. Decision-making by the childbearing person and family as indicated
  c. Family's development of an appropriate birth plan
    (1) Childbirth preparation
    (2) Breastfeeding
    (3) Childrearing classes
  d. Information regarding critical resources in birth site
    (1) Labor and birth procedures and expectations
    (2) Rooming-in
    (3) Breastfeeding support
    (4) Sibling visitation and/or presence at birth
    (5) Family visitation
    (6) Possibility of early discharge

- Perinatal loss and associated grief stages and process
1. Factors associated with the concept of loss and grieving
  a. Perception of the individual(s) experiencing the loss and its severity
  b. Support and assistance in doing grief work
2. Types of maternity losses
  a. Infertility
  b. Loss of a baby
    (1) Miscarriage
    (2) Abortion
    (3) Stillbirth
    (4) Adoption

c. Loss of expectations
  (1) Premature infant
  (2) Congenital deformities
  (3) "Damaged" infant
3. Stages of grief
  a. Shock, manifested by:
    (1) Denial
    (2) Disbelief
    (3) Fear
    (4) Isolation
    (5) Crying
    (6) Hostility
    (7) Bitterness
    (8) Introversion
    (9) Sadness
    (10) Numbness
  b. Physical signs and symptoms
    (1) Weight loss
    (2) Insomnia
    (3) Fatigue
    (4) Restlessness
    (5) Shortness of breath
    (6) Chest pain
  c. Suffering—the reality stage
    (1) Acceptance of the reality
    (2) Adaptation
    (3) Preoccupation with lost person
    (4) Questioning of what happened and why
    (5) Feelings of fear, guilt, and anger persist
  d. Resolution—acceptance and adaptation are complete
    (1) Reinvests in other significant relationships
    (2) Moves on but remembers the lost person
4. Maladaptive grief reactions
  a. Avoidance or distortion of normal grief expression
  b. Agitated depression; psychosomatic conditions
  c. Morbid attachment to possessions of deceased
  d. Persistent loss of self-esteem
5. Healthcare provider's role in helping the normal grieving process
  a. Listen
  b. Facilitate the patient's expression of feelings
  c. Provide nonjudgmental environment
  d. Accept behaviors of grief

Education and Counseling

- Principles of learning that apply to individuals during pregnancy
  1. Factors that facilitate or impede learning
    a. Readiness of the learner; time to discuss
    b. Healthcare provider's knowledge of childbearing person's and family's learning needs
    c. Group teaching—enhances and enriches learning
  2. Factors that critically influence teaching/learning
    a. Alternative lifestyles; different cultures
    b. Disadvantaged social milieus

c. Age and maturity—adolescents, educational level, life experience
- Principles of teaching for the role of parent educator
  1. Individual teaching and counseling—topic and quantity of information need to fit the client
  2. Prioritize information provision
    a. Respond to questions or experiences of the person
    b. Anticipatory guidance of pregnancy realities
    c. Danger signs of critical complications; drug dangers, prescription, over-the-counter, and drugs that can be misused; any other information needed for the health and well-being of the individual and the fetus
- Childbirth education
  1. Preparation for childbearing—ultimately aids in reducing the need for analgesics/anesthetics during labor
    a. Formal or informal
    b. Content to be included
      (1) Bodily changes in pregnancy with associated reproduction anatomy
      (2) Exercises for activities of daily living (ADLs) during pregnancy and for labor
      (3) Nutrition
      (4) Fetal growth and development
      (5) Substance abuse
      (6) Signs of beginning labor
      (7) Information for infant feeding decision making
      (8) Preparation for breastfeeding
      (9) Postpartal course and care
      (10) Preparation of siblings for birth
      (11) Pain coping strategies in labor
      (12) Vaginal birth after cesarean (VBAC) versus elective repeat cesarean section (ERCS) if previous cesarean section
  2. Learning needs of the breastfeeding/chestfeeding/lactating individual
    a. Anticipatory guidance for person with inverted nipples
    b. Principles of milk production
      (1) Caloric needs of mother
      (2) Liquid needs of mother
      (3) Mechanics of proper infant positioning and latching on
      (4) Factors that affect milk supply
  3. Learning needs for parenthood
    a. Plans for the baby's health care
    b. Needs and adaptation for the home
    c. Identification of family/social supports
- Family planning
  1. Pregnancy learning needs for postpartum contraceptive options
  2. Learning needs when considering postpartum bilateral tubal ligation
    a. Expert counseling
    b. Signing consent papers
- Human sexuality and pregnancy
  1. The effects of pregnancy on sexual response
  2. Changes in sexual desire throughout pregnancy—influenced by hormones, energy level, relationship,

body image, fears of hurting the baby, cultural beliefs and practices

3. Concept of body image—may feel awkward, clumsy, ugly, especially in late pregnancy
4. Factors during pregnancy that may alter this image—support or lack thereof for maternal feelings; responses, either positive or negative, from people of importance
5. Variations in sexual practice and their use during pregnancy
   a. Positions for intercourse—alternative positions may enhance comfort with an increase in abdominal size
   b. Cunnilingus
   c. Fellatio
   d. Anal intercourse
6. Sexual activity may be continued throughout a healthy pregnancy
7. The potential relationship between orgasm and uterine contractions
   a. Contraindicated if preterm labor threatens
   b. May help initiate labor

Pharmacologic Considerations in the Antepartum Period

- Teratogens (derived from the Greek word meaning "monster")—any agent that acts during embryonic or fetal development to produce a permanent alteration of form or function
- The Pregnancy and Lactation Labeling Final Rule (PLLR) went into effect on June 30, 2015. By June 29, 2018, all Food and Drug Administration (FDA) risk factor categories were to be removed from drug labels and replaced by narrative sections to include a more comprehensive description of pregnancy and lactation risk and effects. The PLLR includes the following sections: pregnancy exposure registry, risk summary, clinical considerations, and data that describe the information used in the previous sections.
- Prior to the PLLR, the FDA risk factor categories for prescription drugs in pregnancy were used for medication labeling. The old categories are included in this review in case these categories appear in the Women's Health Nurse Practitioner (WHNP)/American Midwifery Certification Board (AMCB) certification exams.
  1. Category A—adequate, well-controlled studies in pregnant individuals have not shown an increased risk of fetal abnormalities; examples: folic acid, levothyroxine
  2. Category B—animal studies have revealed no evidence of harm to the fetus; however, there are no adequate and well-controlled studies in pregnant individuals *or* animal studies have shown an adverse effect, but adequate and well-controlled studies in pregnant individuals have failed to demonstrate a risk to the fetus; examples: ondansetron, amoxicillin

  3. Category C—animal studies have shown an adverse effect, and there are no adequate and well-controlled studies in pregnant individuals *or* no animal studies have been conducted, and there are no adequate and well-controlled studies in pregnant individuals; examples: sertraline, fluconazole
  4. Category D—studies, adequate and well-controlled or observational, in pregnant individuals have demonstrated a risk to the fetus; however, the benefits of therapy may outweigh the potential risk; examples: phenytoin, lithium
  5. Category X—studies, adequate and well-controlled or observational, in animals or pregnant individuals have demonstrated positive evidence of fetal abnormalities; use of the product is contraindicated in individuals who are or may become pregnant; examples: methotrexate, warfarin
- Live vaccines—generally contraindicated in pregnancy because of concerns about the risk of transmitting the virus to a developing fetus; recommendation to give the vaccine 4 weeks prior to pregnancy or to wait until the postpartum period
- Vaccines considered safe in pregnancy
  1. Tetanus/diphtheria/acellular pertussis (Tdap)—Advisory Committee on Immunization Practices (ACIP) recommends Tdap vaccination during each pregnancy whether the patient has received Tdap (or Td) in the past
  2. Hepatitis B—high-risk individuals who are antigen and antibody negative can be vaccinated during pregnancy
  3. Tetanus—vaccination during pregnancy can protect at-risk newborns against neonatal tetanus; in maternal trauma, may be indicated
  4. Influenza—trivalent inactivated influenza vaccine (TIV) recommended for all pregnant individuals during the influenza season; live attenuated nasal influenza vaccine contraindicated during pregnancy
  5. COVID-19—recommended for everyone ages 6 months and older including pregnant and lactating individuals; may be administered on the same day as other routinely recommended vaccines, including influenza vaccine; refer to CDC for updates on booster vaccinations
- Vaccines contraindicated during pregnancy or whose safety has not been established
  1. Rubella (German measles)—attenuated live-virus vaccine contraindicated immediately before or during pregnancy; offer vaccination postpartum
  2. Varicella—attenuated live-virus vaccine (Varivax) contraindicated in pregnancy; offer vaccination postpartum

Techniques Used to Assess Fetal Health

- Ultrasound (US)
  1. Definition—method in which intermittent high-frequency sound waves are transmitted through tissues by way of a transducer placed on the abdomen or in the vagina, and then reflected off the underlying

structures so that tissues, fluid, bones, fetal activity, and vessel pulsations are discernible

2. Types of ultrasound
   a. Abdominal ultrasound—most commonly used method
   b. Transvaginal ultrasound—may be used in early pregnancy
3. Indications for ultrasound use can be found in an earlier section of the chapter

- Doppler velocimetry blood flow assessment
  1. Used in tertiary settings only if uteroplacental insufficiency resulting in FGR is suspected or present
  2. Detects velocity of blood flow through the fetal umbilical artery to the placenta; displayed in a waveform
  3. Normal waveforms produced when the ratio of systolic to diastolic blood flow (S/D ratio) is approximately 3; abnormal ratio is more than 3

- Amniocentesis
  1. Amniotic fluid is aspirated from the amniotic sac and evaluated for genetic well-being or disorders, and fetal lung maturity
  2. Usually performed between 14 and 16 weeks for genetic evaluation or assessment of neural tube defects
  3. Used later in pregnancy—assessment of lung maturity; rule out amnionitis or fetal hemolytic disease (Rh or anti-D)
  4. Risks—infection, bleeding, preterm labor, PROM, fetal loss
  5. Benefits
     a. Provides early diagnosis; may decrease morbidity and mortality if elective abortion (AB) is sought
     b. May decrease psychological stress; support systems can be established prior to delivery
     c. If a lethal anomaly is diagnosed and pregnancy continues, allow parents/care providers to plan (i.e., avoid a cesarean section)
  6. Special precaution—if the mother is Rh negative and at risk for isoimmunization, administer RhoGAM with amniocentesis

- Chorionic villus sampling (CVS)
  1. Sample of chorionic villi from the placenta is aspirated either transabdominally or transcervically; the outer trophoblastic layer is obtained because these tissues have the same genetic makeup as the fetus; the tissue is examined for genetic information
  2. Used for prenatal diagnosis; performed between 10 and 13 weeks
  3. Benefits
     a. Performed 3–4 weeks earlier than amniocentesis
     b. Cultures grow rapidly, resulting in early diagnosis
  4. Risks
     a. Infection, bleeding, miscarriage
     b. Risk of limb deformities (if performed before 9 weeks)
     c. Technically more difficult
     d. Contraindicated in case of maternal blood group sensitization

- Fetal movement counting (FMC)/fetal kick counts (FKC)
  1. FMC/FKC
     a. Maternal self-report of fetal movement to assess fetal wellness

b. Most pregnant individuals are aware of fetal movement between 16 and 22 weeks' gestation; multiparas are generally aware of movement sooner than nulliparas are
c. Fetus has periods of sleep and wakefulness that change according to gestation
d. Fetal movement is strongest between 29 and 38 weeks
e. FMC/FKC is a safe, simple, no-cost, noninvasive fetal assessment technique
f. Research has demonstrated that fetal activity is a good predictor of well-being
g. Dramatic decrease or cessation of movement is cause for concern

2. Methods for performing FMC/FKC—adjusted to client's abilities with instructions to count fetal movements starting at 28 weeks (identifiable risk present) or 34–36 weeks (low risk for uteroplacental insufficiency)
   a. Sanovsky's protocol
      (1) Count FM 30 minutes three times daily; four or more movements in a 30-minute period is reassuring
      (2) If fewer than four movements in a 30-minute period, then continue for 1 hour
      (3) Contact care provider if fewer than 10 movements or if movements become weak
   b. Cardiff "count to 10" method
      (1) A chart to check off 10 fetal movements in one counting session
      (2) Start at approximately the same time daily
      (3) Chart how long it took to count 10 movements
      (4) If fewer than 10 movements in 10 hours or the amount of time to reach 10 movements increases, a nonstress test should be performed

- Nonstress test (NST)
  1. Method to assess fetal well-being by observing the FHR response to fetal movement
  2. 75% of fetuses at 28 weeks experience heart rate accelerations in association with fetal movement
  3. External electronic fetal monitoring (EFM) is used to record FHR accelerations in response to fetal movement
  4. Accelerations may be spontaneous or may be induced by vibroacoustic stimulation (VAS)
  5. Fetal hypoxia depresses the medullary center in the brain that controls FHR response, resulting in depression of frequency or amplitude of the FHR
  6. Indications for assessment of fetal well-being with NST
     a. Decreased fetal movement
     b. Postterm
     c. Diabetes, hypertension, IUGR
  7. Interpretation of results
     a. Reactive—two or more accelerations in FHR of 15 or more beats per minute (bpm), lasting for ≥15 seconds, within a 15- to 20-minute period for >32 weeks GA; if between 28 and 32 weeks, criteria are ≥10 bpm, lasting 10 seconds
     b. Nonreactive—FHR fails to demonstrate the required accelerations within a 40-minute period, requiring further evaluation

c. Unsatisfactory or inconclusive—FHR tracing that is uninterpretable or of poor quality, sometimes caused by a vigorous infant; test should be repeated (individual site protocols vary)

d. Factors potentially affecting NST results
   (1) Fetal sleep
   (2) Smoking within 30 minutes of testing
   (3) Maternal intake of medications
   (4) Fetal central nervous system (CNS) anomalies
   (5) Fetal hypoxia and/or acidosis

e. A nonreactive NST may be followed by a BPP, a contraction stress test, or a repeat NST

f. If indicated, NSTs should be repeated either weekly or biweekly

- Contraction stress test (CST)—assessment of fetal well-being by observing FHR response to uterine contractions
  1. Physiology
     a. During uterine contractions, placental vessels are compressed, and intervillous blood flow to the fetus is decreased
     b. A fetus that is compromised or hypoxic has decreased oxygenation; may result in metabolic acidosis
  2. Method
     a. Test is conducted in the hospital
     b. EFM; monitor the FHR response to uterine contractions
     c. Contractions may be spontaneous, the result of administration of exogenous oxytocin, or from nipple stimulation
     d. Acceptable test—three palpable contractions lasting 40–60 seconds
  3. Results
     a. Negative—no late or variable decelerations
     b. Equivocal or suspicious—presence of nonrepetitive or nonpersistent decelerations, or long-term variability is absent
     c. Positive—persistent late decelerations with 50% or more of the contractions
  4. Contraindications to CST
     a. Absolute—previous classical cesarean section or myomectomy, placenta previa, at risk for preterm labor
     b. Relative—GA less than 37 weeks, multiple gestation

- Amniotic fluid volume (AFV) measurement—several techniques are used to measure the AFV: subjective assessment by an expert examiner, measurement of a single deepest vertical pocket of fluid, and measurement of AFI
  1. Single deepest pocket of fluid—keeping the transducer perpendicular to the floor, the single deepest vertical pocket of fluid that is free of fetal parts of the umbilical cord is measured; normal measurement is between 2 and 8 cm
  2. AFI—virtually divide the uterus into four quadrants and measure the deepest vertical pocket of fluid in each quadrant with ultrasound; AFI is the sum of the four measurements obtained; normal measurement is between 5 and 24 cm

- Biophysical Profile (BPP)—procedure utilizing ultrasound to evaluate five fetal variables to assess fetal risk; prospective studies have demonstrated that BPP is superior to CST as a predictor of fetal well-being or distress
  1. Method
     a. Test is composed of five observable variables—NST, muscle tone, breathing movements, gross body movements, AFV
     b. In addition to NST, the fetus is evaluated via USG for a 30-minute time period to observe the remaining four variables
  2. BPP scoring—each of the five variables is scored from 0 (abnormal) to 2 (normal); the scores for each are totaled
     a. Breathing movements—one or more episodes in 30 minutes; none = 0, present = 2
     b. Body movement—three or more discrete body or limb movements in 30 minutes; none = 0, present = 2
     c. Tone—one or more episodes of extension with a return to flexion; none = 0, present = 2
     d. Qualitative AFV—at least one pocket of amniotic fluid that measures at least 2 cm in two perpendicular planes; none = 0, present = 2
     e. Reactivity—reactive NST; nonreactive scored as 0, reactive = 2
  3. Scoring interpretation criteria
     a. 8–10 is normal (in the absence of oligohydramnios)
     b. 6 is equivocal, repeat testing
     c. 4 or less is abnormal
  4. Modified BBP, NST, and AFI—see the Postterm Pregnancy section in Chapter 7, *Complex Pregnancy Care*

- Percutaneous umbilical blood sampling (PUBS) or cordocentesis
  1. Definition—the process in which a needle is introduced under real-time ultrasound through the gravid abdomen and then into the umbilical cord; blood is aspirated, or blood and/or medications are introduced into the fetus
  2. Usually performed after 20 weeks
  3. Used for prenatal diagnosis—Rh (anti-D) disease, fetal infections, blood factor abnormalities, chromosomal or genetic disease, fetal hypoxia assessment
  4. Used to treat the fetus—fetal transfusion, administer drug therapy
  5. Concerns
     a. Similar to amniocentesis and CVS procedures
     b. Must be performed by a skilled individual who is able to secure immediate delivery and an appropriate level of neonatal care, if necessary

- Methods to assess fetal lung maturity
  1. Respiratory distress syndrome (RDS)—a major neonatal complication associated with preterm birth
  2. Assessment of fetal lung maturity—accomplished by assessing the amniotic fluid
  3. Different tests may be used to assess the factors that help prevent atelectasis
  4. Prior to 39 weeks' gestation, there should be an evaluation of fetal lung maturity if labor induction or

cesarean delivery is electively scheduled to help prevent iatrogenic prematurity and RDS
  a. Lecithin/sphingomyelin ratio (L/S)
    (1) Lecithin is elevated after 35 weeks
    (2) Sphingomyelin remains fairly constant

    (3) Ratio of 2:1 or greater is indicative of fetal lung maturity except in diabetes
    (4) L/S ratio may also not be accurate in hydrops fetalis and nonhypertensive glomerulonephritis

Questions

Select the best answer.

1. A patient's menstrual period is 1 month overdue. The level of pregnancy diagnosis is:
  a. positive
  b. possible
  c. presumptive
  d. probable

2. A patient is trying to get pregnant and had unprotected intercourse on day 14 of the patient's 28-day menstrual cycle. The pregnancy test was negative 3 days later. Appropriate next steps to confirm pregnancy would be to:
  a. order a serum pregnancy test
  b. order an ultrasound
  c. prescribe progesterone
  d. repeat the test in a week

3. Pregnancy tests detect which hormone?
  a. Estrogen
  b. hCG
  c. hPL
  d. Progesterone

4. During the first few weeks of pregnancy, progesterone is secreted by the:
  a. corpus luteum
  b. endometrium
  c. placenta
  d. trophoblasts

5. Blood in the chorionic villi pertains to the circulation of the:
  a. amnion
  b. fetus
  c. placenta
  d. pregnant person

6. The vessels of the umbilical cord consist of:
  a. one vein carrying oxygenated blood and two arteries carrying deoxygenated blood
  b. one vein carrying deoxygenated blood and two arteries carrying oxygenated blood
  c. two veins carrying oxygenated blood and one artery carrying deoxygenated blood
  d. two veins carrying deoxygenated blood and one artery carrying oxygenated blood

7. The uterus is palpable at the symphysis pubis at:
  a. 6 weeks' gestation
  b. 8 weeks' gestation
  c. 12 weeks' gestation
  d. 16 weeks' gestation

8. Implantation occurs _____ after fertilization.
  a. 24–48 hours
  b. 3–4 days
  c. 6–7 days
  d. 9–10 days

9. Placental transport of oxygen and glucose occurs by:
  a. active osmosis
  b. active perfusion
  c. facilitated diffusion
  d. simple perfusion

10. The human zygote has:
  a. 2 pairs of sex chromosomes
  b. 23 pairs of chromosomes
  c. 23 telomeres
  d. 46 chromosomes from each parent

11. The trophoblast will ultimately become the:
  a. blastocyst
  b. embryo
  c. placenta
  d. umbilical cord

12. A grade I systolic murmur is heard at the initial visit of a primigravida patient. The next best step in management would be:
  a. a cardiology consult
  b. chest radiograph
  c. immediate referral
  d. no intervention

13. The drop in diastolic blood pressure that occurs during normal pregnancy is partly the result of:
  a. increased cardiac output
  b. plasma volume expansion
  c. pooling of plasma in the tissues
  d. progesterone's effect on the vessel walls

14. Changes in the respiratory system due to pregnancy may cause:
  a. cough
  b. increased chest diameter
  c. pale nasal mucosa
  d. tachypnea

15. A cis-woman who is a G1P0 at 34 weeks states she is having "a lot of vaginal discharge," but no other symptoms or problems. On exam, a white, odorless discharge of moderate quantity is visible. The next best step is to:
  a. evaluate for trichomoniasis
  b. reassure the patient that this is normal
  c. send a vaginal culture
  d. treat for candida

16. A pregnant patient comes for a 24-week visit and mentions that her interest in sex has increased greatly. Which of the following is accurate guidance about increased libido in pregnancy?
    a. A normal variation of response in pregnancy
    b. An abnormal response to a changing body image
    c. Reflective of repressed desire to disrupt the pregnancy
    d. The early sign of a parenting disorder

17. At the 36-week visit, a pregnant patient is having nightmares that include labor and fears of having an abnormal baby. Which of the following responses demonstrates an understanding of anxiety in pregnancy?
    a. Encourage the patient to tell you more about the nightmares and fears.
    b. Make an appointment for the patient with a mental health nurse practitioner.
    c. Reassure the patient that there are dangers about which we all have to worry.
    d. Tell the patient there is nothing to worry about because most babies are fine.

18. Initial management of constipation in pregnancy should include suggestions for:
    a. decreased protein intake
    b. increased intake of fiber and fluids
    c. limitation of calcium-rich foods
    d. use of a laxative

19. A patient has experienced three spontaneous abortions and is now pregnant for the fourth time. The term that defines this patient's obstetric status is:
    a. multipara
    b. nullipara
    c. primigravida
    d. primipara

20. The calculation of estimated date of birth (EDB) by Naegele's rule is based on a(n):
    a. 28-day menstrual cycle
    b. 32-day cycle
    c. average length of pregnancy of 290 days
    d. length of pregnancy of 270 days

21. Pregnant for the third time, the patient has an obstetric history that indicates two miscarriages at 16 and 18 weeks, respectively, and one twin birth at 36 weeks. One twin died, but the other is alive and well. The four-digit descriptor of parity accurately reflecting this history is:
    a. 0121
    b. 0221
    c. 2021
    d. 2201

22. At a first antepartum visit, a patient with a 6-month-old daughter reports not having had a menstrual period while nursing. The midwife/WHNP diagnoses that the patient is pregnant. How is the estimated date of birth (EDB) best calculated in this scenario?
    a. Determine the expected period date and calculate from there.
    b. Document quickening and extrapolate from there.
    c. Get a good sexual history and use the last coitus as the basis for calculation.
    d. Send the patient to the fetal assessment unit for an ultrasound.

23. A pregnant patient who is a G1P0 at 20 weeks has an abdominal exam that shows the uterine fundus to be halfway between the symphysis and the umbilicus. This finding leads you to consider:
    a. fetal growth restriction
    b. inadequate weight gain
    c. nothing because it is normal
    d. oligohydramnios

24. In an abdominal exam using Leopold's maneuvers, the first step is to determine fetal:
    a. attitude
    b. engagement
    c. lie
    d. position

25. At a first antepartum visit, a patient is found to be 10 weeks pregnant and requests to listen for the FHT. The WHNP has a handheld Doppler available. Of the following, which response reflects a correct understanding of fetal development?
    a. "There is no reason to listen because it cannot be heard until 18 weeks."
    b. "We can try to listen today. But we may not hear the heartbeat yet."
    c. "Yes! We can definitely hear the heartbeat as early as 6.5 weeks."
    d. "You will need a referral for an ultrasound to detect a heartbeat."

26. Normal findings on speculum and pelvic examination of a pregnant person include:
    a. a firm, slightly enlarged cervix
    b. an open cervical os
    c. bluish color of the cervix
    d. pale vaginal mucosa

27. A primigravida at 13.5 weeks has not felt the baby move yet and is concerned. Which of the following is an example of an accurate response?
    a. "I will order an ultrasound just to be sure everything is fine."
    b. "I would like you to return in a week so we can recheck it."
    c. "You are worrying too much—just relax."
    d. "You may not feel movement until around 20 weeks."

28. Maternal serum alpha-fetoprotein screening is performed in what time frame during pregnancy?
    a. 8–12 weeks
    b. 12–15 weeks
    c. 15–19 weeks
    d. 20–24 weeks

29. The CDC recommends screening for GBS:
    a. at the first visit
    b. at 20 weeks
    c. at 35–37 weeks
    d. when labor starts

30. Cell-free DNA screens for the risk of the following chromosomal abnormalities:
    a. Trisomy 13, 18, and 21
    b. phenylketonuria and maple syrup urine disease
    c. Spina bifida, cleft lip, and anencephaly
    d. Cystic fibrosis

31. An NST containing two fetal heart accelerations lasting 15 seconds that are 15 beats per minute above the baseline is considered:
    a. negative
    b. nonreactive
    c. positive
    d. reactive

32. The recommended folic acid supplement for a pregnant person with a history of a baby with a neural tube defect is:
    a. 0.4 mg per day starting with a missed period
    b. 0.4 mg per day throughout pregnancy
    c. 2 mg per day prior to conception
    d. 4 mg per day starting before conception

33. A pregnant patient is 5 ft 4 in and weighs 190 lb (BMI = 33). Per the IOM guidelines for weight gain in pregnancy, which is the most accurate goal:
    a. gain 11–20 lb
    b. gain 25–35 lb
    c. lose 10–15 lb
    d. maintain current weight

34. Exercise guidelines for healthy pregnant people include suggestions to:
    a. begin an intense program of exercise, especially if pre-pregnancy weight was high
    b. discontinue exercise at 20 weeks
    c. limit fluids before exercising
    d. modify the existing program if symptoms occur

35. Which if the following reflects accurate anticipatory guidance concerning sexual activity during pregnancy?
    a. The desire for sex typically wanes after the first trimester.
    b. The pregnant person's sexual desire may change throughout pregnancy.
    c. Limit sexual activity beyond the third trimester in an uncomplicated pregnancy.
    d. With a history of preterm labor, sexual intercourse is contraindicated in pregnancy.

36. Breastfeeding should be discouraged for pregnant patients who:
    a. have inadequate mammary tissue
    b. are HIV positive and untreated
    c. desire to pump and bottlefeed
    d. do not have family support

37. A patient comes in for the first antepartal visit at 8 weeks and reports nausea every morning and an inability to eat and drink in the afternoon. Of the following options, the best first step in management at this point would include:
    a. advising the patient to eat small, frequent meals
    b. a prescription for anti-nausea medicine
    c. recommending a carbonated beverage on rising
    d. vitamin B_6 50 mg twice a day

38. The fatigue of early pregnancy is best managed by:
    a. encouraging increased caffeinated drinks
    b. encouraging increased exercise
    c. reassurance and rest
    d. ruling out a thyroid problem

39. Leg cramps during pregnancy may be relieved by:
    a. hot compresses
    b. flexion of the foot
    c. pointing the toes
    d. hot tub baths

40. At a 36-week visit, a pregnant patient reports somewhat swollen hands and feet. Objective findings include 2 lb weight gain since the last visit 2 weeks ago, blood pressure of 128/76 mm Hg, and no proteinuria. Which of the following is the most appropriate plan?
    a. Normalize the patient's edema and reschedule for 1 week.
    b. Order strict bedrest.
    c. Refer the patient to perinatology for suspected preeclampsia.
    d. Restrict fluid intake.

41. A primigravida patient asks about the value of childbirth preparation classes during a second-trimester visit. Which of the following accurately reflects the evidence related to the benefit of childbirth preparation classes in pregnancy?
    a. Decreased cesarean rates
    b. Improved parenting skills
    c. Less use of IVs in labor
    d. Reduced use of anesthesia

42. Which of the following reflects current recommendations for gestational diabetes screening for pregnant patients with a BMI >30?
    a. Daily fingersticks for blood sugar monitoring
    b. Fasting blood glucose each trimester
    c. Hemoglobin A_{1c} in the first trimester
    d. Screening in early pregnancy and at 24–28 weeks

43. A pregnant patient at 34 weeks' gestation has a fundal height of 39 cm. Abdominal palpation reveals a large uterus and difficulty feeling fetal parts. The most likely diagnosis is:
    a. macrosomic fetus
    b. multiple gestation
    c. polyhydramnios
    d. uterine fibroid

44. During the initial prenatal visit, the patient reports having had a rubella immunization 3 weeks before conceiving this baby. A responsive plan includes:
    a. advising the patient to consider termination of the pregnancy
    b. consulting with an infectious disease specialist
    c. continuing regular antenatal care
    d. referring the patient to a perinatologist

45. A 25-year-old pregnant patient at 14 weeks' gestation has the following physical examination findings: a 1 cm, mobile, well-defined, nontender mass in the upper, outer quadrant of her right breast. Of the following, which is the next best step in management?
    a. Explain that this is a common hormonal change in pregnancy.
    b. Monitor the mass at each visit to assess for any change.
    c. Refer the patient for further evaluation with biopsy.
    d. Schedule a mammogram to be done in the third trimester.

46. The BPP assesses fetal well-being by:
    a. assessing the results of a CST and ultrasound measurement of amniotic fluid
    b. combining the results of an NST and ultrasound evaluation to assess five variables
    c. conducting serial ultrasounds to evaluate fetal breathing, body movement, and tone
    d. evaluating fetal movement with kick counts after exposure to exogenous oxytocin

47. Which of the following is an appropriate plan of care for a patient at 40 weeks' gestation with a BPP score of 8, which includes a score of 2 for amniotic fluid volume (AFV)?
    a. Admit for induction of labor
    b. Order a contraction stress test
    c. Repeat the BPP in 48 hours
    d. Schedule a visit for 1 week

48. Blood glucose monitoring for an antenatal patient with gestational diabetes should be done:
    a. 1 hour after the smallest and largest meals of the day
    b. 1 hour before each meal
    c. fasting and 1 or 2 hours after each meal
    d. once a week, at the same time each week

49. A patient who is 11 weeks pregnant calling from the emergency department has sustained a laceration and is concerned that the hospital clinician wants to administer a tetanus booster. Of the following, which is the most accurate advice regarding receiving the tetanus shot in pregnancy?
    a. Any tetanus vaccine is contraindicated in pregnancy.
    b. In this case, the full vaccination dose is required.
    c. The tetanus booster is safe in pregnancy if needed.
    d. Vaccination should be delayed until the third trimester.

50. A person who is pregnant for the second time and whose first pregnancy ended with a spontaneous abortion at 10 weeks is a:
    a. multigravida
    b. multipara
    c. primigravida
    d. primipara

51. A pregnant patient presents for her 24-week visit, at which time she reports a diminished interest in sex. Which of the following is the most accurate response?
    a. Tell the patient that this is common and not a cause for concern
    b. Reassure the patient that the interest will return in the third trimester
    c. Tell the patient to get more rest and the interest will increase
    d. Discuss the patient's thoughts and feelings about sex

52. The screening test for GBS requires that the specimen be obtained from the:
    a. ectocervix and vaginal sidewalls
    b. ectocervix and endocervical os
    c. endocervical os and rectum
    d. vaginal introitus and rectum

53. Pregnancy loss and the patient's need for appropriate grieving occur across the reproductive spectrum. Maladaptive grief reactions are best addressed by:
    a. telling the patient to put the baby's things away
    b. listening to whatever the patient has to say
    c. encouraging the patient to be strong to get past it
    d. making the patient an appointment with a therapist

54. Recommended routine screening tests at an initial antenatal visit during the first trimester include:
    a. GBS culture
    b. syphilis serology
    c. triple marker screen
    d. ultrasound

55. Which of the following statements concerning influenza vaccination for pregnant patients is true?
    a. Vaccination is recommended for all individuals who will be pregnant during the influenza season.
    b. Pregnant individuals with HIV infection should not receive this vaccination.
    c. The pregnant patient should be offered the option of either the injection or nasal administration of the vaccine.
    d. Vaccination should be given only in the second or third trimester.

56. The RDAs of calories and protein, respectively, during pregnancy are:
    a. 3,000 kcal and 50 g/day
    b. 3,500 kcal and 60 g/day
    c. 3,800 kcal and 60 g/day
    d. 2,500 kcal and 60 g/day

57. A patient presents for her 36-week visit. Abdominal exam reveals a likelihood of polyhydramnios. In response to her question about where the fluid comes from, an accurate answer would be that it comes from:
    a. the pregnant patient's blood volume
    b. a combination of maternal serum and fetal urination
    c. amniotic epithelium and fetal functions
    d. fluid ingested by the mother

58. A 24-year-old primigravida presents for her initial visit and asks how the fetus has genes from both her husband and herself. The best response is based on which of the following concepts?
    a. Mitosis occurs, producing half the number of chromosomes.
    b. Meiosis occurs, producing half the number of chromosomes.
    c. The egg is a somatic cell.
    d. Sperm is a somatic cell.

59. Which of the following are parts of the placenta?
    a. Trophoblasts, chorion, amnion
    b. Trophoblasts, chorion, endometrium
    c. Chorion, amnion, umbilical cord
    d. Intervillous spaces, endometrium, trophoblasts

60. The term conceptus means:
    a. the embryo and placenta
    b. the embryo and membranes
    c. the embryo, membranes, and placenta
    d. the embryo, membranes, placenta, and endometrium

61. Which structure in human reproduction produces the most diverse and greatest quantity of steroid and protein hormones?
    a. Trophoblast
    b. Blastocyst
    c. Chorion laeve
    d. Deciduas basalis

62. At the 32-week visit, a patient asks the clinician to explain what they are looking for or feeling when doing an abdominal exam with Leopold's maneuvers. The best response includes that they are:
    a. determining the placement of the placenta
    b. finding the direction in which the fetus is lying
    c. evaluating the size of the uterus
    d. evaluating the adequacy of fetal growth

63. Appropriate routine screening tests at an 18-week visit include:
    a. gestational diabetes testing
    b. chlamydia and gonorrhea tests
    c. CBC or hematocrit
    d. multiple marker screen

64. A patient at 37 weeks calls to report the feeling that the fetus is moving less. After further inquiry, you decide to send the patient for an NST. When the patient asks what this test is, the clinician explains that it is an assessment of fetal well-being based on:
    a. evaluation of body movements
    b. breathing movements
    c. FHR response to fetal movement
    d. fetal body tone

65. A patient comes for a first visit at 11 weeks' gestation. Her history reveals her concern about sore gums that sometimes bleed. Which of the following reflects the next best steps?
    a. The patient should be referred to a periodontist for further evaluation.
    b. Provide reassurance that gingivitis is common in pregnancy due to increased vascularity.
    c. Initiate antibiotic therapy to prevent systemic infection.
    d. Place the patient on a soft diet until the bleeding resolves.

66. A pregnant patient presents at 32 weeks' gestation with vaginal bleeding for the past 6 hours, back pain, and irregular abdominal cramping pain. The exam reveals diffuse abdominal tenderness and increased uterine tone. Which of the following is the most likely diagnosis?
    a. Marginal placenta previa
    b. Placental abruption
    c. Preterm labor
    d. Pyelonephritis

67. A postterm pregnancy is best diagnosed by:
    a. certain LMP
    b. third-trimester ultrasound
    c. fundal growth
    d. quickening

68. Serial beta hCG levels are done after uterine evacuation for hydatidiform mole to:
    a. ensure that the person is not pregnant in the first year after treatment
    b. monitor for persistent trophoblastic proliferation
    c. identify a pregnancy early so appropriate care can be provided
    d. assess for a possible undetected ectopic pregnancy

69. A patient indicates that they are afraid of oxytocin (Pitocin) because their sister had a uterine rupture when she was induced. Which of the following is the best action?
    a. Reassure the patient because they will not need induction anyway.
    b. Discuss how oxytocin (Pitocin) is given and provide assurance that nothing will go wrong.
    c. Discuss alternative methods to promote uterine readiness and contractions.
    d. Explain that oxytocin (Pitocin) is the best way to get through labor, and it is not a problem.

70. A patient's (G2 P1001) initial visit reveals a healthy pregnant patient. The urinalysis and culture and sensitivity (C&S) report indicates a colony count of greater than 100,000 organisms per milliliter. The next best step includes:
    a. refer the patient to a urologist to evaluate for underlying renal disease
    b. encourage fluids and repeat C&S in 2 weeks
    c. initiate treatment with antibiotics
    d. advise the patient to contact you in case of any UTI symptoms

71. Antepartum care for the patient who is HIV positive should focus mainly on:
    a. ensuring fetal well-being at all cost
    b. frequent drug testing to ensure that the patient is not using IV street drugs
    c. testing the partner and providing treatment if necessary
    d. maintaining the patient's health and preventing neonatal transmission

72. On reviewing the record of a currently pregnant patient, you note the following pregnancy history: P1112. What obstetric history can be derived from this information?
    a. Two previous pregnancies, of which one infant was term and one was a premature stillbirth
    b. You are unable to determine an obstetric history from this information.
    c. Three pregnancies with one term birth and premature twins
    d. Three pregnancies, of which one was term, one premature, and one an abortion

73. Polyhydramnios is defined as:
    a. AFI greater than 10 cm
    b. a single pocket greater than 5 cm
    c. AFI greater than 15 cm
    d. a single pocket greater than 8 cm

74. The etiology of polyhydramnios is associated with:
    a. overhydration
    b. fetal anomalies of the GI tract
    c. fetal anomalies of the cardiovascular system
    d. preeclampsia with edema

75. The fetal system most closely associated with oligohydramnios is the:
    a. GI system
    b. CNS
    c. renal system
    d. cardiovascular system

76. When speaking with a primigravida about the way a baby develops, a clinician would most accurately describe the embryonic stage as the:
    a. period between the 2nd and 8th weeks
    b. time from implantation to 12 weeks into pregnancy
    c. period when drugs are least likely to affect development
    d. period from fertilization to 4 weeks

77. During the embryonic stage, all major organ systems are formed except the:
    a. heart
    b. reproductive organs
    c. liver
    d. lungs

78. Determining an accurate EDB is critical because:
    a. It is the basis for making decisions toward the end of the pregnancy.
    b. Mothers want to know the exact date the baby will be born.
    c. It is all that is needed to plan a 37-week elective cesarean section.
    d. Families want to make plans around the baby's birth.

79. Which of the following would not be a normal physical examination finding during pregnancy?
    a. Blue color of vaginal mucosa and cervix
    b. Hypertrophy of nasal mucosa and gums
    c. Mildly enlarged, nodular thyroid
    d. Thickening of vaginal mucosa

80. During the last 8 weeks of pregnancy, the fetus:
    a. finishes the final formation of the renal system
    b. completes the development of reproductive organs
    c. experiences the closure of the foramen ovale
    d. increases weight through fat accumulation

81. The determination of an accurate EDB is best accomplished by using:
    a. the first day of the LMP
    b. a complete menstrual history
    c. the use of Naegele's rule
    d. the date when symptoms of pregnancy began

82. Dating of pregnancy by USG is most accurate in the first trimester using:
    a. CRL
    b. HC
    c. AC
    d. FL

83. Which of the following statements most accurately reflects the growth of the pregnant uterus?
    a. At 14 weeks, it begins to rise out of the pelvis, and at 24 weeks is at the umbilicus.
    b. At 14 weeks, it is halfway to the umbilicus, and at 20 weeks is at the umbilicus.
    c. At 12 weeks, it begins to rise out of the pelvis, and at 20 weeks is at the umbilicus.
    d. At 10 weeks, it begins to rise out of the pelvis, and at 16 weeks is at the umbilicus.

84. Which of the following is a presumptive sign of pregnancy seen in the vagina?
    a. Softening of the uterine isthmus
    b. Asymmetrical bulge in the uterus
    c. Softening of the cervix
    d. Bluish discoloration of the mucosa

85. A pregnancy is maintained through hormones produced by the:
    a. egg sac and placenta
    b. corpus luteum and chorion
    c. corpus luteum and placenta
    d. ovary and placenta

86. Of the four pelvic types, which is more likely to lead to a posterior position with higher possibility of dystocia?
    a. Android
    b. Platypelloid
    c. Anthropoid
    d. Gynecoid

87. The characteristic gait of pregnancy results from:
    a. a shift in the center of gravity as the uterus enlarges
    b. the effects of relaxin and estrogen
    c. the effects of relaxin and progesterone
    d. the effects of increasing amounts of estrogen and progesterone

88. The effect of pregnancy on the cardiovascular system is most clearly seen in:
    a. lower diastolic blood pressure in the third trimester
    b. a 10% cardiac volume increase that peaks in mid-pregnancy
    c. a resting pulse increase of 10–15 beats in the first trimester
    d. a slight decrease in cardiac output in the second trimester

89. The usual 1 g drop in hemoglobin during pregnancy is due to:
    a. a blood volume increase of 30%–50%
    b. a decrease in iron absorption
    c. decreased production of red blood cells
    d. the increasing iron needs of the fetus

90. Which of the following is considered a risk factor for psychological well-being in pregnancy?
    a. Limited support network
    b. Introversion at any point
    c. Ambivalence any time
    d. Concern about the danger signs

91. The maternal mortality ratio is defined as the number of deaths of childbearing individuals that result from the reproductive process per:
    a. 1,000 live births
    b. 100,000 live births
    c. 100,000 pregnant individuals
    d. 100,000 reproductive-age individuals

92. A patient comes for the first pregnancy visit. The obstetric history includes one spontaneous abortion, one termination of pregnancy, one infant born at 36 weeks, and one infant born at 41 weeks. Both infants are living. This patient's parity is:
    a. 2022
    b. 2122
    c. 1212
    d. 1122

93. The pelvic planes of obstetric significance are the:
    a. inlet, midplane, and outlet
    b. inlet, posterior outlet, and anterior outlet
    c. inlet, posterior midplane, and anterior midplane
    d. linea terminalis, posterior outlet, and anterior outlet

94. Which of the elements of clinical pelvimetry defines the midplane?
    a. Diagonal conjugate
    b. Intertuberous diameter
    c. Ischial spines distance and sacrum
    d. Pubic arch

95. Amniocentesis is used in early pregnancy to:
    a. screen for fetal anomalies
    b. diagnose fetal genetic well-being
    c. evaluate maternal genetic problems
    d. determine AFI and muscle tone

96. CVS has an advantage over amniocentesis because:
    a. It can be done 3–4 weeks earlier.
    b. There is less risk for infection.
    c. There is less risk for limb deformities.
    d. There is greater specificity in test results.

97. When considering the use of fetal movement counting for a particular patient, it is important to know that:
    a. Fetuses move constantly, so the counting can be done at any time.
    b. Fetal movement is strongest at 29–38 weeks.
    c. Most pregnant individuals do not feel the fetus move before 24 weeks.
    d. There is only one way to perform fetal movement counts.

98. The basis for the NST to assess fetal well-being is that:
    a. Fetal movement will increase the patient's heart rate.
    b. The fetus responds to an increase in heart rate by accelerating movement.
    c. Fetal movement should cause no significant change in FHR.
    d. FHR accelerates in association with fetal movement.

99. Contraindications to the CST include:
    a. GA greater than 37 weeks
    b. history of ectopic pregnancy
    c. nonreactive NST
    d. placenta previa

100. A 32-year-old patient (G1 P1001), during a discussion of infant care and breastfeeding, says, "My first baby did not like the breast, then I did not have enough milk, so I stopped breastfeeding after 2 weeks." Which of the following is the best response to her statement?
    a. Suggest that the patient probably misinterpreted what was going on and should not have stopped nursing.
    b. Delve further into what occurred and how the patient decided to stop breastfeeding.
    c. Let the patient know that dehydration is a likely cause of the patient not having enough milk to feed the baby.
    d. Reassure the patient that listening to one's body is the right thing to do for oneself and one's infant.

Answers with Rationales

1. **c.** presumptive
   Amenorrhea is a presumptive sign of pregnancy. *Presumptive signs of pregnancy* refer to signs and symptoms that may be caused by something else. Amenorrhea may be caused by sickness or stress.

2. **d.** repeat the test in a week
   The patient performed the test too early and will need to repeat the test in 1 week. Sensitive urine pregnancy tests can detect pregnancy approximately 1 week after conception.

3. **b.** hCG
   The placenta secretes hCG hormone to help maintain corpus luteum function and production of progesterone; levels found in serum and urine assays of pregnant individuals are detected in pregnancy tests.

4. **a.** corpus luteum
   The corpus luteum secretes progesterone, which is essential in preparing the uterus for implantation of the fertilized ovum and maintaining the pregnancy.

5. **b.** fetus
   The chorionic villi develop from the outer wall of the blastocyst, which establishes an intimate connection with the endometrium and gives rise to the placenta.

6. **a.** one vein carrying oxygenated blood and two arteries carrying deoxygenated blood
   The umbilical cord contains two arteries that carry fetal deoxygenated blood to the placenta and that are smaller in diameter than the vein, and one vein that carries oxygenated blood from the placenta to the fetus and that is characterized by twisting or spiraling to minimize snarling.

7. **c.** 12 weeks' gestation
   The uterus is palpable at the symphysis pubis at 12 weeks. This is also the time that the fetus begins to make spontaneous movements in utero.

8. **c.** 6–7 days
   Implantation occurs 6–7 days after fertilization and usually in the upper, posterior wall of the uterus.

9. **c.** facilitated diffusion
Both oxygen and glucose are transported across the placenta via facilitated diffusion.

10. **b.** 23 pairs of chromosomes
The human zygote contains the haploid number of chromosomes: 23 pairs. It possesses half the diploid or normal number of pairs of chromosomes, 46 pairs, found in somatic, or body, cells.

11. **c.** placenta
The trophoblast is an essential component of the placenta.

12. **d.** no intervention
Approximately 90% of pregnant individuals develop a physiologic systolic heart murmur. They may exhibit exaggerated splitting of S_1, an audible third sound, or a soft transient diastolic murmur.

13. **d.** progesterone's effect on the vessel walls
Diastolic blood pressure is lower in the first two trimesters because of the development of new vascular beds and the relaxation of peripheral tone by progesterone, which results in decreased flow resistance.

14. **b.** increased chest diameter
Thoracic circumference increases by 5–6 cm, and residual volume decreases.

15. **b.** reassure the patient that this is normal
Absent any other symptoms besides increased vaginal discharge in a 34-week pregnant individual, and without odor or other presenting abnormal findings, reassurance may be given to the mother that an increase in vaginal discharge is normal in pregnancy. If there is further concern, rule out pathology.

16. **a.** a normal variation of response in pregnancy
Increased libido is a normal variation of response in pregnancy.

17. **a.** Encourage the patient to tell you more about the nightmares and fears.
It is the healthcare provider's role to listen and facilitate a patient's expression of feelings and to provide a nonjudgmental environment.

18. **b.** increased intake of fiber and fluids
The first line of treatment for constipation is to increase fluids and fiber. Other strategies include recommending prune juice or a warm beverage in the morning and encouraging exercise and stool softeners.

19. **b.** nullipara
Nullipara is the term for a person who has not carried a baby to 500 g or 20 weeks.

20. **a.** 28-day menstrual cycle
The calculation of EDB by Naegele's rule is based on a 28-day menstrual cycle, assuming the average length of pregnancy to be 280 days, or 10 lunar months.

21. **a.** 0121
A. The patient has not had any term pregnancies, which accounts for the first number, 0. The patient had a preterm delivery at 36 weeks of twins, which accounts for the second number; even though these were twins, they still count as one number—thus, the 1. The patient had two miscarriages at less than 20 weeks, which accounts for the third number, a 2. The fourth number is the total number of living children. One of the patient's twins died; therefore, they have only one living child.

22. **d.** Send the patient to the fetal assessment unit for an ultrasound.
If the patient is uncertain about the LMP, an ultrasound may be used to calculate the estimated GA.

23. **a.** fetal growth restriction
The fundus is typically found at the umbilicus at 20 weeks.

24. **c.** lie
The first Leopold's maneuver palpates for the fetal lie, followed by the presentation, position, and attitude.

25. **b.** "We can try to listen today. But we may not hear the heartbeat yet."
FHTs can be auscultated by Doppler as early as 10 weeks, but this is done more commonly at 12 weeks.

26. **c.** bluish color of the cervix
A normal finding in pregnancy is the changing of the color of the cervix to a bluish hue due to the increased vasculature.

27. **d.** "You may not feel movement until around 20 weeks."
Quickening is the maternal perception of fetal movement, which usually occurs between 18 and 20 weeks for primiparas; it occurs earlier for multigravidas, at about 14–18 weeks.

28. **c.** 15–19 weeks
Second-trimester screening (also known as multiple marker screening) is performed between 15 and 20 weeks to detect neural tube defects and trisomies 18 and 21. Serologic testing measuring MSAFP, estriol, and hCG is called a triple screen; with the addition of inhibin A, this becomes a quad screen.

29. **c.** at 35–37 weeks
GBS screening is performed at 35–37 weeks by swabbing the vaginal introitus and rectal specimens.

30. **a.** Trisomy 13, 18, and 21
Cell-free DNA is a screening test that can determine risks for trisomy 13, 18, and 21.

31. **d.** reactive
A reactive NST constitutes two or more accelerations in FHR of 15 or more beats per minute lasting for 15 seconds or more within a 15- to 20-minute period.

32. **d.** 4 mg per day starting before conception
A 0.4-mg daily supplement of folic acid is recommended for individuals of childbearing age, and a 4-mg daily supplement prior to and during pregnancy is recommended for individuals with a history of previous infant with neural tube defect.

33. **a.** gain 11–20 lb
Per the IOM (2009), pregnant people who have a pre-pregnancy BMI >30, the recommended weight gain is 0.4–0.6 lb per week in the second and third trimesters, for a total of 11–20 lb.

34. **d.** modify the existing program if symptoms occur
In the absence of either medical or obstetric complications, 30 minutes or more of moderate exercise per day on most, if not all, days of the week is recommended for pregnant individuals.

35. **b.** The pregnant person's sexual desire may change throughout pregnancy.
Changes in sexual desire throughout pregnancy are influenced by hormones, energy level, the relationship with the sexual partner, body image, fears of hurting the baby, and cultural beliefs and practices.

36. **b.** are HIV positive and untreated
Breastfeeding is recommended for all pregnant people who wish to do so except for individuals who are HIV positive and are untreated, have active tuberculosis (TB), use illicit drugs, or take prescribed cancer chemotherapy agents.

37. **a.** advising the patient to eat small, frequent meals
Nausea and vomiting during pregnancy are most common in the first trimester. It is recommended that patients eat small, frequent meals, with no restriction on the kind of food or how often. Education includes discontinuing prenatal vitamins with iron until nausea and vomiting have resolved but continuing folic acid. Other recommendations may include consuming raspberry tea, peppermint tea, carbonated beverages, or hard candy; using acupressure, including sea bands for wrists; taking ginger 1 g per day in divided doses, pyridoxine (vitamin B$_6$) 25 mg BID or TID orally, doxylamine 12.5 mg BID or QID with pyridoxine orally, metoclopramide 5–10 mg q6–8h orally, or promethazine 25 mg q4h per rectal suppository.

38. **c.** reassurance and rest
Provide patients with reassurance that fatigue is a normal first-trimester problem and will pass. Other recommendations include getting mild exercise and good nutrition, decreasing activities and fluid intake in the evening to decrease nocturia, and planning rest periods.

39. **b.** flexion of the foot
Leg cramps may be relieved by flexing the ankle to stretch the calf, decreasing phosphate in the diet, drinking no more than two glasses of milk per day, massaging the affected leg, keeping the legs warm, walking, exercising, and taking calcium tablets and magnesium tablets.

40. **a.** Normalize the patient's edema and reschedule for 1 week.
The patient is gaining appropriate weight and is normotensive, without protein in the urine, and without any severe features of preeclampsia. The patient can be reassured that edema at this stage in the pregnancy is normal. If the patient exhibits any other symptoms, however, an evaluation by a healthcare provider would be required.

41. **d.** reduced use of anesthesia
Preparation for childbearing ultimately aids in reducing the need for analgesics and anesthetics during labor.

42. **d.** Screening in early pregnancy and at 24–28 weeks
High-risk obstetric patients need to be screened for diabetes as soon as possible using standard diagnostic testing.

43. **c.** polyhydramnios
Polyhydramnios is indicated by uterine size larger than expected for GA, difficulty auscultating FHR and palpating fetal parts, and mechanical pressure exerted by the large uterus.

44. **d.** refer the patient to a perinatologist
There are no documented cases of congenital rubella syndrome from vaccination, but it is recommended to give the vaccine at least 4 weeks before attempting pregnancy or postpartum; the vaccine may be given while breastfeeding.

45. **b.** Monitor the mass at each visit to assess for any change.
This well-defined, nontender mass has benign characteristics, and watching it would be an acceptable approach. A malignant breast mass is usually nontender, firm, irregularly shaped, and fixed to underlying tissue.

46. **b.** combining the results of an NST and ultrasound evaluation to assess five variables
A BPP consists of five parameters: NST, breathing, movement, tone, and AFV.

47. **d.** Schedule a visit for 1 week
A BPP score of 8/10 is a reassuring, normal score. BPP scoring interpretation criteria are as follows: 8–10 is normal; 6 is equivocal, repeat testing; 4 or less is considered abnormal and needs further evaluation.

48. **c.** fasting and 1 or 2 hours after each meal
Based on available data, glucose monitoring for obstetric patients diagnosed with gestational diabetes is to check their blood sugar levels four times daily: fasting, plus 1 or 2 hours after each meal.

49. **c.** The tetanus booster is safe in pregnancy if needed.
Tetanus vaccination during pregnancy can protect at-risk newborns against neonatal tetanus; in maternal trauma, it may be indicated.

50. **a.** multigravida
A multigravida is a person who has been pregnant two or more times, regardless of the result of the pregnancies.

51. **d.** discuss the patient's thoughts and feelings about sex
It is the healthcare provider's role to listen and facilitate the patient's expression of feelings and to provide a nonjudgmental environment.

52. **d.** vaginal introitus and rectum
GBS screening is performed at 35–37 weeks by swabbing the vaginal introitus and rectal specimens.

53. **b.** listening to whatever the patient has to say
It is the healthcare provider's role to listen and facilitate the patient's expression of feelings and to provide a nonjudgmental environment.

54. **b.** syphilis serology
Obtaining syphilis serology is a recommended routine screening for the first initial antenatal visit during the first trimester.

55. **a.** Vaccination is recommended for all individuals who will be pregnant during the influenza season.
The TIV is recommended for all pregnant individuals during influenza season; live attenuated nasal influenza vaccine is contraindicated during pregnancy.

56. **d.** 2,500 kcal and 60 g/day
The recommended dietary allowances for pregnancy are 2,500 kcal/day and 60 g/day of protein.

57. **c.** amniotic epithelium and fetal functions
Amniotic fluid is produced by the amniotic epithelium. Water transfers across the amnion and through the fetal skin. In the second trimester, the fetus starts to swallow, urinate, and inspire amniotic fluid.

58. **b.** Meiosis occurs, producing half the number of chromosomes.
Meiosis is the process of two successive cell divisions, producing cells, egg, or sperm that contain half the number of chromosomes found in somatic cells.

59. **a.** Trophoblasts, chorion, amnion
Parts of the placenta are trophoblasts, chorion, amnion and chorionic villi, intervillous spaces, and decidual plate.

60. **c.** the embryo, membranes, and placenta
A conceptus comprises all tissue products of conception: embryo (fetus), fetal membranes, and placenta.

61. **a.** Trophoblast
Human trophoblasts produce more diverse steroid and protein hormones and in greater amounts than does any endocrine tissue in all of mammalian physiology.

62. **b.** finding the direction in which the fetus is lying
Leopold's maneuvers consist of four abdominal palpation maneuvers used to determine the following fetal characteristics: lie, presentation, position, and attitude.

63. **d.** multiple marker screen
Second-trimester screening (also known as multiple marker screening) is performed between 15 and 20 weeks to detect neural tube defects and trisomies 18 and 21.

64. **c.** FHR response to fetal movement
An NST is a method to assess fetal well-being by observing the FHR response to fetal movement.

65. **b.** Gingivitis is common in pregnancy with increased vascularity of connective tissue.
Gingivitis often occurs during pregnancy and may result in bleeding of the gums.

66. **b.** placental abruption
Placental abruption is the premature separation of the placenta from the uterus; it may be partial or complete. Signs of placental abruption include vaginal bleeding, uterine tenderness and rigidity, contractions or uterine irritability and/or tone, and fetal tachycardia or bradycardia.

67. **a.** certain LMP
Dating a pregnancy is most accurate with a certain LMP.

68. **b.** monitor for persistent trophoblastic proliferation
Weekly serial beta hCG levels are recommended after surgical evacuation for hydatidiform mole to monitor for persistent trophoblastic proliferation and identify metastatic disease, including choriocarcinoma.

69. **c.** Discuss alternative methods to promote uterine readiness and contractions.
Oxytocin (Pitocin) may be utilized to help initiate or facilitate labor by stimulating the contraction of the uterine smooth muscle. Other methods, such as nipple stimulation, may also be employed to promote uterine readiness and contractions.

70. **c.** initiate treatment with antibiotics
A diagnosis of a UTI can be made by finding 100,000 colonies of pathogenic bacteria in a urinary culture. Treatment with appropriate antibiotics is necessary. Untreated asymptomatic bacteriuria may lead to pyelonephritis, which may lead to serious complications for both mother and baby.

71. **d.** maintaining the patient's health and preventing neonatal transmission
Maintaining the health of the patient and preventing vertical transmission to the neonate are the priorities when caring for people with HIV.

72. **d.** Three pregnancies, of which one was term, one premature, and one an abortion
The numbers represent a patient's obstetric history, expressed via TPAL: one term delivery, one preterm delivery, one abortion (spontaneous or elective), and two living children.

73. **d.** a single pocket greater than 8 cm
Polyhydramnios is an excess of amniotic fluid diagnosed as an AFI greater than or equal to 24 cm or a maximum deepest vertical pocket of equal to or greater than 8 cm.

74. **b.** fetal anomalies of the GI tract
The etiology of polyhydramnios may include CNS or GI tract fetal anomalies.

75. **c.** renal system
Oligohydramnios is associated with genitourinary abnormalities in the fetus.

76. **a.** period between the 2nd and 8th weeks
Embryonic development is the period of organogenesis, which begins in the 3rd week after fertilization and spans 8 weeks; around that time, a person may miss her next menstrual period, and pregnancy tests will turn positive by detecting hCG.

77. **d.** lungs
All major organ systems are formed during the embryonic stage except for the lungs.

78. **a.** It is the basis for making decisions toward the end of the pregnancy.
Determining an accurate EDB is critical because an accurate estimation of the date of birth is the basis for making decisions toward the end of the pregnancy.

79. **c.** Mildly enlarged, nodular thyroid
A mildly enlarged, nodular thyroid is an abnormal physical exam finding. The other findings are normal findings in pregnancy.

80. **d.** increases weight through fat accumulation
During 32–36 weeks of gestation, the fetus continues to increase weight as more subcutaneous fat accumulates.

81. **a.** the first day of the LMP
A complete menstrual history, which includes determining the first day of the LMP and the length of menstrual cycles, allows for a more accurate EDB.

82. **a.** CRL
In the first trimester, the most accurate parameter for dating is the CRL measurement.

83. **c.** At 12 weeks it begins to rise out of the pelvis, and at 20 weeks is at the umbilicus.
    At 12 weeks' gestation, the uterus becomes an abdominal organ and rises out of the pelvis. At 20 weeks, the uterus is typically found at the umbilicus.

84. **d.** Chadwick's sign
    Chadwick's sign is a presumptive sign of pregnancy. *Presumptive sign of pregnancy* refers to signs and symptoms that may be caused by pregnancy. Amenorrhea may be caused by sickness or stress.

85. **c.** corpus luteum and placenta
    The corpus luteum secretes progesterone to maintain the endometrium and pregnancy until the placenta takes over production.

86. **a.** Android
    An android pelvic type is commonly known as a male pelvis. Approximately 32.5% of white people and 15.7% of nonwhite people have this type of heavy, heart-shaped pelvis, which leads to increased posterior positions, dystocia, and operative births.

87. **c.** the effects of relaxin and progesterone
    Relaxin and progesterone affect cartilage and connective tissue, resulting in a loosening of the sacroiliac joint and symphysis pubis.

88. **b.** a 10% cardiac volume increase that peaks in midpregnancy
    Cardiac volume increases by approximately 10% and peaks at about 20 weeks, and resting pulse increases by 10–15 beats per minute, with the peak occurring at 28 weeks.

89. **a.** a blood volume increase of 30%–50%
    Blood volume increases 30%–50% from nonpregnant levels, and plasma volume expands, which result in a physiologic anemia.

90. **a.** Limited support network
    Risk factors for psychological well-being include having a limited support network, high levels of stress, psychological/mental health issues, and problem pregnancies.

91. **b.** 100,000 live births
    The maternal mortality ratio is the number of deaths of childbearing individuals that result from the reproductive process per 100,000 live births.

92. **d.** 1122
    TPAL represents a patient's obstetric history. This patient has had one term pregnancy, one preterm pregnancy, two abortions, and two live children.

93. **a.** inlet, midplane, and outlet
    Three planes are of obstetric significance—inlet, midplane, and outlet.

94. **c.** Ischial spines distance and sacrum
    The distance between the ischial spines normally measures 10 cm, which is the smallest diameter of the pelvis, and defines the midplane.

95. **a.** screen for fetal anomalies
    Amniocentesis is used in early pregnancy to obtain amniotic fluid to be sent for chromosomal studies.

96. **a.** It can be done 3–4 weeks earlier.
    An advantage of CVS over amniocentesis is that CVS can be performed between 10 and 13 weeks' gestation, which is 3–4 weeks earlier than amniocentesis is feasible.

97. **b.** Fetal movement is strongest at 29–38 weeks.
    Fetal movement is strongest between 29 and 38 weeks' gestation. Fetal movement counting is a safe, simple, no-cost, noninvasive fetal assessment technique. Research has demonstrated that fetal activity is a good predictor of well-being. A dramatic decrease or cessation of such movement is cause for concern.

98. **d.** FHR accelerates in association with fetal movement.
    The NST is a method to assess fetal well-being by observing the fetal heart rate response to fetal movement.

99. **d.** placenta previa
    Contraindications for a CST include previous classic cesarean section or myomectomy, placenta previa, the mother being at risk for preterm labor, gestational age less than 37 weeks, and multiple gestation.

100. **b.** Delve further into what occurred and how the patient decided to stop breastfeeding.
    It is the healthcare provider's role to listen and facilitate the patient's expression of feelings and to provide a nonjudgmental environment.

Bibliography

American College of Obstetricians and Gynecologists. (2019a). ACOG practice bulletin No. 204: fetal growth restriction. *Obstetrics and Gynecology, 133*(2), e97–e109

American College of Obstetricians and Gynecologists. (2019b). ACOG practice bulletin no. 202: gestational hypertension and preeclampsia. *Obstet Gynecol, 133*(1), e1–e25.

American College of Obstetricians and Gynecologists. (2020). *Repeated miscarriages.* https://www.acog.org/womens-health/faqs/repeated-miscarriages

American College of Obstetricians and Gynecologists. (2021a). Antepartum fetal surveillance: ACOG practice bulletin, number 229. *Obstetrics and Gynecology, 137*(6), e116–e127.

American College of Obstetricians and Gynecologists. (2021b). Anemia in pregnancy: ACOG practice bulletin, number 233. *Obstetrics and Gynecology, 138*(2), e55–e64.

American College of Obstetricians and Gynecologists. (2021c). Prediction and prevention of spontaneous preterm birth: ACOG Practice Bulletin, Number 234. *Obstetrics and Gynecology, 138*(2), e65–e90.

Blackburn, S. (2018). *Maternal, fetal, & neonatal physiology: A clinical perspective* (5th ed.). Elsevier.

Caughey, A. B., & Turrentine, M. (2018). ACOG practice bulletin: Gestational diabetes mellitus. *Obstetrics and Gynecology, 131*(2), E49–E64.

Centers for Disease Control and Prevention. (2016). *Fetal alcohol spectrum disorders (FASDs).* https://www.cdc.gov/fasd/about/?CDC_AAref_Val=https://www.cdc.gov/ncbddd/fasd/facts.html

Centers for Disease Control and Prevention. (2021a). Births: Final data for 2019. *National Vital Statistics Reports, 70*(2). https://www.cdc.gov/nchs/data/nvsr/nvsr70/nvsr70-02-508.pdf

Centers for Disease Control and Prevention. (2021b). Pregnancy and vaccination. https://www.cdc.gov/vaccines/pregnancy/index.html.

Cunningham, F., Leveno, K., Bloom, S., Dashe, J., Hoffman, B. Casey, B., & Spong C. (2022). *Williams obstetrics* (26th ed.). McGraw-Hill.

Dashe, J. S., Pressman, E. K., Hibbard, J. U., & Society for Maternal-Fetal Medicine (SMFM). (2018). SMFM consult series# 46: Evaluation and management of polyhydramnios. *American Journal of Obstetrics and Gynecology, 219*(4), B2–B8.

Erick, M., Cox, J. T., & Mogensen, K. M. (2018). ACOG practice bulletin 189: Nausea and vomiting of pregnancy. *Obstetrics & Gynecology, 131*(5), 935.

Kaimal, A. J., Dugoff, L., Norton, M. E., & American College of Obstetricians and Gynecologists. (2020). Screening for fetal chromosomal abnormalities: ACOG practice bulletin, number 226. *Obstetrics & Gynecology, 136*(4), e48–e69.

Landon, M., Galan, H., Jauniaux, E., Driscoll, D., Berghella, V., Grobman, W., Kilpatrick, S., & Cahill, A. (2020). *Gabbe's Obstetrics: Normal and problem pregnancies* (8th ed.). Elsevier.

Murthy, N., Wodi, A. P., Bernstein, H., McNally, V., Cineas, S., & Ault, K. (2022). Advisory committee on immunization practices recommended immunization schedule for adults aged 19 years or older—United States, 2022. *Morbidity and Mortality Weekly Report, 71*(7), 229.

Pernia, S. & Maagd, G. (2016). The new pregnancy and lactation labeling rule. *Pharmacy and Therapeutics, 41*(11), 713–715.

Phillippi, J. & Kantrowitz-Gordon, I. (Eds.). (2025). *Varney's midwifery* (7th ed.). Jones & Bartlett Learning.

Rhoads, J., Demler, T. L., & Dlugasch, L. (2021). *Advanced health assessment and diagnostic reasoning.* Jones & Bartlett Learning.

Rose, N. C., Kaimal, A. J., Dugoff, L., & Norton, M. E. (2020). Screening for fetal chromosomal abnormalities: ACOG practice bulletin, Number 226. *Obstetrics and Gynecology, 136*(4), e48–e69. https://doi.org/10.1097/AOG.0000000000004084

Schuiling, K. D., & Likis, F. E. (2020). *Gynecologic health care: With an introduction to prenatal and postpartum care: with an introduction to prenatal and postpartum care.* Jones & Bartlett Learning.

Siega-Riz, A. M., Bodnar, L. M., Stotland, N. E., & Stang, J. (2020). The current understanding of gestational weight gain among women with obesity and the need for future research. *NAM Perspectives.* https://doi.org/10.31478/202001a

Tharpe, N., Farley, C., & Jordan, R. (2022). *Clinical practice guidelines for midwifery and women's health* (6th ed.). Jones & Bartlett Learning.

Urato, A. C. (2020). ACOG practice bulletin No. 220: Management of genital herpes in pregnancy. *Obstetrics & Gynecology, 136*(4), 850–851.

Workowski, K. A., Bachmann, L. H., Chan, P. A., Johnston, C. M., Muzny, C. A., Park, I., ... & Bolan, G. A. (2021). Sexually transmitted infections treatment guidelines. *MMWR Recommendations and Reports, 70*(4), 1.

CHAPTER 7

Complex Pregnancy Care

Jamille Nagtalon-Ramos
Melicia Escobar

Substance Use

- Substances with known potential for use, misuse, and/or addiction
  1. To avoid stigma which can adversely affect people with a substance use disorder (SUD), using this type of person-first language instead of terms such as "addict," "user," "drug abuser," "alcoholic," "drunk." Adverse effects include:
     a. Decreased willingness to seek or enter treatment
     b. Isolation
     c. Biased care from healthcare professionals

Alcohol

- Approximately 15.1 million adults ages 18 and older have an alcohol use disorder (AUD)—9.8 million men and 5.3 million women
- One in nine pregnant individuals reported drinking alcohol in the past 30 days; among pregnant individuals, one-third reported binge drinking
- Medical and obstetric complications related to alcohol
  1. Effects on pregnant individual—preeclampsia, placental abruption (also known as abruptio placentae), placenta previa, spontaneous abortion, ectopic pregnancy, premature rupture of membranes (PROM), mental health effects (e.g., depression, anxiety, suicidal thoughts or behavior)
  2. Effects on fetus/infant—alcohol use in pregnancy can cause fetal alcohol spectrum disorders (FASDs)
     a. FASDs are physical, behavioral, and intellectual disabilities that last a lifetime
     b. As many as 1 in 20 U.S. schoolchildren may have FASD
     c. Low birth weight and growth; complications with heart, kidneys, and other organs; damage to parts of the brain, which leads to behavioral and intellectual disabilities, such as difficulty with attention and hyperactivity

- Screening tools for alcohol use
  1. CAGE
     a. *C:* Have you felt the need to *cut* down on your drinking?
     b. *A:* Have people *annoyed* you by criticizing your drinking?
     c. *G:* Have you ever felt bad or *guilty* about your drinking?
     d. *E:* Have you ever had a drink first thing in the morning to steady your nerves or get rid of a hangover (*eye-opener*)?
  2. TWEAK
     a. Tolerance: How many drinks can you hold?
     b. Worried: Have close friends or relatives worried or complained about your drinking in the past year?
     c. Eye-openers: Do you sometimes take a drink in the morning when you first get up?
     d. Amnesia: Has a friend or family member ever told you about things you said or did while you were drinking that you could not remember?
     e. Cut down: Do you sometimes feel the need to cut down on your drinking?

Nicotine

- Prevalence
  1. Approximately 7.2% of pregnant individuals who gave birth in 2016 smoked during pregnancy
  2. Prevalence is highest for pregnant individuals aged 20–24 (10.7%), followed by individuals aged 15–19 (8.5%) and 25–29 (8.2%)
  3. Non-Hispanic American Indian or Alaska Native pregnant individuals had the highest prevalence (16.7%); Non-Hispanic Asian pregnant individuals had the lowest prevalence of smoking during pregnancy (0.6%)
- Obstetric complications related to tobacco/nicotine use
  1. Pregnant individuals who smoke have a 47% increased risk of stillbirth compared to those who do not; risk is higher with heavier smoking

2. Pregnant individuals who are passively exposed to tobacco (secondhand smoke) have a 23% increased risk as compared to those who are not
3. Effects on the pregnant individual—preeclampsia, placental abruption, placenta previa, spontaneous abortion, ectopic pregnancy, PROM
4. Effects on infant—congenital malformation, fetal growth restriction, premature birth, and small for gestational age

Other Substances

- Estimated 5% of pregnant individuals use one or more addictive substances
- Obstetric complications related to substance use
  1. Neonatal abstinence syndrome (NAS)—infant goes through withdrawal at birth due to opioids (prescription pain relievers or heroin), barbiturates, benzodiazepines
  2. Severity of withdrawal symptoms depends on the drug(s) used, quantity of drugs, length of abuse, metabolism of the drugs, and infant's gestational age, and if the infant was born full term or prematurely
  3. Symptoms of drug withdrawal in neonates can develop up to 14 days after birth
     a. Blotchy skin coloring
     b. Diarrhea
     c. Excessive or high-pitched crying
     d. Abnormal sucking reflex
     e. Fever
     f. Hyperactive reflexes
     g. Increased muscle tone
     h. Irritability
     i. Poor feeding
     j. Rapid breathing
     k. Seizures
     l. Sleep problems
     m. Slow weight gain
     n. Nasal congestion and sneezing
     o. Sweating
     p. Trembling
     q. Vomiting
  4. General effects of drugs on infant
     a. Congenital anomalies
     b. Low birth weight
     c. Premature birth
     d. Small head circumference
     e. Sudden infant death syndrome (SIDS)

Marijuana (Cannabis)

- Legal status of cannabis varies from state to state
  1. Due to the legalization of cannabis for medicinal and recreational use in many states across the country, the number of pregnant individuals using cannabis has increased. Cannabis use is higher in pregnant individuals living in states that allow medical and adult recreational use compared to those living in states with use restrictions (Vachhani et al., 2022).
  2. In states with *unregulated* cannabis, there is an increased chance of unknown or undesired polysubstance use with additives (e.g., fentanyl) added to the street supply

3. State regulations may have implications for screening/testing and consequences for pregnant patients who test positive for cannabis use (e.g., incarceration)
- Range of self-reported prevalence of marijuana use during pregnancy is 2%–5% (ACOG, 2017)
- Some individuals report using marijuana to treat severe nausea during the first trimester of pregnancy
- Safety of use not proven. Animal studies suggest disruption of fetal brain development
- Children exposed to marijuana prenatally had poor visual-motor coordination, decreased attention span, and behavioral problems
- American College of Obstetricians and Gynecologists (ACOG, 2017) recommendation is to avoid cannabis use while planning a pregnancy, during pregnancy, and breastfeeding/chestfeeding

Stimulants (Cocaine and Methamphetamine)

- Hard to determine and isolate effects of cocaine in individuals and their children because additional compounding factors may exist, such as alcohol use, poor nutrition, and inadequate prenatal care
- Obstetric complications related to cocaine and methamphetamine use
  1. Maternal effects
     a. Migraines
     b. Seizures
     c. PROM
     d. Placental abruption
     e. Hypertensive crisis
     f. Spontaneous abortion
     g. Preterm labor
     h. Pregnant individuals who use methamphetamine have a greater risk of preeclampsia, premature delivery, placental abruption
  2. Infant effects
     a. Low birth weight
     b. Small head circumference
     c. Shorter in length than babies born to mothers who do not use cocaine
     d. Irritability
     e. Hyperactivity
     f. Tremors
     g. High-pitched cry
     h. Excessive sucking at birth
     i. Children exposed to methamphetamine in utero have increased emotional reactivity and anxiety/depression, more withdrawn, and cognitive problems

MDMA (3,4-Ethylenedioxymethamphetamine; Ecstasy, Molly)

- Insufficient research on the effects of MDMA use during pregnancy
- Limited research shows exposure to MDMA in utero may cause learning, memory, and motor problems

Heroin

- Heroin passes through the placenta to the fetus
- Heroin use can result in NAS

Prescription and Over-the-Counter (OTC) Drugs

- Minimal research for obvious reasons—scientists cannot give potentially dangerous drugs to pregnant individuals, and pregnant individuals are typically excluded from studies on new medications
- Some prescription and OTC medications are safe to take in pregnancy; obtain a thorough medication, supplement, and herbal history and determine safety, risks, and benefits on an individual basis
- Refer to Chapter 11, *Principles of Pharmacology*, for new pregnancy and lactation labeling rule

Factors Associated with Increased Risk for Substance Abuse in Pregnancy

- Lack of education
- Low self-esteem
- Depression
- Personal history of substance abuse
- Low socioeconomic status
- Family history of substance abuse
- Financial problems and poverty
- Being in abusive relationships, history of physical abuse
- Feelings of hopelessness
- Drug-abusing partner

Goals

- Ideal—stop using harmful substances
- If unable to stop completely, reduce the quantity and types of substances used
- Mobilize resources to support and encourage
- Drug rehabilitation

Ethical Considerations—Who Should Be Screened?

- Universal and mandatory versus none for anyone
  1. SBIRT (Screening, Brief Intervention, Referral, Treatment)—identify the severity and level of treatment required; brief intervention with the goal of increasing insight and motivation; referral for more extensive treatment and specialty care
- Screening of those with a positive history or who exhibit signs of use
- Legal implications
  1. Mandatory reporting to child protective services
  2. Possible loss of infant custody to child protective services
  3. Criminal prosecution of a woman for putting the fetus at risk

Intimate Partner Abuse/ Violence Against Women (VAW)

- Prevalence
  1. Annually, an estimated 324,000 pregnant individuals experience abuse
  2. In the United States, homicide is the leading cause of death among pregnant and postpartum individuals
  3. Individuals who experienced abuse/violence prior to pregnancy are more likely to be abused during pregnancy
- Screening techniques for ascertaining the presence of VAW; essential questions asked during history taking include
  1. Have you ever been emotionally or physically abused by your partner or someone important to you?
  2. Within the past year, have you been hit, slapped, kicked, shoved, or otherwise hurt by anyone?
  3. Have you ever been hit, slapped, kicked, or otherwise physically hurt while you were pregnant?
- Definitions of VAW
  1. Physical
     a. Choking (associated with the highest fatality risk), pushes, slaps, punches, etc.
     b. Locks woman in or out of the house
     c. Refuses to buy food
     d. Refuses access to medical care
     e. Destroys property or pets
     f. Abuses children
  2. Emotional
     a. Engages in name calling or insults
     b. Isolates from family and friends
     c. Publicly humiliates
     d. Makes all decisions
     e. Withholds affection
  3. Sexual
     a. Treats women as sex objects
     b. Forces sexual acts with self or others
     c. Jealous anger with accusations
     d. Withholds sex and affection
     e. Engages in sadistic sexual acts
  4. Financial
     a. Withholds money
     b. Runs up bills abused individual must pay
     c. Makes all monetary decisions
     d. Manipulates the relationship through money
  5. Social
     a. Immigrant individuals may not have extended family/support in the United States and consequentially trapped by their partners/abusers
     b. Undocumented immigrants may be threatened by their partners/abusers for reporting them to authorities
- Diagnosis of abuse
  1. History
     a. Depression or suicide attempts
     b. Substance abuse
     c. Childhood abuse (sexual or physical)

d. Multiple injuries
e. Complaints of chronic pain
f. Repeated spontaneous abortions (SAB), threatened abortions (TAB)
g. Sexually transmitted infections (STIs)
2. Physical
a. Assessing for injuries—multiple bruises in various stages of recovery; proximal versus distal: proximal tends to be intentional; hidden injuries: breasts, abdomen, back, and so on
b. Treatment delays—old scars or bruises visible
c. Patterned injuries—with reasonable certainty can determine what kind of object caused injury (e.g., bite marks)
d. Physical findings inconsistent with history
e. Genital trauma, vaginismus
f. Poor weight gain in pregnancy
3. Others
a. Partner appears "overprotective"
b. Missed appointments
- Effect of pregnancy on VAW
- Risks in pregnancy in the situation of violence/abuse, to the individual and fetus
- Management
1. Data collection
2. Forensic examination
3. Safety
4. Counseling
5. Acute intervention
6. Long-term aid
7. Referral
- Community resources for people who have experienced violence/abuse
- Legal and emergency issues related to domestic violence

Infectious Disease in Pregnancy

TORCH Infections
- The most common infections associated with congenital disease
- TORCH acronym stands for *Toxoplasmosis*; *Other*: syphilis, varicella-zoster, parvovirus B19; *Rubella*; *Cytomegalovirus*; *Herpes*

Toxoplasmosis
- Incidence—40% to 50% of adults in the United States have the antibody to toxoplasmosis; about 5% seroconvert during pregnancy
1. Congenital infection—3 in 1,000 infants
2. Severe congenital infection—1 in 8,000 pregnancies
- Clinical manifestation
1. Most infections are asymptomatic
2. 10% of infected infants have damage resulting in lower IQ and deafness
3. Can cause spontaneous abortion, prematurity, and FGR

- Diagnostic tests and laboratory findings
1. Detection of *Toxoplasma*-specific immunoglobulin (IgG, IgM, IgA, IgE) antibodies
2. Diagnosis—direct observation of the parasite in stained tissue sections, cerebrospinal fluid (CSF), or other biopsy material
3. Testing for anti-*Toxoplasma* IgG antibody is difficult to interpret—not a practical test to perform; universal screening of pregnant individuals for toxoplasmosis is *not* recommended in the United States. Screen pregnant individuals who are immunocompromised or infection is suspected
- Management
1. Treatment—in collaboration with maternal–fetal medicine/high-risk obstetrics
a. Spiramycin is recommended for pregnant patients whose infections were acquired and diagnosed before 18 weeks of gestation and infection of the fetus is not documented or suspected
b. Pyrimethamine, sulfadiazine, and leucovorin are recommended for infections acquired at or after 18 weeks of gestation or when infection in the fetus is documented or suspected
2. Prevention
a. Fully cook meat to at least 145°F (63°C) and poultry to 160°F (71°C)
b. Do not drink unpasteurized milk or eat unpasteurized cheese
c. Avoid handling and/or changing kitty litter because toxoplasmosis is found in cat feces
d. Avoid drinking untreated water
e. Proper handwashing following gardening or wear gloves while gardening because soil might be contaminated with cat feces

Syphilis
- Refer to Chapter 5, Gynecologic, Reproductive, and Sexual Disorders

Varicella-Zoster (VZV)
- Herpes virus—causes two common infections
1. Varicella—chickenpox
a. Primary infection is rare in pregnancy
b. Greatest risk for congenital varicella syndrome is when the pregnant person is infected in the first 20 weeks
c. Maternal infection occurring from 6 days before to 2 days after delivery can be passed to the newborn, causing serious infection—5% mortality
d. Varicella infection causes varicella pneumonia in 10%–30% of pregnant adults; this is a medical emergency
2. Herpes zoster—shingles
a. Secondary infection
b. Poses little risk to the pregnant person or baby
- Incidence—5 in 1,000 pregnant individuals
- Pathophysiology and transmission
1. Respiratory inhalation of virus particles

2. Results in a viremia
3. Incubation period is 10–21 days, usually 14–16 days after exposure
4. Virus may be transmitted up to 2 days prior to the rash's appearance
5. VZV is highly contagious; incidence peaks in winter and spring
- Clinical manifestation
  1. Prior to rash, adults experience fever, malaise, myalgias, headache
  2. Rash—maculopapular rash that becomes vesicles
  3. New vesicles continue for 3–4 days
  4. Crusted by 1 week
- Complications
  1. Pneumonia—14% maternal mortality
  2. Increased risk of preterm labor and birth
  3. Maternal varicella onset between 5 days before and 2 days after delivery may result in neonatal infection; fatality rate can be as high as 30% (likely due to fetal exposure to the virus without the benefit of receiving vertical transmission of maternal antibodies)
- Management
  1. Treatment
     a. Antiviral agent—IV acyclovir for severe infection in woman
     b. Infection in pregnant patient within 6 days before delivery—give varicella-zoster immunoglobulin (VZIG), prepare for tocolysis to delay delivery, give VZIG to infant
     c. Infection in a pregnant patient within 3 days postpartum—give infant VZIG
  2. Prevention
     a. Varicella vaccination for all susceptible individuals of reproductive-age preconception or postpartum
        (1) Conception should be delayed for 1 month after the last treatment dose due to a risk of mild varicella infection after vaccination with live, attenuated vaccine
     b. VZIG as early as possible if the pregnant patient exposed and susceptible

Parvovirus B19 (Fifth Disease)

- Prevalence—may affect 1%–5% of pregnant people
- Pathophysiology—single-stranded DNA virus
- Transmission
  1. Through respiratory secretions, such as saliva, sputum, or nasal mucus, when an infected person coughs or sneezes
  2. Through blood or blood products
  3. Rate of vertical transmission from an infected pregnant person to fetus ranges from 17% to 33%
  4. More often in late winter, spring, early summer
  5. Disease transmission to fetus and likelihood of severe complications are highest in second trimester
- Clinical manifestation
  1. Asymptomatic in about 20% of infected people
  2. Healthy adults—mild rash and illness
  3. Immunocompromised adults—reticular rash in the trunk; painful, swollen joints; severe anemia

- Complications
  1. Spontaneous abortion
  2. Severe fetal anemia
  3. Hydrops fetalis
  4. Stillbirth
- Screening, diagnostic tests, and laboratory findings
  1. Routine serologic screening of all pregnant people is not recommended by ACOG
  2. Pregnant patient—if infection suspected, parvovirus B19–specific IgG and IgM serologies
  3. Fetal infection
     a. Histologically
     b. Presence of viral particles by electron microscopy
     c. Viral DNA may be identified by polymerase chain reaction (PCR) of amniotic fluid or fetal blood by cordocentesis
- Management
  1. Treatment
     a. No specific antiviral drug to treat parvovirus B19
     b. Nonsteroidal anti-inflammatory drugs (NSAIDs) and acetaminophen may be used for muscle and joint pain experienced by the pregnant patient; caution with use of NSAIDS in the third trimester
  2. Fetal assessment
     a. Ultrasound exam to evaluate for signs of fetal anemia or hydrops fetalis
     b. Cord blood sampling to determine the degree of fetal anemia
     c. Doppler ultrasound of the fetal middle cerebral artery (MCA) to assess fetal anemia risk
  3. Prevention
     a. No vaccine or medicine can prevent parvovirus B19 infection
     b. Handwashing with soap and water
     c. Avoid touching eyes, nose, or mouth
     d. Avoid contact with sick people

Rubella

- Incidence
  1. Rare in the United States
- Pathophysiology
  1. Single-stranded RNA virus
  2. Acquired respiratory disease
  3. Occurs 2–3 weeks following exposure
  4. Infectious virus is present in respiratory tract 1 week prior to symptom development
- Transmission
  1. Direct contact with nasal or throat secretions of infected individuals
  2. Droplets spread through sneezing or coughing
- Clinical manifestations
  1. Discrete pinkish-red maculopapular rash
  2. Appears first on the face, then on the trunk and extremities
  3. May also have lymphadenopathy, fever, arthralgias
  4. Symptoms last 3 days
  5. As many as 50% of all infections are subclinical
- Complications
  1. Spontaneous abortion

2. Stillbirth
3. Congenital Rubella Syndrome (CRS)—FGR, cataracts, retinopathy, heart defects, such as patent ductus arteriosus, hearing impairment
4. Risk of long-term complications from CRS is highest if the mother is infected in the first trimester
- Diagnostic tests and laboratory findings
  1. Demonstrate serologic conversion
  2. Recent rubella infection results in specific IgM in the fetal blood
  3. Can use CVS to recover virus
- Management
  1. Treatment—no antiviral therapy available
  2. Prevention
     a. Vaccination of susceptible individuals of reproductive age, preconception or postpartum
     b. No documented cases of CRS from the vaccine, but recommend giving at least 4 weeks prior to attempting a pregnancy or postpartum; may be given while breastfeeding

Cytomegalovirus (CMV)

- Incidence
  1. Most common congenital infection
  2. Occurs in 0.2%–2.2% of all neonates
- Pathophysiology—double-stranded DNA herpes virus
- Transmission
  1. Sexual contact
  2. Direct contact with infected blood, urine, or saliva
  3. Vertical transmission due to transplacental infection or exposure to genital secretions at delivery, or breastfeeding
- Clinical manifestation
  1. Adults are usually asymptomatic
  2. May experience mononucleosis-like syndrome: fever, chills, malaise, myalgias; leukocytosis, lymphocytosis, abnormal liver function test, and lymphadenopathy
- Complications
  1. Approximately 30% of infants who are severely infected with CMV die
  2. An estimated 65%–80% of those neonates who survive experience severe neurologic morbidity
- Diagnostic tests and laboratory findings
  1. In adults, CMV-specific IgG and IgM serologies
  2. PCR of infected blood, urine, saliva, cervical secretions, or breastmilk
- Management
  1. Treatment—No treatment available for maternal or fetal CMV infection
  2. Prevention
     a. No vaccine or medicine can prevent CMV infection
     b. Handwashing with soap and water
     c. Avoid touching eyes, nose, or mouth
     d. Avoid contact with sick people

Herpes Simplex Virus (HSV)

- Refer to Chapter 5, Gynecologic, Reproductive, and Sexual Disorders

Human Immunodeficiency Virus (HIV) and Acquired Immunodeficiency Syndrome (AIDS)

- Incidence
  1. In 2021, there were 32,100 new HIV diagnoses in the United States; 51% were among adults and teens in the South (CDC, 2024c)
  2. Rates and incidence from 2012 to 2016
     a. Heterosexual women—decreased 8%
     b. Among individuals who inject drugs—decreased 17%
- Pathophysiology
  1. DNA retroviruses called human immunodeficiency viruses include HIV-1 and HIV-2
  2. Most cases worldwide are HIV-1
  3. Retroviruses have genomes that encode reverse transcriptase, allowing the virus to make DNA copies of itself in the host cells
- Transmission—pregnant person to infant
  1. If a pregnant person with HIV does *not* receive antiretroviral therapy (ART) during pregnancy, the rate of transmission is between 15% and 25%
  2. If a pregnant person with HIV does receive ART during pregnancy, the rate of transmission is less than 1% if multi-agent ART is used and if the viral load is undetectable at delivery
- Clinical manifestation
  1. Initial HIV infection
     a. Incubation period from exposure to clinical disease—days to weeks
     b. Acute viral illness syndrome—lasts 10 days or less
     c. Fever
     d. Night sweats
     e. Fatigue
     f. Rash
     g. Headache
     h. Lymphadenopathy
     i. Pharyngitis
     j. Myalgias
     k. Arthralgias
     l. Nausea
     m. Vomiting
     n. Diarrhea
     o. Becomes asymptomatic and chronic viremia begins
     p. Average time to AIDS is 10 years
  2. Clinical manifestation of AIDS
     a. Generalized lymphadenopathy
     b. Oral hairy leukoplakia
     c. Aphthous ulcers
     d. Thrombocytopenia
     e. Opportunistic infections
     f. Esophageal or pulmonary candidiasis
     g. Persistent herpes
     h. CMV
     i. Molluscum contagiosum
     j. Pneumocystis
     k. Toxoplasmosis
     l. Neurologic disease—50%

- Screening, diagnostic tests, and laboratory findings
  1. Risk assessment—drug use/sexual histories
  2. Universal screening of pregnant people for HIV as part of routine prenatal tests with the option to decline (opt-out screening) recommended
  3. Repeat screening in the third trimester if high risk, high incidence of HIV in individuals of reproductive age in the geographic area, signs or symptoms of acute HIV infection
  4. Separate written consent for HIV testing should not be required; general consent for medical care should be considered sufficient to encompass consent for HIV testing
  5. Rapid HIV testing during labor and delivery if status unknown
  6. HIV testing (refer to **Figure 7-1** for recommended laboratory HIV testing algorithm for serum or plasma specimens)
     a. Antibody testing
        (1) Screening tests—enzyme immunoassay (EIA or ELISA) checks for proteins that the body makes in response to the presence of the virus
        (2) Since 2014, the CDC has recommended discontinuing the Western blot as a form of confirmatory testing
     b. Direct viral screens
        (1) Nucleic acid testing if suspect acute retroviral syndrome or recent infection
        (2) Confirm with subsequent antibody testing to document seroconversion
  7. CD4 counts
     a. CD4 cells are a type of white blood cell that play a vital role in the immune system
     b. HIV attacks CD4 cells and damages the cells; causes the number of CD4 cells in the blood to decline
     c. When the CD4 cell count decreases, the body has a harder time fighting infections
     d. CD4 count <200 cell/mm^3 is definitive diagnosis for HIV
  8. Viral load
     a. High viral load—indicates an increased number of HIV particles in the blood; a recent transmission, untreated, or uncontrolled HIV
     b. Low viral load—only a few copies of HIV in the person's bloodstream

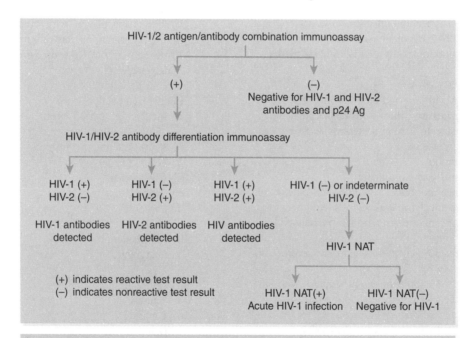

Figure 7-1 Recommended Laboratory HIV Testing Algorithm for Serum or Plasma Specimen. *Abbreviations:* FDA, Food and Drug Administration; HIV, human immunodeficiency virus; NAT, nucleic acid test.

- Management of HIV-positive pregnant patients
  1. Prevention of transmission
  2. Initial evaluation
  3. Complete review of systems (ROS)
  4. Physical examination
  5. Initial labs—HIV antibody, CD4 count, viral load
  6. Follow-up by a team of experts (infectious disease specialists, maternal–fetal medicine); interdisciplinary approach is most effective
  7. Prevention of vertical transmission
     a. Viral load is strongest predictor for vertical transmission
     b. Multi-agent ART during pregnancy—start after the first trimester if the mother does not need treatment
     c. Intravenous zidovudine therapy during labor and delivery
     d. Avoid artificial rupture of membranes if delivery is not imminent
     e. Consider cesarean section at 38 weeks if viral load >1,000 copies/mL
     f. Treat infant with ART—usual regimen is 6 weeks
  8. Prevention of opportunistic infections
  9. Standard precautions for all bloodborne and body fluid–borne pathogens—blood, all body fluid secretions and excretions, nonintact skin, mucous membranes
- Treatment—antepartum
  1. Goals are the treatment of maternal infection and reduction of risk for perinatal transmission
  2. Highly active antiretroviral therapy (HAART)
     a. Two nucleoside analogues—zidovudine, didanosine, zalcitabine, or lamivudine *and*
     b. Protease inhibitor—indinavir, ritonavir, saquinavir, or nonnucleoside analogue (nevirapine, delavirdine, efavirenz)
     c. Start after the first trimester unless the pregnant person needs treatment
- Treatment—intrapartum
  1. Zidovudine IV throughout labor and delivery for vaginal birth
  2. Zidovudine IV starting 3 hours before cesarean section and through delivery
- Counseling
  1. Pretest counseling is important
  2. Informed consent
  3. Post-test counseling is also important
- Legal issues
  1. Confidentiality
  2. Reporting
  3. Discuss with the patient regarding partner treatment
  4. Discrimination
- Concurrent disease concerns for HIV-infected individuals
  1. Syphilis
  2. Tuberculosis
  3. Human papillomavirus (HPV)
  4. Hepatitis B
  5. Pneumococcal infection
- Possible effects on pregnancy outcome
  1. PROM
  2. Preterm labor and birth

  3. LBW
  4. Fetal demise
  5. HIV transmission to the fetus
- Fetal assessment as clinically indicated
  1. Ultrasound (US)
  2. Fetal movement counting (FMC)
  3. Nonstress test (NST) with amniotic fluid index (AFI), biophysical profile (BPP)
- Intrapartum care
  1. Avoid invasive procedures
  2. Maintain universal body fluid precautions for all births
  3. Cleanse maternal secretions from the baby as soon as possible
  4. Drain umbilical cord for cord blood to avoid needles
  5. Provide emotional support
- Postpartum care
  1. HIV can be transmitted through human milk to the infant.
     a. Low risk of transmission (<1%): if taking antiretroviral therapy (ART) and has a sustained, undetectable viral load
     b. Higher risk of transmission: if individuals have detectable viral loads
        (1) Resource: National Perinatal HIV/AIDS hotline (1-888-448-8764) consultation
     c. Consideration must be given if safe infant feeding alternatives are absent; breastfeeding/chestfeeding may be recommended with continued use of ART to reduce transmission (WHO recommendation)

Zika

- Definition—Zika is a virus spread to people primarily through the bite of an infected mosquito and is linked to congenital anomalies
- Transmission
  1. Mosquito bite
  2. Sexual intercourse with an infected person (whether the person is symptomatic or not)
- Clinical manifestations
  1. Symptoms in adults—typically mild, lasting several days to a week; people may not realize that they have been infected
     a. Fever
     b. Rash
     c. Headache
     d. Joint pain
     e. Conjunctivitis
     f. Muscle pain
  2. Infants born to a pregnant person infected with Zika may have microcephaly and severe brain damage
- Screening and testing
  1. Nucleic acid amplification test (NAAT) and IgM antibody testing on a serum specimen
  2. Zika virus NAAT on a urine specimen
- Prevention
  1. No vaccination available
  2. Condom use with people infected with Zika or people who live or have recently traveled to places with a Zika outbreak

3. Avoid travel to areas with a Zika outbreak for people considering pregnancy or who are currently pregnant
4. If travel cannot be avoided, take measures to avoid mosquito bite
   a. Use an Environmental Protection Agency (EPA)–registered insect repellent; these are safe for pregnant and lactating individuals
   b. Wear long-sleeved shirts and long pants
   c. Stay in places with air conditioning or window and door screens to keep mosquitoes out
   d. Remove standing water around the home

Fetal Growth Aberrations

Fetal Growth Restriction (FGR)

- Definitions—Fetal growth restriction (FGR) is the preferred diagnostic term for describing a fetus whose estimated fetal weight or abdominal circumference (AC) falls below the 10th percentile; Small for gestational age (SGA) is the diagnostic term that describes a newborn with a birth weight below the 10th percentile
  1. Clinically significant categorizations
     a. Symmetry—Symmetric or asymmetric
     b. Timing—early (more progressive) or late onset (less severe)
     c. Severity—less or more severe (at or <3rd percentile; increased risk of neonatal mortality and morbidity)
- Differential diagnosis
  1. The genetic design of a constitutionally small infant (parents are also small)
- Incidence—3% to 8%; leads to 18% mortality rate
- Symmetric growth restriction
  1. Insult occurs early in pregnancy, likely in the first trimester → resulting in a decreased in the number and size of cells → affects growth pattern for the body and head → symmetric reduced growth
  2. Causes
     a. Congenital infections
     b. Chromosomal abnormalities
     c. Maternal drug use—tobacco, alcohol, Dilantin (phenytoin), cocaine, heroin
  3. Increased risk of adverse long-term sequelae
- Asymmetric growth restriction
  1. Appears later in the pregnancy
  2. Two main etiologic pathways
     a. Reduced nutrition to fetus → diminished glycogen stores → decreased liver volume → decrease in abdominal circumference
     b. Abnormalities in uteroplacental perfusion → increased right cardiac afterload → cardiac output diverted toward left ventricle → increase in blood and nutrient supply to vital organs of the body → asymmetrical head-sparing appearance
  3. Causes
     a. Maternal factors
        (1) Hypertension
        (2) Anemia
        (3) Collagen disease
        (4) Type-I Diabetes Mellitus
     b. Placental factors
        (1) Previa
        (2) Abruption
        (3) Malformations
        (4) Infarctions
        (5) Single umbilical cord artery
     c. Fetal factors
        (1) Multiple gestation
        (2) Anomalies
  4. Diagnosis
     a. Review history
     b. Physical examination
        (1) Fundal height
        (2) EFW
        (3) Fetal AC
     c. Ultrasound to confirm diagnosis
        (1) Anomalies
        (2) Serial studies for growth
        (3) AFI
        (4) Doppler flow studies
  5. Fetal effects
     a. Fetus adjusts to conditions by conserving energy and decreasing metabolic requirements
     b. Fetus stops growing
     c. Risk of intrauterine fetal demise
  6. Management
     a. Seek consultation
     b. If you can identify a cause, counsel the patient and make adjustments
        (1) Decrease smoking
        (2) Nutrition evaluation
     c. Emotional support and anticipatory guidance
     d. Serial ultrasounds for growth with Doppler studies
     e. Serial NSTs and AFI or BPPs (weekly or twice weekly)
     f. TORCH titer, including Zika testing
     g. Amniocentesis, chromosome evaluation of parents
     h. Consider delivery, if necessary

Large for Gestational Age (LGA)/Macrosomia

- Definition—in the United States, newborns weighing more than 4,000 g at birth (some studies define LGA as >4,500 g) (macrosomia) or over the 90th percentile in weight for gestational age
- Risk factors
  1. Ethnic/racial origins
  2. Obesity
  3. Previous LGA/macrosomic neonate
  4. Previous shoulder dystocia
  5. Size of the father
  6. Birth weights of both the mother and the father
  7. Diabetes or history of gestational diabetes
  8. Previous uterine myomata
  9. Multiparity

- Physical examination
  1. Fundal height
  2. EFW and palpation of fetal parts
  3. Maternal body habitus
- Differential diagnosis
  1. Inaccurate dating
  2. Polyhydramnios
  3. Multiple gestation
  4. Diabetes
  5. Uterine fibroids
- Management
  1. Discuss risks and challenges
  2. Diet counseling
  3. Ultrasound for EFW
  4. Consult
  5. Prepare/Anticipate shoulder dystocia

Multiple Gestation

- Incidence
  1. Twins—114,161 births; birth rate 31.2 per 1,000 U.S. live births in 2021
  2. Triplets or higher-order birth rate—80 per 1,000 U.S. live births in 2021
- Definitions
  1. Zygosity—the condition of zygotes as it relates to twins
     a. Monozygotic (MZ)—4/1,000 worldwide
     b. Dizygotic (DZ)—8/1,000 worldwide
  2. Chorionicity—refers to placentation; most reliable when assessed in the first trimester
  3. Multiple gestation accounts for fewer than 1% of births but more than 10% of perinatal mortality
  4. Incidence varies with race and increases with age, parity, and heredity
- DZ (fraternal)—fertilization of two separate ova by two separate sperm
  1. Use of fertility drugs increases chance
  2. Clomid—1:10 risk
  3. Gonadotropins—1:5 risk
  4. In vitro fertilization (IVF) increases risk
- MZ (identical)—division of a single fertilized egg
  1. Most risk factors are unknown
  2. Time of zygote division determines membrane development
     a. Days 0–3—dichorionic, diamniotic (30%)
     b. Days 4–8—monochorionic, diamniotic (68%)
  3. Between days 9 and 12—monochorionic, monoamniotic (2%)
  4. After day 13—conjoined twins (<1%)
- Family history increases the risk
- Clinical skills are important in identifying multiple pregnancies
- Signs and symptoms
  1. Fundal height greater than dates
  2. Earlier or exaggerated discomforts of pregnancy
  3. Two distinct fetal heartbeats
  4. Outline of more than one fetus
  5. Palpation of multiple small parts
  6. Ultrasound of two or more fetuses

- Differential diagnosis
  1. Macrosomia
  2. Uterine, ovarian, or pelvic mass
  3. Distended bladder
  4. Polyhydramnios
  5. Hydatidiform mole
  6. Inaccurate dates
- Potential complications
  1. Hyperemesis
  2. Preterm labor, PROM, preterm birth
  3. 36% deliver before 36 weeks' gestation
  4. 50% deliver before 37 weeks' gestation
  5. SGA—55% of multiple-gestation infants weigh less than 5 lb
  6. Twin-to-twin transfusion
  7. Oligohydramnios
  8. Perinatal asphyxia
  9. Preeclampsia
  10. Postpartum hemorrhage
  11. Pyelonephritis
  12. Maternal anemia
  13. Placental problems
      a. Previa
      b. Abruption
  14. Fetal anomalies
- Antepartum management
  1. Seek consultation
  2. Discuss the risks and benefits of management, serial ultrasounds, and regular fetal surveillance
  3. Counsel about maternal nutrition, rest, exercise, and stress
     a. Increased nutritional needs
     b. Increased iron
     c. Small, frequent meals
     d. Exercise limitations and bed rest are both controversial
  4. Provide emotional support
  5. Evaluate weekly for weight, fetal growth, signs and symptoms of preterm labor, and elevated blood pressure
  6. Preterm labor monitoring
     a. Possible administration of glucocorticoids for lung maturity
     b. Tocolytic therapy
     c. Birth plan should include the availability of a physician consultant for birth

Blood Incompatibilities: D(Rh) Isoimmunization

- Incidence
  1. Highest incidence found in the Basques of France and Spain—25% to 40%
  2. White Americans—approximately 15%
  3. Black Americans—approximately 5%–8%
  4. American Hispanics—approximately 5%–10%
- Types
  1. ABO incompatibility
     a. Approximately 20%–25% of pregnancies are ABO incompatible

b. Isoimmunization causes 60% of fetal hemolytic disease

2. Maternal serum contains anti-A or anti-B
   a. Rarely causes more than fetal anemia with mild to moderate neonatal hyperbilirubinemia in the first 24 hours of life
   b. Caused by IgM anti-B or IgM anti-A crossing the placenta poorly

3. Sensitization caused by minor antigens
   a. Some cause hemolytic disease, some do not
   b. Believed to be the result of incompatible transfusion, although may be seen in multiparas

4. Kell—may have mild to severe disease with hydrops (K-kills)

5. Duffy—Fy^a may have mild to severe disease with hydrops; Fy^b is not associated with problems

- Pathogenesis for Rh isoimmunization
  1. Three requirements
     a. Fetus must be D+ and the pregnant individual D–
     b. Pregnant individual must be able to be sensitized
     c. Sufficient quantities of fetal cells must gain access to the pregnant patient's bloodstream
  2. Conditions supporting Rh isoimmunization
     a. Transfusion of incompatible blood to the mother, usually before pregnancy
     b. Fetomaternal exchange of blood during:
        (1) Delivery
        (2) Spontaneous or induced abortion (a person may not realize they are pregnant)
        (3) Amniocentesis
        (4) Ectopic pregnancy
        (5) Placental abruption
        (6) Unknown cause

- Implications
  1. Maternal
     a. No significant maternal complications
  2. Fetal
     a. Mother produces anti-D antibodies (IgG), which cross the placenta
     b. Hemolysis of fetal red blood cells (RBCs)
     c. Fetal anemia, hematopoiesis in liver and spleen
     d. Enlargement of fetal liver and spleen
     e. Liver and spleen show degenerative changes
     f. Erythroblastosis fetalis—ascites, cardiac failure, hydrothorax
     g. Hydrops fetalis with generalized edema
     h. Fetal loss/death
  3. Newborn
     a. Pregnant individual's IgG is still present and attacking RBCs
     b. Further RBC breakdown occurs
     c. Fetal liver is immature and unable to clear RBCs
     d. Hyperbilirubinemia results
     e. Elevated bilirubin level causes kernicterus, with central nervous system (CNS) damage and if left untreated, possible death

- Management
  1. Unsensitized pregnancy—pregnant individual Rh negative with negative antibody titer
     a. ABO/D group and antibody titer at first visit
     b. Repeat antibody screen at 28 weeks and give RhoGAM if remains unsensitized
     c. Rho(D) immunoglobulin (RhoGAM) is protective for 12 weeks
     d. If the infant is Rh positive, give the pregnant patient RhoGAM again after delivery
  2. Sensitized pregnancy—mother Rh negative with positive antibody titer (>1:4)
     a. Seek consultation—co-manage or transfer care
     b. Follow the fetus with serial ultrasounds to assess for signs of ascites
     c. Follow titers to assess the need for amniocentesis

Post-Term Pregnancy (Postdates Pregnancy)

- Definition—pregnancy continuing beyond 42 completed weeks of gestation
- Incidence
  1. An estimated 6%–12% of pregnancies go beyond 42 weeks of gestation
  2. Approximately 25% of post-term pregnancies result in babies who have postmaturity syndrome
  3. Associated with increased morbidity and mortality for both pregnant person and fetus
- Diagnosis
  1. Based on careful gestational age assessment
     a. Certain last menstrual period (LMP)
     b. Early examination
     c. Sizing by bimanual examination
     d. Fundal height
     e. Fetal heart tones (FHTs) by Doppler and fetoscope
  2. Report of sexual history
  3. Report of quickening
  4. Early ultrasonography (USG) gestational dating
     a. Crown–rump length (CRL) best; between 6 and 14 weeks
     b. Dating using biparietal diameter (BPD), head circumference (HC), abdominal circumference, femur length (FL); before 26 weeks
- Potential complications
  1. Shoulder dystocia—if the fetus is macrosomic
  2. Problems related to oligohydramnios
  3. Problems related to uteroplacental insufficiency
  4. Neonatal meconium aspiration
  5. Stillbirth
- Management
  1. Continue fetal movement counts between 40 and 41 weeks
     a. At 41 weeks, begin biweekly NST/AFI or BPP
     b. BPP if abnormal NST; contraction stress test (CST) used less frequently
     c. Doppler velocimetry
     d. See consultation
     e. Expectant management and delivery
        (1) Consider induction when cervix is ripe
        (2) Prostaglandins may be used to promote cervical ripening

(3) Methods of labor induction—oxytocin, foley bulb, prostaglandins, membrane stripping, amniotomy, nipple stimulation

(4) Deliver if any indication of fetal compromise or oligohydramnios

(5) Be prepared for possible meconium staining of fluid

Diagnosed Obesity in Pregnancy

- Definition—Classified based on body mass index (BMI); according to the 2009 Institute of Medicine (IOM)/National Research Council recommendations, diagnosed obesity is defined as a BMI ≥30
  1. Weight stigmatization is common in healthcare; biases based on weight and body size can impact clinical care and diagnosis.
- World Health Organization BMI categories (**Table 7-1**)
- Incidence
  1. Among individuals of reproductive age, approximately 27% are diagnosed as overweight and 41% are diagnosed with obesity
- Effects on pregnancy—increases risks for multiple conditions
  1. Continued or increased stigmatization resulting in:
     a. psychological impacts (e.g., low self-esteem, depression, anxiety, disordered eating)
     b. late or misdiagnoses and treatment due to over-attribution of symptoms to high BMI
     c. avoidance behaviors resulting in less prenatal care or screening/testing
  2. Pregnancy loss and stillbirth
  3. Neural tube defects
  4. Hydrocephaly
  5. Cardiovascular, orofacial, and limb reduction anomalies
  6. Gestational diabetes
  7. Macrosomia
  8. Shoulder dystocia
  9. Longer first stage of labor
  10. Labor induction
  11. Preeclampsia

Table 7-1 Weight Category According to BMI

Category	BMI
Underweight	<18.5
Normal weight	18.5–24.9
Overweight	25.0–29.9
Obesity class I	30.0–34.9
Obesity class II	35.0–39.9
Obesity class III	≥40

Modified from World Health Organization. 2018. Obesity and overweight. Retrieved from https://www.who.int/en/news-room/fact-sheets/detail/obesity-and-overweight

12. Cesarean section
13. Venous thromboembolism
14. Postpartum weight retention
15. Metabolic dysfunction
16. Pre-gravid obesity in future pregnancies

- Management
  1. Respectful, person-centered approach to counseling and management should be employed to mitigate adverse impacts due to weight stigmatization
  2. Antepartum
     a. Standard or targeted ultrasound between 18 and 24 weeks to detect anomalies and soft markers for aneuploidy
     b. Ultrasounds every 4–6 weeks to monitor fetal growth
     c. Weekly NSTs (pre-pregnancy BMI 35.0–39.0 kg/m² beginning at 37 weeks; pre-pregnancy BMI greater than 40 kg/m² beginning at 34 weeks)
     d. Patients with obstructive sleep apnea (OSA) should be evaluated by sleep medicine specialist
     e. Early gestational diabetes screening with glucose tolerance test
  3. Intrapartum considerations for pregnant individuals with BMI >50.0 kg/m²
     a. Epidural or spinal anesthesia may be technically difficult due to body habitus and loss of landmarks
     b. Due to excessive tissue and edema, general anesthesia may be potentially difficult; follow recommendations for preoxygenation, proper positioning, and use of fiberoptic equipment
     c. Higher dose of broad-spectrum antibiotics
  4. Postpartum—increased risk for venous thromboembolism
     a. Mechanical thromboprophylaxis via pneumatic compression stockings
     b. Pharmacologic thromboprophylaxis with low-molecular-weight heparin recommended during the postpartum period

Hyperemesis Gravidarum (HG)

- Definition—persistent vomiting during pregnancy unrelated to other causes
- Incidence
  1. Affects 0.3%–3% of pregnancies
  2. Number one reason for hospitalization in the first trimester
  3. Number two reason (after preterm labor) for hospitalization during pregnancy
- Etiology
  1. Cause is unknown
  2. Some have theorized a relation between HG and human chorionic gonadotropin (hCG) given that the peak of hCG coincides with the most severe symptoms
  3. Theoretical link to estrogen; lower levels of estrogen associated with lower incidence of nausea and vomiting in pregnancy

4. Possible evolutionary adaptation to avoid certain foods that may be potentially dangerous to the pregnant person and fetus
- Risk factors
  1. History of HG in previous pregnancy
  2. Possible genetic link; family history of HG
  3. Motion sickness
  4. Migraine headaches
- Diagnosis
  1. Diagnosis of exclusion; no set diagnostic criteria; varies among providers
  2. Typical criteria
     a. Severe and intractable vomiting with unknown etiology
     b. Weight loss of at least 5% of pre-pregnancy weight
     c. Ketonuria
     d. Electrolyte imbalance, thyroid and liver lab abnormalities
  3. Differential diagnosis
     a. Acute fatty liver of pregnancy
     b. Addison's disease
     c. Appendicitis
     d. Diabetic ketoacidosis
     e. Gastroenteritis
     f. Gastroparesis
     g. Hepatitis
     h. Intestinal obstruction
     i. Kidney stones
     j. Migraine headaches
     k. Pancreatitis
     l. Preeclampsia
     m. Pyelonephritis
- Assessment tool of the severity of nausea and vomiting— Pregnancy-Unique Quantification of Emesis and Nausea (PUQE; **Table 7-2**)

- Management
  1. Nonpharmacologic therapies
     a. Multivitamins
     b. Frequent, small meals every 1–2 hours
     c. Avoid spicy or fatty foods
     d. Bland, dry foods; high-protein snacks; crackers before getting out of bed
     e. Avoidance of odors and other stimuli
     f. Ginger 1 g per day in divided doses
     g. Acupressure, acupuncture, acustimulation at P6 or Neiguan point
  2. Pharmacologic therapies
     a. Pyridoxine (vitamin B_6) 10–25 mg QUID or TID orally; maximum dose of 200 mg/day
     b. Diclegis (approved by Food and Drug Administration [FDA] in 2013)—combined pyridoxine 10 mg and doxylamine 10 mg orally; two tablets for moderate nausea or vomiting of pregnancy (NVP) before bedtime; for severe NVP, four tablets (one tablet in the morning, one tablet in the afternoon, two tablets at bedtime)
     c. Metoclopramide 5–10 mg q6–8h orally
     d. Promethazine 25 mg q4h per rectal suppository
     e. Ondansetron—can be considered for severe or refractory NVP; evidence is limited on its safety or efficacy; risk versus benefit should be weighed in each case. Black box warning on this drug—not to be used in pregnancy according to FDA
     f. Rarely, if not responsive to medical therapy and unable to maintain weight, enteral tube feedings
     g. If not able to tolerate liquids without vomiting and no response to outpatient management, hospitalization for IV rehydration, antiemetic therapy, and nutritional support

---

Table 7-2 Modified Pregnancy-Unique Quantification of Emesis and Nausea

Circle the answer that best suits your situation from the beginning of your pregnancy.

1. On average in a day, for how long do you feel nauseated or sick to your stomach?

Not at all	1 hour or less	2–3 hours	4–6 hours	More than 6 hours
(1)	(2)	(3)	(4)	(5)

2. On average in a day, how many times do you vomit or throw up?

7 or more times	5–6 times	3–4 times	1–2 times	I did not throw up
(1)	(2)	(3)	(4)	(5)

3. On average in a day, how many times do you have retching or dry heaves without bringing anything up?

None	1–2 times	3–4 times	5–6 times	7 or more times
(1)	(2)	(3)	(4)	(5)

Total score (sum of replies to 1, 2, and 3): mild NVP, 6 or less; moderate NVP, 7–12; severe NVP, 13 or more.

Abbreviation: NVP, nausea or vomiting of pregnancy.

Reproduced from Lacasse, A., Rey, E., Ferreira, E., Morin, C., & Berard, A. (2008). Validity of a modified Pregnancy-Unique Quantification of Emesis and Nausea (PUQE) scoring index to assess severity or nausea and vomiting of pregnancy. *American Journal of Obstetrics and Gynecology, 198,* 71.e1–71.e7.

Tuberculosis (TB)

- Definition—infection, mostly in the lung, by *Mycobacterium tuberculosis*; clinical disease occurs in 10% of those infected
- Populations at risk for TB
  1. HIV-infected people
  2. Foreign-born people from countries with high TB prevalence
  3. Medically underserved low-income populations
  4. Close contact with persons with active infection
  5. People who use alcohol and illicit intravenous drugs
- Incidence
  1. In 2022, 8,331 reported cases (2.5 cases per 100,000 persons); an estimated 13 million people living with latent TB
- Screening tests for TB—purified protein derivative of tuberculin (PPD) intradermally
  1. If negative (i.e., no induration), no further assessment is needed
  2. Positive test interpreted based on risk factors
     a. 5 mm is positive for very high risk—HIV positive, with abnormal chest radiograph, recent contact with an active case
     b. 10 mm is positive for high risk (i.e., individuals born outside the United States, HIV-negative IV drug users, low-income populations, associated medical problems)
     c. 15 mm is positive for persons with none of these risks
  3. Vaccination with bacillus Calmette–Guérin (BCG) requires special guidance for interpretation
- Signs and symptoms
  1. Cough with minimal sputum production
  2. Low-grade fever
  3. Hemoptysis
  4. Weight loss
- Diagnosis
  1. Chest radiograph
  2. Sputum for acid-fast bacillus
  3. Extrapulmonary disease occurs in any organ; disseminated disease exists in 40% of HIV-positive patients
- Treatment (CDC, 2016e)
  1. Untreated TB poses a higher risk to the fetus than treatment does
  2. Latent TB infection
     a. Isoniazid (INH) daily or twice weekly using directly observed therapy for 9 months
     b. Supplementation with 10–25 mg/day of pyridoxine (vitamin B) recommended
     c. 3HP INH and rifapentine—not recommended for women planning to be pregnant in the next 3 months
  3. TB disease
     a. Initial treatment is INH, rifampin, and ethambutol daily for 2 months; then INH and rifampin daily, or twice weekly for 7 months (for a total of 9 months)

b. Streptomycin and pyrazinamide are contraindicated in pregnancy
  4. HIV-related TB disease
     a. Treatment for pregnant individuals who are HIV-positive with TB disease is the same as for nonpregnant individuals
     b. See the latest CDC guidelines for full information
  5. Potential for increased hepatotoxicity risk during pregnancy and the first 2–3 months postpartum
  6. Breastfeeding is not contraindicated with TB treatment
  7. Precautions
     a. Liver toxicity
     b. Drug resistance

Bleeding in Pregnancy

First-Trimester Bleeding

- Definition—bleeding occurring within the first 12 weeks of pregnancy
  1. 40% of pregnant individuals have some bleeding in the first trimester
  2. 80% of spontaneous abortions occur in the first 12 weeks of gestation
  3. 90% of pregnancies with bleeding continue to term after FHT observed
- Differential diagnosis
  1. Implantation bleeding
  2. Threatened abortion: inevitable, complete, incomplete, missed
  3. Ectopic pregnancy
  4. Cervicitis
  5. Cervical polyps
  6. Vaginitis
  7. Trauma/intercourse
  8. Disappearing twin
  9. Autoantibody/autoimmune disorder
- Diagnosis
  1. Pelvic examination
     a. Speculum examination to visualize the cervix
     b. Bimanual examination to assess uterus and adnexa for size and tenderness
  2. Laboratory diagnosis
     a. Serum hCG is positive 7–9 days after fertilization
     b. Beta-human chorionic gonadotropin (β-hCG) doubles every 1.4–2.0 days with normal intrauterine pregnancy (IUP)
     c. β-hCG increases by only one-third or less when an ectopic pregnancy exists
     d. Rule of 10
        (1) β-hCG = 100 at time of missed menses
        (2) β-hCG = 100,000 at 10 weeks (peak)
        (3) β-hCG = 10,000 at term
        (4) β-hCG elimination half-life = 24 hours
        (5) 90% of ectopic pregnancies have β-hCG less than 6,500
  3. Treatment—depends on etiology

Abortion

- Types of abortion
  1. Spontaneous abortion—occurring without apparent cause
  2. Threatened abortion—the appearance of signs and symptoms of possible loss of the fetus (i.e., vaginal bleeding with or without intermittent pain)
  3. Inevitable abortion—cervix is dilating; uterus will be emptied and cannot be stopped
  4. Incomplete abortion—an abortion in which part of the products of conception has been retained in the uterus
  5. Complete abortion—all the products of conception have been expelled
  6. Missed abortion—the fetus died before completion of 20 weeks' gestation, but products of conception are retained; no bleeding or cramping
  7. Recurrent pregnancy loss—three or more consecutive abortions
- Etiology—fetal factors
  1. Abnormal development of zygote such as from chromosomal abnormalities is responsible for about 50% of spontaneous abortions
  2. Autosomal trisomy is the most frequently identified chromosomal anomaly, followed by Turner's syndrome
- Etiology—maternal factors
  1. Incidence increases with parity and/or short interpregnancy interval
  2. Incidence increases with parental age
- Common causes of spontaneous abortion
  1. Anatomic anomalies
  2. Infections
  3. Immune factors, including autoimmune clotting disorders
  4. Endocrine effects
  5. Recreational drugs/alcohol/environmental toxins
     a. Smoking
     b. Ethanol (EtOH)
     c. Caffeine
     d. Radiation
     e. Cocaine
     f. Anesthetic gases/surgery
  6. Severe malnutrition
  7. Age of gametes
- General management
  1. Obtain blood type if not known
  2. Draw baseline serum β-hCG
  3. Repeat β-hCG in 48 hours
  4. Ultrasound
  5. Should be able to visualize an IUP transabdominally at hCG of 6,500
  6. Should be able to visualize an IUP transvaginally at hCG of 2,000
  7. RhoGAM for unsensitized Rh-negative patients
- Management specific to the type of abortion
  1. Inevitable or incomplete abortion
     a. Surgical dilation and curettage (D&C)
     b. Medical management
     c. Expectant management
     d. Emotional support and anticipatory guidance
  2. Threatened abortion or disappearing twin
     a. Pelvic rest
     b. Emotional support and anticipatory guidance

Ectopic Pregnancy

- Definition—implantation of the blastocyst anywhere other than the endometrium
- Approximately 95% of ectopic pregnancies occur in the oviducts
- Second leading cause of death of pregnant individuals in the United States
- Occurs in about 1 per 85 pregnancies; rate is highest in the 35- to 44-year age group
- Risk Factors
  1. STI—especially chlamydia and gonorrhea
  2. Therapeutic abortion followed by infection
  3. Endometriosis
  4. Previous pelvic surgery
  5. Failed bilateral tubal ligation
  6. Mechanical—problems with tubes, such as scarring
  7. Functional—menstrual reflux, hormonal alteration of tubal motility
- Sites for ectopic pregnancy
  1. Ampulla—78%
  2. Isthmus—12%
  3. Interstitial—2%
  4. Fimbria—less than 1%
  5. Other sites—abdominal, ovarian, and broad ligament
- Symptoms
  1. Amenorrhea but frequently with vaginal spotting
  2. Lower pelvic and/or unilateral abdominal pain
  3. Unilateral tender adnexal mass
  4. Some patients have no symptoms
- Clinical picture
  1. Severe abdominal pain
  2. Cervical motion tenderness
  3. Free fluid on ultrasound
  4. Cul-de-sac fullness
  5. Shoulder pain second to diaphragmatic irritation
  6. Vertigo or fainting
- Diagnosis
  1. Physical examination
  2. Serum β-hCG (90% of ectopics have β-hCG less than 6,500; abnormal interval increases)
  3. Ultrasound
  4. Culdocentesis
  5. Laparoscopy
- Differential diagnosis
  1. Pelvic inflammatory disease (PID)
  2. Ovarian cyst
  3. Appendicitis
- Management
  1. Seek consultation and transfer to medical management
  2. Tubal preservation is the goal
  3. Salpingectomy/salpingostomy/tubal resection
  4. Methotrexate if appropriate
  5. RhoGAM for Rh-negative pregnant individuals

Hydatidiform Mole (Gestational Trophoblastic Disease)

- Incidence—1:1,500 to 1:2,000
- Highest incidence at the beginning and end of reproductive years, with the greatest incidence after age 45
- Clinical manifestations
  1. Abnormal uterine bleeding
  2. Size/dates discrepancy
  3. Lack of fetal activity
  4. HG
  5. Gestational hypertension
  6. Passage of vesicular tissue
- Diagnosis
  1. Ultrasound
  2. Serum β-hCG
- Management
  1. Uterine evacuation by suction curettage
  2. Close surveillance for persistent trophoblastic proliferation or malignant changes
  3. Recommend avoidance of pregnancy for 1 year
  4. Serial β-hCG levels every 2 weeks until normal, then once a month for 6 months, then every 2 months for 1 year

Second-Trimester Bleeding

- Bleeding is less common during this time in pregnancy

Mid-Trimester Spontaneous Abortion

- May be associated with autoimmune disorders
- May be related to cocaine use
- May be related to anatomic or physiologic factors
- Infection in the cervix or vagina

Cervical Insufficiency

- Symptoms
  1. Painless dilation
  2. Bloody show
  3. Spontaneous rupture of membranes
  4. Vaginal/pelvic pressure
- Risk factors
  1. Previous mid-trimester loss
  2. Cervical surgery
  3. Diethylstilbestrol (DES)
- Treatment
  1. Seek consultation with an obstetrician
  2. Cervical cerclage after 12–14 weeks; success rate of 80%–90%
     a. Risk of ruptured membranes or infection
  3. Monitor cervical length via transvaginal ultrasound

Placental Anomalies

- Low-lying placenta
  1. One-third of pregnant patients have a low-lying placenta in the first trimester
  2. Only 1% of pregnant patients have previa in the third trimester
- Partial abruption
  1. May resolve
  2. May reabsorb
  3. Diagnosis—ultrasound
  4. Three predominant locations for placental abruption; size of hemorrhage is predictive of fetal survival
     a. Subchorionic—between the placenta and the membranes
     b. Retroplacental—between the placenta and the myometrium; worse prognosis than for subchorionic hemorrhage
     c. Preplacental—between the placenta and amniotic fluid
  5. Seek consultation as needed

Third-Trimester Bleeding

- Incidence—4% of all pregnancies
- Never perform a digital vaginal examination on a patient's cervix in the presence of third-trimester bleeding unless certain there is no previa
- Placenta previa—responsible for 20% of third-trimester bleeds
  1. Definition—placenta is located over or next to the internal cervical os; may be partial (not totally covering the os), marginal (palpable at margin of os), or complete (completely covering the os)
  2. Incidence
     a. Ranges from 0.4% to 0.6%
     b. Occurs in 1 in 300 pregnancies
  3. Risk factors
     a. Multiparity
     b. Previous cesarean section or other uterine surgery
     c. Smoking
  4. Signs and symptoms
     a. Primary—associated with painless vaginal bleeding
     b. Secondary—unengaged fetal presentation and/or malpresentation
     c. Sometimes bleeding is associated with contractions
  5. Diagnosis
     a. History
     b. Ultrasound
  6. Management
     a. See consultation; in some practices, may necessitate co-management
     b. Observant management until delivery
     c. If bleeding, hospitalize the patient
     d. Tocolytic therapy may be considered for up to 72 hours
     e. If premature, consider corticosteroids to accelerate lung maturity
     f. May be able to deliver vaginally if bleeding is not severe and os is not completely covered
     g. If vaginal birth is considered, will require access to immediate cesarean delivery
     h. If complete previa, medical management and cesarean birth needed

Placental Abruption

- Definition—premature separation of the placenta from the uterus, which may be partial or complete; cause of 30% of third-trimester bleeding
- Risk factors
  1. Hypertension—chronic or gestational
  2. Trauma
  3. Smoking
  4. Cocaine use
  5. Multiparity
  6. Uterine anomalies or tumors
- Signs and symptoms
  1. Vaginal bleeding
  2. Uterine tenderness and rigidity
  3. Contractions or uterine irritability and/or tone
  4. Fetal tachycardia or bradycardia
- Complications
  1. Shock
  2. Fetal compromise or death
  3. Disseminated intravascular coagulation (DIC)
- Diagnosis
  1. Clinical evaluation
  2. Fetal monitoring
  3. Ultrasound
- Management
  1. Need collaboration between high-risk/maternal fetal medicine, obstetricians, anesthesiology, nursing, blood bank
  2. Monitor clotting studies and hemoglobin (Hgb)/hematocrit (Hct), platelets
  3. Stabilize patient
  4. Delivery as indicated by the fetal or maternal condition

Placenta Accreta Spectrum

- Definition—normal trophoblast invasion of part or all the placenta beyond the uterine endometrium and into the myometrium
- Incidence—increasing over the years likely due to increased rate of Cesarean section
  1. 1970s–1980s: studies showed 1 in 2,510 and 1 in 4,017
  2. 1982–2002: 1 in 533
  3. 2016: 1 in 272
- Risk factors
  1. Previous cesarean section; risk increases with the number performed: 0.3% with first cesarean section, 6.74% with 5 or more cesarean sections
  2. Placenta previa—in 3% of patients diagnosed with placenta previa and no history of cesarean section; rate increases exponentially with cesarean section
  3. Advanced maternal age
  4. Multiparity
  5. Prior uterine surgeries
  6. Asherman syndrome
- Signs and symptoms
  1. Often causes no signs or symptoms during pregnancy
  2. Vaginal bleeding
- Diagnosis
  1. By obstetric ultrasound; may be seen in the first trimester but more likely in the second and third trimesters

  2. Color flow Doppler imaging may facilitate the diagnosis
- Management
  1. Antenatal diagnosis is critical to optimize management and outcomes
  2. Multidisciplinary care team accustomed to management of placenta accreta spectrum that includes experienced obstetricians and maternal–fetal medicine subspecialists, pelvic surgeons, urologists, interventional radiologists, obstetric anesthesiologists, critical care experts, general and trauma surgeons, neonatologists, nursing leadership, blood bank
  3. Delivery in maternity centers that have the expertise and can coordinate resources in case of severe hemorrhage

Epilepsy

- Definition—chronic condition resulting in seizures; negatively impacted by reproductive function; conversely, epilepsy poses certain risks in pregnancy
- Effects on the pregnant person
  1. Increase in seizure frequency and severity
  2. Increase in perinatal mortality
  3. Preeclampsia
  4. Preterm labor
  5. Stillbirth
  6. Increased risk of cesarean section
  7. Increased risk of miscarriage
  8. Postpartum hemorrhage
- Effects on the fetus/neonate
  1. Growth restriction; LBW
  2. Congenital disabilities (related to medication exposure)
- Management
  1. Antiepileptic drug (AED) therapy is key, but not always effective
  2. Preconception evaluation is important and may be predictive; 9–12 months seizure-free preconceptually is a good indicator for prenatal course
  3. Pharmacokinetic changes in pregnancy affect AED metabolism
  4. AED monotherapy is preferable to decrease fetal effects
  5. Valproate should be avoided due to teratogenicity
  6. Fears related to genetic inheritance, maternal/fetal outcomes, and the ability to breastfeed should be reviewed preconceptually and prenatally
  7. Folic acid should be recommended prior to conception and prenatally
  8. Adjust the dose of AED postpartum and discuss contraceptive options

Thrombocytopenia

- Definition—serum platelet count $<150 \times 10^9$/L in pregnancy; not necessarily clinically relevant
- Differential diagnosis
  1. Gestational thrombocytopenia (GT); most common etiology
  2. Bone marrow disorders

3. Nutritional deficiencies
4. Drug-related
5. Immune thrombocytopenic purpura (ITP)
6. Congenital thrombocytopenia
7. Fetal–neonatal alloimmune thrombocytopenia
8. Antiphospholipid syndrome
9. Systemic lupus erythematosus
10. Infectious (e.g., HIV, Hep C, cytomegalovirus, H. pylori)
11. In the third trimester:
    a. Gestational hypertension, preeclampsia/eclampsia/HELLP (hemolysis, elevated liver enzymes, low platelet count) syndrome
    b. Thrombotic thrombocytopenic purpura
    c. Hemolytic uremia syndrome
    d. Acute fatty liver
    e. DIC
- Maternal/fetal effects
  1. GT is often asymptomatic
  2. Bleeding events (i.e., cutaneous, mucosal)
  3. Hemorrhagic complications
  4. Generalized petechiae or ecchymosis (with fetal–neonatal alloimmunity)
- Management
  1. No evidence-based guideline for monitoring GT; draw platelet count each prenatal visit and 1–3 months postpartum
  2. Consultation or co-management may be warranted
  3. For idiopathic thrombocytopenic purpura (ITP), corticosteroids and IV immunoglobulin may be required
  4. For ITP, splenectomy should be avoided; safely performed in the second trimester
  5. For acute hemorrhage or in preparation for urgent surgery, platelet transfusion may be warranted
- Education
  1. Educate based on the risk of vaginal bleeding in the intrapartum period (i.e., candidacy for epidural placement, birth)
  2. Epidural or spinal placement acceptable with platelet counts of $>70 \times 10^9$/L
  3. Avoid NSAIDs, salicylates, and potential trauma
  4. Defer IM injections (i.e., vitamin K) and other surgical interventions (i.e., circumcision) until the neonatal platelet count is drawn and evaluated
  5. Observe neonate for 2–5 days after birth due to slight risk for neonatal thrombocytopenia

Gastroesophageal Reflux (GERD) in Pregnancy

- Definition/etiology—movement of gastric contents from the stomach and into the esophagus; see also the Gastroesophageal Reflux Disease (GERD) section in Chapter 3, *Primary Care*, for considerations related to preexisting GERD
  1. Common in pregnancy; affects 40%–80% of pregnant people, most in the third trimester

  2. Related to the effects of increasing estrogen and progesterone on the lower esophageal sphincter and enlarging uterus, which increase thoracic pressure
- Risk factors
  1. Certain foods/beverages (i.e., fatty foods, coffee, caffeine, onion, garlic, spicy foods)
  2. Medications
  3. Overeating or eating quickly
  4. Lying down after eating
- Differential diagnosis—preeclampsia or HELLP syndrome
- Physical exam
  1. Blood pressure to rule out hypertensive disorders
  2. Abdominal exam
- Maternal effects
  1. Burning and pain
  2. Sleep disturbance
  3. May trigger nausea and vomiting of pregnancy
  4. Cough or hoarseness
- Management—offer a stepwise approach
  1. Nonpharmacologic modifications and nonsystemic therapies
     a. Diet and intake modification
     b. Proper body positioning after meals
     c. Loose-fitting clothes
     d. Magnesium hydroxide or trisilicate (i.e., generic: aluminum hydroxide, magnesium hydroxide; brand name: Maalox, Mylanta)
     e. Avoid antacids with sodium carbonate (i.e., generic: aspirin/citric acid/sodium bicarbonate; brand name: Alka-Seltzer), which can cause maternal or fetal alkalosis
  2. Medication therapy
     a. Sucralfate—mucosal protectant; minimally absorbed
     b. Histamine-2-receptor agonists (i.e., famotidine (Pepsid); NOT ranitidine due to safety concerns)
     c. Proton pump inhibitors (i.e., lansoprazole (Prevacid; NOT omeprazole due to safety concerns)—does not work immediately
  3. Use antacids and other medication therapy with caution as they can impede absorption of other medications (e.g., iron or follow acid supplementation)
- Patient education
  1. GERD can be common in pregnancy and typically subsides after pregnancy
  2. Report persistent symptoms despite medication, including interrupted sleep, difficulty swallowing, weight loss, blood in sputum or vomit, or black stools

Stillbirth

- Definition
  1. Fetal death at 20 weeks' gestation or greater *or* weight greater than 350 g (if gestational age unknown)
  2. Does not include fetal loss due to termination or induction of labor for previable fetuses
- Incidence—overall rate is 5.96 per 1,000 live births and stillbirths; occurring in 1 in 160 births or 23,600 stillbirths annually in the United States
- Half occur prior to 28 weeks

- Non-Hispanic Black women are disparately affected; have twice the rate of stillbirth of non-Hispanic white women—10.53 per 1,000 live births and stillbirths
- Risk factors
  1. In developed countries:
     a. Congenital and karyotypic anomalies
     b. Growth restriction and placental anomalies
     c. Medical conditions (i.e., obesity, diabetes, systemic lupus erythematosus [SLE], renal and thyroid disorders, cholestasis)
     d. Hypertensive conditions
     e. Infections
     f. Smoking
     g. Multiple gestation
     h. Advanced maternal age
     i. History of previous stillbirth
     j. Specific to non-Hispanic Black women and birthing people in the United States—disparities in care, resources, and environmental stressors and implicit and explicit biases as a result of structural racism
  2. In developing countries:
     a. Obstructed or prolonged labor and sequelae
     b. Infection
     c. Hypertensive conditions
     d. Congenital and karyotypic anomalies
     e. Poor nutritional status
     f. Malaria
     g. Sickle cell disease
- Physical exam
  1. Patient vital signs
  2. Evaluation of patient perception of fetal movement
  3. Abdominal exam including evaluation of FHTs with Doppler, uterine tenderness, fundal height
  4. Pelvic exam in evaluation of Bishop score and palpation of presenting part
  5. Ultrasound including evaluation of fetal heartbeat (verified by two clinicians), overriding cranial bones, gas in the fetal abdomen
- Diagnosis—cannot detect a fetal heartbeat; may need consulting physician to pronounce the death and/or complete death certificate
- Effects on the pregnant/birthing person
  1. With retained products of conception greater than 2–4 weeks
     a. Fever
     b. DIC
     c. Rupture of membranes
     d. Onset of labor
  2. Psychosocial—grief, depression, anxiety
- Management
  1. Co-management or collaboration may be necessary at any point
  2. Screening of the birthing person
     a. β-hCG levels
     b. Complete blood count (CBC)
     c. Type and screen
     d. Kleihauer–Betke test
     e. HbA$_{1c}$
     f. TORCH panel

3. Expectant management—beyond 2 weeks, and no longer than 4–5 weeks
   a. Consider lab work—CBC, prothrombin time (PT)/ partial thromboplastin time (PTT), fibrinogen)
   b. Monitor for fever and DIC
4. Active management
   a. Second-trimester dilation and evacuation
   b. Induction of labor
      (1) Misoprostol 200–400 mcg vaginally every 4–12 hours prior to 28 weeks' gestation, including in patients with prior uterine scar
      (2) After 28 weeks:
         (a) Cervical ripening—misoprostol, Foley bulb/Cook catheter
         (b) Cervical dilation—laminaria
         (c) Induction—oxytocin IV
   c. Consider pain management options
   d. Cesarean section should be reserved for instances where induction of labor is not an option
5. Coping with loss
   a. Acknowledge loss and grief
   b. Anticipate depression and anxiety
   c. Connect to support services and groups; family support
   d. Use appropriate language; consider religious and cultural beliefs
6. Care of the body of the baby after birth
   a. Fetal screening
      (1) Cord blood
      (2) Placental evaluation and culture
      (3) Fetal karyotyping and other genetic testing
   b. Autopsy, optional
   c. Religious support (i.e., priest, pastor, rabbi, imam), if desired
   d. Creating a keepsake box
   e. Burial, cremation; other funeral/memorial services
   f. Facilitate for the patient to hold fetus, if desired
7. Postpartum care and follow-up
   a. Routine immediate postpartum care
   b. RhoGAM if indicated
   c. Lactation suppression
   d. Referral to bereavement support and services; consider other mental health services
   e. Consider contraception
   f. Follow-up outpatient appointment 3–6 weeks postpartum

Thromboembolic Disorders

- See also the Thromboembolic Disease section in Chapter 3, *Primary Care*, for non-pregnancy-related considerations
- Definition—venous thromboembolism (VTE) results from physical and anatomic changes associated with pregnancy and postpartum that create an increased thrombotic state, thereby increasing the risk of blood
  1. Hypercoagulability
  2. Increased venous stasis

3. Decreased venous outflow
4. Compression of vena cava and pelvic veins by enlarging uterus
5. Decreased maternal mobility

- Types
  1. Deep vein thrombosis (DVT)—most common (75%–80%); typically in the lower extremities, proximal, iliac, and iliofemoral veins
  2. Pulmonary embolism (PE)—infrequent (20%–25%); results when a DVT breaks loose and travels to the lungs, interfering with respiration
- Risk factors
  1. Pregnancy and postpartum
  2. Personal or family history of VTE
  3. Inherited thrombophilia
  4. Sickle cell disease
  5. Autoimmune disorders
  6. Diabetes
  7. Hypertension and preeclampsia
  8. Heart disease
  9. BMI >30
  10. Advanced maternal age
  11. Varicose veins
  12. Smoking
  13. Multiple gestation
  14. Cesarean birth
  15. Hospitalization
- Physical exam
  1. Signs and symptoms:
     a. DVT—pain, swelling, change in color, change in calf circumference
     b. PE—dyspnea, tachypnea, tachycardia, chest pain, cough, fever, anxiety, cyanosis, hemoptysis
  2. Imaging—ultrasound (compression and with flow Doppler), magnetic resonance imaging (MRI), computed tomography (CT) with contrast (where ultrasound and MRI are not available)
- Differential diagnosis
  1. Muscle strain
  2. Cellulitis or phlebitis
  3. Myocardial infarction
  4. Pneumothorax
- Perinatal effects
  1. Recurrent thrombosis
  2. Ulceration
  3. Post-thrombotic syndrome (chronic pain or swelling)
  4. Death
  5. Fetal compromise or death
- Management
  1. Medical management for treatment or prophylaxis
     a. Heparin (unfractionated; low-molecular-weight [LMW])
        (1) Does not cross the placenta
        (2) Increased renal excretion and protein binding in pregnancy
        (3) Shorter half-lives and lower peak plasma concentrations
        (4) Higher dose and more frequent administration typically required; adjusted based on activated partial thromboplastin time (aPTT) (unfractionated) or maternal weight (LMW)
     b. Warfarin (vitamin K agonist)
        (1) Not safe in pregnancy due to harmful fetal effects; consider switching to heparin prior to conception or in the third trimester when fetal risk is greatest
        (2) Rarely used outside of individuals with mechanical heart valves
     c. Avoid oral direct thrombin inhibitors and factor Xa inhibitors as maternal, fetal, and neonatal theoretical adverse effects exist; switch to heparin prior to conception
  2. Endovascular management
     a. Inferior vena cava (ICV) filter and pharmacomechanical catheter-directed thrombolysis (PCDT)
     b. Invasive procedure; may be useful in individuals at risk for PE for whom anticoagulant therapy is ineffective; more research required
     c. Exposure risk to the fetus related to radiation exposure exists with placement
- Patient education
  1. For individuals already on anticoagulant therapy, consider the risks and benefits of continued therapy in the preconception period or as indicated
  2. Consider the risk of VTE and the need for prophylaxis
  3. Prevention measures such as ambulation/exercise, support hose, hydration
  4. Smoking cessation
  5. Travel precautions including prevention measures adapted for travel

Malpresentations

- Malpresentation of the fetus may be of significance during the prenatal period—breech and shoulder (transverse lie)
- Concept—the presenting part determines the presentation
  1. Breech—longitudinal lie with buttocks in the lower pole
     a. Incidence
        (1) Between 29 and 32 weeks—14%
        (2) At term—3.4%
     b. Variations
        (1) Frank—legs are extended up over the fetal abdomen and chest
        (2) Complete—legs are flexed at the hips and knees
        (3) Footling or incomplete—one or both feet or knees are lowermost
     c. Etiology—some situation that distorts the shape of the fetus or the uterus
        (1) Uterine septum
        (2) Fetal anomaly (e.g., hydrocephaly)
        (3) Fetal attitude (e.g., extension of spinal column or neck)
        (4) Placenta previa
        (5) Conditions resulting in abnormal fetal movement or muscle tone

d. Diagnosis
   (1) Abdominal examination—Leopold's maneuvers findings (four maneuvers)
      (a) Fetal part in the fundus is round, hard, freely movable, and ballotable
      (b) Find back and small parts
      (c) Part in the lower pole is large, nodular body
      (d) Determine the degree of engagement and reaffirm previous findings by confirming the lack of cephalic prominence in the lower pole
   (2) Vaginal findings compared to vertex findings
      (a) No fetal skull sutures or fontanels
      (b) Round indentation (anus)
      (c) Tissue texture is softer than head, if completely breech; toes, feet, or knees may be palpated if footling
e. Risks—short-term benefits to maternal and neonatal mortality and morbidity with planned cesarean birth; long-term benefits are less clear.
   (1) Labor dystocia
   (2) Cord prolapse
   (3) Fetal head entrapment
f. Treatment
   (1) External cephalic version (ECV)
      (a) Success rate—35% to 86%
      (b) Consider maternal Rh status
      (c) Antenatal monitoring post-ECV
      (d) Criteria
         i. Normal amniotic fluid volume
         ii. Reactive NST
         iii. EFW between 2,500 and 4,000 g
   (2) Moxibustion
   (3) Anticipatory guidance regarding the plan for version as well as plans for persistent breech
   (4) Webster chiropractic maneuvers
2. Shoulder—transverse lie in which the shoulder or arm is found in the lower pole; contraindication to vaginal birth
  a. Incidence—0.4%
  b. Etiology
   (1) Multiparity
   (2) Placenta previa
   (3) Polyhydramnios
   (4) Uterine anomalies
  c. Treatment—similar to breech in terms of correcting the lie with ECV and preparation for persistent transverse lie

Hypertensive Disorders of Pregnancy

- Definitions
  1. Chronic hypertension—blood pressure ≥140/90 mm Hg diagnosed before pregnancy, before 20 weeks' gestation, or after 12 weeks' postpartum
  2. Gestational hypertension (GHTN)—new-onset blood pressure elevation after 20 weeks' gestation, without proteinuria; if blood pressure does not return to normal in the postpartum period, consider changing diagnosis to chronic hypertension
  3. Chronic hypertension with superimposed preeclampsia—chronic hypertension with new-onset proteinuria at greater than 300 mg in 24 hours, but no proteinuria before 20 weeks' gestation; *or* sudden increase in proteinuria or blood pressure or platelet count of less than 100,000/mm³ in women with hypertension and proteinuria before 20 weeks' gestation
  4. Preeclampsia—pregnancy-specific hypertensive disorder; associated with symptoms such as headaches, visual disturbances, epigastric pain, and rapid edema development; includes blood pressure ≥140/90 mm Hg on two occasions at least 4 hours apart after 20 weeks' gestation *or* blood pressure >160/100 mm Hg (confirmed within a few minutes) in a woman who was previously normotensive and proteinuria ≥300 mg per 24-hour urine collection or protein/creatinine ratio ≥0.3 *or*, if other quantitative methods are unavailable, a dipstick result of 2+ *or* in the absence of proteinuria, new-onset hypertension with the new onset of the following severe features:
     a. Thrombocytopenia—platelet count <100,000/mcL
     b. Renal insufficiency—serum creatinine >1.1 mg/dL or doubling of serum creatinine concentration without renal disease
     c. Impaired liver function—doubling of normal levels of liver transaminases
     d. Pulmonary edema
     e. Cerebral or visual symptoms
  5. HELLP syndrome—*H*emolytic anemia, *E*levated *L*iver enzymes, and *L*ow *P*latelet count; may occur antepartum or postpartum
  6. Eclampsia—seizures that cannot be attributed to other causes in a patient with preeclampsia
- Management of hypertension in pregnancy
  1. Seek consultation; will need to co-manage and/or transfer care
  2. In many cases, swift intervention lowers the severity; while delayed treatment can increase morbidity
  3. Chronic hypertension is treated with antihypertensive medications; blood pressure levels be maintained between 120/80 and 160/105 mm Hg
  4. Chronic hypertension with a risk for adverse pregnancy outcomes should be treated with low-dose aspirin (60–80 mg) PO daily starting in the late first trimester
  5. Chronic hypertension, without other perinatal or fetal complications, expectant management is recommended until 38 weeks; with superimposed preeclampsia without severe features and without perinatal complications, expectant management until 37 weeks is recommended; with severe features, expectant management until 34 weeks recommended.
  6. Recommended first-choice antihypertensives—labetalol, nifedipine, and hydralazine

7. For preeclampsia without severe, antenatal surveillance includes assessment of maternal symptoms, daily fetal movement counts, twice-weekly blood pressure monitoring, weekly serologic assessment of platelets and liver enzymes

8. For patients with preeclampsia with severe features, magnesium sulfate for the prevention of eclampsia is recommended in the intrapartum–postpartum period

- Risk factors
  1. Nulliparity
  2. Adolescent or advanced maternal age (>35 years)
  3. Multiple gestation
  4. Family history of preeclampsia or eclampsia
  5. Obesity and insulin resistance
  6. Chronic hypertension
  7. Limited exposure to father of baby's sperm—new partner, donor insemination
  8. Antiphospholipid antibody syndrome and thrombophilia

- Theory of causes
  1. Abnormal trophoblast invasion
  2. Coagulation abnormalities
  3. Vascular endothelial damage
  4. Cardiovascular maladaptation
  5. Immunologic phenomena
  6. Genetic predisposition
  7. Dietary deficiencies or excesses
  8. Chronic stress (i.e., experiences of racism, impacts of systemic racism, inequitable distribution of SDoH)

- Antepartum management of preeclampsia
  1. Conduct diet assessment related to nutrient density
  2. Adequate fluids
  3. Restricted activities (some experts advise)
  4. Monitor blood pressure, proteinuria, edema, weight, intake and output, deep tendon reflexes (DTRs), subjective symptoms

- Laboratory tests
  1. Serum AST and ALT
  2. Serum creatinine
  3. Complete blood count
  4. Serum electrolytes
  5. Blood urea nitrogen
  6. Spot urine protein/creatinine ratio (or collection and testing of 24-hour urine sample for total protein and creatinine for creatinine clearance)
  7. Electrocardiogram or echocardiogram as appropriate

- Assessment of fetus
  1. Daily fetal movement assessment
  2. NST
  3. AFI/BPP
  4. Ultrasound with Doppler studies for growth

- Intrapartum and postpartum management
  1. Goal is to prevent seizures
  2. Magnesium sulfate
     a. Given IV
     b. Used as an anticonvulsant
     c. Side effects—flushing, somnolence
     d. Overdosage signs and symptoms
        (1) Loss of patellar reflex
        (2) Muscular paralysis

(3) Respiratory arrest
(4) Aggravated by decreased urine output (MgSO$_4$ is excreted by kidneys)
     e. Antidote is calcium gluconate
  3. Valium (diazepam)—rarely used as anticonvulsant
  4. Antihypertensives with BP of 160/110 or higher that is confirmed as persistent (15 minutes or longer)
     a. First-line therapies: IV labetalol, IV hydralazine, immediate-release (IR) oral nifedipine
     b. IR nifedipine is most appropriate where IV access has not been established
     c. Sodium nitroprusside is reserved for extreme cases where hypertension is resistant to other medications; administered by anesthesia, maternal–fetal medicine, or critical care specialist
  5. Diuretics are *not* recommended—pregnant person is already volume depleted

- HELLP syndrome—affects 10% of patients with preeclampsia with severe features
  1. Diagnosis
     a. Hemolysis
     b. Abnormal peripheral blood smear
     c. Increased bilirubin ≥1.2 mg/dL
     d. Elevated liver enzymes—aspartate transaminase (AST), alanine aminotransferase (ALT), lactic acid dehydrogenase (LDH)
     e. Platelet count <100,000
  2. Treatment
     a. Magnesium sulfate
     b. Bed rest
     c. Crystalloids
     d. Albumin 5%–25%
     e. Delivery as indicated
     f. Plasma volume expansion

- Eclampsia
  1. Signs and symptoms—same as for preeclampsia with seizures
  2. Management—medical management
     a. Magnesium sulfate
     b. Administer oxygen
     c. Safety—prevent injuries and minimize aspiration during seizures
     d. Stabilize and deliver

- Prevention of pregnancy-induced hypertension
  1. Calcium and vitamin D supplementation if at risk and has low dietary intake
  2. Low-dose aspirin

Diabetes

- Definition—endocrine disorder of abnormal carbohydrate metabolism resulting in inadequate production and/or utilization of insulin

- Gestational diabetes (GDM)
  1. Diabetes occurs in 7% of pregnancies; 86% of these cases are gestational diabetes mellitus
  2. Results from the diabetogenic effect of pregnancy
  3. Human placental lactogen (hPL) acts as an insulin antagonist

4. Estrogen and progesterone may also act as insulin antagonists
- Diagnosis
  1. Risk assessment at the initial prenatal visit
  2. High risk
     a. Pre-pregnancy diagnosis of obesity
     b. Physical inactivity
     c. Prior history of GDM
     d. Prior LGA infant weighing more than 9 lb
     e. Age >25 years
     f. Strong family history of type 2 diabetes
     g. Black, Hispanic, American Indian, Alaska Native, Native Hawaiian, or Pacific Islander
     h. Hypertension and/or history of cardiovascular disease
     i. High levels of high-density lipoprotein (HDL) and triglycerides
     j. Polycystic ovary syndrome (PCOS) and other conditions associated with insulin resistance
     k. Hemoglobin 1c ≥5.7%
     l. Being treated for HIV infection
  3. Low risk
     a. Age <25 years
     b. Normal weight before pregnancy
     c. Member of an ethnic group with a low prevalence of diabetes
     d. No known diabetes in first-degree relatives
     e. No history of abnormal glucose tolerance
     f. No history of poor obstetric outcome
- Screening
  1. High risk—screen as soon as possible using standard diagnostic testing to exclude preexisting diabetes
  2. All pregnant patients regardless of risk—screen at 24–28 weeks
     a. Two-step approach
        (1) Screen with a 1-hour 50-g glucose challenge test (GCT)
        (2) If 130 mg/dL (90% sensitivity) or more, or greater than 140 mg/dL (80% sensitivity), perform a diagnostic 100-g 3-hour diagnostic oral glucose tolerance test (OGTT) on another day after an overnight 8-hour fast
        (3) Diagnosis of GDM can be made if two of the results from the 3-hour testing are abnormal utilizing either the Carpenter and Coustan or the National Diabetes Data Group criteria
     b. One-step approach
        (1) Perform a 75-g 2-hour OGTT after an overnight 8-hour fast
        (2) Measure fasting plasma glucose at 1 and 2 hours post-OGTT
        (3) Diagnostic criteria for one-step approach for GDM—presence of any abnormal number of the following plasma glucose values:
     c. Fasting—95 mg/dL or greater
     d. 1 hour—180 mg/dL or greater
     e. 2 hours—155 mg/dL or greater
- Presence of three or more of the following risk factors increases the chance of perinatal mortality
  1. Uncontrolled hyperglycemia

2. Ketonuria, nausea, vomiting
3. GHTN, edema, proteinuria
4. Pyelonephritis
5. Lack of compliance with care
6. Patient age >35 years
- Management—objective is to maintain strict levels of maternal glucose for optimal perinatal outcomes
  1. Co-manage or transfer to the perinatal center
  2. Diet
     a. 30 kcal/kg of actual or ideal body weight
     b. Breakfast—25%
     c. Lunch—30%
     d. Dinner—30%
     e. Snack—15%
  3. Distribution of calories
     a. Protein—20% of calories
     b. Fat—30% to 35% of calories
     c. Carbohydrates—45% to 50% of calories
  4. Medications
     a. Insulin—does not cross the placenta; first-line therapy
     b. Oral hypoglycemics—metformin and glyburide; cross the placenta, not FDA-approved treatment of GDM; metformin may be a safe and reasonable first-line alternative to insulin
  5. Maternal monitoring
     a. GHTN
     b. Changing insulin requirements
     c. Decreased need in the first trimester because of low hPL levels
     d. Increased need in the second trimester because of increasing hPL levels
     e. HgbA$_{1c}$/fasting plasma
  6. Fetal monitoring
     a. Increased risk of neural tube defects and cardiac anomalies in patients with nongestational diabetes
     b. Ultrasound for FGR, macrosomia, polyhydramnios
     c. FMC beginning at 28 weeks
     d. Antenatal testing is not indicated if nutritional modification and glucose monitoring alone are effective
     e. Antenatal testing (i.e., NST, BPP) beginning at 32 weeks if poorly controlled or requiring medication therapy without other comorbidities
  7. Immediate postpartum—monitor insulin requirements; usually decrease 24–48 hours after delivery of the placenta
  8. Perform 75-g 2-hour OGTT at 6–12 weeks postpartum—screen for diabetes and then follow with subsequent screening for diabetes or prediabetes

Thyroid Disease

- Definition—most common thyroid diseases in pregnancy are nontoxic goiter, hyperthyroidism, hypothyroidism, and thyroiditis
- Impact of pregnancy on maternal thyroid physiology is great; structural and functional changes related to pregnancy can cause confusion in defining abnormalities

- Thyroid enlarges somewhat because of hyperplasia and increased vascularity but does not cause serious thyromegaly
- Thyroid hormones in pregnancy—total serum thyroxine (TT_4) and triiodothyronine (TT_3) concentrations increase; thyroid-stimulating hormone (TSH) and free thyroxine (FT_4) levels are not affected
- Thyrotoxicosis or hyperthyroidism
    1. Incidence—1/2,000 pregnancies
    2. Signs and symptoms
        a. Tachycardia—more than normal in pregnancy
        b. Elevated sleeping pulse rate
        c. Thyromegaly
        d. Exophthalmos
        e. Failure to gain weight with normal or increased food consumption
    3. Diagnosis
        a. Elevated serum FT_4 or free thyroxine index (FTI) levels
        b. Decreased TSH levels
    4. Treatment
        a. Control with thioamide drugs; propylthiouracil or methimazole
        b. Thyroidectomy if medical approach unsuccessful; more easily done outside pregnancy because of increased vascularity
    5. Maternal and fetal outcomes
        a. Good if treatment successful
        b. If not, higher incidence of preeclampsia and heart failure as well as preterm birth, FGR, and stillbirth

Acquired Anemias

- Iron-deficiency anemia
    1. Definition—hemoglobin less than 11.0 g/dL in the first trimester, 10.5 g/dL in the second trimester, 11.0 mg/dL in the third trimester and postpartum
    2. Etiology—related to poor nutrition resulting in inadequate iron stores; the consequence of the expansion of blood volume with inadequate expansion of maternal hemoglobin mass
    3. Signs and symptoms
        a. May not be apparent unless severely anemic due to the body compensating for a chronic low hemoglobin state
        b. Associated with LBW, premature delivery, perinatal mortality
    4. Differential diagnosis
        a. Anemia associated with chronic disease
        b. Blood loss effect
    5. Diagnostic tests
        a. CBC including hemoglobin and hematocrit
        b. Serum ferritin levels lower than normal
        c. Microcytic, hypochromic erythrocytes
        d. Serum iron-binding capacity elevated; not a significant finding because it is elevated in pregnancy in the absence of iron deficiency
    6. Management and treatment—correct the hemoglobin mass deficit and rebuild iron stores

    7. Iron replacement therapy
    8. Ferrous sulfate, ferrous gluconate, ferrous fumarate
    9. Include vitamin C and folic acid
    10. Intramuscular or intravenous therapy if the patient is unable to take orally or if severely anemic
    11. Iron therapy for 3 months after anemia is corrected
- Anemia from acute blood loss
    1. Definition—drop in hemoglobin due to moderate to severe blood loss, which can occur at any time in pregnancy
    2. Etiology—abortion, ectopic pregnancy, hydatidiform mole, placenta previa, abruptio placenta, placenta implantation anomalies, and postpartum hemorrhage
    3. Management and treatment
        a. Massive hemorrhage requires restoration of volume and cells to maintain perfusion of vital organs
        b. Treat residual iron depletion (Hgb ≥7 g/dL) with oral iron for 3 months as long as the individual is afebrile and able to ambulate
- Megaloblastic anemia
    1. Definition—group of hematologic disorders characterized by blood and bone marrow abnormalities caused by impaired DNA synthesis
    2. Prevalence—rare in the United States
    3. Etiology—in the United States, during pregnancy, most always results from folic acid deficiency due to lack of consumption of green leafy vegetables, legumes, and animal protein
    4. Signs and symptoms—nausea, vomiting, and anorexia that worsen as deficiency increases
    5. Diagnosis—laboratory tests showing hypersegmentation of neutrophils, macrocytic erythrocytes, bone marrow megaloblastic erythropoiesis
    6. Risks to the fetus—neural tube defects
    7. Prevention
        a. Folic acid—0.4 mg daily for individuals of childbearing age; 4 mg daily prior to and during pregnancy for patients with a history of previous infant with neural tube defect
        b. Nutritious diet
        c. Iron

Inherited Anemias: Hemoglobinopathies

- Sickle cell hemoglobinopathies
    1. Types
        a. Sickle cell anemia (SS disease)
        b. Sickle cell–hemoglobin C disease (SC disease)
        c. Sickle cell–beta-thalassemia disease (S–β-thalassemia disease)
    2. Etiology—individual inherits a gene for S hemoglobin from each parent, or an S and a C gene from each, or an S and β-thalassemia gene from each
    3. Incidence
        a. SS disease—1 in 12 Black Americans has sickle cell trait—SA hemoglobin; theoretical incidence is 1 in 576 but is actually less common

b. SC disease—1 in 40 Black Americans has hemo-globin C gene; incidence of SC disease in Black pregnant individuals is 1 in 2,000
c. S–β-thalassemia disease—1 in 2,000 Black women

4. Signs and symptoms—SS is the worst of hemoglob-inopathies in pregnancy
a. Sickle cell crisis occurs more frequently in pregnancy
b. Infections and pulmonary complications are more common
c. Contributes to maternal mortality

5. Differential diagnosis
a. Thalassemia
b. Glucose-6-phosphate dehydrogenase (G6PD) deficiency

6. Physical findings
a. Hgb ≤7 g/dL
b. Intense pain of crisis particularly in the third trimester, in labor, and in postpartum
c. Fever due to dehydration or infection
d. Acute chest syndrome—pleuritic pain, cough, fever, lung infiltrate, and hypoxia

7. Management
a. Consult and co-manage with obstetrician
b. Weekly fetal surveillance after 32–34 weeks
c. Pain medication
d. Follow-up, including possible need for paternal blood screening and genetic counseling
e. Counseling for current and future pregnancies

Questions

Select the best answer.

1. One of the screening tools for alcohol use in pregnancy is the CAGE tool. This tool asks a set of questions including:
   a. Have you felt the need to cut down on your drinking?
   b. How many drinks can you hold?
   c. Has a friend or family member ever told you about things you said or did while you were drinking that you could not remember?
   d. Do you often engage in drinking games?

2. Which population of women has the lowest prevalence of smoking during pregnancy?
   a. Black
   b. Non-Hispanic American Indian
   c. Hispanic
   d. Non-Hispanic Asian

3. Maternal obstetric complications related to tobacco use may include:
   a. hypotension
   b. gestational diabetes
   c. placental abruption
   d. postterm pregnancy

4. Neonatal complications related to maternal tobacco use include:
   a. LGA infants
   b. post-term birth
   c. fetal growth restriction (FGR)
   d. rebound hypoglycemia

5. The neonatal condition in which an infant is in with-drawal from opioids at birth is called:
   a. neonatal abstinence syndrome (NAS)
   b. gestational diabetes
   c. fetal alcohol syndrome (FASD)
   d. Ballard's score

6. A pregnant patient states that she has been using mar-ijuana (cannabis) to help with her nausea during the first trimester. What is the best advice to give to the patient?
   a. "Given that marijuana has been legalized in many states, you have every right to use marijuana at your leisure."
   b. "You should wait until the second trimester to use marijuana in pregnancy."
   c. "As long as you are obtaining the marijuana from a dispensary, you should not have to worry."
   d. "The safety of marijuana use during pregnancy has not been proven."

7. Infant effects of maternal cocaine use may include:
   a. large for gestational age
   b. hypotonia
   c. high-pitched cry
   d. sweating

8. Preventive strategies against toxoplasmosis infection include:
   a. fully cooking meat to at least 98.6°F
   b. avoiding pasteurized milk and cheeses
   c. avoiding handling kitty litter
   d. fully cooking poultry to 72.5°F

9. A pregnant nurse who had previously received the var-icella vaccine works at a nursing home caring for older adults. The nurse was exposed to one of the nursing home residents who had shingles. What next steps should this pregnant nurse take?
   a. Obtain an obstetric ultrasound as soon as possible.
   b. Ask the provider to be swabbed for varicella.
   c. Get a varicella vaccine within 72 hours of exposure.
   d. Use universal precautions only since shingles pose lit-tle risk to the pregnant patient or baby.

10. The varicella vaccine is recommended for:
    a. all susceptible patients of reproductive age prior to conception
    b. all pregnant patients in their first trimester
    c. all pregnant patients in their last trimester
    d. all postpartum patients regardless of when their last varicella vaccine was given

11. A patient receiving the varicella vaccine at a preconcep-tion visit should wait how many weeks before attempting pregnancy?
    a. No wait is required.
    b. 1 week
    c. 4 weeks
    d. 12 weeks

12. Parvovirus is spread through:
    a. contaminated food
    b. cat feces
    c. respiratory secretions
    d. touch

13. Preventive measures to avoid the spread of the parvovirus include:
    a. vaccination prior to conception
    b. B19 oral medication
    c. handwashing with soap and water
    d. vaccination postpartum

14. Rubella is spread through:
    a. contaminated food
    b. cat feces
    c. respiratory secretions
    d. infected mosquitoes

15. Congenital rubella syndrome may lead to:
    a. hearing impairment
    b. large for gestational age
    c. gestational diabetes
    d. sandal toe gap

16. A patient receiving the rubella vaccine at a preconception visit should wait how many weeks before attempting pregnancy?
    a. There is no waiting period.
    b. 1 week
    c. 4 weeks
    d. 12 weeks

17. Clinical manifestations of CMV in adults include:
    a. a discrete pinkish-red maculopapular rash
    b. a maculopapular rash that evolves into vesicles
    c. a rash along the dermatomes
    d. CMV is usually asymptomatic.

18. If a pregnant person with HIV does not receive antiretroviral therapy during the pregnancy, the rate of transmission to the neonate is:
    a. less than 1%
    b. between 15% and 45%
    c. between 55% and 75%
    d. more than 80%

19. If a pregnant person with HIV and an undetectable viral load receives antiretroviral therapy during the pregnancy and intrapartum, the rate of transmission to the neonate is:
    a. less than 1%
    b. between 5% and 15%
    c. between 15% and 25%
    d. more than 80%

20. The Zika virus is primarily transmitted through:
    a. contaminated food
    b. infected mosquitoes
    c. respiratory secretions
    d. cat feces

21. Infants born to a pregnant person infected with the Zika virus may have:
    a. microcephaly
    b. rebound hypoglycemia
    c. hydrocephaly
    d. vesicular lesions

22. Symmetric fetal growth restriction can be caused by:
    a. abnormalities in uteroplacental perfusion
    b. hypertension
    c. anemia
    d. maternal drug use

23. Asymmetric fetal growth restriction can be caused by:
    a. abnormalities in uteroplacental perfusion
    b. phenytoin use during the first trimester
    c. tobacco use
    d. cocaine use

24. Which person has the greatest risk of having a macrosomic infant?
    a. A person with a prepregnancy BMI of 19
    b. A person with a partner who is 5 ft 8 in. tall and weighs 140 lb
    c. A person with a previous history of gestational diabetes
    d. A person and a partner who both weighed less than 6 lb at birth

25. A pregnant patient who is at 42 weeks' gestation is in the office to obtain a nonstress test. She states, "I don't even know why I'm here getting this monitoring thing. I should be enjoying my last days of freedom before this baby comes. Why do I even need to get monitored?" The best answer is:
    a. "Being pregnant beyond 42 weeks has been associated with increased morbidity and mortality. We want to assess the fetus to make sure everything is going well."
    b. "It's a pain, I know. We just need you to not complain about it so much anymore. We are just doing our best to take care of you."
    c. "You should be thankful that you made it this far with this pregnancy."
    d. "We want to see if we can get this baby out as soon as possible."

26. When faced with a patient who manifests clear evidence of having experienced violence, your first goal is to:
    a. evaluate the patient's safety
    b. get the patient to a shelter
    c. tell the patient to press charges
    d. get photos of all injuries

27. Cordocentesis may be used:
    a. as an adjunct to chorionic villus sampling
    b. to obtain blood samples for a fetal fibronectin test
    c. to provide fetal blood transfusion
    d. to relieve pressure on a prolapsed cord

28. Substances classified as addictive:
    a. include only illegal drugs
    b. include only drugs that are inhaled or injected
    c. include both legal and illegal drugs
    d. do not include alcohol

29. Which of the following behaviors is most common during pregnancy?
    a. Binge drinking
    b. Cigarette smoking
    c. Marijuana smoking
    d. Occasional alcohol use

30. Correct information concerning pregnancies with first-trimester bleeding includes which of the following?
    a. Approximately 10% of pregnant patients have some bleeding in the first trimester.
    b. Bleeding that occurs between 10 and 12 weeks is often caused by implantation.
    c. Cervical incompetence is a common cause of first-trimester bleeding.
    d. Approximately 90% of pregnancies in which FHT are heard will continue to term after early bleeding.

31. A patient presents with an LMP of 8 weeks ago and a positive urine pregnancy test. The patient has been having a small amount of bleeding for the past 12 hours, along with some mild abdominal cramping. A pelvic exam reveals a closed cervix and a slightly enlarged uterus. The differential diagnosis for this patient includes:
    a. complete abortion and threatened abortion
    b. ectopic pregnancy and inevitable abortion
    c. ectopic pregnancy and threatened abortion
    d. incomplete abortion and inevitable abortion

32. An example of an autosomal recessive disease is:
    a. *BRCA2* breast cancer
    b. cystic fibrosis
    c. hemophilia
    d. trisomy 21

33. A pregnant patient at 34 weeks' gestation tells you that she noticed a small amount of blood on her underwear this morning about an hour after having sexual intercourse. She is not having any pain or contractions. Your initial differential diagnosis for this patient would include:
    a. cervicitis
    b. incompetent cervix
    c. placental abruption
    d. premature rupture of membranes

34. Risks to the fetus in a postterm pregnancy are related to all the following except:
    a. fetal macrosomia
    b. meconium aspiration
    c. polyhydramnios
    d. uteroplacental insufficiency

35. Symmetric growth restriction is more likely than asymmetric growth restriction to:
    a. be related to multiple gestation
    b. become apparent first in late pregnancy
    c. occur as a result of maternal medical illness
    d. result from maternal cigarette smoking

36. Loss of a fetus in the second trimester is most frequently related to:
    a. hydatidiform mole
    b. inevitable abortion
    c. ectopic pregnancy
    d. incompetent cervix

37. As a result of an early USG, a low-lying placenta is verified. What do you tell the patient?
    a. Approximately 30% of pregnant individuals with a low-lying placenta in early pregnancy will have placenta previa in the third trimester.
    b. Approximately 30% of pregnant individuals have a low-lying placenta in the first trimester.

    c. Regular vaginal examinations will be done in the third trimester to monitor any obstruction of the cervix.
    d. Vaginal delivery is contraindicated if the patient has a marginal placenta previa.

38. A pregnant patient has the following history: vaginal delivery at 38 weeks; spontaneous abortion at 8 weeks; elective abortion at 13 weeks; vaginal delivery at 34 weeks; two living children; now 28 weeks' pregnant. This patient's gravity and parity are:
    a. G5 P1122
    b. G5 P0222
    c. G3 P2002
    d. G3 P2112

39. Which of the following tests is diagnostic rather than screening?
    a. MSAFP
    b. Nuchal translucency US
    c. Amniocentesis
    d. USG at 10 weeks

40. An elevated maternal AFP result is associated with which of the following?
    a. Down syndrome
    b. Neural tube defect
    c. An autosomal recessive gene
    d. X-linked recessive inheritance

41. Which of the following factors would predispose a pregnant patient to having a baby with GBS disease?
    a. History of previous GBS-positive infant
    b. Bacterial vaginosis in current pregnancy
    c. Frequent urinary tract infections (UTIs) prior to pregnancy
    d. Streptococcal pharyngitis in the third trimester

42. When a patient comes for her 38-week visit, she reports that a friend gave birth last week and had a placental abruption. The patient is now concerned that she might have the same experience. What information would you share with the patient about this condition?
    a. In the event of bleeding near term, 50% of cases are related to placental abruption.
    b. In the third trimester, pregnant patients have a 30% chance of having a placental abruption.
    c. The likelihood of having a placental abruption occur is basically zero at this time.
    d. A placental abruption is associated with risk factors such as hypertension, smoking, and trauma.

43. *Genotype* refers to the:
    a. expression of genes present in an individual
    b. dominant genes that will be inherited by a fetus
    c. pair of genes for each characteristic inherent in an individual
    d. recessive genes that will be passed on to a fetus

44. Which of the following patients should receive RhoGAM postpartum?
    a. Nonsensitized Rh-negative mother with a Rh-negative baby
    b. Nonsensitized-Rh negative mother with a Rh-positive baby
    c. Sensitized Rh-negative mother with a Rh-negative baby
    d. Sensitized Rh-negative mother with a Rh-positive baby

45. Aneuploidy describes which of the following situations?
    a. Down syndrome
    b. *BRCA1* and *BRCA2* inheritance
    c. Cystic fibrosis genes
    d. Sickle cell anemia

46. A patient, G2 P0010, comes for the first antepartal visit. The history indicates that the patient had a pregnancy loss at 18 weeks. She is gravely concerned that it will happen again in this pregnancy. Discussion of cervical cerclage needs to include which of the following points?
    a. It will be done after 12–14 weeks and is successful 80%–90% of the time.
    b. It will be done after 16–20 weeks and is successful 80%–90% of the time.
    c. It will be done after 16–20 weeks and is successful 50%–60% of the time.
    d. It will be done after 12–14 weeks and is successful 50%–60% of the time.

47. The CDC's recommended treatment for primary syphilis in a 10-week-pregnant patient is benzathine penicillin G 2.4 units IM:
    a. × 1 dose after the first trimester
    b. × 2 doses at the time of diagnosis
    c. × 3 doses weekly
    d. × 1 dose at the time of diagnosis

48. At an initial prenatal visit, a pregnant patient is diagnosed with bacterial vaginosis. She does not have any symptoms of vaginal infection. You tell the patient that:
    a. All pregnant patients should be treated as if they have asymptomatic bacterial vaginosis.
    b. Pregnant patients who are at risk for preterm delivery should be treated if they have asymptomatic bacterial vaginosis.
    c. Only pregnant patients at risk for preterm delivery should be treated for symptomatic bacterial vaginosis.
    d. Pregnant patients who are at risk for preterm delivery should be tested for asymptomatic bacterial vaginosis early in the third trimester.

49. The CDC's recommended treatment for trichomoniasis during pregnancy is:
    a. metronidazole 2 g orally
    b. clindamycin 300 mg orally BID × 7 days
    c. azithromycin 1 g orally
    d. ceftriaxone 125 mg IM

50. Symmetric intrauterine growth restriction:
    a. generally becomes evident in midpregnancy
    b. is usually associated with placental abnormalities
    c. is caused by conditions that result in a reduction in cell size
    d. is a neonatal diagnosis made when the infant falls below the 10th percentile

51. The result of a 1-hour 50-g GCT at 28 weeks for a 34-year-old G5 P4004 was 154 mg/dL. Follow-up 100-g glucose tolerance test produced the following results: 100, 192, 185, and 160 mg/dL. The plan for this patient should include:
    a. obtaining fasting glucose tests at 32 and 36 weeks to ensure that levels stay at or below 100 mg/dL
    b. referring the patient to a nutritionist to help her limit further weight gain to no more than 10 lb

    c. referring the patient to a perinatologist for periumbilical blood sampling to determine fetal blood glucose levels
    d. screening for diabetes at 6–12 weeks postpartum

52. The fundal height for a pregnant patient at 20 weeks' gestation was 1 cm below the umbilicus. At today's 24-week visit, fundal height is at the umbilicus. The patient is feeling regular fetal movement, and the fetal heart rate is 140 bpm. The most appropriate management for this patient is:
    a. ordering a biophysical profile
    b. ordering an ultrasound
    c. performing a nonstress test at this visit
    d. scheduling the next visit for 4 weeks from today

53. Ectopic pregnancy is consistent with no intrauterine sac on transvaginal ultrasound and an hCG titer of less than:
    a. 100 IU/L
    b. 1,500 IU/L
    c. 6,500 IU/L
    d. 10,000 IU/L

54. An 18-year-old female patient is 16 weeks pregnant. She has a positive chlamydia test. Appropriate management includes:
    a. erythromycin base 500 mg orally QID for 7 days and ceftriaxone 125 mg IM
    b. azithromycin 1 g orally in a single dose and perform a test of cure in 3–4 weeks
    c. ofloxacin 300 mg orally BID for 7 days and rescreen in the third trimester
    d. spectinomycin 2 g IM now and repeat in 1 week

55. A 29-year-old (G4 P2012) patient is at 41 weeks today. She reports occasional cramping, denies leaking/bleeding, and states she passed a "mucus plug" yesterday. The patient asks how she will know if she is in labor because both her previous births were induced. The correct response is:
    a. True labor occurs when contractions are 7–8 minutes apart and last for 45 seconds.
    b. Real labor is when contractions are 2–3 minutes apart and are very painful.
    c. Labor contractions usually become more regular and more intense over time.
    d. Contractions begin slowly; once they are 4–5 minutes apart, it is real labor.

56. Hyperthyroidism in pregnancy is diagnosed by:
    a. elevated FT_4 levels
    b. low free T_3 levels
    c. elevated TSH
    d. elevated TT_4 levels

57. ABO incompatibility occurs in which percentage of pregnancies?
    a. 15%
    b. 20%–25%
    c. 25%–40%
    d. 5%–8%

58. A 32-year-old patient (G2 P1001) is Rh negative. Her first pregnancy was uneventful, and she received RhoGAM after the birth. The patient read on the Internet that problems are much more likely with the second pregnancy. The correct response is:
    a. Because the patient reports that she has had no transfusions since the previous birth, there is no problem.

b. The RhoGAM the patient received in the last pregnancy will prevent any problems in this pregnancy.

c. The patient was not sensitized in the first pregnancy, and you will provide monitoring and treatment to prevent it in this pregnancy.

d. It is likely that the fetus is Rh negative, so there is no real concern that she will have any problems related to this factor.

59. At 28 weeks' gestation, a patient's Hgb is 12.4. g/dL. At the initial first-trimester visit, the Hgb was 12.8 g/dL. Management will include:
    a. obtaining a CBC and ferritin level
    b. asking if the patient is having difficulty tolerating the iron supplement and changing to a different type if needed
    c. rechecking the history to see if the patient may be at risk for an inherited anemia
    d. encouraging the patient to continue getting dietary iron and taking the iron supplements

60. Folic acid deficiency anemia is characterized by:
    a. hemoglobin of 9 g/dL or less
    b. low ferritin levels
    c. elevated serum iron-binding capacity
    d. macrocytic erythrocytes

61. Which of the following statements is *true* concerning sickle cell hemoglobinopathies?
    a. Having the sickle cell trait means that one parent has sickle cell disease.
    b. Disease is present when the person inherits a sickle cell gene from each parent.
    c. G6PD deficiency is a potential complication of sickle cell disease.
    d. One in 100 Black Americans has sickle cell trait.

62. Normal changes in pregnancy may confound a diagnosis of appendicitis. With this possibility in mind, which of the following are critical signs or symptoms pointing to possible appendicitis in pregnancy?
    a. Persistent abdominal pain and tenderness
    b. Intermittent lower abdominal cramping
    c. Elevated WBC level
    d. Nausea and vomiting

63. A patient (G1 P0) comes for her 36-week visit with a piece of paper in hand: "I am really confused about this birth plan business. What am I supposed to do about my birth? Don't I just show up when I am in labor?" How will you counsel her today?
    a. "It really does not matter what you write because the hospital has its own plan."
    b. "You will need to be very detailed about each element of the birth experience so you get what you want."
    c. "The plan provides the opportunity for you to make choices about events associated with the birth."
    d. "The healthcare provider who is there when you are in labor will tell you what is best for you and how to do it."

64. A patient (G2 P1001) comes for her first visit. She is concerned about the possibility of a UTI because her sister was recently hospitalized for pyelonephritis. What facts would you share to enhance her understanding?
    a. UTIs do occur in approximately 10% of pregnancies.
    b. Approximately 25% of pregnant individuals who experience UTI in pregnancy will develop pyelonephritis.
    c. If the patient has a history of UTIs before pregnancy, she will be screened with a urine culture each trimester.
    d. Pregnant individuals are typically screened for asymptomatic bacteriuria in early pregnancy.

65. Which of the following groups is at greatest risk for developing a UTI in pregnancy?
    a. Adolescents
    b. Pregnant individuals with twins
    c. Pregnant individuals older than 35 years
    d. Pregnant individuals with diabetes

66. A patient returns for the reading of the PPD injection that was placed during the first prenatal visit. You read the result as 10 mm of induration. The patient is American-born and healthy and has no known history of contact with the disease. How do you interpret this result?
    a. It is positive, and the patient needs a referral to an infectious disease specialist.
    b. It is unclear, and the patient should have a chest radiograph to be certain.
    c. It is positive, and you should give the patient a prescription for INH.
    d. It is negative because the patient has no high-risk characteristics for the disease.

67. Which of the following statements concerning HIV in pregnancy is *true*?
    a. The main route of acquiring the infection is IV drug use.
    b. Viral load is the strongest predictor for transmission of infection to the infant during the birth process.
    c. Cesarean section is the recommended route of delivery for all HIV-infected patients to reduce the risk of transmission of infection to the infant.
    d. Breastfeeding/chestfeeding should be recommended only if the patient's viral load is less than 200 copies/mL.

68. A patient who is 32 weeks pregnant has had symptoms of preterm labor and has a history of preterm delivery at 34 weeks. A fetal fibronectin test is negative. You advise her that:
    a. She has a 60% chance of going into labor within the next week.
    b. It is really too early in the pregnancy for this test to be of much value.
    c. The result offers some reassurance that the patient will not go into labor in the next 2 weeks.
    d. It is really too late in the pregnancy for this test to be of much value.

69. A decision is made to start tocolytic therapy for a patient at 30 weeks' gestation with preterm labor. Betamethasone IM has also been ordered because the administration of corticosteroids:
    a. decreases the respiratory side effects of tocolytic drugs
    b. decreases the incidence of premature rupture of membranes
    c. enhances the effects of tocolytic drugs
    d. reduces the incidence of newborn respiratory distress syndrome

70. A patient comes for the 32-week visit, and you determine that the fetus is in a breech presentation. Your plan is to:
    a. send the patient to the maternal–fetal medicine unit for an external cephalic version
    b. refer the patient to a perinatologist for a care decision and treatment
    c. send the patient for an ultrasound to confirm breech presentation
    d. wait until 36 weeks to see if a spontaneous version has occurred

71. A pregnant patient presents for the 32-week visit with no complaints. All findings from previous visits have been normal. Today she has a blood pressure of 145/95 mm Hg. An expected additional finding if she has mild preeclampsia would include:
    a. lower-extremity edema
    b. serum creatinine >1.1 mg/dL
    c. right upper epigastric pain
    d. elevated liver function tests

72. Iron-deficiency anemia in the second trimester is most commonly due to:
    a. blood volume expansion
    b. degradation of erythrocytes
    c. folate deficiency
    d. poor nutrition

73. A CBC in a Black pregnant patient reveals a hemoglobin concentration of 8.5 g/dL and hypochromic, microcytic erythrocytes. The most likely diagnosis is:
    a. β-thalassemia
    b. iron deficiency
    c. folate deficiency
    d. sickle cell anemia

74. Pregnancy-induced megaloblastic anemia can be treated with:
    a. folic acid
    b. iron supplementation
    c. a protein-rich diet
    d. vitamin B_{12}

75. Which of the following is the most common risk factor when sickle cell anemia complicates pregnancy?
    a. Hypertension
    b. Miscarriage
    c. Perinatal mortality
    d. UTI

76. In the management of anemia following placental abruption, which of the following is the most appropriate treatment strategy?
    a. Administration of anticoagulant
    b. Replacement of platelets
    c. Restoration of volume and blood cells
    d. Transfusion of iron

77. Diabetogenic effects in pregnancy are in part related to levels of:
    a. hPL
    b. estrogen
    c. placental insulinase
    d. progesterone

78. Which of the following individuals is at the lowest risk for developing gestational diabetes in pregnancy?
    a. A 17-year-old white patient with a BMI of 30
    b. A 24-year-old white patient who is pregnant for the first time
    c. A 25-year-old Latinx patient with a history of PCOS
    d. A 32-year-old Black patient who is a vegan

79. Gestational diabetes places the fetus at risk for which of the following outcomes?
    a. Cardiac anomalies
    b. Neural tube defects
    c. Polyhydramnios
    d. Preterm birth

80. Which of the following is the most appropriate screen for a patient who is at the end of the postpartum period and whose pregnancy was affected by gestational diabetes?
    a. 50-g 1-hour oral glucose screen
    b. 100-g 3-hour OGTT
    c. 75-g 2-hour OGTT
    d. Fasting glucose levels

81. Which of the following is an FDA-approved first-line treatment for gestational diabetes?
    a. Acarbose
    b. Glyburide
    c. Insulin
    d. Metformin

82. Which of the following is considered a severe feature of preeclampsia?
    a. Abdominal pain
    b. Blood pressure of 140/90 mm Hg
    c. Light sensitivity
    d. Thrombocytopenia

83. Which of the following is a risk factor for hypertensive disorders of pregnancy?
    a. Adolescence
    b. Multiparity
    c. Singleton pregnancy
    d. Thyroid disorder

84. Which of the following is the most appropriate strategy for antepartum management of preeclampsia?
    a. Fluid restriction
    b. Increased physical activity

c. Referral to a registered dietician
d. Weekly fetal movement assessment

85. When IV access has not been established in the intrapartum setting and the need for immediate treatment related to preeclampsia exists, which of the following is the most appropriate therapy?
 a. Hydralazine
 b. Labetalol
 c. Nifedipine
 d. Nitroglycerine

86. Magnesium toxicity is best managed by:
 a. administering calcium gluconate
 b. dialysis
 c. administering diazepam
 d. observation

87. Which of the following steps can help prevent preeclampsia from occurring in pregnancy among individuals at high risk who do not have a preexisting hypertensive disorder?
 a. Prescribe oral labetalol
 b. Recommend daily low-dose aspirin
 c. Suggest reducing dietary sodium
 d. Supplement with magnesium

88. Which of the following physiological and anatomic changes is associated with an increased risk of venous thrombosis in pregnancy?
 a. Compression of the uterine artery
 b. Decreased venous outflow
 c. Decreased venous stasis
 d. Hypocoagulability

89. A 26-year-old nulliparous white cis woman is being admitted to the hospital in labor. She has been previously diagnosed with opioid use disorder and has been taking Subutex during her pregnancy. Her prenatal course has been otherwise uncomplicated. For this patient, which of the following is a risk factor for thromboembolism?
 a. Age
 b. Pregnancy
 c. Race/ethnicity
 d. Subutex use

90. Which of the following is a first-line imaging tool to diagnose DVT in pregnancy?
 a. CT
 b. MRI
 c. Ultrasound
 d. X-ray

91. Which of the following anticoagulants is NOT safe in pregnancy?
 a. Heparin
 b. Lovenox
 c. Low-dose aspirin
 d. Warfarin

92. Of the following factors, which is the most characteristic of pruritic urticarial papulae and plaques of pregnancy (PUPPP)?
 a. Elevated estrogen
 b. Family history
 c. Inflammation
 d. Multigravidity

93. Which of the following is associated with the most severe neonatal outcome?
 a. Impetigo
 b. Primary herpes simplex virus
 c. Pruritis gravidarum
 d. PUPPP

94. A pregnant 28-year-old woman who is a G1P0 presents at her first antenatal visit at 12 weeks' gestation with a variable reddish-brown rash on her torso, hands, and feet. The rash does not itch. The patient reports fatigue and a recent sore throat. Which of the following laboratory tests may be the most helpful in determining a diagnosis?
 a. CBC
 b. Quantiferon Gold
 c. RPR
 d. Serum bile acid

95. What is the most accurate way to confirm a diagnosis of herpes simplex virus upon visualization of a vesicular vulvar lesion?
 a. Draw a blood sample
 b. Perform a punch biopsy
 c. Swab the lesion
 d. View with a colposcope

Answers with Rationales

1. **a.** Have you felt the need to cut down on your drinking? The CAGE tool includes the following questions:
 • C: Have you felt the need to cut down on your drinking?
 • A: Have people annoyed you by criticizing your drinking?
 • G: Have you ever felt bad or guilty about your drinking?
 • E: Have you ever had a drink first thing in the morning to steady your nerves or get rid of a hangover (eye-opener)?

2. **d.** Non-Hispanic Asian
 Non-Hispanic Asian women have the lowest prevalence of smoking during pregnancy (0.6%), whereas non-Hispanic American Indian or Alaska Native women have the highest prevalence (16.7%).

3. **c.** placental abruption
 Maternal risks for tobacco use include preeclampsia, placental abruption, placenta previa, spontaneous abortion, ectopic pregnancy, and PROM.

4. **c.** fetal growth restriction (FGR)
 Infant effects of maternal tobacco use include FGR, premature birth, and SGA.

5. **a.** neonatal abstinence syndrome (NAS)
 NAS is a condition in which an infant goes through withdrawal at birth due to fetal exposure to opioids (prescription pain relievers or heroin), barbiturates, or benzodiazepines.

6. **d.** "The safety of marijuana use during pregnancy has not been proven."
Because the safety of using marijuana has not been proven, ACOG recommends avoiding use of this drug while planning a pregnancy, during pregnancy, and breastfeeding.

7. **c.** high-pitched cry
Infant effects of maternal cocaine use include low birth weight, small head circumference, shorter length than babies born to mothers who do not use cocaine, irritability, hyperactivity, tremors, high-pitched cry, and excessive sucking at birth.

8. **c.** avoiding handling kitty litter
Preventive strategies against toxoplasmosis infection include the following:
   • Fully cook meat to at least 145°F (63°C) and poultry to 160°F (71°C).
   • Do not drink unpasteurized milk or eat unpasteurized cheese.
   • Avoid handling and/or changing kitty litter.
   • Avoid drinking untreated water.
   • Perform good handwashing following gardening or wear gloves while gardening because soil might be contaminated with cat feces.

9. **d.** Use universal precautions only since shingles poses little risk to the pregnant patient or baby.
There is no reason to be alarmed given that shingles poses little risk to the pregnant patient or baby with prior maternal vaccination.

10. **a.** all susceptible patients of reproductive age prior to conception
Varicella vaccination is recommended for all susceptible reproductive-age individuals prior to conception (at least 4 weeks before attempting pregnancy) or postpartum.

11. **c.** 4 weeks
Varicella vaccination is recommended for all susceptible reproductive-age individuals prior to conception (at least 1 month before attempting pregnancy).

12. **c.** respiratory secretions
Parvovirus spreads through respiratory secretions, such as saliva, sputum, or nasal mucus; when an infected person coughs or sneezes; through blood or blood products; and vertically from pregnant person to infant.

13. **c.** handwashing with soap and water.
There is no vaccine or medication to prevent parvovirus B19 infection. However, handwashing with soap and water and avoiding touching one's eyes, nose, and mouth and avoiding contact with sick people may be helpful preventive measures.

14. **c.** respiratory secretions
Rubella is an acquired respiratory disease and can be spread through respiratory secretions.

15. **a.** hearing impairment
Infants affected with congenital rubella syndrome may exhibit the following effects: IUGR, cataracts, retinopathy, heart defects such as patent ductus arteriosus, and hearing impairment.

16. **c.** 4 weeks
Although there are no documented cases of CRS from vaccine, the recommendation is to wait at least 4 weeks prior to attempting a pregnancy following rubella vaccination. The vaccine may be given to mothers postpartum and while breastfeeding.

17. **d.** CMV is usually asymptomatic.
Adults with CMV are usually asymptomatic. However, some may experience mononucleosis-like syndrome: fever, chills, malaise, myalgias; leukocytosis, lymphocytosis, abnormal liver function test, and lymphadenopathy.

18. **b.** between 15% and 45%
Without intervention, HIV transmission rate during pregnancy is anywhere from 15% to 45%.

19. **a.** less than 1%.
2008 data from the United Kingdom and Ireland showed that pregnant individuals receiving ART had transmission rates of about 1%.

20. **b.** infected mosquitoes
The Zika virus is primarily transmitted through bites of infected mosquitoes and sexual intercourse with an infected person.

21. **a.** microcephaly
Infants born to a pregnant person infected with Zika may have microcephaly and severe fetal brain damage.

22. **d.** maternal drug use
Maternal use of tobacco, alcohol, phenytoin (Dilantin), cocaine, and heroin can cause asymmetrical fetal growth restriction, along with congenital infections and chromosomal abnormalities.

23. **a.** abnormalities in uteroplacental perfusion
Asymmetrical growth restriction is caused by two main factors: reduced nutrition to the fetus and abnormalities in uteroplacental perfusion.

24. **c.** A person with a previous history of gestational diabetes
The person who has the greatest risk for having a macrosomic infant is an individual with a previous history of gestational diabetes. Other risk factors relate to ethnic/racial origins, obesity, previous LGA/macrosomic neonate, previous shoulder dystocia, size of the father, birth weights of both the mother and the father, diabetes or history of gestational diabetes, previous uterine myomata, and multiparity.

25. **a.** "Being pregnant beyond 42 weeks has been associated with increased morbidity and mortality. We want to assess the fetus to make sure everything is going well."
A pregnancy continuing beyond 42 weeks is called postterm. Being pregnant past 42 weeks is associated with increased morbidity and mortality.

26. **a.** evaluate the patient's safety
The healthcare provider's primary goal when caring for a patient who is abused is to evaluate the patient's safety.

27. **c.** to provide fetal blood transfusion.
Cordocentesis is the process in which a needle is introduced under real-time ultrasound through the maternal abdomen and then into the umbilical cord. Blood is then aspirated or blood and/or medications are introduced into the fetus.

28. **c.** include both legal and illegal drugs
Both legal and illegal substances have the potential to be addicting.

29. **b.** Cigarette smoking
According to the Safe Passage Study (Dukes, 2018) 15.4% of pregnant individuals use tobacco, compared to 5.4% who use illicit drugs, 9.4% who drink alcohol, 2.3% who engage in binge drinking, and 0.4% who engage in heavy drinking.

30. **d.** Approximately 90% of pregnancies in which FHT are heard will continue to term after early bleeding.
Approximately 90% of pregnancies with bleeding will continue to term after FHTs are observed. Other information to discuss with the patient includes the following: 40% of pregnant individuals have some bleeding in the first trimester, and 80% of spontaneous abortions occur in the first 12 weeks of pregnancy.

31. **c.** ectopic pregnancy and threatened abortion
The differential diagnosis for bleeding in the first trimester includes implantation bleeding, threatened abortion, ectopic pregnancy, cervicitis, cervical polyps, vaginitis, trauma/intercourse, disappearing twin, and autoantibody/autoimmune disorder.

32. **b.** cystic fibrosis
An autosomal recessive trait is expressed only when both copies of the gene are the same. For example, cystic fibrosis and sickle cell anemia are genetic disorders associated with autosomal recessive traits.

33. **a.** cervicitis.
Painless bleeding after sexual intercourse at 34 weeks' gestation may be due to irritation of the cervix from cervicitis. Placental abruption is usually associated with painful bleeding, whereas premature rupture of membranes is typically characterized by loss of fluid.

34. **c.** polyhydramnios
Postterm pregnancy is typically associated with decreased amniotic fluid rather than an excess of such fluid.

35. **d.** result from maternal cigarette smoking
Symmetric growth restriction is associated with maternal use of drugs, such as tobacco, alcohol, Dilantin (phenytoin), cocaine, and heroin.

36. **d.** incompetent cervix
Second-trimester fetal loss is most likely due to an incompetent cervix. The other stated causes of fetal loss—hydatidiform mole, inevitable abortion, and ectopic pregnancy—are related to first-trimester loss.

37. **b.** Approximately 30% of pregnant individuals have a low-lying placenta in the first trimester.
One-third of pregnant individuals have a low-lying placenta in the first trimester. Most cases will resolve, however, so that only 1% have previa in the third trimester.

38. **a.** G5 P1122
This patient has had five total pregnancies, including her current pregnancy, one term delivery, one preterm delivery, two abortions, and two living children.

39. **c.** Amniocentesis
Amniocentesis is a diagnostic test for genetic evaluation or assessment of neural tube defects.

40. **b.** Neural tube defect
An elevated maternal serum alpha-fetoprotein (AFP) is associated with neural tube defects, multiple gestation, and placental abruption.

41. **a.** History of previous GBS-positive infant
Risk factors for group B *Streptococcus* (GBS) disease include history of previous GBS-positive infant, delivering early (before 37 weeks' gestation), developing fever during labor, having a long period between water breaking and delivery, and having a previous infant with early-onset disease.

42. **d.** A placental abruption is associated with risk factors such as hypertension, smoking, and trauma.
Risk factors for placental abruption include hypertension (chronic or gestational), trauma, smoking, cocaine use, multiparity, and uterine anomalies or tumors.

43. **c.** pair of genes for each characteristic inherent in an individual
Genotype refers to the total hereditary information present in an individual—that is, the pair of genes for each characteristic.

44. **b.** Nonsensitized Rh-negative mother with a Rh-positive baby
A nonsensitized Rh-negative postpartum patient with a Rh-positive baby needs RhoGAM postpartum to prevent future sensitization. A sensitized Rh-negative postpartum patient does not need RhoGAM because she is already sensitized. Likewise, a nonsensitized Rh-negative postpartum patient with a Rh-negative baby does not need RhoGAM.

45. **a.** Down syndrome
Aneuploidy is an abnormal number of chromosomes in a cell. An abnormal number of chromosomes—specifically, the presence of an extra chromosome 21—can be found in individuals with Down syndrome.

46. **a.** It will be done after 12–14 weeks and is successful 80%–90% of the time.
Cervical cerclage is done after 12–14 weeks and has a success rate of 80%–90%. There is a risk of ruptured membranes or infection. There is a need to monitor cervical length via transvaginal ultrasound.

47. **d.** × 1 dose at the time of diagnosis
The treatment for early syphilis in pregnant individuals is one dose of benzathine penicillin G 2.4 million units IM.

48. **b.** pregnant patients who are at risk for preterm delivery should be treated if they have asymptomatic bacterial vaginosis.
The following treatment is recommended for all pregnant patients with symptoms of bacterial vaginosis: metronidazole 500 mg PO BID × 7 days *or* metronidazole 250 mg PO TID × 7 days *or* clindamycin 300 mg PO BID × 7 days. Treatment of asymptomatic BV among pregnant women at low risk for preterm delivery has not been reported to reduce adverse outcomes of pregnancy.

49. **a.** metronidazole 2 g orally
The treatment for trichomoniasis in pregnancy is metronidazole 2 g PO × 1 at any stage of pregnancy.

50. **a.** generally becomes evident in midpregnancy
Symmetric growth restriction appears around 18–20 weeks and may be caused by congenital infections, chromosomal abnormalities, or maternal drug use (tobacco, alcohol, Dilantin [phenytoin], cocaine, heroin). It has an increased risk of adverse long-term sequelae.

51. **d.** screening for diabetes at 6–12 weeks postpartum
The patient's 1-hour OGTT results are abnormal, and a diagnosis of gestational diabetes can be made. Thus, a screening for pregestational diabetes at 6–12 weeks postpartum is necessary.

52. **b.** ordering an ultrasound
Ordering an ultrasound is the most appropriate management of the patient to evaluate fetal size and gestation. The patient is too early in gestation for a biophysical profile and a nonstress test. Waiting 4 weeks for an evaluation is too long to wait—the patient needs to be evaluated much sooner.

53. **c.** 6,500 IU/L
Ninety percent of ectopic pregnancies are associated with β-hCG levels less than 6,500 IU/L.

54. **b.** azithromycin 1 g orally in a single dose and perform a test of cure in 3–4 weeks
The recommended treatment for chlamydia is azithromycin 1 g PO × 1 *or* amoxicillin 500 mg orally TID × 7 days.

55. **d.** Contractions begin slowly; once they are 4–5 minutes apart, it is real labor.
Labor usually begins with slow contractions that gradually become more regular and closer together. When contractions are 4–5 minutes apart, this is a sign of real labor.

56. **a.** elevated FT_4 levels
Elevated serum-free thyroxine FT_4 or FTI levels indicate hyperthyroidism in pregnancy.

57. **b.** 20%–25%
An estimated 20%–25% of pregnancies are ABO incompatible.

58. **c.** The patient was not sensitized in the first pregnancy, and you will provide monitoring and treatment to prevent it in this pregnancy.
The patient is Rh negative and received RhoGAM postpartum with her first pregnancy. She was not sensitized in the first pregnancy. The patient can be monitored and provided RhoGAM to prevent sensitization in this pregnancy.

59. **d.** encouraging the patient to continue getting dietary iron and taking the iron supplements
The average hemoglobin level in pregnancy is 12.5 g/dL. The patient's hemoglobin level is slightly below normal, and she can be encouraged to continue getting dietary iron and taking the iron supplements.

60. **d.** macrocytic erythrocytes
Folic acid–deficiency anemia is characterized by laboratory tests showing macrocytic erythrocytes, hypersegmentation of neutrophils, and bone marrow megaloblastic erythropoiesis.

61. **b.** Disease is present when the person inherits a sickle cell gene from each parent.
Sickle cell anemia is present when the person inherits a sickle cell gene from each parent.

62. **a.** Persistent abdominal pain and tenderness
Persistent abdominal pain and tenderness are the most critical symptoms of appendicitis.

63. **c.** "The plan provides the opportunity for you to make choices about events associated with the birth."
It is the healthcare provider's role to listen and facilitate the patient's expression of feelings and to provide a nonjudgmental environment.

64. **d.** Pregnant individuals are typically screened for asymptomatic bacteriuria in early pregnancy.
UTI occurs in 2%–7% of all pregnancies. UTI may be asymptomatic (asymptomatic bacteriuria), and 25%–30% of cases will progress to pyelonephritis if left untreated.

65. **d.** Pregnant Individuals with diabetes
Pregnant individuals with diabetes are at greatest risk for UTI. Other risk factors include sickle cell trait and pregnancy.

66. **d.** It is negative because the patient has no high-risk characteristics for the disease.
PPD test interpretation is based on risk factors.

67. **b.** Viral load is the strongest predictor for transmission of infection to the infant during the birth process.
Viral load is the strongest predictor for vertical transmission of HIV.

68. **c.** The result offers some reassurance that the patient will not go into labor in the next 2 weeks.
A negative result on a fetal fibronectin test is useful in ruling out imminent (within 14 days) preterm birth before 37 weeks' gestation; its predictive value can be as high as 94%.

69. **d.** reduces the incidence of newborn respiratory distress syndrome
Corticosteroids, such as betamethasone and dexamethasone, are commonly used in women/pregnant individuals at risk for preterm delivery to reduce the risk of respiratory distress and cerebral hemorrhage in the newborn.

70. **d.** wait until 36 weeks to see if spontaneous version has occurred
The incidence of breech presentation is 14% between 29 and 32 weeks' gestation and 3.5% at term. Anticipatory guidance regarding a plan for version as well as plans for persistent breech should be reviewed with the patient.

71. **b.** serum creatinine >1.1 mg/dL
Preeclampsia is the development of blood pressure higher than or equal to 140/90 mm Hg on two occasions at least 4 hours apart after 20 weeks' gestation, and proteinuria greater than or equal to 300 mg per 24-hour urine collection or protein/creatinine ratio greater than or equal to 0.3 or, if other quantitative methods are unavailable, a dipstick result of 1^+. In the absence of proteinuria, diagnosis parameters for preeclampsia include new-onset hypertension with any of the following: Thrombocytopenia—platelet count <100,000/mcL, renal insufficiency—serum creatinine >1.1 mg/dL or doubling of serum creatinine concentration without renal disease, impaired liver function—doubling of normal levels of liver transaminases, pulmonary edema, cerebral or visual symptoms

72. **a.** blood volume expansion
Iron-deficiency anemia in the second trimester is most commonly a consequence of the expansion of blood volume with inadequate expansion of maternal hemoglobin mass.

73. **b.** iron deficiency
Microcytic, hypochromic erythrocytes, and low hemoglobin are typical findings with iron-deficiency anemia.

74. **a.** folic acid
The underlying etiology of pregnancy-induced megaloblastic anemia is blood and bone marrow abnormalities caused by impaired DNA synthesis. Folic acid supplementation is necessary to correct this type of anemia.

75. **d.** UTI
Infections and pulmonary complications are common in pregnancies complicated by sickle cell anemia.

76. **c.** Restoration of volume and blood cells
Massive hemorrhage requires restoration of volume and cells to maintain perfusion of vital organs.

77. **a.** hPL
Diabetogenic effects in pregnancy are in part related to hPL, which acts as an insulin antagonist.

78. **b.** A 24-year-old white person who is pregnant for the first time
The following are risk factors for gestational diabetes: overweight or obesity, physical inactivity, history of GDM, prior LGA infant, age >25 years, strong family history of type 2 diabetes, race/ethnicity (Black, Hispanic, American Indian, Alaska Native, Native Hawaiian, or Pacific Islander), hypertension, elevated HDL and triglycerides, PCOS, elevated HbA_{1c}, being treated for HIV.

79. **c.** Polyhydramnios
GDM places the fetus at risk for IUGR, macrosomia, and polyhydramnios.

80. **c.** 75-g 2-hour OGTT
A 75-g 2-hour OGTT should be drawn at 6–12 weeks postpartum to screen for diabetes, followed by subsequent screening for diabetes or prediabetes as part of routine primary care.

81. **c.** Insulin
Insulin is FDA-approved as a first-line treatment during pregnancy, as it does not cross the placenta. Although metformin may be a safe first-line treatment, it is not FDA-approved for this indication. Metformin, glyburide, and acarbose all cross the placenta and can enter the fetus.

82. **d.** Thrombocytopenia
Severe features of preeclampsia include thrombocytopenia, renal insufficiency, impaired liver function, pulmonary edema, and cerebral or visual symptoms.

83. **a.** Adolescence
The following are risk factors for hypertensive disorders of pregnancy: nulliparity, adolescent or advanced maternal age (>35 years), multiple gestation, family history of preeclampsia or eclampsia, obesity and insulin resistance, chronic hypertension, limited exposure to father of baby's sperm (new partner), donor insemination, and antiphospholipid antibody syndrome and thrombophilia.

84. **c.** Referral to a registered dietician
Antepartum management may include dietary assessment, adequate hydration, restricted activity, monitoring (blood pressure, weight, edema, intake, output, DTRs, patient symptoms), and daily fetal movement assessment.

85. **c.** Nifedipine
Immediate-release nifedipine is most appropriate where IV access has not been established.

86. **a.** administering calcium gluconate.
The antidote for magnesium toxicity is calcium gluconate 1 g intravenous.

87. **b.** Recommend daily low-dose aspirin
Low-dose aspirin, calcium, and vitamin D supplementation may be useful in preventing preeclampsia among high-risk individuals who do not have a preexisting hypertensive disorder.

88. **b.** Decreased venous outflow
Physiological and anatomic changes associated with an increased risk of venous thrombosis in pregnancy include hypercoagulability, increased venous stasis, decreased venous outflow, compression of the vena cava and pelvic veins by the enlarging uterus, and decreased maternal mobility.

89. **b.** Pregnancy
This woman has the following risk factors for thromboembolism: pregnancy and hospitalization. Advanced maternal age, smoking, complications related to hypertension, and personal or family history are among risk factors generally.

90. **c.** Ultrasound
Ultrasound is a first-line imaging tool to diagnose DVT in pregnancy. MRI can be used if ultrasound is not conclusive and the symptoms suggest DVT. CT with contrast can be used where ultrasound and MRI are not available. X-ray is not helpful for imaging thrombosis.

91. **d.** Warfarin
Warfarin is not safe in pregnancy due to its harmful effects on the fetus. If a patient is already using warfarin, consider switching to heparin in the preconception period or in the third trimester when fetal risk is greatest.

92. **c.** Inflammation
PUPPP is characterized by perivasculitis.

93. **b.** Primary herpes simplex virus
A primary infection with HSV-2 during pregnancy is associated with preterm birth, low birth weight, and neonatal sequelae including local or disseminated infection and encephalopathy.

94. **c.** RPR
An RPR test is part of the standard initial antepartum visit lab set and will confirm a suspected diagnosis of secondary syphilis that aligns with this presentation.

95. **c.** Swab the lesion
Swabbing the lesion will provide for the most accurate diagnosis of a visualized lesion. Drawing a serum HSV level is not specific to that lesion. A punch biopsy should not be performed on an open wound. Visualization will not necessarily yield a diagnosis.

Bibliography

American College of Obstetricians and Gynecologists (ACOG). (2014, reaffirmed in 2020). Practice bulletin no. 142: Cerclage for the management of cervical insufficiency. *Obstetrics and Gynecology, 123*(2), 372–379.

American College of Obstetricians and Gynecologists (ACOG). (2015, reaffirmed 2020). Practice bulletin no. 151: Cytomegalovirus, parvovirus B19, varicella zoster, and toxoplasmosis in pregnancy. *Obstetrics and Gynecology, 125*, 1510–1525.

American College of Obstetricians and Gynecologists (ACOG) (2017, reaffirmed 2021); Committee Opinion No. 722: Marijuana Use During Pregnancy and Lactation. *Obstetrics & Gynecology.* 130 (4): e205–e209. doi: 10.1097/AOG.0000000000002354.

American College of Obstetricians and Gynecologists (ACOG). (2018, reaffirmed 2021). Practice bulletin no. 189: Nausea and vomiting in pregnancy. *Obstetrics and Gynecology, 131*(1), e15–e30.

American College of Obstetricians and Gynecologists (ACOG). (2018, reaffirmed 2022). Practice bulletin no. 196: Thromboembolism in pregnancy. *Obstetrics and Gynecology, 132*(1), e1–e17.

American College of Obstetricians and Gynecologists (ACOG). (2018, reaffirmed 2021). Obstetric care consensus no. 7: Placenta accreta spectrum. *Obstetrics and Gynecology, 132*(6), e259–e275.

American College of Obstetricians and Gynecologists (ACOG). (2018). Practice bulletin no. 190: Gestational diabetes mellitus. *Obstetrics and Gynecology, 131*(2), e49–e64.

American College of Obstetricians and Gynecologists (ACOG). (2018). SMFM statement: Pharmacological treatment of gestational diabetes. *Obstetrics and Gynecology, 218*(5), B2–B4.

American College of Obstetricians and Gynecologists (ACOG). (2019a). Committee opinion no. 767: Emergent therapy for acute-onset, severe hypertension during pregnancy and postpartum period. *Obstetrics and Gynecology, 133*(2), e174–e180.

American College of Obstetricians and Gynecologists (ACOG). (2019b). Practice bulletin no. 202: Gestational hypertension and preeclampsia. *Obstetrics and Gynecology, 133*(1), e1–e25.

American College of Obstetricians and Gynecologists (ACOG). (2019c). Practice bulletin no. 207: Thrombocytopenia in pregnancy. *Obstetrics and Gynecology, 133*(3), e181–e193.

American College of Obstetricians and Gynecologists (ACOG). (2019d). Practice bulletin no. 204. Fetal growth restriction. *Obstetrics and Gynecology, 133*(2), e97–109.

American College of Obstetricians and Gynecologists (ACOG). (2020). Practice bulletin no. 223: Thyroid disease in pregnancy. *Obstetrics and Gynecology, 135*, e261–74.

American College of Obstetricians and Gynecologists (ACOG). (2021a). Committee opinion no. 818: Medically indicated late-preterm and early-term deliveries. *Obstetrics and Gynecology, 137*(2), e29–e33.

American College of Obstetricians and Gynecologists (ACOG). (2021b). Practice bulletin no. 233: Anemia in pregnancy. *Obstetrics and Gynecology, 138*, e55–64.

American College of Obstetricians and Gynecologists (ACOG). (2021c). Practice bulletin no. 10: Management of stillbirth. *Obstetrics and Gynecology, 135*(3), e110–e132. doi: 10.1097/AOG.0000000000003719

American College of Obstetricians and Gynecologists (ACOG). (2021d). Practice bulletin no. 230: Obesity in pregnancy. *Obstetrics and Gynecology, 137*, e128–e144.

American College of Obstetricians and Gynecologists. (2021e). Seizures: Clinical updates in women's health care primary, *Obstetrics and Gynecology, 137*(1), 204.

American College of Obstetricians and Gynecologists. (2022). Practice bulletin no. 196. Thromboembolism in Pregnancy. *Obstetrics and Gynecology, 132*, e1–e17.

American College of Obstetricians and Gynecologists (ACOG), Committee on Obstetric Practice, & Society for Maternal-Fetal Medicine. (2021). Indications for outpatient antenatal fetal surveillance: ACOG committee opinion no. 828. *Obstetrics and Gynecology, 137*(6), e177–e197.

American Diabetes Association Professional Practice Committee. (2022). Classification and diagnosis of diabetes: Standards of medical care in diabetes. *Diabetes Care, 45*(1), S17–S38. https://doi.org/10.2337/dc22-S002

American Diabetes Association Professional Practice Committee. (2022). Management of diabetes in pregnancy: Standards of medical care in diabetes—2022. *Diabetes Care, 45*(1), S232–S423. https://doi.org/10.2337/dc22-S015

Bradford, H., Olson, S., Muñoz, E., & Solis, E. (2024). Appendix: 4A Skillful communication to mitigate clinician bias. In J. Phillippi & I. Kantrowitz-Gordon (Eds.), *Varney's midwifery* (7th ed., pp. 154–168). Jones & Bartlett Learning.

Centers for Disease Control and Prevention. (2018). *Parasites: Toxoplasmosis (Toxoplasma infection): Prevention and control.* https://www.cdc.gov/toxoplasmosis/prevention/?CDC_AAref_Val=https://www.cdc.gov/parasites/toxoplasmosis/prevent.html

Centers for Disease Control and Prevention. (2019a). *Cytomegalovirus (CMV) and congenital CMV infection.* https://www.cdc.gov/cytomegalovirus/hcp/clinical-overview/?CDC_AAref_Val=https://www.cdc.gov/cmv/clinical/index.html

Centers for Disease Control and Prevention. (2019b). Estimated HIV incidence and prevalence in the United States, 2010–2016. *HIV Surveillance Supplemental Report, 24*(1). https://www.cdc.gov/hiv/group/gender/pregnantwomen/index.html

Centers for Disease Control and Prevention. (2019c). Zika virus. Retrieved from https://www.cdc.gov/zika/hcp/diagnosis-testing/?CDC_AAref_Val=https://www.cdc.gov/zika/hc-providers/testing-guidance.html

Centers for Disease Control and Prevention. (2020). *Pregnancy and rubella.* https://www.cdc.gov/rubella/pregnancy/?CDC_AAref_Val=https://www.cdc.gov/rubella/pregnancy.html

Centers for Disease Control and Prevention. (2021). Diagnoses of HIV infection in the United States and dependent areas, 2020. *HIV surveillance report*, 2021, 33.

Centers for Disease Control and Prevention. (2022a). *Chickenpox (varicella).* https://www.cdc.gov/chickenpox/hcp/clinical-overview/?CDC_AAref_Val=https://www.cdc.gov/chickenpox/hcp/index.html

Centers for Disease Control and Prevention. (2023). *Parvovirus B19 and fifth disease.* https://www.cdc.gov/parvovirusb19/index.html

Centers for Disease Control and Prevention. (2023). *Tuberculosis (TB); Data and statistics.* https://www.cdc.gov/tb/statistics/default.htm

Centers for Disease Control and Prevention. (2024). *About Toxoplasmosis.* Retrieved from https://www.cdc.gov/toxoplasmosis/about/index.html

Centers for Disease Control and Prevention. (2024). *Fetal alcohol spectrum disorders (FASDs): Data and statistics.* Retrieved from https://www.cdc.gov/fasd/data/index.html#:~:text=Up%20to%201%20in%2020,FASDs%20can%20experience%20lifelong%20issues.

Centers for Disease Control and Prevention. (2024). Understanding the Impact of Data: HIV, Diagnoses, Incidence, and Prevalence. Retrieved from: https://www.cdc.gov/hiv-data/about/impact.html#:~:text=CDC%20estimates%20that%2032%2C100%20people,in%20the%20U.S.%20during%202021.&text=CDC%20estimates%20that%201%2C212%2C400%20people,at%20the%20end%20of%202021.

Devis, P. & Knuttinen, M. G. (2017). Deep vein thrombosis in pregnancy: Incidence, pathogenesis and endovascular management. *Cardiovascular Diagnostic Therapy, 7*(3), S309–S319.

Dukes, K., Tripp, T., Willinger, M., Odendaal, H., Elliott, A. J., Kinney, H. C., ... & Li, C. M. (2017). Drinking and smoking patterns during pregnancy: Development of group-based trajectories in the Safe Passage Study. *Alcohol, 62*, 49–60.

Ellsworth Bowers, E. R. & Kitzman, M. E. (2024). Pregnancy-related conditions. In J. Phillippi & I. Kantrowitz-Gordon (Eds.), *Varney's midwifery* (7th ed., pp. 907–956). Jones & Bartlett Learning.

HIV.gov. (2023). *Maternal HIV testing and identification of perinatal exposure.* https://clinicalinfo.hiv.gov/en/guidelines/perinatal/maternal-hiv-testing-identification-exposure

Jordan, R. G., & Cockerham, A. Z. (2024). Common discomforts of pregnancy. In K. Trister Grace, C. L. Farley, N. K. Jeffers, & T. Tringali (Eds.), *Prenatal and postnatal care: A person-centered approach* (3rd ed., pp. 223–262). Wiley Blackwell.

Jordan, R. G. & White, H. (2024). Perinatal loss and grief. In K. Trister Grace, C. L. Farley, N. K. Jeffers, & T. Tringali (Eds.), *Prenatal and postnatal care: A person-centered approach* (3rd ed., pp. 223–262). Wiley Blackwell.

Martin, J. A., Osterman, M. J. K., & Driscoll, A. K. (2023). Declines in cigarette smoking during pregnancy in the United States, 2016–2021. *National Center for Health Statistics Data Brief No. 458.* https://www.cdc.gov/nchs/data/databriefs/db458.pdf

National Institutes of Health's Office of AIDS Research. (2024). Recommendations for the Use of Antiretroviral Drugs During Pregnancy and Interventions to Reduce Perinatal HIV Transmission in the United States. https://clinicalinfo.hiv.gov/en/guidelines/perinatal/introduction

Osterman, M. J. K., Hamilton, B. E., Martin, J. A., Driscoll, A. K., & Valenzuela, C. P. (2023). *Births: Final data 2021.* National Center for Health Statistics. https://www.cdc.gov/nchs/data/nvsr/nvsr72/nvsr72-01.pdf

Society for Maternal Fetal Medicine. (2018). SMFM statement: Pharmacologic treatment of gestational diabetes. *American Journal of Obstetrics and Gynecology, 218*(5), B2–B4.

Substance Abuse and Mental Health Services Administration. (2023). Key substance use and mental health indicators in the United States: Results from the 2022 National Survey on Drug Use and Health (HHS Publication No. PEP23-07-01-006, NSDUH Series H-58). Center for Behavioral Health Statistics and Quality, Substance Abuse and Mental Health Services Administration. https://www.samhsa.gov/data/report/2022-nsduh-annual-national-report

Tsakiridis, I., Mamopoulos, A., Athanasiadis, A., & Dagklis, T. (2019). Management of breech presentation: a comparison of four national evidence-based guidelines. *American Journal of Perinatology, 37*(11), 1102–1109.

U.S. Department of Health and Human Services. (2018). *2018 quick reference guide: Recommended laboratory HIV testing algorithm for serum or plasma specimens.* https://stacks.cdc.gov/view/cdc/50872

Vachhani, K., Simpson, A. N., Wijeysundera, D. N., Clarke, H., & Ladha, K. S. (2022). Cannabis use among pregnant women under different legalization frameworks in the United States. *The American Journal of Drug and Alcohol Abuse, 48*(6), 695–700.

World Health Organization. (2021). Obesity and overweight. https://www.who.int/en/news-room/fact-sheets/detail/obesity-and-overweight

CHAPTER 8

Intrapartum

Melicia Escobar

Initial Assessment

- Reason for visit (chief concern)
- Sociodemographic/social determinants of health information
  1. Age—opposite ends of the age spectrum associated with risks
     a. Adolescents
        (1) Prone to receiving poor social support resulting in barriers to accessing care
        (2) At risk for low birth weight and prematurity
        (3) Increased risk for:
            (a) Hypertensive disorders of pregnancy
            (b) Premature labor
            (c) Preterm birth
            (d) Fetal growth restriction (FGR)
            (e) Infant mortality
        (4) Risk likely multifactorial with associated distribution of the social determinants
     b. Advanced maternal age in pregnancy is considered 35 years of age and greater
        (1) Higher incidence of infertility and first-trimester spontaneous abortion and ectopic pregnancy
        (2) Proportional increase in rates of chromosomal abnormalities with advancing age
        (3) Increased rates of complications
            (a) Hypertensive disorders of pregnancy
            (b) Preterm delivery
            (c) Gestational diabetes
            (d) Dysfunctional labor leading to cesarean birth
            (e) Relationship to underlying disease processes
            (f) Placenta previa and abruption
  2. Ethnicity—Certain genetic disorders are increased within specific ethnic groups
  3. Impacts of racism and other forms of bias on social determinants of health
     a. Lower socioeconomic status directly proportional to poor obstetric outcomes, including low birth weight and premature labor and delivery, especially among Black birthing people
     b. Can be related to limited access to prenatal care and necessary resources, such as whether one lives in a food-desert area or in an area with ample resources
- Gravidity and parity
  1. Length of labor
     a. Nullipara average longer labors
     b. Multipara average shorter labors
     c. Grand multiparous patients (parity >5) can have prolonged dysfunctional labors
  2. Obstetric complications
     a. Increased parity associated with increased rates of:
        (1) Abruptio placenta
        (2) Placenta previa
        (3) Multifetal pregnancy
        (4) Postpartum hemorrhage (PPH)
     b. Grand multiparity can contribute to abnormal presentation, including transverse lie
- Estimated gestational age (EGA)—based on the determination of the estimated date of delivery (EDD); synonymous terms for EDD include estimated date of birth (EDB) and estimated date of confinement (EDC); latter term was traditionally used but is now less frequently used because of negative connotations of the word *confinement*
  1. Menstrual dating (using Naegele's rule)—add 7 days to the first day of the last menstrual period and subtract 3 months
  2. Ultrasound dating—most accurate if performed in the first trimester
  3. Anatomic dating by fundal height measurement; accuracy may be affected by parity and body habitus
- Review of the antepartum course—preferably using prenatal chart
  1. History of prenatal visits
     a. Timing of first visit
     b. Compliance with the visit schedule
     c. Unscheduled visits/consults

2. Weight gain
   a. Prepregnancy weight/body mass index (BMI)
   b. Appropriateness of interval weight gain
   c. Total weight gain
3. Blood pressure
   a. Initial blood pressure
   b. Changes in blood pressure values throughout pregnancy
4. Fundal height growth
5. Ultrasound results
6. Current medications
7. Obstetric complications/unscheduled visits
- Laboratory data
1. Blood type and Rh factor
2. Hemoglobin/hematocrit
3. Hepatitis B surface antigen status
4. Rubella status
5. Pap test result
6. Sexually transmitted infection (STI) screening results (including human immunodeficiency virus [HIV], rapid plasma reagin [RPR]), hepatitis C
7. Glucose screening
8. Group B *Streptococcus* (GBS) culture
9. Genetic screening and testing results
   a. Chorionic villus sampling (CVS)
   b. Amniocentesis
   c. Multiple marker screening (quad or penta)
   d. Nuchal translucency combined with human chorionic gonadotropin (hCG) and pregnancy-associated plasma protein-A (PAPP-A) levels
   e. Cell-free fetal DNA (also known as noninvasive prenatal screening [NIPS])
   f. Carrier screening
- Obstetric history
1. Gravidity—total number of pregnancies
2. Parity—outcome of previous pregnancies
   a. Expressed as a four-digit number (TPAL)
   b. First digit is the number of full-term infants (T); second digit is number of preterm infants (P); third digit is number of abortions (spontaneous/elective) (A); fourth digit is number of living children (L)
3. Description of previous pregnancies
   a. Duration of gestation
   b. Birth weight
   c. Duration of labor
   d. Type of delivery
   e. Analgesia/anesthesia
   f. Complications of the antepartum, intrapartum, or postpartum period
   g. Place of delivery
   h. Birth attendant
- Family history
1. Obstetric complications
2. Genetic diseases, including chromosomal abnormalities and ethnicity-based disorders
3. Congenital defects or syndromes
4. Medical disorders
   a. Hypertension (HTN)
   b. Diabetes
   c. Thyroid disorder

d. Cardiac disease
e. Asthma
   (1) Level of severity
   (2) History of hospitalization, intubation, or use of oral steroids
- Past medical history
1. Allergies
2. Medical conditions
3. Previous surgeries
4. Medication (over-the-counter and prescription) and herb/supplement use
- Review of systems
1. Genitourinary
2. Respiratory
3. Cardiovascular
4. Gastrointestinal
5. Neurologic, psychological, and mental health
6. Musculoskeletal
- Labor status
1. Onset of contractions
2. Description of contractions
   a. Frequency
   b. Duration
   c. Intensity
3. Status of membranes
   a. Time of rupture
   b. Amount
   c. Color
   d. Odor
4. Frequency of fetal movements
5. Presence or absence of bloody show
6. Other subjective symptoms
   a. Nausea and vomiting
   b. Rectal pressure

Physical Examination

- Vital signs
- Abdominal examination
1. Abdominal palpation for estimated fetal weight, fetal presentation, and position during labor
   a. Determination of attitude is more difficult secondary to fetal descent
   b. Location of fetal back provides best determination of fetal position without pelvic examination
2. Palpation of contraction intensity and uterine resting tone
3. Presence of fetal movement
4. Location of fetal heart tones
- Pelvic examination
1. External perineal inspection
   a. Presence of bloody show
   b. Presence of amniotic fluid
   c. Presence of lesions
2. Internal examination
   a. Sterile speculum examination—*before digital examination* if ruptured membranes are suspected, frank bleeding is present, or inspection for herpetic lesions is necessary

b. Digital examination
(1) Dilation of the cervix (0–10 cm)
(2) Effacement of the cervix (0%–100%)
(3) Consistency of the cervix (firm, medium, soft)
(4) Position of the cervix (anterior, midposition, posterior)
(5) Station—relationship of the leading edge of the fetal presenting part to the ischial spines (in centimeters) (**Figure 8-1**)
(a) 0 station—the presenting part is at the level of the spines
(b) –3, –2, –1 station—number of centimeters of the presenting part above the level of the ischial spines
(c) +1, +2, +3 station—number of centimeters of the presenting part below the level of the ischial spines
(6) Presenting part—the anatomic part of the fetus that first descends into the pelvis
(7) Position—relationship between the denominator of the presenting part and the maternal pelvis
(a) Cephalic presentation—the denominator is the occiput
(b) Breech presentation—the denominator is the sacrum
(c) Shoulder presentation—the denominator is the scapula
(d) Face presentation—the denominator is the mentum
(e) Brow presentation—the denominator is the browline
(8) Status of membranes

(9) Clinical pelvimetry—assessment of the adequacy of the bony pelvis
(a) The pelvis is composed of four bones
i. Two innominate bones
ii. Sacrum
iii. Coccyx
(b) Symphysis pubis joins the two innominate (pubic) bones anteriorly
(c) True pelvis defines the birth canal (**Figure 8-2**)
i. Inlet boundaries are at the level of the sacral promontory (posteriorly), the linea terminalis (laterally), and the upper margins of the pubic bones (anteriorly)
ii. Midplane of the pelvis is known as "the plane of least dimensions"; the boundaries are the sacrum at the junction of the fourth and fifth sacral vertebrae (posteriorly), the ischial spines (laterally), and the inferior border of the symphysis pubis (anteriorly)
iii. Outlet boundaries are the sacrococcygeal joint (posteriorly), the inner surface of the ischial tuberosities (laterally), and the lower border of the symphysis pubis (anteriorly)
• Fetal heart rate (FHR) assessment
1. Continuous—by external electronic fetal monitor or cardiotocography
a. Determination of the FHR baseline
b. Assessment of variability
c. Determine the presence or absence of periodic changes, including accelerations, decelerations, tachycardia, or bradycardia

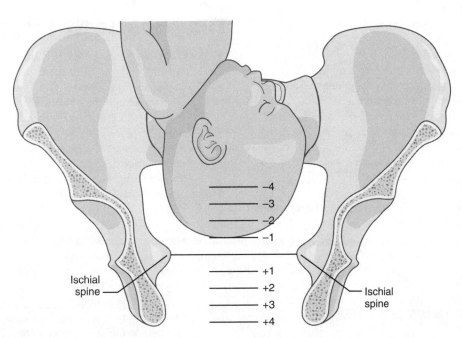

Figure 8-1

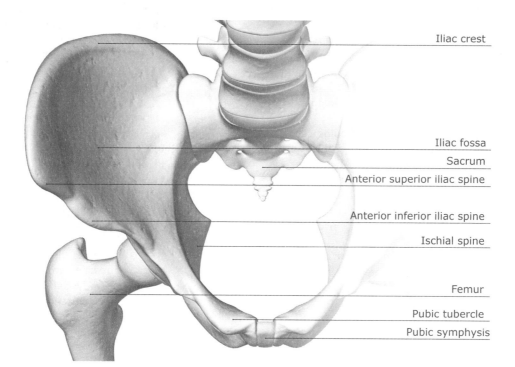

Iliac crest

Iliac fossa
Sacrum
Anterior superior iliac spine

Anterior inferior iliac spine

Ischial spine

Femur
Pubic tubercle
Pubic symphysis

Figure 8-2

© MedicalRF.com/Getty Images

2. Continuous—by internal monitoring via fetal scalp electrode (FSE)
   a. Measures the actual R-to-R interval of the fetal QRS complex; provides more accurate surveillance
   b. Increased risk of infection with internal monitoring; most frequently used if unable to obtain clear tracing with an external monitor
3. Intermittent by Doppler
   a. Auscultation of FHR at prescribed intervals based on the stage of labor to assess fetal tolerance of labor
   b. Unable to determine variability or isolated decelerations
   c. Reserved for patients without a priori risk for fetal acidemia
4. FHR tracings classification
   a. Category I: Normal; no action required
   b. Category II: Indeterminate; require continued evaluation and close monitoring
   c. Category III: Associated with abnormal fetal acid–base status; prompt action required
- Head-to-toe examination
  1. General affect and coping abilities
  2. Head, eyes, ears, nose, and throat
     a. Absence of facial edema
     b. Absence of upper respiratory infection (URI) signs
  3. Heart and lungs
     a. Heart sounds without murmurs, rubs, or gallops—may have split S_1, I–II/VI systolic murmur, audible S_3
     b. Respiratory effort and rate; lungs clear to auscultation
  4. Abdomen
     a. Fundal height and appropriateness given gestational age

  b. Abdominal palpation for estimated, fetal position, presentation, and attitude if not performed previously
  c. Presence of scars or lesions
  d. Intensity of contractions by palpation
  e. Location of fetal heart tones
  5. Pelvic examination—described in detail in this chapter
  6. Extremities
     a. Presence or absence of edema
     b. Presence or absence of varicosities
     c. Reflexes

Diagnostic Studies

- Type of studies—depends on the policies of the birthing facility
  1. Complete blood count (CBC)
  2. Blood type and Rh—may need to type and screen or cross-match depending on the pregnant patient's risk status
  3. Repeat testing for HIV, syphilis, or hepatitis if indicated by history, examination findings, or required by law (varies by state and local municipalities)
- Urine testing
  1. Protein
  2. Glucose
  3. Ketones
- Cervical/vaginal/perineal cultures performed during sterile speculum examination if indicated
  1. Cervical culture if suspect active infection
  2. Culture of any suspicious lesions
  3. Vaginal and rectal cultures for GBS if rupture of membranes before 37 weeks and unavailable

Management and Teaching

- Based on the birthing facility's policies; patient desire; and risk status for discussion, consultation, and management options
- Admission versus outpatient management
  1. May admit during active labor; patient may desire outpatient management
  2. If admitted in the latent phase, the patient incurs increased risk for medical interventions
  3. Factors to consider in decision-making
     a. Stable condition of birthing person and fetus
     b. Stage of labor
     c. Fetal position
     d. Membrane status (intact or ruptured)
     e. Nullipara versus multipara
     f. Functional versus prodromal labor
     g. Pain status
     h. Labor support at home
     i. Need for increased fetal surveillance
     j. Birthing person's desires and sense of safety
- Intravenous access
  1. If intravenous access is necessary via a saline lock or IV catheter, the most common IV fluids are:
     a. Lactated Ringer's solution
     b. 5% dextrose with lactated Ringer's solution (D5LR)
     c. 0.9% NaCl solution
  2. Factors to consider in decision-making
     a. Hydration status, including the presence of ketonuria
     b. Need for oxytocin induction or augmentation
     c. Need for antibiotics
     d. Predisposing factors for PPH, such as an overdistended uterus
     e. Abnormal placentation
     f. Grand multiparity
     g. Need for pain medication or regional anesthesia
- Limitations of activity level
  1. Patients can be encouraged to ambulate to help labor progress and increase coping abilities
  2. Factors to consider in decision-making
     a. Birthing person's desires
     b. Unstable lie or malpresentation
     c. Need for increased fetal surveillance and monitoring
     d. Membrane status and station of the presenting part
     e. Hypertensive disorders of pregnancy
     f. Exhaustion level
- Nutrition and fluid status
  1. Energy levels can be positively influenced by oral intake
  2. Factors to consider in decision-making
     a. Gastrointestinal motility/absorption
     b. Potential need for anesthesia during labor
     c. Birthing facility policy
  3. Can consider gastrointestinal (GI) protective agents such as magnesium/aluminum hydroxide, calcium carbonate/magnesium hydroxide, and sodium citrate/citric acid combinations

- Monitoring of vital signs
  1. Dependent on the stage of labor and risk status
  2. Patients with ruptured membranes require more frequent vital signs, especially temperature
- Pain management/coping during labor and delivery
  1. Nonpharmacologic methods
     a. Can allow the birthing person to feel more in control of the birth process
     b. Can be used without significant risk of side effects—especially helpful in latent labor
        (1) Ambulation and movement; use of birthing ball
        (2) Hydrotherapy
        (3) Breathing and relaxation/hypnotherapy
        (4) Music
        (5) Position changes
        (6) Acupuncture/acupressure
        (7) Intracutaneous sterile water injections
        (8) Touch and massage; warm compresses such as a heating pad or rice sock
        (9) Aromatherapy
        (10) Continuous labor support from a doula or support person
  2. Analgesia
     a. Used to ameliorate the pain sensation; may change and alter consciousness; some medications have an amnesiac effect
     b. Can be used in latent and active phases
     c. Avoid within 1 hour of birth because of the potential respiratory depressant effect on the fetus
        (1) Hypnotics—rarely used in current practice; these drugs do not possess analgesic qualities; benzodiazepines may cause amnesia and disrupted thermoregulation in the newborn (even after one IV dose)
        (2) Opioids
        (3) Sedatives—may be used in conjunction with opioids for therapeutic rest
        (4) Nitrous oxide—self-administered inhaled gas in 50:50 mix with oxygen via face mask
           (a) Safe for mother and fetus, administered before and during contraction
           (b) Does not diminish uterine contractility
  3. Anesthesia
     a. Provides complete neurologic block
     b. Can interfere with muscular action
     c. Possible effect on the labor progress; may cause an increase in need for obstetric intervention
     d. Can have systemic effects, including hypotension (most common) and fever
     e. Inadvertent dural puncture can cause a spinal headache
        (1) Spinal/intrathecal
        (2) Epidural
  4. Local blocks—provide pain blockade at the site of pain for brief periods of time
     a. Paracervical
     b. Pudendal
     c. Local infiltration

- Fetal well-being monitoring—method used depends on the risk status of mother, the policy of the birthing facility, and clinician preferences in combination with the mother's desires
  1. Intermittent auscultation
     a. Facilitates increased mobility
     b. Increased patient comfort
     c. Equivalent to continuous fetal monitoring when performed at appropriate intervals for patients without prior risk for fetal acidemia
     d. Requires one-to-one labor attendance
     e. Associated with decreased rates of intervention
  2. Continuous fetal monitoring
     a. May be indicated for antepartum or intrapartum risk factors
     b. Reactive fetal monitor tracing (Category I) is predictive of a well-oxygenated fetus
     c. Interpretation of fetal well-being can be equivocal in the presence of Category II FHR tracings
- Support people and their roles
  1. Labor support can improve a laboring patient's perception of labor
  2. One-to-one labor support can assist the laboring patient to cope better with labor
  3. Especially when provided by a doula (someone who is there solely to support the laboring patient and who has no medical responsibilities), dedicated labor support has been found to decrease the use of obstetric interventions and promote physiologic birth
- Management of membranes
  1. Intact membranes provide a barrier to the introduction of bacteria into the uterus
  2. Intact membranes can facilitate rotation of the head during pelvic descent
  3. Early rupture of membranes with unengaged vertex can increase the risk of cord prolapse
  4. Artificial rupture of membranes (AROM) may assist in the augmentation of labor if dysfunctional or arrested
- Physician role
  1. Clarify with the patient the role of the certified nurse–midwife (CNM) in relation to the consulting physician
  2. Review indications for physician involvement
- Birth preferences
  1. Birth preferences, ideally reviewed in the prenatal period, should be revisited/reviewed with the patient on admission and discussed in relation to status at that time
  2. Recognize that birth preferences may be limited by a variety of factors—health-related complications, financial, insurance, workforce-related, political, etc.
  3. Must center respect for the whole person, promoting physical, emotional, cultural, environmental health and wellness

Mechanisms of Labor

- The 4 Ps of labor
  1. Power of contractile efforts
     a. Adequacy of strength
     b. Assess the need for augmentation of labor

  2. Passenger
     a. Lie
     b. Presentation
     c. Position
     d. Size
     e. Synclitism versus asynclitism
        (1) The relationship of the sagittal suture line to the maternal sacrum and symphysis pubis
        (2) Synclitism denotes that the sagittal suture is midway between these two bones; biparietal diameter is parallel to the planes of the pelvis
        (3) Asynclitism denotes that the sagittal suture is oriented toward the pubis or the sacrum (**Figure 8-3**)
            (a) Posterior asynclitism—the sagittal suture is closer to the symphysis pubis
            (b) Anterior asynclitism—the sagittal suture is closer to the sacrum
            (c) Can be the cause of labor dystocia
            (d) Lax abdominal musculature contributes to asynclitism
  3. Passageway
     a. Clinical pelvimetry
     b. Classification of the pelvic structure
  4. Psyche
     a. Laboring the patient's view of labor/birth and the patient's ability to handle it
     b. Appropriateness of emotional support
     c. Education or preparation of labor
     d. Meaning of the pregnancy
     e. Ability to achieve the birth plan
     f. History of sexual abuse
- Labor assessment and progress
  1. Evolving Evidence
     a. Friedman's curve (1972) conflicts with more recent findings by Zhang et al. (2010). Among

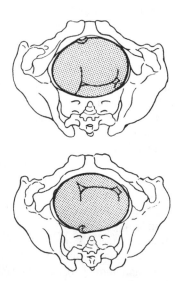

Figure 8-3

spontaneous labors with normal neonatal outcomes, Zhang et al. found that:
   (1) Nulliparous birthing people demonstrated no clear inflection point in cervical dilation in labor; while multiparous birthing people's cervical dilation accelerated after 6 cm.
   (2) There was not a deceleration period in either group.
   b. Labor progress and patterns may also vary based on other factors such as patient BMI or induction
   c. Labor progress must be taken in context
2. Stages of Labor
   a. First stage—from onset of regular contractions through full dilation (10 cm)
      (1) Latent labor—from the onset of regular contractions until 6 cm
         (a) Contraction pattern
            i. May be irregular
            ii. Mild to moderate intensity
         (b) Length
            i. Variable; may be shorter in duration for multiparous patients
      (2) Active labor—from 6 to 10 cm
         (a) Contractions pattern
            i. Become more frequent, regular, and intense
            ii. In active labor, typically every 2–3 minutes lasting at least 60 seconds
            iii. Moderate to strong by palpation
         (b) Length
            i. Variable; may be shorter in duration for multiparous patients
            ii. May also be impacted by augmentation methods
         (c) Strength of contractions
            i. Externally measured by palpation
            ii. Internally
               a. By intrauterine pressure catheter (IUPC)
               b. Adequacy in the active phase is considered 200–250 Montevideo units (mVu) in 10 minutes averaged over a 30-minute period
         (d) Descent
            i. Variable; May be influenced by the 4Ps
   b. Second stage of labor—from full dilation until the birth of the baby; pushing or expulsive phase
3. Labor progress abnormalities—Expectations for cervical dilation must be based on a nonlinear, hyperbolic curve as opposed to Friedman's linear model.
   a. May be overdiagnosed when admission occurs early in labor prior to 4–6 cm
   b. Based on Consortium of Safe Labor (CSL) data, the following parameters for dilation have been proposed and are supported by ACOG, SMSF, and consistent with WHO guidelines:
      (1) Latent phase—nulliparas and multiparas have varying labor progression before 6 cm
      (2) Active phase—nulliparas ($<$0.5–0.7 cm/hour) and multiparas ($<$0.5–1.3 cm/hour)

Management of the First Stage of Labor

- Assessment of maternal status
   1. Patient's psychological status
      a. Perception of pain/coping
      b. Coping ability and coping strategies
      c. Presence and support of people
      d. Patient's perception of the need for admission to the birthing facility
   2. Patient's physical status
      a. Vital signs
         (1) Temperature
            (a) Slightly elevated ($<$100°F) during labor, highest in the time preceding and immediately following the birth
            (b) Epidural anesthesia and other medications (e.g., misoprostol) can artificially elevate temperature
         (2) Blood pressure
            (a) Systolic blood pressure may increase 10–20 mm Hg during contractions
            (b) Diastolic blood pressure may increase 5–10 mm Hg during contractions
            (c) Blood pressure returns to prelabor levels between contractions
            (d) Pain and fear can contribute to elevations in blood pressure
         (3) Pulse
            (a) Because of the increased metabolic rate during labor, pulse rate is slightly elevated
            (b) Inversely proportional to the action of the contraction; increases during increment and decreases at acme
            (c) For this reason, if the fetus is having recurrent accelerations during contractions, it is important to place a pulse oximeter to distinguish the FHR from the maternal pulse
         (4) Respiration
            (a) Slightly increased rate during labor
            (b) Hyperventilation is common and related to pain response; can lead to alkalosis
- Assessment of labor progress
   1. Vaginal examinations
      a. Allows assessment of labor progress related to cervical dilation and/or fetal descent
      b. Frequency of vaginal examinations depends on the phase of labor, the clinician's choice, the patient's wishes, and the status of membranes
   2. Partographs—graph of labor curve
      a. Designed by Dr. Emmanuel Friedman (1972) to chart labor progress to ensure adequacy; no longer utilized as the standard measure of progress
      b. Research by Philpott and Castle (1972) suggests that aggressive management interventions (such as oxytocin augmentation) should not be initiated unless dilation averages less than 0.56–0.64 cm/hour in active labor

c. Recent evidence on the normal progress of the first stage of labor (Zhang et al., 2010) supports the use of an individualized approach

- Pain management
  1. Basis of labor pain
     a. Physiologic
        (1) Intensity of contractions
        (2) Degree of cervical dilation
        (3) Descent of the fetus causing pressure on pelvic structures
        (4) Fetal size
        (5) Fetal position
        (6) Hypoxia of uterine muscle cells during the action of contractions
     b. Psychological
        (1) Fear
        (2) Anxiety
        (3) Lack of knowledge regarding the labor process
        (4) Lack of support
        (5) Cultural influences
  2. Negative physiologic responses related to labor pain
     a. Hyperventilation
     b. Stress responses—related psychological effect causes increased cortisol and decreased placental perfusion
     c. Increased cardiac output and blood pressure
  3. Factors influencing pain management decisions
     a. Patient choice or birth plan
     b. Stage of labor
     c. Fetal status
     d. Other factors contributing to pain response
     e. Possible routes of medication administration
     f. Availability of pain medication modalities
     g. Nursing staff availability
  4. Pain management methods
     a. Nonpharmacologic pain relief
        (1) Relaxation and breathing techniques
        (2) Hydrotherapy—tub, shower, Jacuzzi
        (3) Position changes; ambulation
        (4) Massage
        (5) Environmental measures (i.e., quiet surroundings, aromatherapy, music)
        (6) Acupuncture/acupressure
        (7) Hypnosis
     b. Pharmacologic pain relief
        (1) Opioid analgesics given in early/latent labor but should be avoided close to birth as this can adversely affect newborn transition
           (a) Morphine sulfate for prodromal labor 10–15 mg IM *or*
           (b) Fentanyl 50–100 μg IV or IM *or*
           (c) Meperidine 50–75 mg IM or 25–50 mg IV—rarely used in current practice because the metabolite normeperidine accumulates in the fetus and potentiates depressant effects on the newborn
        (2) Mixed agonist–antagonist opioid analgesics
           (a) Butorphanol 1–2 mg IV or 2 mg IM
           (b) Nalbuphine 10–20 mg IM or 5 mg IV
     c. Anesthesia
        (1) Spinal/intrathecal
        (2) Epidural
        (3) Pudendal
        (4) Nitrous oxide—combination of 50% nitrous oxide and 50% oxygen self-administered via inhalation mask

- Assessment and evaluation of fetal well-being
  1. Physiology of FHR regulation
     a. Parasympathetic/sympathetic nervous system—responsible for the variability of the FHR
     b. Baroreceptors
        (1) Increased pressures can cause a vagal response in the fetus
        (2) Located in the carotid arteries and vessels in the periphery
     c. Chemoreceptors
        (1) Located in the aortic arch and carotid sinus
        (2) Sensitive to changes in the fetal pH, O_2 level, and CO_2 level; respond by increasing fetal blood pressure and heart rate
     d. Sympathetic nervous system activation increases the baseline FHR
     e. Parasympathetic nervous system activation decreases the baseline FHR
  2. Evaluation of the FHR in labor
     a. Baseline
        (1) Normal range for a fetus at term is 110–160 beats per minute (bpm)
        (2) FHR between 110 and 120 bpm can be normal at term with appropriate variability
        (3) Assessed over approximately 10 minutes, the mean FHR in the absence of periodic changes rounded to the nearest five beats should be documented
     b. Bradycardia
        (1) FHR <110 bpm for 10 or more minutes
        (2) Marked bradycardia—FHR <100 bpm for 10 or more minutes
        (3) Causes
           (a) Cord compression
           (b) Rapid descent
           (c) Vagal stimulation
           (d) Medications
           (e) Anesthesia or medications
           (f) Placental insufficiency
           (g) Fetal cardiac anomalies
           (h) Fetal acidemia
           (i) Terminal condition of the fetus
     c. Tachycardia
        (1) FHR >160 bpm for more than 10 minutes
        (2) Causes
           (a) Perinatal fever
           (b) Maternal dehydration
           (c) Infection
           (d) Medications, especially beta sympathomimetics
           (e) Chronic fetal hypoxia
           (f) Can be compensatory after a temporary fetal hypoxia event
           (g) Undiagnosed prematurity
           (h) Excessive fetal movement

d. Variability
   (1) Combination of influences between the sympathetic and parasympathetic nervous systems
   (2) Baseline variability—fluctuations in the baseline of the FHR
      (a) Absent—undetectable amplitude
      (b) Minimal—amplitude range ≤5 bpm
      (c) Moderate—amplitude range 6–25 bpm
      (d) Marked—amplitude ≥25 bpm
e. Accelerations—sign of fetal well-being; cannot be produced by acidotic fetus (indicates fetal pH of more than 7.20)
   (1) Greater than 32 weeks—a peak of ≥15 bpm above the baseline lasting ≥15 seconds but <2 minutes from beginning to end of acceleration
   (2) ≤32 weeks—a peak of ≥10 bpm above the baseline lasting ≥10 seconds but <2 minutes from beginning to end of acceleration
f. Periodic changes
   (1) Variable decelerations (**Figure 8-4**)
      (a) Abrupt (onset to nadir <30 seconds) periodic or nonperiodic decrease in the FHR that differs in shape from one deceleration to another; decrease in FHR from the baseline is ≥15 bpm lasting ≥15 seconds but <2 minutes

      (b) FHR deceleration does not reflect the shape of the contraction
      (c) Can occur at any time in relation to the contractions
      (d) Inconsistent shape; can look like a U, V, or W
      (e) Generally occurs as an abrupt drop below the FHR baseline and a rapid return to baseline
      (f) Generally caused by cord compression
      (g) Implications
         i. With rapid recovery to baseline and good variability, generally considered an uncompromised fetus
         ii. Suspect fetal compromise with slow recovery to baseline, increasing length or depth of decelerations, absent variability, or increasing frequency of decelerations
      (h) Management
         i. Position change
         ii. IV fluid bolus
         iii. Pelvic examination, to rule out cord prolapse
         iv. Contact consulting physician if warranted
         v. Consider amnioinfusion

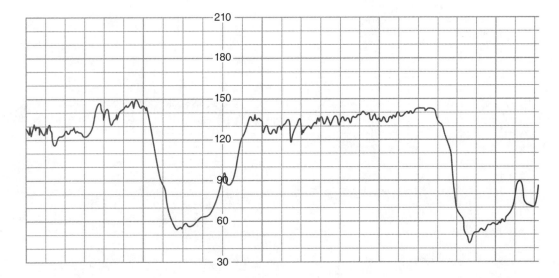

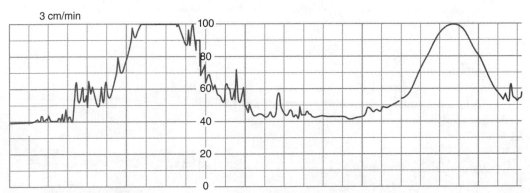

Figure 8-4

(2) Early decelerations (**Figure 8-5**)
  (a) Uniformly shaped slowing of the FHR that mirrors the contractions
  (b) Gradual descent to the nadir (≥30 seconds) with gradual return
  (c) FHR usually remains within the normal range and deceleration usually less than 90 seconds
  (d) Deceleration begins, peaks, and ends with the contraction
  (e) Generally caused by head compression with fetal descent, vagal stimulation
  (f) Generally considered a benign pattern—not a reflection of fetal acidosis
  (g) Management—surveillance; may indicate the onset of the second stage of labor
(3) Late decelerations (**Figure 8-6**)
  (a) Uniformly shaped gradual (≥30 seconds) slowing of the FHR that begins with the peak of the contraction and does not return to baseline until after the completion of the contraction
  (b) FHR may or may not remain within the normal fetal heart range

  (c) Can occur in an isolated fashion; more ominous when occurs repetitively
  (d) Possible causes
    i. Uteroplacental insufficiency
    ii. Fetal hypoxia
    iii. Uterine tachysystole
    iv. Decreased placental blood flow
    v. Maternal hypotension
    vi. Abruptio placenta
    vii. Medication effect
  (e) Management
    i. Left lateral position
    ii. IV fluid bolus
    iii. Attempt to correct the underlying cause
    iv. Consult with physician
3. Fetal monitoring techniques
  a. All patients require some method of fetal monitoring in labor
  b. Modality is based on risk status (pregnant person or fetal), birth site, and patient desire
  c. For low-risk patients, intermittent auscultation is equivalent to continuous fetal monitoring to detect fetal compromise
  d. FHR monitoring techniques

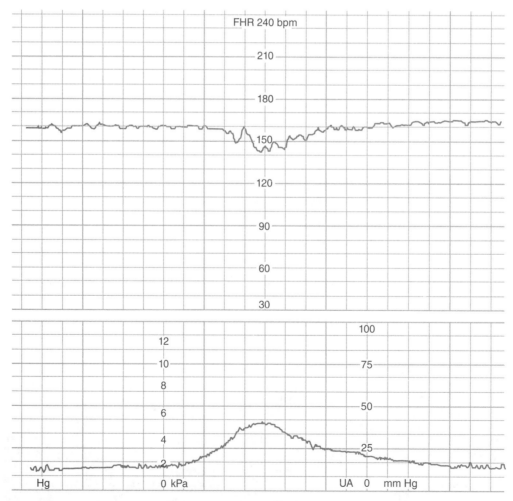

Figure 8-5

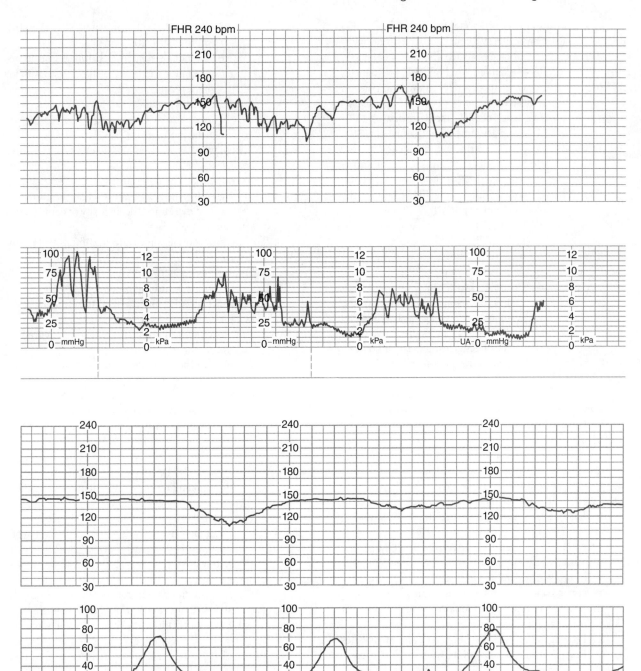

Figure 8-6

(1) Intermittent FHR auscultation by fetoscope or Doppler
   (a) Should be considered for term, low-risk pregnancies
   (b) Frequency of auscultation—also depends on facility's protocol
   (c) American College of Nurse–Midwives (ACNM) recommends:
      i. Active labor—auscultate starting at the peak of a contraction to 30–60 seconds after a contraction, every 15–30 minutes
      ii. Second stage—auscultate starting at the peak of a contraction to 30–60 seconds after a contraction, every 5 minutes
      iii. Frequency should be increased at any point given changes in the labor that could potentially impact fetal well-being
   (d) Can only be classified as Category I and II (Category III tracing cannot be assessed without variability data)

(2) Continuous fetal monitoring
  (a) Can be done with traditional electronic monitors or wireless patch system (e.g., Novii)
  (b) Recommended for high-risk pregnancies or when intermittent monitoring is not indicated
  (c) Frequency of FHR tracing review
    i. Every 15 minutes in the first stage
    ii. Every 5 minutes in the second stage
  (d) Modalities for continuous fetal monitoring
    i. External FHR—ultrasound detection and tracing of the FHR through the abdominal wall
    ii. Internal FHR
      a. Via FSEs
      b. Directly measures fetal heartbeat by measuring the R-to-R interval during heartbeats
      c. Indications include inability to monitor externally (such as inability to maintain an external tracing in the patients living in larger bodies)

- FHR tracing classifications—the assessment of the fetal heart rate evaluation
  1. Category I—normal tracing; associated with normal acid–base balance
    a. Normal baseline
    b. Moderate FHR variability
    c. Absent late or variable decelerations
    d. Present or absent early decelerations
    e. Present or absent accelerations
  2. Category II—indeterminate tracing; not predictive of fetal acid–base status; requires continued monitoring and evaluation
    a. Baseline rate of either bradycardia or tachycardia
    b. Minimal, absent with no recurrent decelerations, or marked variability
    c. No accelerations despite fetal stimulation
    d. Recurrent variable decelerations with minimal or moderate baseline variability
    e. Prolonged decelerations between 2 and 10 minutes
    f. Recurrent late decelerations with moderate baseline variability
    g. Variable decelerations that have "overshoots" or "shoulders"
  3. Category III—abnormal tracings; associated with abnormal fetal acid–base status; prompt corrective action or facilitation of birth required; characterized by absent FHR variability in conjunction with any of the following:
    a. Bradycardia
    b. Recurrent variable decelerations
    c. Recurrent late decelerations
    d. Sinusoidal pattern
    e. Direct fetal testing
      (1) Fetal scalp stimulation
        (a) During vaginal examination, fetal head is stimulated
        (b) Expected result should be FHR acceleration of more than 15 beats off baseline for more than 15 seconds
        (c) Expected result correlates to fetal pH of more than 7.20
        (d) Cannot be reliably performed during deceleration or bradycardia; must wait for FHR recovery
        (e) Validity and reliability are not well-established
  4. External uterine monitoring
    a. Tocodynameter—senses the changes in pressures against the strain gauge resulting from the change in abdominal wall contour
      (1) Records contraction interval and duration
      (2) Cannot determine the intensity of contractions
    b. Palpation
  5. IUPC—can accurately measure the intensity of contractions in mm Hg so that the adequacy of contractions can be calculated in mVu

- Fetal positions during birthing process
  1. Mechanisms of labor and cardinal movements based on occiput anterior (OA) position
    a. Left occiput anterior (LOA)—most common position of birth
    b. Position and appropriate cardinal movements are facilitated in the gynecoid pelvis
    c. Cardinal movements of labor (**Figure 8-7**)
      (1) Descent—usually in the left occiput transverse (LOT) position if engagement occurs during labor with rotation to LOA
      (2) Flexion—vertex begins partially flexed; is completely flexed when reaches the pelvic floor, changing presenting diameter to suboccipitobregmatic of 9.5 cm
      (3) Internal rotation—rotation of 45 degrees to OA allows the head to maximize the anterior–posterior (AP) diameter of the gynecoid pelvis
      (4) Extension—fulcrum of the neck under the symphysis pubis allows the birth of the head
      (5) Restitution—vertex rotates 45 degrees as the shoulders begin entering the AP diameter
      (6) External rotation—as the head rotates another 45 degrees, shoulders complete the remainder of the rotation to allow delivery in direct AP diameter
  2. Mechanisms of labor and cardinal movements with occiput posterior (OP) position
    a. Incidence of OP presentation is 15%–30%
    b. Right occiput posterior (ROP) is five times more common than left occiput posterior
    c. Approximately 90% of OP presentations rotate to OA via long arc rotation of 135 degrees (ROP to right occiput transverse [ROT] to right occiput anterior [ROA] to OA)
    d. Short arc rotation of 45 degrees results in the direct OP (or deep transverse pelvic arrest if failure to rotate completely)
    e. Cardinal movements for persistent OP position (short arc rotation)
      (1) Descent—head enters pelvis at an oblique angle (more often ROP than left occiput posterior [LOP])

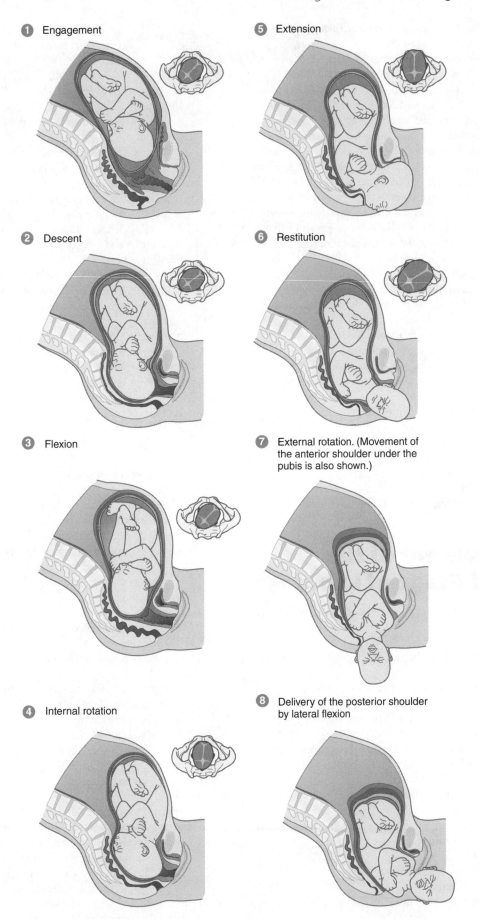

1 Engagement

2 Descent

3 Flexion

4 Internal rotation

5 Extension

6 Restitution

7 External rotation. (Movement of the anterior shoulder under the pubis is also shown.)

8 Delivery of the posterior shoulder by lateral flexion

Figure 8-7

(2) Flexion presents a smaller diameter through the pelvis

(3) Internal rotation—head rotates 45 degrees to OP position

(4) Flexion/extension—once rotation is complete; birth of the head occurs by movements of flexion until the sinciput impinges beneath the symphysis pubis and then the remainder of the head is born by extension

(5) Restitution—fetal head rotates 45 degrees to either ROP or LOP position

(6) External rotation—head rotates another 45 degrees as shoulders complete the remainder of rotation to the anterior–posterior diameter of the outlet to facilitate birth

- Emotional support
  1. Psychological
     a. Calm environment
     b. Perception of safety and support for birthing person and baby
     c. Maintenance of privacy and modesty
     d. Participation in the plan of care
  2. Role of the labor support person
     a. Reinforcement of and positive encouragement for the laboring patient
     b. Participation in the birth process
        (1) Providing nourishment or oral fluids and/or ice chips
        (2) Encouraging position changes
        (3) Relaxation techniques
        (4) Massage
        (5) Coaching with breathing techniques

Management of the Second Stage of Labor

- Begins with complete dilation and ends with the birth of the infant
- Patient status
  1. Vital signs (may be dictated by institutional protocols/parameters)
     a. Blood pressure (BP)—every 5–15 minutes
        (1) BP must be taken between contractions
        (2) BP can be elevated 10 mm Hg in the second stage of labor because of pushing effort
     b. Temperature—every 2 hours if membranes intact; every 1 hour if membranes ruptured
  2. Hydration and fluid status
     a. IV or oral fluids should be encouraged because of:
        (1) Increased metabolism
        (2) Increased respiratory efforts/hyperventilation of transition
        (3) Diaphoresis
        (4) Nausea and vomiting
     b. Bladder status
        (1) Bladder distention can compromise pelvic capacity
        (2) Inability to void may require catheterization

(3) Prevent the problem by having the patient void (or catheterize) when full dilation approaches

3. Behaviors and coping ability
   a. Assessment of fatigue
   b. Coping ability
   c. Response to pain and pressure
4. Pain control
   a. Evaluate the level of sensation in a patient with an epidural to determine whether the anesthetic level is hindering pushing efforts
   b. Pudendal anesthesia is occasionally used in patients without epidural as fetal descent occurs, causing perineal distention and pain, who request anesthesia at this point
5. Expulsive effort
   a. Patient should be coached to achieve effective pushing effort when the fetal head has reached +1 station to avoid adverse events to the patient and fetus.
   b. A resting period of passive descent or "laboring down" before active pushing may be appropriate for where the fetal station is at or above 0 stations without an urge to push. Fetal well-being should always be considered.
   c. Types of pushing
      (1) In recent studies, open-glottis, physiologic pushing and closed-glottis Valsalva pushing were found to have no difference in effectiveness or outcome.
      (2) Directive and spontaneous pushing efforts—limited data; no harm through spontaneous, patient-controlled efforts
      (3) Pushing efforts should be guided by the patient
   d. Close communication at the point of crowning of the fetal head can facilitate a birth that both protects the perineum and acknowledges any overwhelming pressure
6. Integrity of the perineum
   a. Patient preference is generally avoidance of episiotomy
   b. Increased risk of obstetric anal sphincter injuries (OASIS)
   c. Indications for episiotomy: to expedite birth secondary to fetal or maternal indication
   d. Types of episiotomy
      (1) Midline—incision of the posterior fourchette and perineal body centrally; greater risk of third- and fourth-degree laceration and damage to the anal sphincter, which threatens fecal continence
      (2) Mediolateral—incision from the posterior fourchette at a 45-degree angle through the transverse perineal and bulbocavernosus muscles; greater risk of perineal and posterior labial nerves and other vaginal muscles and glands central to sexual health functions.

- Fetal status
  1. Vaginal examination
     a. Evaluation of descent with pushing effort

b. Normalcy of fetal position and adaptation to the maternal pelvis
  (1) Molding (oblong shaping of the fetal head in the birth canal; an expected variation)/caput succedaneum (edema of the fetal head assessed during the second stage)
  (2) Synclitism versus asynclitism
  (3) Appropriate rotation to facilitate delivery

2. FHR monitoring
  a. Need for increased frequency of FHR evaluation
    (1) Evaluation at least every 15 minutes
    (2) More commonly every 5 minutes or after each contraction
  b. Periodic changes (early and variable decelerations) in FHR common—decelerations secondary to head compressions

- Pain relief
  1. Breathing techniques
    a. Controlled breathing as contraction begins and ends assists in focusing efforts
    b. Promote relaxation between pushing efforts
  2. Opioid analgesia
    a. Avoid giving within 1 hour of birth
    b. Can cause respiratory depression in the neonate
  3. Regional anesthesia
    a. Effectively lessens the pain and pressure sensations of the second stage
    b. Can lengthen the second stage secondary to pelvic musculature relaxation and decreased pressure sensations
    c. Pudendal—lidocaine 1% up to 10 mL on each side
      (1) Provides dense nerve block to the perineum
      (2) Does not inhibit pushing efforts
      (3) Needs to be timed well for the best anesthetic effect
        (a) Primipara—when vertex is at +2
        (b) Multipara—shortly before complete dilation
  4. Local anesthesia
    a. Perineal infiltration—lidocaine 1% with and without epinephrine to 2%, usually 10 mL in divided dosing (up to 30 mL maximum of 1% solution)
    b. Used before cutting an episiotomy
    c. For repair of episiotomy or laceration(s)

- Emotional support
  1. Encouragement
  2. Participation of labor support persons
  3. Adherence to the birth plan

- Cardinal movements of labor—eight basic movements that take place to allow birth in vertex presentation
  1. Engagement—biparietal diameter of fetal head passes through the pelvic inlet
  2. Descent—occurs secondary to forces of uterine contractions; change in the tone of pelvic musculature and pushing
  3. Flexion—occurs when the fetal head meets the resistance of the pelvic floor during descent and forces the smaller suboccipitobregmatic diameter to enter the pelvis first
  4. Internal rotation—causes the fetal head to rotate to the anteroposterior diameter of the maternal pelvis, most

commonly causing the occiput to rotate to the anterior portion of the pelvis
5. Extension—mechanism by which the birth of the fetal head occurs; the fetal head follows the curve of Carus; the suboccipital region of the fetal head pivots under the maternal pubic symphysis
6. Restitution—rotation of the head 45 degrees and realignment to the shoulders
7. External rotation—occurs as the shoulders rotate 45 degrees, bringing the shoulders into the anteroposterior diameter of the pelvis; the head also rotates another 45 degrees
8. Birth of the body occurs by lateral flexion of the shoulders via the curve of Carus

Birth Management

- Maintenance of pelvic integrity
  1. Anatomy
    a. Pelvic floor musculature
      (1) Function to support pelvic organs
      (2) Aids in the anterior rotation of the fetus during pelvic descent and birth
      (3) Consists of two muscle groups
        (a) The levator ani, made up of:
          i. Pubococcygeus, made up of:
            a. Pubovaginalis
            b. Puborectalis
            c. Pubococcygeus proper
          ii. Iliococcygeus
    b. Coccygeus
    c. Perineal musculature
      (1) Perineum is more superficial than the pelvic floor musculature
      (2) Perineum is divided into two triangles
        (a) Anteriorly as the urogenital triangle
          i. Superficial transverse perineal muscle
          ii. Ischiocavernosus muscle
          iii. Bulbocavernosus
          iv. Deep transverse perineal muscle
        (b) Posteriorly as the anal triangle
          i. Sphincter ani externus
          ii. Anococcygeal body
  2. Factors interfering with perineal integrity
    a. Size of fetus
    b. Distensibility of perineum
    c. Control of expulsive efforts
    d. Operative delivery modalities (i.e., forceps or vacuum extraction)
    e. Occiput posterior position
    f. Use of lubricants
    g. Birth position
    h. Episiotomy (median or mediolateral)
    i. History of OASIS
  3. Strategies to minimize perineal trauma
    a. Antepartum perineal massage
      (1) Begin at 36–37 weeks
      (2) Increases elasticity and tolerance to perineal stretching

b. External perineal massage from the time of perineal distension—vigorous massage and stretching of the perineum in the second stage of labor has not been shown to be effective and may actually predispose the laboring patient to an increased risk of lacerations

c. Warm compresses during second stage
    (1) Increases circulation to perineum
    (2) Promotes elasticity
    (3) Assists in the relaxation of the musculature

d. Lateral positioning for birth

e. Counterpressure to maintain flexion of the fetal head during birth

f. Education of the mother regarding the importance of controlled delivery of the head

g. Support of the perineum at the time of birth (this is controversial; some clinicians adopt a hands-off approach to birth)

- Episiotomy—surgical incision performed to enlarge the vaginal opening to allow delivery of the fetal head
    1. Technique
        a. Median episiotomy
            (1) Place index and middle fingers, slightly separated and palm side down, in vagina
            (2) Insert scissors into the introitus in an up-and-down position with one blade placed externally and one blade placed internally
            (3) Depth of insertion should correspond to the length of intended episiotomy
            (4) Incise tissue in one motion deliberately and purposefully
            (5) Evaluate adequacy of incision; repeat if indicated
        b. Mediolateral episiotomy—generally used if patient has a short perineum to avoid a laceration into the anal sphincter
            (1) Same procedure except that the direction of the scissors is a 45-degree angle from the base of the introitus directed either right or left
            (2) The angle of the incision should be aimed toward the corresponding ischial tuberosity
            (3) Much more difficult to repair
    2. Lacerations (**Figure 8-8**)
        a. First degree—involves the vaginal mucosa, posterior fourchette, and perineal skin
        b. Second degree—involves the same structures as first-degree laceration plus perineal muscles
        c. Third degree—involves the same structures as second-degree laceration plus tearing through the entire thickness of the rectal sphincter
        d. Fourth degree—involves all the structures as third-degree laceration plus tearing of the rectal mucosa
    3. Repair
        a. Fundamentals of repair
            (1) Use of aseptic technique
            (2) Adequate anesthesia
            (3) Visibility through good hemostasis
            (4) Appropriate suture material, including needle size

(5) Minimize local tissue trauma through gentle and limited blotting
(6) Minimize the amount of suture used
(7) Good approximation of tissues decreasing dead space and restores the normal anatomy

b. Suture material
    (1) Vicryl is the most common suture material
    (2) Chromic catgut—alternative used for repair
    (3) Suture gauge
        (a) 3-0
            i. Vaginal mucosa
            ii. Subcutaneous tissue
            iii. Subcuticular tissue
        (b) 4-0 for finer repairs
            i. Periurethral
            ii. Periclitoral
            iii. Anterior wall of the rectum
        (c) 2-0 for areas requiring more tensile strength
            i. Vaginal wall lacerations
            ii. Cervical lacerations
            iii. Deep interrupted sutures for repair of pelvic musculature
    (4) Needle selection
        (a) Atraumatic general closure needles are preferable
        (b) Small, fine GI needles should be used for fine stitching
        (c) Cutting needles should not be used

c. Mechanisms of repair of median episiotomy or second-degree laceration
    (1) Inspection of tissues to assess depth and extent of laceration
    (2) Identify all appropriate anatomic structures
    (3) Begin repair approximately 1 cm beyond the apex of the laceration to the vaginal mucosa
    (4) Close the mucosa using continuous locked stitches to the level of the hymenal ring
    (5) Pass needle under the hymenal ring and continue using blanket stitches (nonlocked) to the level of the bulbocavernosus muscle
    (6) Repair bulbocavernosus muscle with a crown stitch using a separate 2-0 suture if desired
    (7) If laceration is deep, consider several deep interrupted stitches using 2-0 suture
    (8) Using the 3-0 suture again, repair the subcutaneous layer with continuous stitching to the perineal apex
    (9) Using mattress stitches, perform subcuticular closure
    (10) At the level of the hymenal ring, bury the suture and tie it off

- Management decisions for birth
    1. Birth setting
        a. Hospital
        b. Birthing center
        c. Home
    2. Timing for the preparation of the birth related to location (i.e., setting up instrument table and donning personal protective equipment)

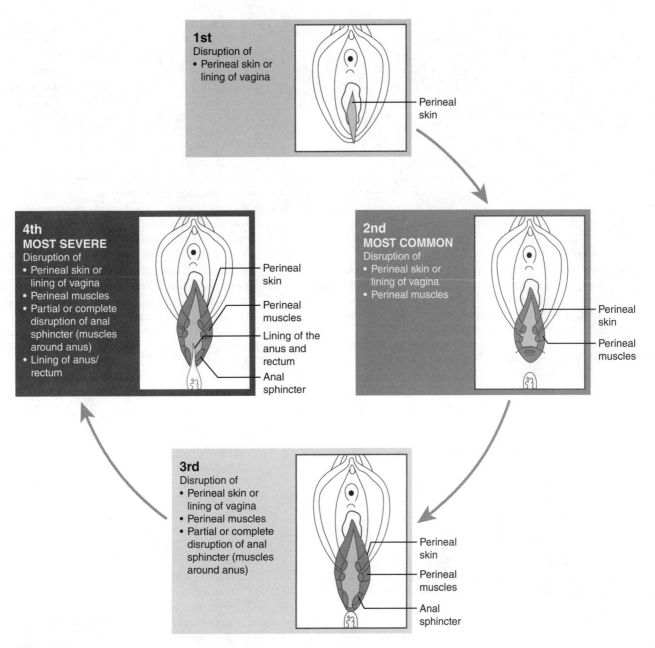

Figure 8-8

3. Delivery position for birth
   a. Semi-sitting
   b. Squatting
   c. Lateral
   d. Hands and knees
   e. Supine or lithotomy (least appropriate but commonly used)
4. Need for an episiotomy
5. Need for/type of additional anesthesia/analgesia
6. Use of perineal support during birth
7. Use of the Ritgen maneuver—assistance, if needed, in delivering fetal head by applying upward pressure to the fetal chin through the rectum during extension

8. Need for additional personnel (i.e., nurse, second midwife, consulting physician, pediatric physician or practitioner)
9. Placement of newborn upon delivery
10. Timing of umbilical cord cutting
- Hand maneuvers for birth in the OA position
   1. Apply counterpressure to the fetal head during crowning to maintain flexion and control extension using the nondominant hand
   2. If using perineal support, place the thumb and index finger laterally on the distended perineum, with the palmar surface supporting the perineal body
   3. Control birth of head during extension

4. After the birth of the head, slide the fingers of the dominant hand around the fetal head to the posterior neck to feel for the umbilical cord
5. If the nuchal cord is present
   a. Gently slip over baby's head if loose
   b. If not easily reduced over the head, slip the cord over the baby's shoulders as the baby is born
   c. If tight
      (1) Somersault maneuver—direct baby's head toward the birthing person's thigh *or*
      (2) Doubly clamp and cut and unwind the cord before delivery of the shoulders (this is to be avoided)
6. Wipe fluid from the baby's face, nose, and mouth with a soft cloth; routine suctioning with a bulb syringe is not necessary
7. After restitution and external rotation, place the palmar surface of each hand laterally on the baby's head
8. With gentle downward traction, and pushing effort, deliver the anterior shoulder; some sources recommend waiting for the next contraction
9. With upward traction, lift the baby's head toward the ceiling to deliver the posterior shoulder while observing the perineum
10. Glide the posterior hand along the head and posterior shoulder to control the baby's posterior arm as it delivers
11. As the baby delivers, maintain the posterior hand under the baby's head with support from the wrist and forearm
12. The anterior hand follows the body of the baby during birth and grasps the baby's lower leg
13. Rotate the baby into the football hold, with the head in the palm and the legs between what was the posterior arm and the attendant's body
14. Keep the baby's head below its hips, and slightly to the side, to facilitate drainage and suctioning
15. If desired and appropriate, place on the birth person's abdomen for delayed cord clamping, drying, and stimulation

- Suctioning
  1. Routine suctioning of nasal and oral passages is no longer recommended because it can cause physical injury to the nares or oropharynx
  2. Most healthy babies can clear their airways with no additional help
  3. Bulb syringe
     a. Generally sufficient to clear oral and nasal passages of fluid and mucus after birth if suctioning is indicated
     b. Minimizes pharyngeal stimulation and tissue trauma (compared to suction catheters)

Management of the Third Stage of Labor

- Begins with the delivery of the infant and ends with the delivery of the placenta

1. Physiologic management versus active management of the third stage of labor (AMTSL) shown to decrease the risk of PPH in the general population
2. Three components of AMTSL per the International Confederation of Midwives (ICM) and International Federation of Gynecology and Obstetrics (FIGO)
   a. Controlled cord traction (once pulsation stops)—World Health Organization (WHO) recommends this step only with a skilled birth attendant, citing evidence of possible harm
   b. Use of a uterotonic agent (such as oxytocin)
   c. Fundal massage after delivery of the placenta

- Delivery of the placenta
  1. Timing—generally 5–30 minutes after the birth
  2. Method of placental separation
     a. Placenta separates from the uterine wall because of a change in uterine size
     b. Hematoma forms behind the placenta along the uterine wall
     c. Separation of the placenta completes
     d. Descent of the placenta to the lower uterine segment or vagina
     e. Expulsion
  3. Signs and symptoms of placental separation
     a. Sudden increase in vaginal bleeding
     b. Lengthening of the umbilical cord
     c. Uterine change in shape from discoid to globular
     d. Uterus rises in the abdomen
  4. Mechanisms of birth of the placental
     a. Schultz
        (1) Presents at the introitus with the fetal side showing
        (2) More common than Duncan
        (3) Separation is thought to occur centrally first
        (4) Majority of bleeding is contained
     b. Duncan
        (1) Presents at the introitus with the maternal side showing
        (2) Less common
        (3) Separation occurs initially at the placental margin
        (4) Bleeding is more visible
        (5) Higher incidence of hemorrhage due to incomplete separation of placenta
  5. Management of birth of the placenta
     a. Obtain cord blood or cord gasses (as needed) after clamping the cord
     b. Inspect the cord for the number of vessels
     c. Guard the uterus while waiting for placenta separation
        (1) No fundal massage before separation
        (2) No traction on the umbilical cord until separation
     d. Use modified Brandt–Andrews maneuver to assess for separation
     e. When separation has occurred, use the Brandt–Andrews maneuver to stabilize the uterus and apply controlled cord traction to assist in the expulsion of the placenta
     f. May have mother push to assist expulsion
     g. Deliver placenta via the curve of Carus

h. If membranes are trailing behind the placenta, carefully deliver membranes

    (1) Use a Kelly clamp or sponge stick clamp onto membranes; gently apply lateral and outward traction

    (2) Hold the bulk of the placenta and twist the placenta over and over until the membranes are delivered

    (3) Inspect the placenta and membranes for completeness

- Appropriate diagnostic tests
  1. Cord blood
     a. Cord blood gasses (arterial, venous)
     b. Fetal blood type and Rh
     c. Direct Coombs's testing
  2. Maternal blood
     a. Kleihauer–Betke test if pregnant individual is Rh negative
     b. CBC, if hemorrhage suspected

- Use of oxytocics
  1. Oxytocin
     a. Used prophylactically against PPH
     b. Causes intermittent uterine contractions to decrease uterine size and the placental bed exposure
     c. Administration
        (1) Intravenous
            (a) Give 20–40 units in 500–1,000 mL of IV fluid (normal saline or lactated Ringer's), with the first liter running rapidly with the birth of the anterior shoulder, second liter at 150 mL/hour
            (b) Can use up to 40 units per liter
            (c) Never give undiluted as a bolus injection
        (2) Intramuscular—10 units intramuscularly if no IV access
  2. Methylergonovine (Methergine)
     a. Causes a sustained, tetanic uterine contraction
     b. Can be used emergently as a one-time dosing or as a series of doses for sustained effect
     c. Contraindicated in hypertensive patients because it causes peripheral vasoconstriction
     d. Administration
        (1) Intramuscular—0.2 mg IM
        (2) Oral
            (a) Generally given as a series of six doses over the first 24 hours postpartum
            (b) 0.2 mg orally every 6 hours
  3. Misoprostol
     a. Administration: 600–1,000 mcg per rectum, or buccally, is usual dose
     b. Side effects—shivering, fever, diarrhea, and abdominal pain possible
  4. 15-Methyl-F_2alpha-prostaglandin (Hemabate)
     a. Administration
        (1) 250 mcg
        (2) Can be given IM or intramyometrially
        (3) Contraindicated in patients with asthma or with active cardiac, pulmonary, renal, or hepatic disease

  5. Tranexamic Acid (TXA)
     a. Administration: 1 g IV over 10 minutes; a second dose may be administered after 30 minutes if needed
     b. Should be used as an adjunctive, not a primary treatment
     c. Use cautiously in patients with renal concerns

- Placental abnormalities and variations
  1. Battledore placenta—peripheral cord insertion, at placental margin
  2. Succenturiate lobe
     a. Most common abnormality—3% incidence
     b. Accessory placental lobe within the fetal sac that had continuous vascular connections with the main placenta
     c. Can cause retained placenta or hemorrhage
  3. Velamentous cord insertion
     a. Cord insertion into the fetal sac, not directly into the placental bed, generally 5–10 cm away from the placenta
     b. Can cause shearing of blood vessels during labor or delivery of the placenta, in turn causing hemorrhage
     c. More common in multiple gestations
  4. Circumvallate placenta
     a. Opaque ring of fibrous-appearing tissue on the fetal side of the placenta, caused by a double layer of chorion and amnion
     b. Can be seen in IUGR pregnancies but usually of no clinical significance

- Cord abnormalities and variations
  1. Single umbilical artery
     a. Only one of two umbilical arteries is present; cause unknown
     b. Can be associated with heart, kidney, or digestive tract anomalies and other genetic conditions
  2. Vasa previa
     a. Umbilical cord vessels run across the cervical os; cause unknown
     b. Pressure on or tearing of the vessel(s) in labor that can lead to nonreassuring fetal status or exsanguination
     c. Associated with velamentous cord insertion, placenta previa, and multiple gestation
  3. Umbilical cord cysts
     a. Fluid-filled sacs present on the cord
        (1) True cysts—contain fluid from the embryo, located proximal to the fetus; resolve on their own
        (2) Pseudocysts—most common; contain fluid from Wharton's jelly, located anywhere on the cord. Associated with genetic conditions.
  4. True knot
     a. A knot in the cord as a result of fetal movement
     b. Most common with long cords and in multiple gestation
     c. Can cause miscarriage or stillbirth if tight and prevents the flow of oxygen to the fetus

Management of Immediate Newborn Transition

- Apgar scoring
  1. Devised in 1952 by Dr. Virginia Apgar to identify infants requiring assistance adapting to the extrauterine environment
  2. Significance of scoring
     a. One-minute Apgar scoring reflects initial stabilization
     b. Five-minute Apgar scoring has a relationship to neonatal morbidity and mortality
        (1) Apgar score of less than 7 at 5 minutes indicates need for pediatric/neonatal involvement
        (2) Apgar score of less than 4 at 5 minutes correlates with neonatal mortality
        (3) Low Apgar scores by themselves are not predictive of later neurologic dysfunction
     c. Not as valid an assessment for preterm infants
- Indications for pediatric/neonatal involvement—any condition or circumstance that may compromise the adaptation of the neonate to extrauterine life
  1. Obstetric conditions
     a. Known fetal growth restriction
     b. Birth before 37 weeks
     c. Oligohydramnios
     d. Systemic disease of the birthing person
     e. Congenital abnormalities
  2. Intrapartum conditions
     a. Opioid analgesia at less than 1 hour before birth
     b. Use of sedatives or hypnotics at any point in labor
     c. Chorioamnionitis
     d. Operative delivery, including cesarean birth
     e. Category III FHR tracings

Special Considerations and Deviations from Normal

- Premature labor
  1. Definitions
     a. Premature labor—onset of regular uterine contractions between 20 and 37 weeks' gestation with spontaneous rupture of membranes or progressive cervical changes
     b. Premature birth—delivery before 37 weeks' gestation
        (1) Very preterm: <32 0/7 weeks of gestation
        (2) Moderately preterm: 32 0/7 weeks of gestation through 33 6/7 weeks of gestation
        (3) Late preterm: 34 0/7 weeks of gestation through 36 6/7 weeks of gestation

     c. Term birth—birth between 37 and 42 weeks' gestation
        (1) Early term: 37 0/7 weeks of gestation through 38 6/7 weeks of gestation
        (2) Full term: 39 0/7 weeks of gestation through 40 6/7 weeks of gestation
        (3) Late term: 41 0/7 weeks of gestation through 41 6/7 weeks of gestation
        (4) Post-term: 42 0/7 weeks of gestation and beyond
     d. Small for gestational age (SGA)—birth weight at less than 10th percentile for gestational age; corresponds to fetal growth restriction
  2. Incidence—approximately 10% of all births in the United States
  3. Etiology
     a. Idiopathic and multifactorial; in most cases the cause of premature labor is unknown
     b. Maternal factors
        (1) Systemic diseases
            (a) Hypertensive disorders of pregnancy
                i. Gestational hypertension
                ii. Chronic hypertension
                iii. Preeclampsia with and without severe features
                iv. Chronic hypertension with superimposed preeclampsia
            (b) Renal disease
            (c) Autoimmune disease
            (d) Infection
        (2) Structural uterine abnormalities
            (a) Müllerian defects
            (b) Fibroids
        (3) Overdistended uterus
            (a) Multiple gestations
            (b) Polyhydramnios
        (4) Short cervix
        (5) History of premature labor
        (6) Low socioeconomic factors
     c. Fetal factors
        (1) Preterm premature rupture of membranes—implicated in 30% of all premature labor cases
        (2) Fetal anomalies
        (3) Placental insufficiency
        (4) Infection
  4. Signs and symptoms
     a. Menstrual-like cramping with increasing frequency and intensity
     b. Pelvic pressure, especially suprapubic
     c. Backache, especially low backache
     d. Passage of amniotic fluid
     e. Change in the character of vaginal secretions
     f. Bloody show/spotting
     g. Progressive cervical dilation
  5. Physical findings
     a. Uterine contractions documented by electronic fetal monitoring (EFM) or palpation
     b. Cervical dilation on digital examination
     c. Documented ruptured membranes

6. Differential diagnosis
   a. Urinary tract infection/pyelonephritis
   b. Round ligament pain
   c. Braxton Hicks contractions
   d. Renal colic
   e. Appendicitis
7. Diagnostic tests to consider
   a. Fern and/or nitrazine test if suspect rupture of membranes
   b. Urinalysis with culture and sensitivity
   c. Other tests for suspected infections—chlamydia, gonococcal infection (GC), wet prep
   d. Fetal fibronectin—collect before digital examination; recent sexual activity or blood may affect results
   e. Ultrasound—cervical length and funneling, placental location and status, biophysical profile, and amniotic fluid index
   f. Amniocentesis—fetal surfactant and lecithin/sphingomyelin (L/S) ratio
   g. CBC with differential
8. Management—consultation with the physician regarding the need for transfer of care versus co-management
   a. Nonpharmacologic
      (1) Hydration
      (2) Left-lateral position
   b. Tocolysis—generally used to delay birth more than 48 hours; allows the clinician to give steroids to hasten lung maturity
      (1) Contraindications to tocolysis—any conditions causing a hostile uterine environment
         (a) Placental abruption
         (b) Chorioamnionitis
         (c) Severe preeclampsia
         (d) Placenta previa
         (e) Category III FHR tracing
         (f) Lethal fetal anomalies
         (g) FGR without interval growth
      (2) Most effective tocolytics—calcium channel blockers (nifedipine)
         (a) Drug action—nonspecific smooth muscle relaxant; prevents the influx of extracellular calcium ions into myometrial cells; effect not specific to the uterus
         (b) Side effects
            i. Hypotension
            ii. Flushing
            iii. Nausea, vomiting
         (c) Drug interactions
            i. Beta-agonists
            ii. Magnesium sulfate
         (d) Contraindications
            i. Do not use in the presence of intrauterine infection, gestational or chronic hypertension, or cardiac disease
            ii. Do not use in combination with beta-agonists or magnesium sulfate
         (e) Administration and dosing
            i. Route—PO
            ii. Initial dose of 10 mg

            iii. If contractions continue, repeat doses every 20 minutes for a total of 30 mg in 1 hour
            iv. Once contractions decrease, may give 10 mg every 6 hours or 30–60 mg sustained-release dose per day
      (3) Magnesium sulfate (MgSO$_4$)
         (a) Drug action—acts on vascular smooth muscle, causing vasodilation
         (b) Side effects
            i. Flushing
            ii. Palpitations
            iii. Feeling of warmth
            iv. Lethargy
            v. Muscle weakness
            vi. Dizziness
            vii. Nausea, vomiting
            viii. Respiratory depression
            ix. Pulmonary edema
         (c) Drug interactions—calcium channel blockers
         (d) Contraindications
            i. Do not use concurrently with calcium channel blockers
            ii. Toxic effects at serum level of more than 7 mg/dL
            iii. Antidote is calcium gluconate
         (e) Administration and dosing
            i. Generally IV; can be given IM
            ii. Loading dose 4–6 g in 100 mL intravenous fluid over 20–30 minutes
            iii. Initial maintenance dose 2 g/hour
            iv. If contractions continue, increase by 0.5 g/hour every 30 minutes to a maximum dose of 4 g/hour
            v. Maintain at an effective level for 12–24 hours after contractions stop
            vi. No benefit for weaning when discontinued
   c. Other management decisions
      (1) GBS prophylaxis
         (a) Penicillin G 5 million units IV loading dose followed by 2.5 million units every 4 hours until birth
         (b) Ampicillin is an alternative—2 g IV loading dose followed by 1 g every 4 hours until birth
         (c) Alternative therapy in case of penicillin allergy
            i. Low risk—Cefazolin 2 g IV load followed by 1 g every 8 hours until birth
            ii. High risk—medication selection done based on clindamycin susceptibility requested with initial GBS culture.
               • Clindamycin 900 mg IV every 8 hours until birth
               • Vancomycin—weight-based dosage of 20 mg/kg every 8 hours (max dose 2 g; min infusion time is 1 hour)

(2) Corticosteroid administration
  (a) Stimulates fetal lung maturity; potentially protects against intraventricular hemorrhage
  (b) Betamethasone 12 mg IM in two doses 24 hours apart *or*
  (c) Dexamethasone 6 mg IM every 12 hours for four doses
  (d) Should attempt to delay birth until 24 hours post administration

- Umbilical cord prolapse
  1. Definition—umbilical cord lies below or beside the presenting part; danger is compression of the umbilical cord, which then compromises the blood supply to the fetus
  2. Etiology/incidence
    a. Presenting part does not fill the pelvic inlet; can occur with the rupturing of membranes
    b. Incidence—1 in 400 pregnancies
  3. Signs and symptoms/physical findings
    a. Umbilical cord visible at or outside introitus
    b. Palpation of the cord during vaginal examination
    c. Presumptive diagnosis of occult prolapse if prolonged fetal heart rate deceleration occurs immediately following the rupture of membranes
  4. Management
    a. Elevate presenting part off cord without removing the hand, announce the emergency, and call for physician and other emergency staff support
    b. Assist mother into knee–chest position or steep left-lateral Trendelenburg position
    c. Do not attempt to manipulate the cord, as this may cause cord spasm; if protruding, wrap loosely with warm, normal saline-soaked gauze
    d. Do not rely on cord pulsations as an indicator of fetal status—obtain ultrasound if unable to detect fetal heart tones
    e. Discontinue oxytocin infusion, if applicable
    f. Provide O_2 at 10 L/min
    g. Administer intravenous fluid bolus
    h. Monitor FHR
    i. Consider terbutaline for tocolysis
    j. Prepare for cesarean birth
- Placenta previa
  1. Definition—placenta is located over or very near the internal os
    a. Complete placenta previa—placenta completely covers the cervical os
    b. Partial placenta previa—cervical os partially covered by the placenta
    c. Marginal placenta previa—edge of the placenta within 1 cm of the cervical os
  2. Etiology/predisposing factors
    a. Increased parity
    b. Advanced maternal age
    c. Previous cesarean birth or uterine scar
    d. Multiple gestation
    e. Smoking
  3. Signs and symptoms
    a. *Painless* vaginal bleeding during the third trimester—70% to 80% of cases

b. Bleeding with contractions—10% to 20% of cases
c. Can be diagnosed before hallmark bleed with ultrasound
4. Physical findings—do not perform a digital vaginal examination until placenta location is known; contraindicated with placenta previa
5. Differential diagnosis—placental abruption, preterm labor
6. Diagnostic testing—ultrasound confirmation
7. Management
  a. Acute bleeding requires emergency cesarean birth
  b. Otherwise depends on severity of symptoms and gestational age
  c. Bed rest and/or hospitalization usually indicated
  d. RhoGAM for unsensitized Rh-negative mother
  e. Delivered by cesarean section

- Placental abruption
  1. Definition—premature separation of the placenta from the uterine wall before delivery of the fetus
  2. Etiology
    a. Chronic or gestational hypertension (including preeclampsia, HELLP, or eclampsia)
    b. Severe abdominal trauma
    c. Sudden decrease in uterine volume, such as rupture of membranes with polyhydramnios or multiple gestation
    d. Cocaine use in pregnancy
    e. Tobacco use
    f. Uterine infection
    g. Previous abruption
    h. Advanced maternal age (over 40 years old)
  3. Incidence
    a. One in 100 births
    b. Can be a marginal abruption and not catastrophic
  4. Signs and symptoms/physical findings
    a. With complete abruption, *painful* vaginal bleeding, uterine rigidity, shock
    b. Marginal abruptions have less severe presentations
    c. Bleeding can be concealed
  5. Differential diagnosis—placenta previa, preterm or term labor
  6. Laboratory testing—abnormal clotting factors and decreasing hemoglobin
  7. Diagnostic testing—ultrasound confirmation if placenta previa; ultrasound is not very sensitive for placental abruption
  8. Management
    a. Complete abruption
      (1) Notify consulting physician
      (2) Insert two large-bore IV catheters
      (3) Prepare for immediate cesarean birth
      (4) Obtain blood type and cross-match for blood products, including clotting factors
      (5) Trendelenburg position
      (6) O_2 at 10 L/min if O_2 saturation abnormal
      (7) Monitor fetal status
    b. Partial abruption—management dependent on gestational age
      (1) IV access
      (2) Monitor fetal status

(3) Preparation if immediate surgical intervention is required

- Shoulder dystocia
  1. Definition—Need for additional obstetric maneuvers to deliver the fetal shoulders; difficulty in delivery of shoulders secondary to anterior shoulder becoming impacted on the pelvic rim or posterior shoulder being impacted on the sacral promontory
  2. Etiology/risk factors
     a. Gestational diabetes
     b. LGA fetus
     c. History of macrosomic babies
     d. High prepregnancy BMI
     e. Increased weight gain during pregnancy
     f. Small/abnormal/contracted pelvis
     g. Prior history of shoulder dystocia
     h. Estimated weight of the fetus 1 lb larger than previous infants in a multiparous patient
  3. Incidence—less than 1% of all births
  4. Morbidity and mortality
     a. Maternal—extensive vaginal, perineal lacerations, hemorrhage, trauma
     b. Fetal
        (1) Fractured clavicle
        (2) Brachial plexus injury
        (3) Hypoxia/anoxia
        (4) Fetal death
  5. Signs and symptoms
     a. Turtle sign—the immediate retraction of the fetal head against the perineum after extension
     b. Delayed restitution or need for facilitated restitution without descent
     c. Inability to deliver anterior shoulder with usual traction effort
  6. Management (assuming the patient is in recumbent or semi-Fowlers)
     a. Anticipation of shoulder dystocia is an indication or signal of need for emergency preparedness
     b. Immediately have any physician paged STAT
     c. Notify other staff, including anesthesia and the pediatrics team
     d. Instruct patient to stop pushing until a maneuver has been successful (discussed next)
     e. Perform McRoberts maneuver—place birthing person in exaggerated lithotomy position (knees to shoulders)
     f. Apply suprapubic pressure (*not* fundal pressure) while exerting downward traction on the fetal head while the birth person is pushing
     g. Cut or extend episiotomy—controversial (and if performed, the intent is to increase space for hands to perform necessary maneuvers); catheterize the birthing person's bladder to empty
     h. Begin internal maneuvers—no evidence or consensus regarding the order
        (1) Deliver posterior arm
            (a) Insert hand behind the posterior shoulder
            (b) Splint the arm and sweep across the abdomen and chest until the hand can be grasped externally

(2) Shoulder shrug
    (a) Hand placed under the posterior shoulder, attempt to pull the posterior shoulder toward the vaginal opening by capturing the axillary fossa using a pincer grasp
(3) Posterior axilla sling traction
    (a) A sling is created using a neonatal suction catheter folded in half.
    (b) It is threaded under the posterior shoulder and gentle traction is used to release the posterior arm, sweep the posterior arm, or rotate the shoulders.
(4) Rubin's maneuver
    (a) Collapse the shoulders by inserting a hand onto the back of the anterior shoulder and attempting to rotate the shoulder forward into the oblique position
    (b) Can be combined with suprapubic pressure
(5) Wood's screw maneuver
    (a) Use the same techniques
    (b) Rotate the fetus 180 degrees (keeping the back anterior)
    (c) If still impacted, continue rotation another 180 degrees
  i. Have the birthing person turn to knee–chest position (Gaskin maneuver)—may be difficult for patients with an epidural
  j. Break the anterior fetal clavicle—place thumbs along clavicle and force clavicle outward; controversial because it comes with the possibility of puncturing the lung or injuring subclavian vessels
  k. Cephalic replacement (i.e., Zavanelli maneuver)—rotate and flex head while replacing fetus into the pelvic cavity, followed by immediate cesarean section; controversial because it is associated with significant risk of infant morbidity and mortality

- Breech delivery
  1. The elective vaginal birth of singleton infants in the breech presentation is not recommended by the American College of Obstetricians and Gynecologists (ACOG); vaginal birth of a singleton breech presentation is usually reserved only for breeches that present emergently and when birth is essentially inevitable
  2. B extraction of a second twin is a relatively safe alternative to cesarean birth, assuming the clinician is skilled in vaginal breech births
  3. Definition—birth of infant presenting with buttocks, feet, or knees
     a. Complete breech—legs and thighs are flexed with buttocks presenting
     b. Frank breech—legs extended on abdomen with flexed thighs and buttocks presenting; most common type of breech presentation
     c. Footling breech—one or both feet presenting
     d. Knee presentation—single or double knees are presenting (most rare)
     e. Spontaneous vaginal breech birth—birth without additional external assistance

f. Assisted vaginal birth (partial breech extraction)—spontaneous delivery to the umbilicus; remainder of the body delivered with assistance

g. Total breech extraction—entire body extracted by birth attendant

4. Incidence
   a. Term—3% to 4%
   b. At 28 weeks, 25% of all fetuses are breech
   c. Most convert to cephalic by 34 weeks' gestation

5. Etiology/risk factors
   a. Presentation possibly related to the fetus accommodating to the shape of the uterus
      (1) Preterm fetuses position the head in the upper portion of the uterus because the head is the larger portion of a fetus's body
      (2) At term, the largest part of the fetus is the head, so it descends into the pelvis
   b. Maternal indications
      (1) Gestational age
      (2) Fibroids
      (3) Uterine anomalies
      (4) Abnormal placentation
         (a) Placenta previa
         (b) Cornual fundal implantation
      (5) Oligohydramnios/polyhydramnios
   c. Fetal factors
      (1) Congenital anomalies—threefold increase in anomalies with breech presentation
      (2) Short umbilical cord

6. Morbidity/mortality
   a. Cord prolapse (1.5% of frank breeches; 10% of other breech presentations)
   b. Traumatic vaginal delivery
      (1) Largest part of the fetus is delivered last
      (2) Head entrapment causes injury to organs, the brain, and the skull
   c. Increased perinatal morbidity and mortality

7. Management and treatment
   a. Vaginal breech birth is a co-management situation
   b. Criteria for candidates of vaginal breech birth
      (1) Frank breech presentation
      (2) Estimated fetal weight (EFW) of 2,500–3,800 g
      (3) Flexion of the fetal head
   c. Management decisions
      (1) Continuous fetal monitoring
      (2) IV access
      (3) Use of oxytocin for protraction disorders very controversial; generally cesarean birth is indicated
      (4) Generous episiotomy if indicated (see section on episiotomy)
      (5) Empty bladder before the second stage of labor
      (6) Should deliver as a double setup in the operating room

8. Delivery sequence for partial breech extraction
   a. "Hands off the breech" until the body is born to the umbilicus
   b. Second clinician should maintain head flexion through the abdominal wall during the entire descent

c. Pull down the loop of the cord

d. From this point on, the mother is instructed to push continuously

e. If the legs have not delivered spontaneously, they should be gently guided out of the vagina

f. Apply downward traction with the hands to baby's hips, with thumbs in the sacroiliac region, to encourage delivery of the anterior scapula

g. Primary clinician delivers the anterior arm by moving the hand up the infant's back and over the top of the anterior shoulder, sweeping the arm down across the chest and under the pubis with the clinician's finger

h. Raise the infant so the posterior arm can be delivered in the same manner

i. The back should spontaneously rotate anteriorly; it is important *not* to let the head rotate to the OP position

j. Maintain flexion of the head if needed through the Ritgen maneuver, manual flexion with a fingertip on each side of the baby's head, or Mauriceau-Smellie-Veit maneuver
   (1) With the dominant hand palmar side up, place the index and middle fingers on either side of the nose on the maxilla, with the chest and body resting on the palm and the legs straddling the forearm
   (2) Place the other hand on top of the baby, with the index finger on one side and the middle finger on the other side of the neck extending over the shoulder for traction

k. Again, apply downward traction until the suboccipital region (the hairline is seen coming under the pubic symphysis)

l. Now apply upward traction while elevating the body to deliver the head via the curve of Carus

- Face presentation
  1. Definition—cephalic presentation with an attitude of the head in complete extension, with occiput proximal to the spine; usually begins labor as a brow presentation
  2. Incidence—1 in 250 births; higher rate in multiparas
  3. Etiology
     a. Can be an indicator of cephalopelvic disproportion
     b. Multiple loops of nuchal cord
     c. Tumors of the neck
     d. Anencephalic fetus
  4. Risk factors—if the mentum is not anterior, the fetus is unable to pass under the pubic symphysis
  5. Diagnosis
     a. During Leopold's maneuver, the occipital bone is easily palpated and prominent; the head feels larger than expected, cephalic prominence located on the same side as the fetal back
     b. During vaginal examination, facial landmarks can be palpated
  6. Management
     a. Review clinical pelvimetry to ensure pelvic adequacy
     b. Confirm position is mentum anterior; mentum posterior is contraindicated for vaginal birth

c. Collaborate with consulting physician if protraction disorder occurs

d. Pediatric attendance at the birth

- Twin gestation—intrapartum twins are always a collaborative management situation

  1. Definitions—multiple gestation with two fetuses in the uterus

     a. Monozygotic twins (**Figure 8-9**)—zygotic division between 4 and 8 days
        (1) Identical twins
        (2) One placenta
        (3) Generally one chorion, two amnions

     b. Dizygotic twins (**Figure 8-10**)
        (1) Fraternal twins
        (2) Two placentas
        (3) Two chorions, two amnions

  2. Incidence

     a. Monozygotic twinning rate—stable at 1 per 250 births

     b. Dizygotic twinning rates—increasing as a result of assisted reproductive technologies

  3. Predisposing factors

     a. Family history

     b. Ovulation induction/in vitro fertilization

     c. Sub-Saharan African descent

  4. Diagnosis

     a. Size larger than dates

     b. Auscultation of more than one fetal heartbeat

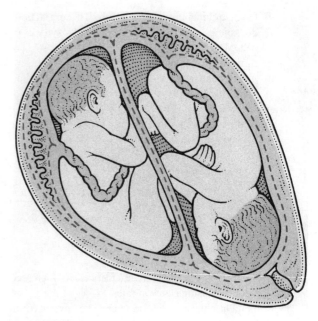

Figure 8-10

© Dorling Kindersley/Getty Images

c. Abnormal Leopold's maneuver findings

d. Ultimate diagnosis by ultrasound

5. Morbidity

   a. Premature labor and birth
   b. Premature rupture of membranes
   c. Malpresentation of the second twin
   d. Cord prolapse
   e. Operative delivery for the second twin
   f. SGA and FGR babies
   g. Twin-to-twin transfusion

6. Management decisions

   a. Physician should be collaborating for all intrapartum decisions and present for the birth
   b. Ultrasound confirmation of presentation
   c. Intravenous catheter insertion
   d. Type and screen blood on admission; some facilities require type and cross-match
   e. Continuous fetal monitoring
   f. Anesthesia presence for birth
   g. Neonatology physician or practitioner attendance for birth
   h. Ultrasound machine in the delivery room
   i. Bladder should be emptied before pushing

7. Management

   a. Birth of the first twin in the usual fashion—if nuchal cord is present, do *not* cut the cord; attempt birth with the cord intact
   b. Upon delivery, clamp the cord and transfer the baby to the pediatric team
   c. Assistant can guide the second twin into the pelvis depending on the presentation
   d. Confirm presentation of the second twin based on ultrasound
   e. Timing of delivery depends on fetal status

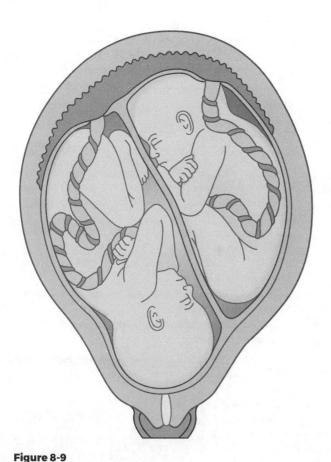

Figure 8-9

© Dorling Kindersley/Getty Images

f. Labor augmentation can be used if contractions do not resume via administration of oxytocin or AROM

g. Birth of second twin

h. Active management of the third stage of labor, observing for PPH

- Retained placenta

1. Definition—placenta that has not separated from the uterine wall after 60 minutes

2. Predisposing factors
   a. Premature delivery
   b. Chorioamnionitis
   c. Prior cesarean birth
   d. Placenta previa
   e. Grand multiparity

3. Etiology
   a. Structurally abnormal uterus
   b. Abnormal placentation—incidence has increased with increasing cesarean rates
      (1) Placenta accreta—adherence to myometrium due to partial or total absence of decidua
      (2) Placenta increta—further extension into the myometrium with penetration into the uterine wall
      (3) Placenta percreta—further extension through the uterine wall to the serosa layer

4. Management
   a. Facilitate usual methods of placental separation
      (1) Allow baby to nurse; nipple stimulation
      (2) Assist mother into squatting position
      (3) Empty patient's bladder
   b. If the third stage is more than 30 minutes, consider that the placenta is retained; notify the consulting physician
   c. Management in preparation for consulting physician
      (1) Monitor for bleeding or shock
      (2) Secure a bedside ultrasound
      (3) Insert IV if none in place
      (4) Prepare mother for manual placenta removal
      (5) Notify anesthesia

Questions

Select the best answer.

1. A patient at 38 weeks' gestation presents to your birth center complaining of a small amount of watery, clear-to-whitish vaginal discharge for the past 8 hours. She has been having Braxton Hicks contractions for a couple of days. The baby is moving on a regular basis, but now she just "does not feel right." Which option represents the best initial assessment action related to her presenting symptoms?
   a. Obtain a 20-minute fetal monitor strip to ensure reactivity.
   b. Perform a sterile speculum exam to rule out rupture of membranes.
   c. Contact the consulting physician regarding the premature rupture of membranes protocol.
   d. Discharge the patient to home to await a better labor pattern.

2. A 37-year-old patient, G4 P0, at 35 weeks, presents saying that she has been having bright red bleeding and clots for 2 hours since vaginal intercourse with her husband. She has saturated two pads in 2 hours. She is *not* having any pain. The most probable diagnosis is:
   a. placenta previa.
   b. cervical irritation from intercourse.
   c. placental abruption.
   d. normal bloody show.

3. Tocolysis of premature labor contractions is most effectively achieved by:
   a. an NSAID.
   b. nifedipine.
   c. intravenous fluids.
   d. an oxytocic.

4. Which one of the following profiles places a patient most at risk for placental abruption?
   a. A 19-year-old G2 P0010 in preterm labor at 35 weeks
   b. A 28-year-old G1, smoker, twin gestation, spontaneous rupture of membranes at 37 weeks
   c. A 28-year-old G3 P2002, induced labor at 41 weeks
   d. A 41-year-old G1, low-lying placenta at 10 weeks

5. Which of the following is the major risk of multifetal gestation?
   a. Eclampsia
   b. Gestational diabetes
   c. Cephalopelvic disproportion
   d. Preterm birth

6. Which of the following sequences represents the cardinal movements of labor and birth for the occiput anterior position?
   a. Flexion, descent, internal rotation, extension, restitution, external rotation
   b. Descent, flexion, extension, internal rotation, external rotation, restitution
   c. Descent, flexion, internal rotation, extension, restitution, external rotation
   d. Descent, flexion, internal rotation, extension, external rotation, restitution

7. The cardinal movement responsible for the birth of the fetal head in the cephalic presentation is:
   a. flexion.
   b. restitution.
   c. extension.
   d. external rotation.

8. The definition of postpartum hemorrhage is blood loss:
   a. greater than 750 mL during a vaginal birth.
   b. greater than or equal to 1,000 mL regardless of method of birth.
   c. of more than 500 mL after a cesarean section.
   d. of 750 mL or more after the third stage of labor.

9. Which of the following statements concerning Apgar scores is correct?
   a. Scoring is especially useful in the assessment of the preterm infant.
   b. Scoring is less useful when the infant is post-term.
   c. A score of less than 7 at 1 minute correlates with increased neonatal morbidity.
   d. Five-minute scoring has a relationship to neonatal morbidity and mortality.

10. Infants born to patients with gestational diabetes are at increased risk for:
    a. hypothermia.
    b. IUGR.
    c. hyperglycemia.
    d. shoulder dystocia.

11. A patient who is a G3 P2002 at 38 weeks presents with regular uterine contractions every 4–6 minutes for 60 seconds for the past 8 hours. The patient's vaginal exam is 2 cm/30%/–2, vertex with intact membranes. The patient is very uncomfortable with the contractions and declines discharge to home at this time. Which of the following best describes the stage of labor the patient is currently in?
    a. in transitional labor
    b. in latent labor
    c. in active labor
    d. not in labor

12. A patient who is a G3 P2002 at 38 weeks presents with regular uterine contractions every 4–6 minutes for 60 seconds for the past 8 hours. The patient's vaginal exam is 2 cm/30%/–2, vertex with intact membranes. The patient is very uncomfortable with the contractions and declines discharge to home at this time. Which of the following is the most appropriate plan of care at this time?
    a. Admit the patient immediately.
    b. Have the patient ambulate for 2 hours and then reassess the patient.
    c. Contact the consulting physician for augmentation of labor.
    d. Defer to the patient's birth plan.

13. A patient who is a G6 P5005 at 39 weeks presents with regular uterine contractions that are every 4 minutes for 60 seconds. The patient's exam is 3 cm/50%/–2, vertex with intact membranes. The FHR is 150 bpm with audible accelerations by Doppler. Which of the following best describes the stage of labor the patient is currently in?
    a. A prolonged latent phase of labor
    b. The latent phase of labor
    c. The active phase of labor
    d. An unknown phase of labor because you cannot make a determination based on this information

14. A patient who is a G6 P5005 at 39 weeks was admitted to the labor floor 9 hours ago. The patient continues to have the same contraction pattern every 4 minutes for 60 seconds. The patient's exam is now 3 cm/100%/0, vertex with intact membranes. The FHR remains in the range of 140–159 bpm with audible accelerations. The patient is exhausted and is no longer coping well with the contractions and "just wants it over." Which of the following is the most accurate diagnosis at this time?
    a. The latent phase of labor
    b. A prolonged latent phase of labor
    c. Arrested labor
    d. A protracted active phase of labor

15. A patient who is a G6 P5005 at 39 weeks was admitted to the labor floor 9 hours ago. The patient continues to have the same contraction pattern every 4 minutes for 60 seconds. The patient's exam is now 3 cm/100%/0, vertex with intact membranes. The FHR remains in the range of 140–159 bpm with audible accelerations. The patient is exhausted and no longer coping well with the contractions and "just wants it over." Which of the following is the next best step?
    a. Discharge to home with encouragement to return with frequent contractions.
    b. Begin labor augmentation with rupture of membranes and pitocin.
    c. Encourage her to continue with her original plan for an unmedicated childbirth.
    d. Offer morphine 10 mg IM for rest to correct this dysfunctional labor pattern.

16. A patient presents to your office stating that she is pregnant and wants to know her due date. The first day of her last period was February 4. Her due date by menstrual dating (Naegele's rule) is:
    a. November 11
    b. October 28
    c. May 11
    d. November 4

17. The denominator of breech presentation is the:
    a. symphysis pubis
    b. sacrum
    c. feet
    d. shoulders

18. Your patient is in active labor and is making appropriate progress. Currently, the patient's exam is 6 cm/100%/2, vertex with intact membranes. During your exam, you notice the position of the vertex is LOT, and the sagittal suture of the fetus is closer to the maternal sacrum. The most likely diagnosis at this time is:
    a. deep transverse pelvic arrest.
    b. anterior asynclitism.
    c. failure to descend.
    d. posterior asynclitism.

19. The patient is in active labor and is making appropriate progress. Currently, the patient's exam is 6 cm/100%/2, vertex with intact membranes. During your exam, you notice the position of the vertex is LOT and the sagittal suture of the fetus is closer to the maternal sacrum. Which of the following is the next best step in labor management?
    a. artificial rupture of membranes
    b. epidural anesthesia
    c. Pitocin augmentation
    d. to encourage movement and position change

20. Your patient is in active labor and is making appropriate progress. Currently, the patient's exam is 6 cm/100%/2, vertex with intact membranes. During your exam, you notice the position of the vertex is LOT and the sagittal suture of the fetus is closer to the maternal sacrum. On the fetal monitor strip, you notice the FHR has intermittently been 100–110 bpm for 20–30 seconds at a time for the past 10–15 minutes with good return to the baseline of 140 bpm. Which of the following elements should be included in the clinical documentation?
    a. Variable decelerations
    b. Late decelerations
    c. Fetal bradycardia
    d. You cannot determine how to document from this information.

21. The most favorable diameter of the fetal head to present in labor is the:
    a. verticomental.
    b. submentobregmatic.
    c. occipitofrontal.
    d. suboccipitobregmatic.

22. Intermittent auscultation of the FHR during labor is:
    a. inferior to continuous fetal monitoring.
    b. acceptable only for out-of-hospital birth.
    c. acceptable for the fetal evaluation of certain patients.
    d. correlated with lower Apgar scores than continuous fetal monitoring.

23. Your patient does not want an episiotomy no matter what happens. Which of the following is the most appropriate way to respond to the patient's concern?
    a. Discuss the indications for episiotomy and how consent is obtained.
    b. Teach the patient perineal massage antenatally.
    c. Explain that skilled midwives never perform episiotomies.
    d. Explain that, as a G1, the patient will likely need an episiotomy.

24. A patient presents while you are covering labor and delivery. The patient is a 33-year-old G3 P2002 at term and in labor with ruptured membranes. Your exam reveals 5 cm/90% effaced/0 station, but you are unable to palpate fontanels or sutures. You suspect that you feel the orbital ridge in the anteroposterior diameter and the chin at 3 o'clock. If this is the case, what is the presentation?
    a. ROT
    b. LMT
    c. RMT
    d. ROA

25. A 33-year-old patient, G3 P2002 at term, presents in labor with ruptured membranes. Your exam reveals 5 cm/90% effaced/0 station, but you are unable to palpate fontanels or sutures. You suspect that you feel the orbital ridge in the anteroposterior diameter and the chin at 3 o'clock. Three hours later, the patient is completely dilated/100% effaced/0 station with an urge to push. Your exam now reveals that the presentation is mentum anterior (MA). What is the next best step?
    a. Prepare the patient for an urgent cesarean section.
    b. Manually attempt to flex the fetal head.

    c. Encourage the patient to push as effectively as possible.
    d. Allow the patient to push only in the hands-and-knees position.

26. If a nuchal arm is encountered during an assisted breech birth, which of the following is the appropriate management?
    a. Exert steady downward traction on the entire fetus.
    b. Slowly rotate the infant 180 degrees to attempt to dislodge the arm.
    c. Raise the baby in a warm towel above the plane of the vagina.
    d. Sweep the arm down by hooking the elbow and pulling the arm down.

27. The most common cause of postpartum hemorrhage is:
    a. sulcus tears.
    b. episiotomy extensions to third- and fourth-degree lacerations.
    c. uterine atony.
    d. cervical lacerations.

28. The process of involution takes place over which of the following time frames?
    a. The first 6 weeks postpartum
    b. The first 24 hours postpartum
    c. The first 2 weeks postpartum
    d. The first year postpartum

29. The following is the clinical picture of your patient. The patient is a G1 P0 at 39 weeks with an uncomplicated pregnancy. The patient's labor started at 4:00 a.m. with regular contractions. The patient was admitted at 8:00 a.m. when the patient's exam was 2–3 cm/100%/–2 station, vertex, membranes intact.
    - At 12:00 p.m., the patient's exam was 3–4 cm/100%/–2, intact.
    - At 4:00 p.m., the patient's exam was 4 cm/100%/–2, intact.
    - At 7:30 p.m., the patient's exam was 5–6 cm/100%/–1, intact.
    - At 8:15 p.m., the patient ruptured membranes, producing light meconium-stained fluid.
    - At 10:00 p.m., the patient's exam was 8 cm/100%/0 station.

    Based on the information provided, at 12:00 p.m. what was the most appropriate diagnosis related to this patient's labor progress?
    a. Latent phase
    b. Protracted latent phase
    c. Unable to determine with this information
    d. Active labor

30. The following is the clinical picture of your patient. The patient is a G1 P0 at 39 weeks with an uncomplicated pregnancy. The patient's labor started at 4:00 a.m. with regular contractions. The patient was admitted at 8:00 a.m. when the patient's exam was 2–3 cm/100%/–2 station, vertex, membranes intact.
    - At 12:00 p.m., the patient's exam was 3–4 cm/100%/ –2, intact.
    - At 4:00 p.m., the patient's exam was 4 cm/100%/–2, intact.

- At 7:30 p.m., the patient's exam was 5–6 cm/100%/–1, intact.
- At 8:15 p.m., the patient ruptured membranes, producing light meconium-stained fluid.
- At 10:00 p.m., the patient's exam was 8 cm/100%/0 station.

What was the most appropriate diagnosis at 7:30 p.m.?

a. Unable to determine based on the information provided
b. Active phase of labor
c. Latent phase of labor
d. Arrest of labor in the active phase

31. The following is the clinical picture of your patient. The patient is a G1 P0 at 39 weeks with an uncomplicated pregnancy. The patient's labor started at 4:00 a.m. with regular contractions. She was admitted at 8:00 a.m. when her exam was 2–3 cm/100%/–2 station, vertex, membranes intact.

- At 12:00 p.m., the patient's exam was 3–4 cm/100%/–2, intact.
- At 4:00 p.m., the patient's exam was 4 cm/100%/–2, intact.
- At 7:30 p.m., the patient's exam was 5–6 cm/100%/–1, intact.
- At 8:15 p.m., the patient ruptured membranes, producing light meconium-stained fluid.
- At 10:00 p.m., the patient's exam was 8 cm/100%/0 station and requested something for pain because the increased pelvic pressure was intolerable.

Which of the following would be the best option indicated for pain relief at this time?

a. Nitrous oxide
b. Intravenous opioids
c. Intravenous diphenhydramine (Benadryl)
d. Spinal block

32. The following is the clinical picture of your patient: She is a G1 P0 at 39 weeks with an uncomplicated pregnancy. Her labor started at 4:00 a.m. with regular contractions. She was admitted at 8:00 a.m. when her exam was 2–3 cm/100%/–2 station, vertex, membranes intact.

- At 12:00 p.m., her exam was 3–4 cm/100%/–2, intact.
- At 4:00 p.m., her exam was 4 cm/100%/–2, intact.
- At 7:30 p.m., her exam was 5–6 cm/100%/–1, intact.
- At 8:15 p.m., she ruptured membranes, producing light meconium-stained fluid.
- At 10:00 p.m., her exam was 8 cm/100%/0 station.
- At 10:50 p.m., you notice early decelerations on the fetal monitor strip that occur with every contraction. The baseline heart rate is in the 140s with average variability.

The most likely cause of these decelerations is:

a. maternal hypotension.
b. head compression.
c. uteroplacental insufficiency.
d. fetal distress related to the meconium fluid.

33. One benefit of placing an internal scalp electrode on a fetus in labor is:

a. the ability to have continuous tracing when external monitoring is insufficient.
b. the ability to detect decelerations.

c. that it keeps the patient in bed.
d. the ability to assess variability.

34. If you are performing scalp stimulation, what is the fetal response that indicates fetal well-being?

a. An FHR deceleration to 100 bpm for 2 minutes
b. An FHR acceleration of 5 bpm over baseline for 5 seconds
c. An immediate variable FHR deceleration
d. An FHR acceleration of 15 bpm for 15 seconds

35. What is the most common position in which the fetus enters the pelvis for birth?

a. ROA
b. LOA
c. ROP
d. LOP

36. The long arc rotation is most commonly performed by babies beginning labor in which presentation?

a. LOP
b. LSA
c. ROA
d. LOA

37. In the second stage of labor, how frequently should the blood pressure of low-risk patients be checked?

a. Every 30 minutes
b. Every 2 minutes
c. Every 60 minutes
d. Every 15 minutes

38. When is the most optimal time to administer pudendal anesthesia for perineal pain relief in a multiparous patient?

a. For the repair of any laceration or episiotomy
b. When the head distends the perineum and the patient complains of the "ring of fire"
c. When the vertex is at +2
d. At approximately 8–9 cm dilated

39. What is the largest group of muscles in the pelvic musculature?

a. Levator ani
b. Pubococcygeus
c. Bulbocavernosus
d. Sphincter ani

40. A third-degree laceration is diagnosed by identification of which of the following structures?

a. Vaginal mucosa
b. Deep transverse perineal muscles
c. Rectal sphincter
d. Hymenal ring

41. The Ritgen maneuver is used to:

a. slow down the descent of the fetal head during birth.
b. control expulsion of the fetal head at the time of birth.
c. avoid lacerations or the need for an episiotomy.
d. assist in the delivery of the fetal head during extension.

42. What complication may be encountered if a placenta is delivered by the Duncan mechanism?

a. Increased perineal lacerations
b. Increased bleeding
c. Increased hemorrhoids due to extra maternal pushing effort
d. Uterine inversion

43. When diagnosed, which of the following would rule out a risk of preterm labor?
    a. Urinary tract infection
    b. Appendicitis
    c. Renal colic
    d. Heartburn

44. The FHR variability is predominantly controlled by the:
    a. parasympathetic/sympathetic nervous system.
    b. baroreceptors.
    c. chemoreceptors.
    d. central nervous system.

45. During uterine contractions, intervillous blood flow to the placenta:
    a. increases.
    b. decreases.
    c. remains unchanged.
    d. has not been studied in humans.

46. Moderate variability of the FHR is a change in how many beats per minute (bpm) from the baseline?
    a. Fewer than 2 bpm
    b. 2–6 bpm
    c. 6–25 bpm
    d. >25 bpm

47. Which of the following is associated with normal variability of the fetal heart rate?
    a. Medications
    b. Congenital cardiac anomalies of the fetus
    c. Placenta previa
    d. Fetal activity patterns

48. Your patient, who you are co-managing with your consulting physician, is 33 weeks and 4 days pregnant. The patient is admitted with premature labor, with a cervical exam of 2–3 cm/80%/–1, vertex, intact. The patient is currently on MgSO$_4$ at 3.0 g/hour with occasional contractions. During rounds, the patient reports feeling flushed and hot, lethargic, and short of breath, with this sensation usually getting better when she changes position. Which response would be best to address the patient's complaints?
    a. "These symptoms are normal with MgSO$_4$, but hopefully we will start weaning the medication today."
    b. "Because you are almost 34 weeks, we can likely discontinue the medication now."
    c. "We will evaluate your shortness of breath with a chest radiograph."
    d. "Being a little uncomfortable is so much better than giving birth to a 33-week-old infant."

49. Which of the following conditions is appropriate for intermittent fetal monitoring?
    a. Labor at 41 weeks and 1 day
    b. Thick, meconium-stained fluid
    c. Nonreactive nonstress test (NST) and now in labor
    d. IV narcotics

50. Birthing people in premature labor are given glucocorticosteroids to:
    a. help stop the uterine contractions
    b. prevent infections, especially chorioamnionitis

    c. speed the maturation of the fetal respiratory system, including the production of surfactant
    d. prevent the muscle wasting commonly seen in patients on bed rest

51. A patient, G3 P2002 at 37 weeks and 1 day, presents to the labor and delivery service with regular contractions every 2–3 minutes for 5 hours. Your vaginal exam reveals 6 cm/100%/–2, LSA position with ruptured membranes positive for light meconium. Which of the following is the best next step?
    a. Admit the patient for expectant management.
    b. Discuss the birth plan with the patient.
    c. Await a reactive tracing before making a management plan.
    d. Notify the consulting physician and prepare for a cesarean section.

52. In a complete breech presentation:
    a. one or both feet are the presenting part.
    b. both hips and knees are flexed, with buttocks presenting.
    c. the baby is flexed at the hips.
    d. the knees are the presenting part.

53. Your patient, who is 41 weeks and 5 days pregnant, presents for postdates testing, including an NST. When you assess the tracing after 20 minutes, the FHR is 140–145 bpm, there are no decelerations, and the variability is moderate, but the tracing does not meet the criteria for reactivity. Which of the following is the best next step?
    a. Admit the patient and induce labor.
    b. Begin a contraction stress test.
    c. Use the vibroacoustic stimulator.
    d. Continue the NST for another 20 minutes.

54. A patient who is at 41 weeks and 6 days' gestation is in labor, at 4 cm/100%/+1, vertex, is having contractions every 3–5 minutes for 50–70 seconds, which are moderate to palpation. The FHR baseline is still in the 140s, but the patient is having variable decelerations to the 110s with good return to baseline and average variability. Which of the following actions is contraindicated at this time?
    a. Allow the patient to get into the Jacuzzi
    b. Begin oxytocin augmentation
    c. Insert an intravenous catheter
    d. Provide expectant management

55. Engagement occurs when the:
    a. fetal head reaches the pelvic floor.
    b. widest diameter of the presenting part descends to or below the pelvic inlet.
    c. biparietal diameter is just above the pelvic inlet.
    d. head is on the perineum.

56. When an IUPC is used for the assessment of uterine contractions, the adequacy is quantified:
    a. in millimeters of mercury.
    b. as mild, moderate, and strong.
    c. in Montevideo units.
    d. in centimeters.

57. With internal monitoring of uterine contractions, which of the following levels must be achieved in 10 minutes to be considered adequate contractile strength to dilate the cervix?
    a. 80–100 mVu
    b. 80–100 mm Hg
    c. 200–250 MVU
    d. 200–250 mm Hg

58. Which of the following would represent a contraindication to the use of an IUPC?
    a. Desired birth plan
    b. Breech presentation
    c. HIV infection of the laboring patient
    d. Lack of labor progress

59. In the first stage of labor for low-risk laboring women, the interval for intermittent FHR auscultation is:
    a. 15 minutes
    b. 20 minutes
    c. 30 minutes
    d. 60 minutes

60. Of the following, which factor places a patient at risk for preterm labor?
    a. Age of the patient
    b. Nicotine patches
    c. Cervical length of 3.5 cm
    d. Sex of the fetus

61. A patient is seen in labor and delivery at 33 weeks and 1 day complaining of menstrual-type cramping for the past 3 hours. The patient denies vaginal bleeding or ruptured membranes. The fetus is active. The EFM reveals occasional uterine contractions approximately every 8–12 minutes. The FHR is 135–140 bpm. Which of the following tests would be most important in formulating a management plan?
    a. Complete blood count
    b. Cervical culture
    c. Urine culture
    d. Ultrasound

62. A patient is seen in labor and delivery at 33 weeks and 4 days reporting menstrual-type cramping for the past 5 hours. The patient denies vaginal bleeding or ruptured membranes. The fetus is active. The EFM reveals occasional uterine contractions approximately every 8–12 minutes. The FHR is 120–140 bpm. Which of the following is the best next step in the management plan for this patient?
    a. Expectant management until the lab results are back.
    b. Tocolysis
    c. Pain management
    d. Additional information is necessary to formulate the management plan.

63. Which of the following findings in a laboring person represents a risk factor for shoulder dystocia?
    a. Age over 40 years
    b. Epidural anesthesia
    c. Polyhydramnios
    d. BMI over 30

64. Which of the following presentation types is least likely to result in vaginal birth and, therefore, no longer recommended?
    a. Brow presentation
    b. Face presentation
    c. Breech presentation
    d. Vertex presentation

65. During the birth of twins, a tight nuchal cord is noted after the birth of the first twin's head. Which of the following reflects ideal cord management at this point?
    a. Use of a somersault maneuver
    b. Clamping and cutting of a nuchal cord
    c. Reducing the cord manually
    d. Collect cord blood

66. Which of the following represents a risk factor for retained placenta?
    a. Preterm delivery
    b. Multiple gestation
    c. Multiparity
    d. Postterm pregnancy

67. While repairing a first-degree laceration, the clinician notices a continual trickle of bright red blood from the vagina. As they continue their repair, the bleeding becomes slightly more brisk. What would be the next step after fundal massage in the management plan?
    a. Bimanual compression
    b. Administering 20 additional units of oxytocin via the IV
    c. Discussion with the consulting physician regarding the management plan
    d. Methylergonovine IM if the blood pressure is normotensive

68. During the second stage of labor for the high-risk patient, the fetal heart rate should be monitored:
    a. every 5 minutes.
    b. every 15 minutes.
    c. every 30 minutes.
    d. continuously.

69. A sudden bradycardia seen in the second stage of labor after an uneventful labor course and previously normal fetal heart tracing is commonly caused by:
    a. a vagal response in the fetus related to descent.
    b. fetal hypoxia related to length of labor.
    c. cord prolapse.
    d. uteroplacental insufficiency.

70. Which of the following FHR tracings are indicative of a Category III FHR tracing?
    a. A prolonged deceleration with recovery to baseline and with moderate variability
    b. Variable decelerations that become more pronounced during the second stage but with normal FHR between pushing efforts
    c. Late decelerations and an absence of variability
    d. Late decelerations with return to baseline and moderate variability between decelerations

71. The risk factor that is most predictive of a preterm birth during a current pregnancy is:
    a. uterine contractions.
    b. prior preterm labor.

c. prior preterm birth.

d. gestational hypertension.

72. Which of the following mechanisms best describes the cause of pain in the second stage of labor?
    a. Uterine muscle hypoxia with lactic acid build-up
    b. A full bladder being compressed by the fetus
    c. Pressure on the bony pelvis, urethra, bladder, and rectum
    d. Fundal uterine displacement and extension of the fetal lie

73. Hemodynamic changes during the initial postpartum period include:
    a. elevated cardiac output for as long as 48 hours after the birth.
    b. decreased white blood count (WBC) during the first 72 hours after the birth.

c. elevated blood pressure for 48 hours after the birth.

d. decreased urine output for the first 24 hours after the birth.

74. In the initial newborn period, a 10-minute Apgar score is performed:
    a. routinely.
    b. if the 1-minute Apgar score is less than 7.
    c. if the 5-minute Apgar score is less than 7.
    d. if the combined Apgar score at 1 and 5 minutes is less than 16.

75. The bluish discoloration of the baby's hands and feet within the first 24–48 hours after birth is:
    a. acrocyanosis.
    b. circumoral cyanosis.
    c. central cyanosis.
    d. Mongolian spots.

Answers with Rationales

1. **b.** Perform a sterile speculum exam to rule out rupture of membranes versus vaginal infection.
   A sterile speculum examination should be performed if ruptured membranes are suspected.

2. **a.** placenta previa
   With placenta previa, painless vaginal bleeding occurs 70%–80% of the time.

3. **b.** nifedipine
   Recent research has determined that calcium channel blockers are most effective for tocolysis.

4. **b.** A 28-year-old G1, smoker, twin gestation, spontaneous rupture of membranes at 37 weeks
   Tobacco use is a significant risk factor for placental abruption.

5. **d.** Preterm birth
   Preterm labor and birth are major risks in multifetal gestations.

6. **c.** Descent, flexion, internal rotation, extension, restitution, external rotation
   The cardinal movements of labor are descent, flexion, internal rotation, extension, restitution, and external rotation.

7. **c.** extension
   The fetal head is born by the process of extension.

8. **b.** greater than or equal to 1,000 mL regardless of method of birth
   As per ACOG guidelines, the current definition of PPH is greater than or equal to 1,000 mL regardless of method of birth, or blood loss accompanied by signs or symptoms of hypovolemia within 24 hours after the birth process

9. **d.** Five-minute scoring has a relationship to neonatal morbidity and mortality.
   The 5-minute Apgar score is more predictive of neonatal morbidity and/or mortality than is the 1-minute score.

10. **d.** shoulder dystocia
    Gestational diabetes is one of the risk factors for shoulder dystocia.

11. **b.** in latent labor
    The latent phase of labor is from the onset of labor until cervical dilation reaches 4–6 cm.

12. **b.** Have the patient ambulate for 2 hours and then reassess the patient.
    Ambulation for 2 hours allows the clinician to evaluate for cervical change (definition of labor). The patient's perception of need for admission to the birthing facility is also important in clinical decision-making.

13. **b.** the latent phase of labor
    The latent phase of labor is from the onset of labor until cervical dilation reaches 4–6 cm.

14. **b.** a prolonged latent phase of labor
    The patient is exhausted from the abnormal latent phase.

15. **d.** Offer medication of morphine 10 mg IM so she can get some sleep and potentially correct this dysfunctional labor pattern.
    Morphine is quite effective for patient exhaustion due to a prodromal/prolonged latent phase of labor.

16. **a.** November 11
    Naegele's rule is to add 7 days to the first day of the last menstrual period and subtract 3 months.

17. **b.** sacrum
    The sacrum is the denominator for breech presentations.

18. **b.** anterior asynclitism
    Anterior asynclitism is noted when the sagittal suture is closer to the sacrum.

19. **d.** to encourage movement and position change
    Movement and position change can encourage the fetus to descend into a favorable position for birth.

20. **a.** Variable decelerations
    Variable decelerations are abrupt in nature with a decrease in FHR from a baseline of ≥15 bpm lasting ≥15 seconds but <2 minutes.

21. **d.** suboccipitobregmatic
    When the fetal head meets the resistance of the pelvic floor, flexion is encouraged so that the most favorable diameter (suboccipitobregmatic) presents.

22. **c.** acceptable for the fetal evaluation of certain patients
Intermittent auscultation is an acceptable method of assessing fetal well-being in low-risk patients.

23. **a.** Discuss the indications for episiotomy and process for obtaining obtain.
Although episiotomy is no longer a routine procedure, there are specific indications for its use, which should be discussed with the patient.

24. **b.** LMT
LMT is face presentation—the denominator is the mentum.

25. **c.** Encourage the patient to push as effectively as possible.
More than 90% of anterior face presentations deliver vaginally without complications.

26. **d.** Sweep the arm down by hooking the elbow and pulling the arm down.
It is important to remain calm and guide the arm in a physiologic range of motion.

27. **c.** uterine atony
Uterine atony is the most common cause of PPH.

28. **a.** The first 6 weeks postpartum
Normal postpartum involution takes a full 6 weeks to be complete.

29. **a.** Latent phase
The latent phase of labor is from the onset of labor until cervical dilation reaches 4–6 cm.

30. **b.** Active phase of labor
The active phase of labor is from cervical dilation of 4–6 cm until complete dilation.

31. **a.** Nitrous oxide
Nitrous oxide is appropriate for use in second stage and can be controlled by the patient. Intravenous opioids should not be used when birth is anticipated within an hour because of the risk for respiratory depression in the newborn. IV Benadryl would not be effective for pain management and may also run the risk of respiratory depression in the newborn. A spinal block is not indicated for laboring patients.

32. **b.** head compression
Early decelerations are due to a vagal response from head compression and are considered benign.

33. **a.** the ability to have continuous tracing when external monitoring is insufficient
An internal scalp electrode allows for accurate, continuous fetal monitoring when an external monitor is not producing reliable continuous tracing.

34. **d.** An FHR acceleration of 15 bpm for 15 seconds
An FHR acceleration indicates a fetal pH ≥7.20.

35. **b.** LOA
LOA is the more common position for the fetus to enter the pelvis for birth.

36. **a.** LOP
Most babies who are in the posterior position undergo a long arc rotation to an anterior position before birth.

37. **d.** Every 15 minutes

Blood pressure should be evaluated every 15 minutes in the second stage of labor for low-risk patients.

38. **d.** At approximately 8–9 cm dilated
The optimal timing for administration of pudendal anesthesia is just before complete dilation in a multiparous patient because it provides coverage for the birth as well as any repair needed.

39. **a.** Levator ani
The largest group of muscles in the pelvic musculature is the levator ani.

40. **c.** Rectal sphincter
A second-degree laceration involves the vaginal mucosa, posterior fourchette, perineal muscles, and perineal skin.

41. **d.** assist in the delivery of the fetal head during extension
The Ritgen maneuver can be used to expedite the delivery of the fetal head when necessary.

42. **b.** Increased bleeding
Bleeding is more visible and likely to be increased because of incomplete separation of the placenta.

43. **d.** Heartburn
The other conditions—urinary tract infection, appendicitis, and renal colic—may mimic the signs and symptoms of preterm labor, whereas heartburn does not.

44. **a.** parasympathetic/sympathetic nervous system.
FHR variability is controlled predominantly by the autonomic nervous system (parasympathetic/sympathetic).

45. **b.** decreases
During a uterine contraction, the intramyometrial pressure exceeds that of the spiral arteries, resulting in decreased intervillous blood flow.

46. **c.** 6–25 bpm
Moderate variability is defined by an amplitude range of 6–25 bpm.

47. **c.** Placenta previa
The other choices—medications, congenital cardiac anomalies, and fetal activity—are known factors that influence FHR variability.

48. **c.** "We will evaluate your shortness of breath with a chest radiograph."
Shortness of breath is not a typical side effect of magnesium sulfate and should be investigated.

49. **a.** Labor at 41 weeks and 1 day
Forty-one weeks and 1 day is normal gestation (i.e., not preterm or postdates). The other choices entail risk factors that would necessitate continuous fetal monitoring.

50. **c.** speed the maturation of the fetal respiratory system, including the production of surfactant.
Corticosteroid administration accelerates fetal lung maturity.

51. **d.** Notify the consulting physician and prepare for a cesarean section.
LSA indicates that the fetus is in breech presentation. At 6 cm, delivery is not imminent; thus, a cesarean birth is indicated.

52. **b.** both hips and knees are flexed, with buttocks presenting
A complete breech has both hips and knees flexed (like a cannonball dive) and is the most common type of breech presentation.

53. **d.** Continue the NST for another 20 minutes.
The fetus has sleep/wake cycles, so nonreactivity may be due to fetal sleep. Extending the time of the test is common practice to account for this possibility.

54. **a.** Allow the patient to get into the Jacuzzi
Variable decelerations are an indication for continuous monitoring, which cannot be accomplished in the Jacuzzi.

55. **b.** widest diameter of the presenting part descends to or below the pelvic inlet
The widest diameter of the fetal head is the biparietal diameter. The definition of engagement is when the biparietal diameter has cleared the pelvic inlet. Once the head is engaged, the leading edge of the fetal head is at the level of the ischial spines (0 station).

56. **c.** in Montevideo units
Whereas the IUPC quantifies the strength of the contractions in millimeters of mercury, adequacy is determined by the average number of Montevideo units (MVU) over a 10-minute period.

57. **c.** 200–250 MVU
Adequate contraction strength is indicated by 200–250 MVU over a 10-minute period.

58. **c.** HIV infection of the laboring person
Attempts should be made to minimize possible transmission of maternal blood to the fetus, which could occur with the placement of an IUPC.

59. **c.** 30 minutes
This is the low-risk protocol for auscultation of the FHR.

60. **a.** Age of the patient
Patient age over 40 years is an independent risk factor for preterm birth and is found to be iatrogenic in nature. The other risk factors do not place a patient at risk for preterm labor.

61. **c.** Urine culture
A urinary tract infection can mimic—and is a risk factor for—preterm labor.

62. **d.** Additional information is necessary to formulate the management plan.
The information listed is incomplete to formulate a management plan.

63. **d.** BMI over 30

A BMI over 30 is a risk factor for a macrosomic infant. Such infants are at greater risk for shoulder dystocia.

64. **c.** Breech presentation
Vaginal delivery of breech presentations should be reserved only for breeches that present emergently and when birth is essentially inevitable. Brow presentations often convert to vertex as labor advances and the head encounters the pelvic floor.

65. **a.** Use of a somersault maneuver
If a nuchal cord is present, it should not be cut, and birth should be attempted with the cord intact.

66. **a.** Preterm delivery
Preterm birth is a predisposing factor for retained placenta.

67. **d.** Methylergonovine IM if the blood pressure is normotensive
Methylergonovine causes sustained, tetanic uterine contractions but is contraindicated in hypertensive patients. Bimanual compression would be indicated if bleeding is very brisk—for example, like "a fire hose."

68. **d.** continuously
Continuously monitoring in the second stage, per ACOG's recommendations for the high-risk patient.

69. **a.** a vagal response in the fetus related to descent
With rapid descent, a vagal response can occur.

70. **c.** Late decelerations and an absence of variability
A Category III tracing shows an absence of FHR variability.

71. **c.** prior preterm birth
Prior preterm birth is a very strong risk factor for subsequent preterm birth.

72. **c.** Pressure on the bony pelvis, urethra, bladder, and rectum
The descent of the fetus causes pressure on pelvic structures.

73. **a.** elevated cardiac output for as long as 48 hours after the birth
Within the first hours post-delivery, cardiac output increases from 60% to 80%.

74. **c.** if the 5-minute Apgar score is less than 7
Apgar scores are performed routinely at 1 and 5 minutes, with a 10-minute Apgar scoring usually performed only if the 5-minute Apgar score is less than 7.

75. **a.** acrocyanosis.
Bluish discoloration of the baby's hands and feet, known as acrocyanosis, is normal in the first 24–48 hours after birth.

Bibliography

American College of Obstetricians and Gynecologists (ACOG). Committee on practice Bulletins—Obstetrics. (2019). ACOG practice bulletin no. 203: Chronic hypertension in pregnancy. *Obstetrics and Gynecology, 133*(1), e26–e50. https://doi.org/10.1097/AOG.0000000000003020

Cunningham, F. G., Leveno, K., Dashe, J. S., Hoffman, B., Spong, C. Y., & Casey, B. (Eds.). (2022). *Williams obstetrics* (26th ed.). McGraw-Hill.

Friedman, E. A. (1972). An objective approach to the diagnosis and management of abnormal labor. *Bulletin of the New York Academy of Medicine, 48*(6), 842–858.

Landon, M. B., Galan, H. L., Jauniaux, E. R. M., Driscoll, D. A., Berghella, V., Grobman, W. A., Kilpatrick, S. J., & Cahill, A. G. (Eds.). (2021). *Obstetrics: Normal and problem pregnancies* (8th ed.). Mosby Elsevier.

Macones, G. A., Hankins, G. D., Spong, C. Y., Hauth, J., & Moore, T. (2008). The 2008 National Institute of Child Health and Human Development workshop report on electronic fetal monitoring: Update on definitions, interpretation, and research guidelines. *Obstetrics & Gynecology, 112*(3), 661–666.

Phillippi, J. & Kantrowitz-Gordon, I. (Eds.). (2025). *Varney's midwifery* (7th ed.). Jones & Bartlett Learning.

Philpott, R. H., Castle, W. M. (1972) Cervicographs in the management of labour in primigravidas. *Br J Obstet and Gynaecol, 72*, 592.

Posner, G. D., Dy, J., Black, A. Y., Jones, G. D., & Dy, J. (2022). *Oxorn–Foote human labor and birth* (7th ed.). McGraw-Hill.

Tharpe, N., Farley, C., & Jordan, R. G. (2022). *Clinical practice guidelines for midwifery and women's health* (6th ed.). Jones & Bartlett Learning.

Wambach, K., & Spencer, B. (2021). *Breastfeeding and human lactation* (6th ed.). Jones & Bartlett Learning.

Zhang, J., Troendle, J., Mikolajczyk, R., Sundarum, R., Beaver, J., & Fraser, W. (2010). The natural history of the normal first stage of labor. *Obstetrics & Gynecology, 1154*, 705–710.

Zipori, Y., Grunwald, O., Ginsberg, Y., Beloosesky, R., & Weiner, Z. (2019). The impact of extending the second stage of labor to prevent primary cesarean delivery on maternal and neonatal outcomes. *American journal of obstetrics and gynecology, 220*(2), 191–e1.

CHAPTER 9

Postpartum and Lactation

Jamille Nagtalon-Ramos
Michele LaMarr-Suggs

Postpartum

- Also known as the "puerperium" or "fourth trimester"
- Traditionally defined as the first 6 weeks after birth; however, the time frame to recovery and transition to parenting is much longer (up to 1 year postpartum).
- Newer models have been adapted for postpartum women/individuals to access care sooner than traditional models.

Initial Postpartum Period

Review of Patient History

- Pregnancy highlights
  1. Gravidity/parity
  2. Obstetric history
  3. Pertinent medical history
  4. Antepartal issues/problems
  5. Pertinent pregnancy diagnostic tests
     a. Blood type and Rh status
     b. Rubella titer status
     c. Hepatitis B status
     d. HIV status
     e. Rapid plasma reagin (RPR)
     f. Genetic testing
     g. Group B *Streptococcus* (GBS) status
- Labor information
  1. Gestational age at delivery
  2. Presentation to care
     a. Rupture of membranes; if so, what time
     b. Active labor versus induction versus augmentation
     c. Induction of labor and indication (e.g., hypertension, diabetes, post-term)
  3. Complications during labor
     a. Dysfunctional labor
        (1) Prolonged labor

        (2) Precipitous labor
        (3) Shoulder dystocia
        (4) Labor dystocia
        (5) Tachysystole
     b. Chorioamnionitis—treated with antibiotics
        (1) Type
        (2) Number of doses
     c. Uterine rupture
     d. Placental abnormalities
     e. Prolapsed cord
  4. Type of anesthesia/analgesia
- Birth information
  1. Type of birth
     a. Type of delivery
     b. Type of episiotomy/laceration
     c. Type of operative birth
     d. Reason for interventions
     e. Quantitative blood loss (QBL) or estimated blood loss (EBL) if QBL unavailable
  2. Sex of infant
  3. Weight of infant
  4. Apgar scores
  5. Method of feeding

Postpartum Assessment

Early Postpartum Period

- General
  1. Normal—tired but happy
  2. Deviation from normal—unhappy, dissatisfied
- Vital signs
  1. Temperature
     a. Stabilizes during the first 24 hours postpartum
     b. Normal range—98.6 to 100.4°F
     c. Deviation from normal
        (1) Greater than 100.4°F
        (2) Consider differentials—infection, pulmonary embolism

2. Pulse
   a. Normal range—65 to 100 bpm
   b. Deviation from normal
      (1) Greater than 100 bpm
      (2) Consider differentials—infection, increased blood loss, pulmonary embolism
3. Respiratory rate
   a. Normal range—12 to 16/min
   b. If <12/min, consider differentials—overuse of narcotic pain medication, atelectasis, pneumonia
   c. If >16/min, consider differentials—anxiety, pain
4. Blood pressure
   a. Transient increase in blood pressure of as much as 5% of baseline in first 4 days after delivery
   b. If blood pressure >140/90 mm Hg, evaluate for postpartum hypertensive disorder
   c. If blood pressure <90/60 mm Hg, evaluate the causes of hypotension
      (1) Blood loss
      (2) Medication reaction
5. Neurologic
   a. Normal—oriented to person, place, time
   b. Deviation from normal—disoriented, excessive sedation, sudden onset or severe headache
6. Cardiovascular
   a. Normal—no chest pain, regular rate, and rhythm
   b. Deviation from normal—chest pain, palpitations, tachycardia
7. Lungs
   a. Normal—no shortness of breath, able to breathe without difficulties, clear to auscultation
   b. Deviations from normal—shortness of breath; adventitious sound upon auscultation
8. Breasts
   a. Normal
      (1) Nipples may be sore from nursing but not painful
      (2) Nipples erect when stimulated
      (3) Colostrum and breast fullness for 3–5 days
   b. Deviation from normal
      (1) Painful, cracked, bruised, blistered, bleeding nipples
      (2) Erythema
      (3) No breast filling by day 5
9. Abdomen/gastrointestinal
   a. Normal
      (1) Eating and drinking without difficulties
      (2) Return of bowel movement 2–3 days postpartum
      (3) Presence of bowel sounds
      (4) Decreased muscle tone
      (5) Diastasis recti is expected
      (6) Firm fundus and midline; level of fundus appropriate according to process of involution
      (7) Surgical scar is well-approximated, nontender, and without signs and symptoms of infection
   b. Deviation from normal
      (1) Nausea and vomiting, abdominal pain, constipation or diarrhea, no flatus, absent bowel sounds
      (2) Distended abdomen, unable to palpate the uterus
      (3) Fundal height not midline and level increasing not according to postpartum day
      (4) Surgical scar not well-approximated, showing signs of infection and dehiscence
10. Urinary
    a. Normal
       (1) Voiding spontaneously without difficulties
       (2) Diuresis
       (3) Mild external burning, retention, incontinence, lack of sensation or urge to void—common in the first 2 days
       (4) Bladder nondistended and nonpalpable
    b. Deviation from normal
       (1) Dysuria
       (2) Persistent retention or incontinence
       (3) Distended bladder
       (4) Costovertebral angle tenderness
11. Perineum
    a. Normal
       (1) Mild erythema, bruising, edema
       (2) Laceration/episiotomy repair is well-approximated without drainage; mild soreness and tenderness at sight of repair.
       (3) Lochia decreasing in amount each day (mean duration 30 days) and color (rubra→ serosa→ rubra)
       (4) Lochia without foul odor
    b. Deviations from normal
       (1) Worsening perineal tenderness, erythema, edema, bruising
       (2) Presence of hematoma
       (3) Laceration/episiotomy repair is not well-approximated, showing signs of separation
       (4) Malodorous lochia; excessive amounts with clots, soaking pads every 1–2 hours
12. Anus
    a. Normal—hemorrhoids may be present, pink in appearance
    b. Deviation from normal—hemorrhoids deep blue or purple
13. Lower extremities
    a. Normal
       (1) Muscle soreness from positioning during labor
       (2) Bilateral, symmetric mild edema
       (3) Normal reflexes
    b. Deviation from normal
       (1) Unilateral leg pain
       (2) Unilateral calf tenderness
       (3) One leg more edematous than the other

Anatomic and Physiologic Changes

- Uterus
  1. Involution—process of the uterus returning to the prepregnant state
     a. Involves three steps: starts at the time of birth to 6 weeks postpartum
        (1) Contraction of the uterus

(2) Autolysis of myometrial cells

(3) Regeneration of the epithelium

b. Results from reduction in cell size, not reduction in cell number

2. Location of the uterus is determined with respect to the umbilicus

a. Descends about 1 cm per day

b. Noted as "fundus at umbilicus" or "fundus at U"

c. Upon descent, noted as "fundus at U-1"—indicates that the fundus is located at 1 cm below the umbilicus

d. Location of the fundus should be the midline of the abdomen; if displaced to the side, may indicate sub-involution, likely due to a full bladder

e. Immediately after delivery, the uterus contracts to about the size of a grapefruit, located halfway between the umbilicus and symphysis pubis

f. By 12 hours postbirth, uterus is at the level of the umbilicus

g. By 2 weeks, no longer palpated abdominally

h. By 6 weeks, returns to slightly larger than prepregnant size

- Lochia

1. Consists of the breakdown of myometrial placental bed, eschar, and decidual cells

2. Three stages of discharge

a. Rubra

(1) First 3–7 days

(2) Red or red-brown

(3) Fleshy odor

(4) Contains a superficial layer of decidua that has sloughed off the uterus, debris (e.g., cellular remains from vernix, lanugo, and meconium, and necrotic remains of the placenta)

b. Serosa

(1) From day 14 to 21 postpartum

(2) Pinkish-brown color

(3) Serous to serosanguinous secretion

(4) Discharge contains blood, cervical mucus, erythrocytes, leukocytes, decidual tissue

c. Alba

(1) Until cessation of flow in about 4–6 weeks postpartum

(2) Yellowish-to-white discharge

(3) Flow increases with additional activity initially but decreases progressively over the puerperium

(4) Total amount—150 to 400 cc

- Cervix, vagina, and perineum

1. Cervix

a. Immediately after a vaginal birth, appears edematous, dilated 3–4 cm, and bruised; may have lacerations

b. Days 2–3 postpartum, continues to be dilated 2–3 cm

c. By day 7, dilation down to 1 cm

d. By 4 weeks, cervix is no longer dilated

e. Multiparous—at the completion of involution, external os does not return to its prepregnant appearance; remains somewhat wider with a transverse opening, resembling a fish mouth

2. Vagina

a. Initially edematous, relaxed, sometimes bruised with decreased tone

b. By 3–4 weeks postpartum, rugae return, edema, vascularity, and bruising decrease

c. By 6–10 weeks postpartum, vaginal epithelium

d. Decreased lubrication; can lead to pain during sexual intercourse, especially in a lactating person

3. Perineum

a. Edematous with decreased tone immediately after birth

b. Laceration and episiotomy repair should be well-approximated

c. Skin should appear healed at 7 days with only linear scarring at 6 weeks

- Breasts

1. Colostrum is produced upon the birth of the baby; may even have colostrum production during the third trimester

2. Engorgement occurs approximately 72 hours after birth

a. Human milk production begins in the upper-outer milk glands

b. Filling then occurs medially and inferiorly

c. Distention and stasis of vascular and lymphatic circulation cause engorgement as the ducts, lobules, and alveoli fill with milk

3. Milk ejection reflex ("let-down reflex") develops within the first 1–2 weeks

- Hematologic

1. Within the first hours postbirth, cardiac output increases by 60%–80%

2. Over the first 48 hours, as diuresis occurs, plasma volume decreases; cardiac output normalizes by 2 weeks

3. Transient bradycardia may occur in the first 1–2 days postpartum

4. Pulse elevated during pregnancy and may continue to be elevated for up to an hour postbirth

5. Can have transient leukocytosis in the initial 48 hours

6. Pregnancy-related hematologic changes usually return to baseline by 12 weeks postpartum.

- Renal system changes

1. Diuresis occurs within the first 5 days as a result of extravascular fluid shifts

2. Bladder can be hypotonic and edematous immediately after the birth; resolves within 24 hours

3. Prolonged labor, trauma to the vulva, urethra, or bladder, use of anesthesia during cesarean section may result in urinary retention

- Weight loss

1. Caloric intake should at least be 1,800 kcal/day; should be adjusted according to the level of activity of the postpartum patient, whether the patient is lactating, and if the patient is breastfeeding/chestfeeding a singleton or multiples

2. The recommended weight loss after the first month postbirth is a maximum of 4.5 lb/month

3. Exercise can be resumed gradually after delivery depending on the mode of delivery with the absence of medical complications

- Gastrointestinal changes
  1. Peristalsis decreased in first 24 hours; increases the risk of ileus after cesarean birth
  2. Liver enzymes, including aspartate transaminase (AST) and alanine aminotransferase (ALT), return to prepregnant values within 2 weeks
- Abdominal changes
  1. Diastasis recti found in 75%–80% of postpartum women/postpartum patients—if diastasis after the postpartum period, future pregnancies will lack sufficient abdominal support, leading to back pain
  2. Striae are common in most postpartum women/persons
- Endocrine
  1. Lactating/Breastfeeding/Chestfeeding
     a. Lactation is stimulated and prolactin and oxytocin secreted
     b. By negative feedback mechanism, ovulation and menstruation are inhibited by increased prolactin and resulting estrogen suppression
     c. Resumption of menses is variable with supplementation or food introduction
        (1) Generally, ovulation occurs 14–30 days after weaning
        (2) First menses 14 days later
        (3) Mean time to ovulation is 190 days
        (4) If exclusively breastfeeding/chestfeeding, there is a 1%–3% chance of ovulation within the first 6 months postpartum
  2. Nonlactating/Nonbreastfeeding/nonchestfeeding
     a. Prolactin levels fall after initial engorgement
     b. Hormonal shifts to stimulate ovulation begin approximately 3–4 weeks postpartum
     c. First menses at 6–8 weeks postpartum, 70% by 12 weeks

Diagnostic Tests

- Complete blood count
  1. Typically ordered for postoperative patients, patients who had complications intrapartum or in the immediate postpartum period (e.g., hemorrhage), or patients who are symptomatic
  2. Commonly performed the first morning after birth
  3. Acute anemia (Hgb <9 g/dL or 3g Hgb from baseline/prebirth Hgb level) and/or if the patient becomes hemodynamically unstable
- Cord blood testing for blood type, Rh, and Coombs's test
- Kleihauer–Betke screen if Rh negative

Immunizations

- Anti-Rho(D) immune globulin (RhoGAM)—give within 72 hours of birth, if the mother's Rh status is negative and the infant is positive
- Rubella—without evidence of immunity to rubella, offer measles/mumps/rubella (MMR) vaccine prior to discharge
- Tetanus/diphtheria/acellular pertussis (Tdap)
  1. If not received during pregnancy, offer Tdap vaccine before discharge; no minimum interval between receipt of Tdap and of the last tetanus/diphtheria (Td) booster
  2. Immunizing the mother with Tdap will help protect the newborn during the first few months of life when the newborn is most vulnerable to pertussis
- Varicella
  1. Without evidence of immunity to varicella, offer varicella vaccine prior to discharge; second dose should be given 6–8 weeks after the first dose
  2. This vaccine contains a live virus; postpartum patients should be counseled to avoid pregnancy for 4 weeks after the last dose
- Influenza—depending on the season, offer influenza vaccine prior to discharge
- Human papillomavirus (HPV)
  1. Postpartum patients ages 9 through 26 years (can be given up to age 45) who have not completed a primary series should receive three doses of HPV vaccine at 0, 2, and 6 months
  2. If the HPV series was started prior to pregnancy, the series can be completed postpartum without repeating the initial dose(s)
  3. HPV vaccines can and should be given to breastfeeding/chestfeeding women/individuals 26 years and younger who have not previously been vaccinated
- COVID-19
  1. Recommended for all pregnant individuals who were not vaccinated prior to pregnancy.
  2. Pregnant and recently pregnant people up to 6 weeks postpartum should receive a bivalent mRNA COVID-19 vaccine booster dose following the completion of their last COVID-19 primary vaccine dose or monovalent booster.
  3. COVID-19 vaccines are recommended for postpartum and lactating individuals who were not vaccinated prior to or during pregnancy

Postpartum Discomforts

- Involutional pain
  1. Likely to increase in intensity with each subsequent birth
  2. Increases with nursing
  3. Nonpharmacologic relief
     a. Maintain empty bladder and bowels
     b. Relaxation and breathing techniques
     c. Changing positions, sitting up, walking, applying heat, using an abdominal support binder, lying flat on the abdomen
  4. Pharmacologic relief—acetaminophen, ibuprofen
  5. Opioids such as codeine—use with caution because some people are ultra-metabolizers, which puts their infants at risk for respiratory depression due to rapid maternal conversion of codeine to morphine
- Diuresis—maintain fluids to prevent dehydration
- Breast engorgement
  1. Initiate breastfeeding/chestfeeding early and often
  2. Assess that the infant is positioned correctly and properly latched
  3. At times, infants are unable to latch on to severely engorged breasts

4. Instruct the patient to express a small amount of milk manually before each feeding to soften the areola and allow the infant to latch properly
5. The patient can use a breast pump to assist with softening the breasts before feeding by releasing enough milk for the infant to be able to latch on to the mother's breasts
6. Avoid excessive pumping—increases breast milk production and worsens the engorgement
7. Supportive brassiere
8. Warm compress or a warm shower right before feeding
9. If bottle feeding, tight brassiere, ice packs, analgesics, reassurance about time limitation, cold cabbage leaves in brassiere for comfort

- Perineal pain
  1. Evaluate by REEDA (Redness, Edema, Ecchymosis, Discharge, Approximation)
  2. Topical medications/treatments
     a. Witch hazel pads
     b. Dibucaine, benzocaine
     c. Ice packs for the first 24 hours
     d. Sitz baths after 24 hours
     e. Topical anesthetics
     f. Squirt bottle usage when toileting
- Constipation
  1. Risk factors
     a. Lack of ambulation in labor and postpartum period (especially after cesarean/operative delivery)
     b Decreased intestinal peristalsis due to anesthesia
     c. Narcotic use for pain relief
  2. Increase fluids and fiber; stool softener
  3. Encourage frequent ambulation
  4. Laxatives, if needed
- Hemorrhoids
  1. Prevention with bowel regimen of scheduled use of stool softeners to avoid constipation
  2. Avoid straining when moving bowels
  3. Ice packs
  4. Topical anesthetics
  5. Referral if thrombosed

Postpartum Mental Health and Well-Being

Psychological Response to Childbearing

- Positive reactions
  1. Sense of achievement in giving birth
  2. Sense of empowerment and strength
  3. Thrill of a new baby
- Negative reactions
  1. Sense of loss regarding individual self
  2. Feeling of mistrust of body if unable to complete the birth process or if the birth was premature
  3. Feeling of disappointment if labor and delivery did not go as planned
  4. Feeling of frustration if having great difficulty with breastfeeding/chestfeeding

Bonding and Attachment with Infant

- Bonding is different from attachment
  1. Reva Rubin introduced the concept in the 1960s
  2. Bonding is the connection between mother to infant
  3. Most studies refer to this maternal–infant bond as an affective, behavioral, and chemical link
  4. Bonding theory states that to achieve optimal development outcomes, a "sensitive period" of bonding between mother and infant should be allowed in the immediate postpartum period; this sensitive period means close contact is necessary and avoidance of separation is a goal
  5. Early skin-to-skin contact at birth or soon afterward promotes maternal–infant bonding
- Attachment
  1. Mother infant interaction, typically face-to-face, skin-to-skin
  2. Infant's attachment to mother is developed through the mother's responsiveness to the infant's needs

Postpartum Blues and Depression

- Postpartum blues
  1. Affects as many as 80% of all postpartum individuals
  2. Begins within 3–5 days of birth; concurrent with profound hormonal shifts
  3. Very labile emotions (giddiness through sadness and crying); usually defy explanation
  4. Generally, time-limited over 1–2 weeks
  5. Supportive, sensitive care is usually all that is required
- Postpartum depression
  1. Prevalence: Approximately 6.5%–12%; may be higher in lower- and middle-income countries
  2. *Diagnostic and Statistical Manual of Mental Disorders* (*DSM-5*) defines a major depressive disorder: "with peripartum onset or onset of mood symptoms occurs during pregnancy or within 4 weeks following delivery"
  3. Clinical practice and research—define postpartum depression as occurring any time within 4 weeks after childbirth, or 3, 6, or 12 months after childbirth
  4. Risk factors
     a. History of mood and anxiety problems, particularly untreated depression and anxiety during pregnancy
     b. Likely rapid decline and shift of hormones in postpartum period
     c. Genetic
     d. Social factors—intimate-partner violence, prior abuse, lack of social support, negative life events, single parenting, poor relationship status,
     e. Difficulty getting pregnant
     f. Breastfeeding/chestfeeding issues
     g. Adolescent pregnancy
     h. Multiple gestation
     i. Preterm (before 37 weeks) labor and birth
     j. Pregnancy or birth complications/traumatic birth experiences
  5. Symptoms

a. Onset of symptoms around 4–6 weeks; generally worsen over time
b. Symptoms are the same as for major depression in a non-postpartum individual
   (1) Sleep disturbance
   (2) Crying more than usual
   (3) Feeling overwhelmed
   (4) Anxiety
   (5) Irritability
   (6) Anger
   (7) Withdrawing from loved ones
   (8) Feeling disconnected from the infant
   (9) Unable to perform activities of daily living
c. Symptoms can be incapacitating to patients
d. Preoccupation and obsession with the infant's health
e. Can have suicidal, infanticidal, and/or homicidal thoughts or behavior
f. Apathy toward self and/or the infant
g. Symptoms do not improve over time; more likely to worsen
6. Screening
   a. Screen all postpartum individuals for depression
   b. Utilize validated tools—Edinburgh Postnatal Depression Scale (EPDS)
   c. Rule out other illnesses or factors that may cause similar symptoms as postpartum depression
      (1) Postpartum thyroiditis
      (2) Anemia
      (3) Infection
      (4) Sleep deprivation
7. Diagnostic criteria as per *DSM-5*
   a. At least one of the following two symptoms:
      (1) Depressed mood
      (2) Loss of interest or pleasure
   b. In addition, four or more of the following symptoms:
      (1) Depressed mood most of the day, nearly every day (e.g., feels sad, empty, hopeless)
      (2) Marked diminished interest or pleasure in all, or almost all, activities
      (3) Significant unintentional weight loss or decrease or increase in appetite
      (4) Insomnia or hypersomnia
      (5) Psychomotor agitation
      (6) Fatigue or loss of energy
      (7) Feelings of worthlessness or excessive or inappropriate guilt
      (8) Diminished ability to think or concentrate
      (9) Suicidal thoughts or behavior, with or without a plan for attempting suicide
8. Consult
   a. Psychiatry team for proper diagnosis, management, treatment of psychiatric illness
   b. Treatment/management
      (1) Ensure the safety of postpartum patient and infant
      (2) Psychosocial strategies including peer support and counseling
      (3) Complementary and alternative therapies—rigorous evidence has not shown efficacy of these methods

         (a) Omega-3 fatty acids
         (b) Folate
         (c) St. John's wort
         (d) Bright-light therapy
         (e) Exercise
         (f) Massage
         (g) Acupuncture
      (4) Pharmacotherapy
         (a) Selective serotonin reuptake inhibitor (SSRI) as a first-line treatment
         (b) Most SSRIs pass into human milk but are usually compatible with breastfeeding/chestfeeding healthy, full-term infant
         (c) Severe depression may indicate need for benzodiazepine agents

Postpartum Psychosis

- Prevalence—1 to 2 cases per 1,000 births
- Symptoms
   1. Disorganized thinking, bizarre behavior, and speech
   2. Hallucinations with auditory or visual perceptual disturbances
   3. Delusions
- Psychiatric emergency
   1. Need psychiatry team for management of acute episode
   2. Usually requires hospitalization
   3. Patient may be a danger to self, infant, or others
   4. Once the patient is stable, coordination between obstetric providers, nursing, and psychiatry is essential for the patient's recovery

Grief

- Can be related to losing a pregnancy, losing a loved one around the time of pregnancy, birth, or during the immediate postpartum period, having a viable fetus/infant but not meeting expectations (i.e., congenital anomalies or organic cause, such as postpartum depression)
- Stages of grief (Elizabeth Kübler-Ross model)
   1. Denial
   2. Anger
   3. Bargaining
   4. Depression
   5. Acceptance
- Other models of grief are also available

Postpartum Contraception

- Factors to consider when discussing contraceptive options
   1. Return to ovulation
      a. Nonbreastfeeding/chestfeeding patients—around 39 days postpartum
      b. Breastfeeding/chestfeeding patients—varies depending on frequency and duration of breastfeeding/chestfeeding

2. Return to sexual activity—even though clinicians commonly recommend complete pelvic rest for 4–6 weeks, studies have shown that 50% of postpartum patients have resumed sexual activity by the postpartum visit
3. Hypercoagulable state
   a. Postpartum patients continue to be in a state of hypercoagulability for 3–4 weeks after birth as a physiologic adaptive mechanism to prevent postpartum hemorrhage
   b. Estrogen-containing contraceptive methods should be avoided during this early postpartum period
4. Lactation status
   a. Impact of hormonal contraception on lactation is controversial
   b. Combined hormonal contraceptives (those containing estrogen) are typically avoided in the first 21 days

- U.S. Medical Eligibility Criteria for Postpartum Contraception (**Table 9-1**)
- onhormonal forms of contraception
   1. Barrier methods
      a. Cervical cap/diaphragm—cannot be fit until involution is complete
      b. Male and female condoms—can be used immediately
   2. Spermicides
   3. Foam, cream, vaginal contraceptive film, sponge
- Lactation amenorrhea method
   1. Full or nearly full breastfeeding/chestfeeding
      a. Feeding an average of every 4 hours during the day
      b. Feeding an average of every 6 hours at night
      c. Has not substituted solid foods for breastfeeding/chestfeeding for any meals
   2. Infant less than 6 months old
   3. No menses

Table 9-1 U.S. Medical Eligibility Criteria for Postpartum Contraception

Condition	Subcondition	Cu-IUD	LNG-IUD	Implant	DMPA	POP	CHC
Postpartum (in breastfeeding or nonbreastfeeding women, including cesarean delivery)	a. 10 min after delivery of the placenta						
	i. Breastfeeding	2	2				
	ii. Nonbreastfeeding	2	2				
	b. 10 minutes after delivery of placenta to <4 weeks	2	2				
	c. >4 weeks	1	1				
	d. Postpartum sepsis	4	4				
Postpartum (breastfeeding)	a. <21 days postpartum			2	2	2	4
	b. 21 to <30 days postpartum						
	i. With other risk factors for VTE			2	2	2	3
	ii. Without risk factors for VTE			2	2	2	3
	c. 30–42 days postpartum						
	i. With other risk factors for VTE			1	2	1	3
	ii. Without risk factors for VTE			1	1	1	2
	d. >42 days postpartum			1	1	1	2
Postpartum (nonbreastfeeding)	a. 21 days			1	1	1	4
	b. 21–42 days						
	i. With other risk factors for VTE			1	2	1	3
	ii. Without risk factors for VTE			1	1	1	2
	c. >42 days			1	1	1	1

Key:
1: No restriction (method can be used)
2: Advantages generally outweigh the theoretical of proven risks
3: Theoretical or proven risks usually outweigh the advantages
4: Unacceptable health risk (method not to be used)

Abbreviations: CHC, combination hormonal methods (pills, patch, vaginal ring); Cu-IUD, copper IUD; DMPA, depot medroxyprogesterone acetate; IUD, intrauterine device; LNG-IUD, levonorgestrel IUD; POP 5 progestin-only pill; VTE, venous thromboembolism.

4. Choose alternative method if postpartum patient and infant do not fit all three criteria
- Tubal ligation
    1. Permanent method of contraception
    2. Most easily accomplished during hospital stay
    3. Need to obtain consent before birth

Postpartum Follow-Up Care

- Return to care
    1. Traditionally, a postpartum visit was scheduled at 6 weeks postpartum. But new ACOG recommendations recommend scheduling a follow-up visit sooner than 6 weeks for postpartum patients. This may include telehealth visits by phone or videoconferencing tools
    2. If postpartum patient is high-risk (e.g., hypertensive during antepartum, intrapartum, and/or postpartum period/s; gestational or pregestational diabetic, at risk for postpartum mood disorder), follow-up in 1–2 weeks after discharge
- Chart review
    1. Review of pertinent medical, surgical, social, and obstetric history
    2. Review of prenatal care course
    3. Review of the intrapartum period
    4. Infant data
- Physical examination and assessment
    1. General appearance and affect
    2. Vital signs
    3. Breasts
        a. Condition of breasts and nipples
        b. Status of milk production
    4. Abdomen
        a. Abdominal musculature
        b. Assess for the presence of diastasis recti
        c. Uterine fundal examination—uterus should have completed the involution process and has returned to the pelvis
    5. Urinary
        a. Assess for urinary incontinence
        b. If persists, refer to urology
    6. Perineum
        a. Assess the status of lacerations/episiotomy—expect to be well-approximated and healed
        b. Hemorrhoids—may persist
    7. Extremities
        a. Legs are back to normal prepregnancy state
        b. Assess for calf tenderness and warmth
        c. Varicosities
    8. Pain assessment
    9. Emotional status
        a. Complete a full assessment of mood and emotional well-being
        b. Utilize validated tools such as the Edinburgh Postnatal Depression Scale
- Follow-up to complications/issues
    1. Gestational diabetes—fasting 2-hour, 75-g glucose tolerance test

2. Hypertension (pregestational or gestational)
    a. Follow-up with primary care provider
    b. For severe hypertensive status, additional referral to cardiology
3. Fetal demise
    a. Review autopsy report, if indicated and/or patient preference
    b. Emotional support
    c. Refer to local community/hospital support group
4. Separated symphysis pubis
    a. Physical therapy
    b. Occupational therapy
5. Transition to primary, long-term health care—identify a primary healthcare provider who will assume the main responsibility for the patient's ongoing primary care
- Anticipatory guidance
    1. Vaginal bleeding
        a. Lochia—at 4–6 weeks, may continue to have a scant amount of lochia (alba) but typically resolved by this time
        b. Resumption of menses
    2. Diet and nutrition
        a. Many postpartum patients desire to lose weight to return to prepregnancy weight
        b. Advise patient on exercise/physical activity and healthy nutrition; caution against rapid weight loss
    3. Physical activity and exercise
        a. Pelvic floor exercise could be initiated immediately postpartum
        b. Resumption of aerobic exercise is typically safe but varies with each patient depending on prepregnancy and pregnancy activity, type of birth, presence of medical and surgical complications
    4. Sexual activity
        a. Typically advised to avoid sexual intercourse for 4–6 weeks postpartum or until postpartum evaluation
        b. Vaginal dryness during lactation and laceration/episiotomy may contribute to dyspareunia
    5. Returning to work
        a. May need to fill out family leave paperwork for the patient
        b. Patient may be feeling anxious regarding returning to work, coordinating child care for the infant, and finding balance with the transition as a working parent and expanded responsibilities with the family
    6. Sleep and fatigue
        a. Discuss fatigue and sleep disruption
        b. Assess the availability of support

Postpartum Complications

Urinary Retention

- Diagnosis
    1. Inability to void spontaneously within 6–8 hours after birth or after removal of urinary catheter after delivery
    2. Postvoid residual > 150 mL

3. Palpable bladder
4. Fundus of the uterus displaced and not midline to the abdomen
- Risk factors
  1. Epidural anesthesia
  2. Operative vaginal delivery
  3. Episiotomy/laceration, particularly periurethral laceration
  4. Large-for-gestational-age infant
  5. Primiparity
- Complications
  1. Urinary tract infection
  2. Bladder dysfunction
- Management
  1. Nonpharmacologic—effectiveness has not been shown in studies, but are low-risk interventions
     a. Give the patient privacy in the toilet to relax and not feel the pressure to void
     b. Few drops of peppermint oil in the toilet water or bedpan
     c. Sound of running water
     d. Place hand in warm water
  2. Intermittent catheterization
  3. Indwelling catheter
  4. Consult urology

Postpartum Fever and Infection

- Postpartum fever defined as ≥100.4°F × 2 during postpartum days 2–10
- Differential diagnoses
  1. Most common
     a. Endometritis
     b. Wound infection
     c. Urinary tract infection
     d. Mastitis or breast abscess
  2. Less common
     a. Transfusion reaction
     b. Drug reaction
     c. Septic pelvic thrombophlebitis (SPT)
- Clinical manifestations
  1. General malaise/flu-like symptoms
  2. Tachycardia
  3. Abdominal pain
  4. Malodorous lochia
- Uterine infection/endometritis
  1. Risk factors
     a. Prolonged rupture of membranes
     b. Prolonged labor
     c. Multiple cervical exam
     d. Cesarean section
     e. Chorioamnionitis
     f. Lower genital infection with BGS, *Chlamydia trachomatis*, *Mycoplasma hominis*, *Ureaplasma urealyticum*, *Gardnerella vaginalis*
  2. Treatment
     a. Gold standard—clindamycin and gentamicin
     b. Vancomycin—added to regimen if *Staphylococcus aureus* suspected
- Abdominal incision infection

3. Risk factors
   a. Obesity
   b. Diabetes
   c. Corticosteroid therapy
   d. Immunosuppression
   e. Anemia
   f. Hypertension
   g. Hematoma
4. Treatment
   a. Antimicrobials
   b. Surgical drainage
- Wound dehiscence
  1. Risk factors
     a. Wound infection
     b. Obesity
  2. Management
     a. Treat underlying infection
     b. Secondary closure of the incision in the operating room
- Perineal infection
  1. Due to infected episiotomy or laceration
  2. Infection of the perineum may lead to dehiscence of the repair
  3. Management and treatment
     a. Drain and debridement
     b. Antimicrobial therapy
     c. Wound care
     d. Secondary repair when episiotomy/laceration has healed
- Septic pelvic thrombophlebitis
  1. Septic phlebitis along the venous route and then causing thrombosis
  2. Clinical manifestation
     a. Patient has pain in one or both lower abdominal areas
     b. Chills
  3. Diagnosis
     a. Pelvic computed tomography (CT) scan
     b. Magnetic resonance imaging (MRI)

Postpartum Hemorrhage (PPH)

- Leading cause of maternal mortality worldwide
- ACOG definition
  1. Estimated blood loss (EBL) of 1,000 mL regardless of route of delivery
  2. Blood loss accompanied by signs or symptoms of hypovolemia within 24 hours after birth
- Traditional definition
  1. EBL of 500 mL after vaginal delivery
  2. EBL of 1,000 mL after a cesarean section
- Risk factors
  1. Prolonged labor/prolonged use of oxytocin
  2. Chorioamnionitis
  3. High parity
  4. Twins, multiple gestation
  5. Polyhydramnios
  6. Macrosomia
  7. Operative vaginal delivery
  8. Precipitous delivery

- Etiology
  1. Primary
     a. Uterine atony
        (1) Accounts for 70%–80% of cases of PPH
        (2) Soft, boggy uterus
        (3) Management and treatment
            (a) Empty bladder
            (b) Bimanual exam
            (c) Removal of intrauterine clots
            (d) Fundal/uterine massage
            (e) Uterotonics
            (f) Intrauterine tamponade
     b. Obstetric trauma
        (1) Identification of the source of bleeding
            (a) Vaginal
            (b) Vulvar
            (c) Periclitoral
            (d) Perineal
            (e) Cervical
            (f) Genital tract hematoma
        (2) Clinical manifestation
            (a) Patient may complain of labial, rectal, pelvic pressure or pain
            (b) Abnormal vital signs
        (3) Management and treatment
            (a) Hematoma may need incision and drainage
            (b) Arterial embolization
     c. Lacerations
     d. Retained placenta
        (1) Diagnosis
            (a) Visual inspection of the placenta
            (b) Ultrasonography
            (c) Intrauterine manual examination
        (2) Management
            (a) Manual removal of retained placenta
            (b) Curettage with ultrasound guidance
     e. Placenta accreta
     f. Coagulation defects
     g. Inversion of the uterus
- Secondary
  a. Subinvolution
  b. Retained products of contraception
  c. Infection
  d. Coagulation defects
     (1) Acute coagulopathy
         (a) Etiology
             ◦ Placental abruption
             ◦ Amniotic fluid embolism
             ◦ Disseminated intravascular coagulation (DIC)
         (b) Management
             ◦ Volume replacement
             ◦ Initiate transfusion protocol

Lactation

Anatomy of the Mammary Gland

- Suspensory ligaments/fibrocollagenous septa (also known as Cooper's ligaments)—connective tissue in the breast that supports the shape of the breasts
  1. Milk ducts—each breast contains 4–18 primary milk ducts that converge at the nipple
  2. Basic glandular unit—contains 4–18 lobules, each containing alveoli responsible for milk ejection
  3. Nipples and areola—become darker during pregnancy; it is theorized that this darkening of the nipples and areola provides the infant with a visual marker for latching
  4. Areolar glands (also known as Montgomery tubercles)—located in areola; sebaceous glands that provide protective secretion and lubrication to the nipple

Physiology of Lactation

- Mammary changes during pregnancy
  5. Increase in breast size
  6. Darkening of areola pigmentation
  7. Areola tubercles enlarge and become more prominent
  8. Nipples become more erect
  9. Colostrum leakage in the third trimester
  10. Skin over the breast appears more translucent; blood vessels are more visible
- Lactogenesis I
  1. Early pregnancy to third day postpartum
  2. Dependent on hormonal changes
  3. Secretion of small amounts of colostrum
     a. Approximately 100 mL of breast milk produced on postpartum day 1
     b. Contains high concentrations of immunoglobulins, lactoferrin, and oligosaccharides
- Lactogenesis II
  1. Days 2–4 postpartum
  2. Second stage of lactogenesis initiated by:
     a. Delivery of placenta
     b. Decrease in progestin hormone concentration
     c. Increase in prolactin hormone concentration
  3. Volume increases
     a. Approximately 500 mL of breast milk produced on postpartum day 4
     b. Copious milk production begins
     c. Patient will typically refer to the "milk coming in" during this stage
- Lactogenesis III
  1. Begins between 7 and 14 days postpartum
  2. Mature milk is established
  3. Maintenance of milk supply
  4. Milk production depends on supply–demand relationship
     a. Frequent milk transfer
     b. Suckling stimulates the nipple and areola; message sent to the hypothalamus to secrete prolactin and oxytocin hormones
     c. Prolactin stimulates milk production (PROlactin = milk PROduction)
     d. Oxytocin—hormone responsible for stimulating the contraction of myoepithelial cells; this contraction of cells causes milk ejection, also referred to as the "let-down reflex"
- Breastfeeding/Chestfeeding promotion
  1. Immediate skin-to-skin contact after birth
  2. Baby-led and parent-guided physiologic breastfeeding/chestfeeding
  3. Healthcare provider's role is to support the dyad

- Barriers to breastfeeding/chestfeeding
  1. Anatomical variation in breasts
     a. Nipple issues
     b. Mammary gland hypoplasia
     c. History of breast implants
     d. History of breast reduction surgery
  2. Suctioning at birth
  3. Operative vaginal birth
     a. Patient is exhausted and in pain
     b. Vacuum-assisted birth may result in an infant with cephalohematoma
     c. Forceps-assisted birth may result in bruising of the newborn's facial muscles or nerves
  4. Cesarean section
     a. More blood loss with surgery versus vaginal birth
     b. Abdominal incision pain may make positioning difficult
     c. Transient tachypnea
  5. Separation of pregnant patient and baby
  6. Supplementation of formula
  7. Pacifier use
- Contraindications to breastfeeding/chestfeeding
  1. Neonatal conditions
     a. classical galactosemia (galactose 1-phosphate uridyltransferase deficiency)
  2. Maternal infection
     a. Human immunodeficiency virus (HIV) in industrialized nations
        (1) In low- and middle-income nations, risks may outweigh the benefits
     b. Human T-lymphotropic virus 1
     c. Ebola virus
     d. Herpes, active lesion on nipples and breasts
     e. Untreated tuberculosis (TB)
     f. Varicella infection developed 5 days prior to birth to 2 days after birth
  3. Substance use including illicit drugs (illegal or controlled)
     a. Narcotic-dependent patients enrolled in a methadone maintenance program should be *encouraged* to breastfeed/chestfeed with negative screening for HIV and illicit drug use
     b. Alcoholic beverages should be minimized and appropriately timed (>2 hours after ingestion)
     c. Smoking should not occur in the presence of an infant
  4. Specific medications
     a. Antiretrovirals
     b. Anticonvulsants
     c. Chemotherapy agents
     d. Radiation therapy
     e. Retinoids
     f. Statins
- Drugs and lactation
  1. Review patient's medication list of prescribed, over-the-counter, and complementary and alternative medications
  2. Check the LactMed database for information on the levels of such substances in breast milk and infant

blood, and the possible adverse effects on the nursing infant
- Common breastfeeding/chestfeeding problems
  1. Breast engorgement
     a. Prevention is key
        (1) Proper breastfeeding/chestfeeding positioning and attachment
        (2) Emptying one breast at each feeding
        (3) Alternating which breast is offered first
        (4) Frequent milk transfer
     b. Treatment
        (1) Acupuncture
        (2) Hot/warm pack prior to feeding, followed by cold packs after feeding
        (3) Cabbage leaves—inexpensive and soothing, but evidence is inconclusive
        (4) Breast massage
        (5) Hand expression
  2. Insufficient milk supply
     a. Evaluate for medical causes of low milk supply
     b. Assess the frequency and effectiveness of milk removal and transfer
     c. Herbal products, foods, and beverages used as galactagogues
        (1) No scientific evidence for effectiveness and safety
        (2) No standardized dosing
        (3) Fenugreek
        (4) Goat's rue
        (5) Milk thistle
        (6) Oats
        (7) Dandelion
        (8) Seaweed
        (9) Blessed thistle
        (10) Fennel seeds
        (11) Beer
     d. Used in some cultures
     e. Hops and barley in beer are the active ingredients
     f. Alcohol may reduce milk production
     g. Pharmaceutical galactagogue
        (1) Domperidone—warning: increases QT interval and implicated in ventricular arrhythmias and sudden cardiac death
        (2) Metoclopramide—warning: central nervous system (CNS) effects, including sedation, depression, extrapyramidal symptoms
  3. Plugged ducts
- Complications
  1. Mastitis
     a. Affects 1 in 5 women
     b. Diagnostic criteria
        (1) Erythematous, edematous, wedge-shaped area in the breast, typically unilateral
        (2) Fever ≥101.3°F
        (3) Flu-like symptoms
     c. Risk factors
        (1) Damaged nipples
        (2) Infrequent feedings
        (3) Ineffective milk transfer and removal
        (4) Poor latch, attachment

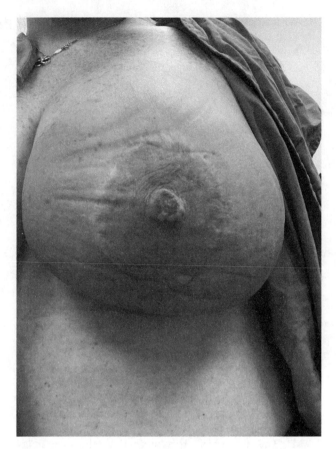

Figure 9-1 Mastitis of the left breast.

f. Alleviating pain may help the patient relax and facilitate the let-down reflex
  (1) First-line antibiotics
g. Dicloxacillin or flucloxacillin 500 mg PO QID × 10–14 days
h. Cephalexin (Keflex) 500 mg QID × 10–14 days
i. If penicillin allergic, clindamycin 300 mg QID or erythromycin 250 mg or 500 mg QID × 10–14 days
  (1) Typically improve/resolve within 48 hours of initiation of antibiotics
2. Breast abscess
a. Collection of pus in the breast, surrounded by inflammation
b. Diagnosis based on physical exam and ultrasound
c. Infecting organism most likely *S. aureus*
d. Management and treatment
  (1) Surgical drainage
  (2) Needle aspiration
  (3) Antibiotics
3. Raynaud's phenomenon
a. Vasospasm of the nipple after breastfeeding/chest-feeding or when the nipples are exposed to cool air
b. Nipple color changes to purple or blanches; may be unilateral or bilateral
c. Severe pain; sharp, burning sensation
d. Treatment with nifedipine
e. Avoidance of exposure to cold air
4. Fungal infection
a. Infecting organism due to candida
b. Diagnosis based on history and physical exam
c. Infant may have signs of thrush or diaper rash
d. Clinical manifestation
  (1) Shiny and red nipple and areola
  (2) Flaky skin around the nipple
  (3) Burning, itching, stabbing pain like "shards of glass" in the breasts
  (4) Treatment
e. Topical nystatin, miconazole, or clotrimazole
f. Gentian violet 1% in 10% alcohol applied to nipple × 4 days
g. APNO cream (Dr. Newman's formula): mupirocin 2% ointment (not cream), betamethasone 0.1% ointment (not cream), miconazole 2%

  (5) Uncoordinated suck
  (6) Oversupply of milk
  (7) Rapid weaning
  (8) Use of bra that is too tight
  (9) Maternal fatigue
  (10) Previous mastitis
d. Treatment
  (1) Analgesia
e. Nonsteroidal anti-inflammatory drugs (NSAIDs), such as ibuprofen—reduce inflammation to help with better latching

Questions

Select the best answer.

1. During postpartum rounds, your multiparous patient is very pleased with her birth and is clearly bonding with her new baby girl. The patient is successfully nursing her baby every 3 hours for 5 minutes. The patient is asking about early discharge and wants to go home as soon as possible. The patient's only complaint is that her left leg is sore because she needed to deliver in stirrups. What would be the most important piece of your assessment?
   a. Availability of assistance at home with her two other children to ensure that she can rest
   b. Breast exam and assessment to check for milk production to ensure adequacy of feeding before discharge
   c. Dietary recall to ensure adequate kilocalories and fluids to produce adequate human milk
   d. Examination of the lower legs to be sure that the muscle strain that she is complaining about is simply related to positioning

2. A 22-year-old postpartum patient had a baby 2 days ago. The patient would like to resume contraception before discharge from the hospital. Which method would be most appropriate for this patient?
   a. DMPA
   b. IUD
   c. Combination oral contraceptive pills
   d. Diaphragm with spermicidal cream

3. A postpartum patient delivered a baby vaginally 4 days ago. The patient's vital signs on the morning of discharge are as follows: heart rate 102, temperature 102.4°F, blood pressure 124/70 mm Hg. The patient reports having enlarged breasts and a feeling of being uncomfortably full. The patient has given up on breastfeeding/chestfeeding because of the nipple pain experienced while feeding. The patient also reports having a partner who is unsupportive with breastfeeding/chestfeeding. The next step includes:
   a. physical assessment of the patient to examine the nipples and breasts
   b. starting broad-spectrum antibiotics immediately
   c. prescribing analgesics to help with the pain and discomfort
   d. providing formula and artificial nipples

4. A patient who is chestfeeding a 15-month-old infant is in the office asking for a nonhormonal contraceptive method that provides protection from STIs. What is the best method for this patient?
   a. Copper IUD
   b. Lactational amenorrhea method
   c. Tubal ligation
   d. Female condom

5. A normal exam for a postpartum patient who had a baby 3 days ago includes:
   a. a firm fundus 3 cm below the umbilicus
   b. a firm fundus 3 cm above the umbilicus
   c. a firm fundus 1 cm below the umbilicus
   d. a firm fundus 1 cm above the umbilicus

6. A postpartum patient comes to the office 3 weeks after having a baby. What is an expected examination finding?
   a. Fundus at the umbilicus
   b. Uterus about the size of a grapefruit
   c. Firm fundus 1 cm above the umbilicus
   d. Uterus no longer palpated abdominally

7. A patient who had a baby 14 days ago calls the office concerned about her bleeding. The patient states, "The bleeding is bright red, and I am filling up the pad about every hour." What instructions should be given to the patient?
   a. "That sounds like the normal amount and type of bleeding that is to be expected. Call when the bleeding gets worse."
   b. "That amount and type of bleeding is normal. Change your pads often to prevent infections."
   c. "That amount and type of bleeding is concerning. Monitor your bleeding over the next 24 hours and call back if it gets worse."
   d. "That amount and type of bleeding is abnormal. Have someone drive you to the triage unit at the hospital, and I will meet you there as soon as possible."

8. On day 2 postpartum, the cervix continues to be dilated at how many centimeters?
   a. 0–1 cm
   b. 0.5–1 cm
   c. 1–1.5 cm
   d. 2–3 cm

9. What is the appearance of a multiparous individual's cervix?
   a. It is the same as the cervix of a nulliparous individual.
   b. The external os appears to be a pinpoint circle.
   c. Only the external os is the same as that of a nulliparous individual.
   d. The external os appears to be a slit resembling a fish mouth.

10. During the postpartum period, normal vaginal findings include:
   a. edema, relaxed-appearing, and sometimes bruised at 8 weeks postpartum
   b. decreased lubrication, especially for lactating patients
   c. increased bruising at 12 weeks postpartum, but only for patients who are lactating
   d. well-lubricated with the return of rugae at 1 week postpartum

11. A patient at 39 weeks' gestation reports colostrum production. The patient states, "I am concerned about this leaking. Is this normal? What should I do?" The correct response should be:
   a. "Soon your breasts will feel engorged, and you'll have copious milk right in time for when the baby is born."
   b. "This is too early for colostrum production. Place ice packs on your breasts to prevent any more milk from being produced."
   c. "This is normal. Colostrum may be produced prior to the birth of your baby."
   d. "This is normal. This process is called the milk-ejection reflex."

12. The process of involution takes place over which time frame?
   a. The first 6 weeks postpartum
   b. The first 24 hours postpartum
   c. The first 2 weeks postpartum
   d. The first year postpartum

13. Thirty-six hours after the patient gave birth, a 16-year-old is crying quietly with the baby in the room as you perform morning rounds. What would be the most helpful response?
   a. Prescribe an SSRI because adolescents are prone to postpartum depression.
   b. Encourage the patient to focus on the baby's needs as the first priority now.
   c. Explain that it is normal to have a combination of sadness and euphoria so close to the time of the birth.
   d. Conduct a screening test for possible postpartum depression.

14. Hemodynamic changes during the initial postpartum period include:
   a. elevated cardiac output for up to 48 hours after the birth
   b. decreased white blood count (WBC) during the first 72 hours postpartum
   c. elevated blood pressure for 48 hours after the birth
   d. decreased urine output for the first 24 hours postpartum

15. A patient is home from a normal spontaneous vaginal delivery 12 hours ago. The patient calls the triage unit concerned about frequent urination. The patient denies having fever, chills, or dysuria. The patient states, "I have been going to the bathroom constantly to pee. I don't have any pain when I go. Is this normal?" The right response is:
    a. "Antibiotics need to be started immediately to prevent the infection from getting worse."
    b. "During the immediate postpartum period, it is common to have increased urination."
    c. "Sounds like you have a urinary tract infection. Try some cranberry juice to help make it better."
    d. "Avoid drinking too many fluids to allow for your bladder some rest."

16. A patient comes to the postpartum visit 4 weeks after the vaginal birth of a 10-pound baby. The patient states that her abdomen feels separated. What should be the next step?
    a. Assess for diastasis recti
    b. Consult general surgery for possible uterine myoma
    c. Obtain liver function tests
    d. Send the patient immediately for an X-ray

17. Postpartum ovulation and menstruation are inhibited by:
    a. increased prolactin
    b. maintenance of prolactin levels
    c. increased estrogen
    d. maintenance of estrogen levels

18. Postpartum patients who are not breastfeeding/chestfeeding typically have their first menses:
    a. around the same time as a person who is breastfeeding/chestfeeding
    b. later than someone who is exclusively breastfeeding/chestfeeding
    c. after 6 months postpartum
    d. sooner than breastfeeding/chestfeeding individuals

19. Anti-Rho(D) immune globulin is:
    a. necessary for postpartum patients whose Rh status is negative and whose infant's Rh status is positive
    b. necessary for postpartum patients whose Rh status is negative and whose infant's Rh status is negative
    c. necessary for postpartum patients whose Rh status is positive and whose infant's Rh status is negative
    d. necessary for postpartum patients whose Rh status is positive and whose infant's Rh status is positive

20. Which postpartum patient should be offered the Tdap vaccine?
    a. A patient who received the Tdap vaccine during a previous pregnancy
    b. A patient who received the Tdap vaccine during the second trimester of pregnancy
    c. A patient who did not receive the Tdap vaccine during pregnancy
    d. A patient who received the Tdap vaccine during the last trimester only

21. The flu vaccine:
    a. is unsafe during pregnancy and the postpartum period
    b. is unsafe for breastfeeding/chestfeeding patients
    c. should be offered to pregnant and postpartum patients
    d. is safer in the nasal spray form than in the injectable form

22. The current recommendation for the HPV vaccine includes:
    a. offering the vaccine to postpartum patients between 11 and 26 years old, who have not been previously vaccinated
    b. offering the vaccine to postpartum patients older than age 18 years
    c. avoiding the vaccine for postpartum individuals who are breastfeeding/chestfeeding
    d. offering the vaccine to pregnant patients who are at least 26 years old

23. Common pharmacologic pain relief options for postpartum patients include:
    a. acetaminophen 650 mg every 4 hours as needed for pain
    b. acetaminophen 1,200 mg every 4 hours as needed for pain
    c. ibuprofen 650 mg every 4 hours as needed for pain
    d. ibuprofen 1,200 mg every 4 hours as needed for pain

24. Management of breast engorgement includes:
    a. pumping to increase milk production
    b. waiting at least 6 hours between feedings
    c. offering formula until the nipples completely heal and engorgement decreases
    d. assessing that the infant is positioned correctly and properly latched

25. Postpartum blues:
    a. may begin within 3–5 days after birth
    b. may happen 12 months after birth
    c. includes symptoms that do not improve over time
    d. requires the immediate start of an SSRI

26. Postpartum depression:
    a. may begin within 3–5 days after birth
    b. may happen 12 months after birth
    c. includes symptoms that improve within a few days after birth
    d. requires the immediate start of an SSRI

27. What is the best contraceptive option for a patient who is asking to start a method 2 weeks after the birth of an infant?
    a. Patch
    b. Vaginal ring
    c. Combined hormonal oral pills
    d. Progestin-only injectable

28. What is the best contraceptive option for a breastfeeding patient who is asking to start a method immediately after the birth of an infant prior to discharge from the hospital?
    a. Patch
    b. Vaginal ring
    c. Combined hormonal oral pills
    d. Progestin-only injectable

29. A patient who had a vaginal birth 1 day ago desires a contraceptive method to use prior to the patient's postpartum visit in 6 weeks. The patient had a fourth-degree laceration that was repaired, and the patient is currently breastfeeding. What is the best choice for this patient?
    a. Diaphragm
    b. Vaginal ring
    c. Combined hormonal oral contraceptive pills
    d. Etonogestrel implant

30. A postpartum patient's concerned partner calls the OB/GYN office stating that the patient had a baby 6 months ago and is acting erratic and bizarre. The caller states that the patient has been "acting off" for a few weeks and has not been wanting to care for herself or the infant. The patient's partner states, "My partner is hearing things that I do not hear. Is that a weird thing to say? What should we do?" What is the best response?
    a. The patient should be brought to the nearest emergency room to be evaluated for postpartum psychosis.
    b. Reassure the partner that this is a normal transition to parenthood and ask the partner to monitor the patient at home for the next few days for postpartum depression.
    c. Check for allergies and call in a prescription for an SSRI to the patient's pharmacy.
    d. Encourage the partner to help the patient start a self-care routine that will have longer-lasting effects.

31. The lactational amenorrhea contraceptive method is most effective:
    a. if the infant is younger than 18 months
    b. if the birth person is breastfeeding/chestfeeding at least every 4 hours during the day
    c. if the birth person is breastfeeding/chestfeeding an average of 8 hours during the night
    d. if the parents are feeding the infant solid foods for at least two-thirds of the meals

32. Contraceptive counseling for tubal ligation includes a discussion regarding:
    a. the permanence of the procedure
    b. its excellent protection from STIs
    c. the convenience of discontinuing this option at any time
    d. the fact that consent is not necessary

33. Risk factors for urinary retention include:
    a. a small-for-gestational-age infant
    b. multiparity
    c. and intact perineum
    d. use of epidural anesthesia during labor and delivery

34. What is the gold-standard treatment for postpartum endometritis?
    a. Clindamycin and gentamycin
    b. Fluconazole and pyridium
    c. Diflucan and terconazole vaginal
    d. Methergine and misoprostol

35. What part of the breasts supports the shape of the breasts?
    a. Milk ducts
    b. Suspensory ligaments

    c. Basic glandular unit
    d. Areolar glands

36. Mammary changes during pregnancy include:
    a. hypopigmentation of the areola
    b. the blood vessels become less visible
    c. the areolar tubercles become enlarged
    d. breast size typically remains the same

37. The first stage of lactogenesis typically occurs during:
    a. the second trimester only
    b. the latter part of the third trimester until 6 weeks postpartum
    c. early pregnancy to the third day postpartum
    d. days 2–4 postpartum

38. The second stage of lactogenesis occurs during:
    a. the second trimester only
    b. the latter part of the third trimester until 6 weeks postpartum
    c. early pregnancy to the third day postpartum
    d. days 2–4 postpartum

39. The second stage of lactogenesis is initiated by all the following mechanisms *except*:
    a. delivery of the placenta
    b. decreased progestin hormone concentration
    c. increased prolactin hormone concentration
    d. initiation of exogenous estrogen

40. Which stage of lactogenesis happens between 7 and 14 days postpartum and is the state in which mature milk is established and the milk supply is maintained?
    a. Lactogenesis I
    b. Lactogenesis II
    c. Lactogenesis III
    d. Lactogenesis IV

41. Which hormone is responsible for stimulating the milk-ejection reflex?
    a. Oxytocin
    b. Prolactin
    c. Human placental lactogen
    d. Renin

42. A potential contraindication to breastfeeding/chestfeeding is:
    a. herpes, where an active lesion is present on the vulva
    b. HIV infection
    c. the birth person's experience of having chickenpox as a toddler
    d. Tylenol use

43. A postpartum patient is breastfeeding a 2-week-old infant and is feeling extremely tired with a fever of 102°F. The patient notices an erythematous, edematous, wedge-shaped area in the left breast. What is the likely diagnosis?
    a. Plugged duct
    b. Mastitis
    c. Engorgement
    d. Breast cancer

44. A patient states that she experiences extreme nipple pain as soon as the infant unlatches from the breast and the nipples become exposed to the cold air. According to the

patient, the nipples then turn a dark purple. What is this patient's likely diagnosis?
   a. Raynaud's phenomenon
   b. Mastitis
   c. Plugged duct
   d. Herpetic lesions on the breast

45. During postpartum rounds, a patient who delivered an infant 6 hours prior states, "I notice that when I breastfeed the baby, I feel fairly strong contraction-like pain. Labor is over. Why am I having contractions now?" Which response would be most appropriate?
   a. "Your body is responding to the events of labor, just like after a tough workout."
   b. "Your uterus sometimes enlarges during the postpartum period; that's why you're having pain."
   c. "The baby's suckling releases a hormone that causes the uterus to contract."
   d. "Let me check your vaginal discharge just to make sure everything is okay."

46. A new parent wants to nurse her infant for only 5 minutes at each breast to avoid sore nipples. Which of the following is appropriate education to provide the patient?
   a. Nipple stimulation will help to reduce engorgement.
   b. Keeping early feedings long will delay the let-down.
   c. Keeping early feedings short lessens nipple trauma.
   d. Reposition the infant to have a better latch.

47. The postpartum patient presents to the office complaining of "feeling ill." The patient is noted to have a temperature of 101.8°F and reports that the symptoms came on "suddenly." The patient is breastfeeding. During examination of the patient's left breast, the clinician identifies a localized area of swelling, redness, and warmth. This area is intensely painful upon palpation. The right breast, by comparison, demonstrates no abnormal findings. From the history and physical exam, the correct diagnosis for this patient is:
   a. engorgement
   b. mastitis
   c. galactocele
   d. cancer

48. A postpartum patient who is breastfeeding is concerned about mastitis because the patient experienced this condition while breastfeeding her last baby. Which of the following would be appropriate for the nurse to suggest as a preventive measure?
   a. Switch to formula
   b. Frequent breastfeeding
   c. Wear a tight-fitting bra
   d. Limit feedings to every 6 hours

49. A new parent asks, "If formula is prepared to meet the nutritional needs of a newborn, what is in breast milk that makes it better?" The proper response is that breast milk contains:
   a. more calcium
   b. important antibodies
   c. essential amino acids
   d. more calories

Answers with Rationales

1. **d.** Examination of the lower legs to be sure that the muscle strain that she is complaining about is simply related to positioning
   It would be important to examine her lower extremities to assess for possible deep vein thrombosis (DVT).

2. **a.** DMPA
   DMPA is an acceptable contraceptive method that can be administered before discharge.

3. **a.** physical assessment of the patient to examine the nipples and breasts
   Prior to making a diagnosis, developing a plan, and implementing treatment, assessment of the patient is necessary.

4. **d.** Female condom
   Female and male condoms are nonhormonal forms of contraception that provide some protection against STIs. The lactational amenorrhea method is not reliable past 6 months postpartum and does not provide protection against STIs. The tubal ligation and copper IUD also do not provide protection against STIs.

5. **a.** a firm fundus 3 cm below the umbilicus
   At 3 days postpartum, the fundus can be found 3 finger-breadths or 3 cm below the umbilicus.

6. **d.** Uterus no longer palpated abdominally
   By 2 weeks postpartum, the uterus is no longer palpated abdominally and has descended into the pelvis.

7. **d.** "That amount and type of bleeding is abnormal. Have someone drive you to the triage unit at the hospital, and I will meet you there as soon as possible."
   At 14 days postpartum, lochia should be turning pinkish in color and not bright red. The amount should also be decreasing, and the patient should not be soaking pads every hour. The patient should be advised to come to the triage unit to be evaluated for postpartum hemorrhage.

8. **d.** 2–3 cm
   It is normal for the cervix to be dilated to 2–3 cm at days 2–3 postpartum.

9. **d.** The external os appears to be a slit resembling a fish mouth.
   For multiparous women, at completion of involution, the external os does not return to its prepregnant appearance. Instead, it remains somewhat wider, with a transverse opening resembling a fish mouth.

10. **b.** decreased lubrication, especially for lactating patients.
    During the postpartum period, the vagina may have decreased lubrication, which can lead to dyspareunia during sexual intercourse.

11. **c.** "This is normal. Colostrum may be produced prior to the birth of your baby."
    The body starts making colostrum during the third trimester of pregnancy.

12. **a.** The first 6 weeks postpartum
Normal postpartum involution takes a full 6 weeks to be complete.

13. **c.** Explain that it is normal to have a combination of sadness and euphoria so close to the time of the birth.
It is important to acknowledge the mother's feelings and provide nonjudgmental support. Provide the patient with an explanation of normal psychological responses to childbirth.

14. **a.** elevated cardiac output for up to 48 hours after the birth
Within the first hours postdelivery, the mother's cardiac output increases by 60%–80%.

15. **b.** "During the immediate postpartum period, it is common to have increased urination."
Diuresis occurs within the first 5 days as a result of extravascular fluid shifts.

16. **a.** Assess for diastasis recti
The patient had a 10-lb infant and feels the abdomen has separated. Although the patient may need a consult with general surgery for possible diastasis recti, the first step is to assess the patient.

17. **a.** increased prolactin
Through a negative feedback mechanism, ovulation and menstruation are inhibited by increased prolactin and the resulting estrogen suppression.

18. **d.** sooner than breastfeeding/chestfeeding individuals
Postpartum patients who are not breastfeeding/chestfeeding typically resume their first menses between 6 and 8 weeks postpartum, whereas exclusively breastfeeding/chestfeeding people may not have their first menses until 6 months postpartum.

19. **a.** necessary for postpartum patients whose Rh status is negative and whose infant's Rh status is positive.
Anti-Rho(D) immune globulin needs to be given within 72 hours of birth if the patient's Rh status is negative and the infant is Rh-positive.

20. **c.** A patient who did not receive the Tdap vaccine during pregnancy
All pregnant patients should be offered the Tdap vaccine during each pregnancy. Although this vaccine is safe during any trimester, ACOG recommends that it be given between 27 and 36 weeks' gestation to provide the most protection for newborns. If a patient does not receive the Tdap vaccine during pregnancy, she should be offered the vaccine during the immediate postpartum period.

21. **c.** should be offered to pregnant and postpartum patients.
The flu vaccine in injectable form should be offered to pregnant and postpartum patients. The flu vaccine in nasal spray form is a live attenuated vaccine and should not be offered to pregnant patients.

22. **a.** offering the vaccine to postpartum patients between 11 and 26 years old, who have not been previously vaccinated.
Individuals ages 9 through 26 who have not completed a primary series should receive three doses of HPV vaccine at 0, 2, and 6 months. If the HPV series was started prior

to pregnancy, the series can be completed postpartum without repeating the initial dose(s).
HPV vaccines can and should be given to breastfeeding/chestfeeding individuals 26 years and younger who have not previously been vaccinated.

23. **a.** acetaminophen 650 mg every 4 hours as needed for pain
The maximum dose for acetaminophen is 4,000 mg per day; for ibuprofen, the maximum dose is 3,200 mg per day.

24. **d.** assessing that the infant is positioned correctly and properly latched.
Breast engorgement is a common postpartum discomfort. Engorgement can worsen with an incorrect latch and infrequent feedings.

25. **a.** may begin within 3–5 days after birth
Concurrent with profound hormonal shifts, postpartum blues begins within 3–5 days of birth.

26. **b.** may happen 12 months after birth
Postpartum depression may happen within the immediate postpartum period or even after a year after giving birth.

27. **d.** Progestin-only injectable
Combined hormonal contraceptive methods are not recommended prior to 21 days postpartum. The best option would be a progestin-only method, such as Depo-Provera.

28. **d.** Progestin-only injectable
Combined hormonal contraceptive methods are not recommended prior to 21 days postpartum due to the patient's hypercoagulable state. Additionally, the patient is breastfeeding and should not use estrogen-containing contraceptives that may affect milk production. The best option would be a progestin-only method, such as Depo-Provera, an implant, or a progestin-only injectable.

29. **d.** Etonogestrel implant
Combined hormonal contraceptive methods are not recommended prior to 21 days postpartum due to the patient's hypercoagulable state. Additionally, the patient is breastfeeding and should not use estrogen-containing contraceptives that may affect milk production. Lastly, this patient has a fourth-degree laceration and should wait a few weeks to be fitted for a diaphragm after giving birth.

30. **a.** The patient should be brought to the nearest emergency room to be evaluated for postpartum psychosis.
The patient is showing signs and symptoms of psychosis, such as hallucinations and erratic behavior.

31. **b.** if the person is breastfeeding/chestfeeding at least every 4 hours during the day
The lactational amenorrhea method is most effective if the patient is fully or nearly fully breastfeeding (i.e., averaging every 4 hours during the day and 6 hours at night), the infant is younger than 6 months, and the parents have not substituted solid foods into the infant's diet.

32. **a.** the permanence of the procedure
Tubal ligation is considered a permanent procedure. This contraceptive method does not provide protection against STIs, and the clinician must obtain consent for the surgery.

33. **d.** use of epidural anesthesia during labor and delivery
Risk factors for urinary retention during the postpartum period include large-for-gestational-age infants, nulliparity, and having a laceration or episiotomy.

34. **a.** Clindamycin and gentamycin
The gold-standard treatment for postpartum endometritis is to use clindamycin and gentamycin to ensure adequate coverage.

35. **b.** Suspensory ligaments
Cooper's ligaments provide support to the breasts. The milk ducts and areolar glands do not provide support and shape to the breasts.

36. **c.** the areolar tubercles become enlarged
Mammary changes during pregnancy include enlargement of the areolar glands, darkening of the areola, enlargement of the breasts, and blood vessels appearing more visible.

37. **c.** early pregnancy to the third day postpartum
The first stage of lactogenesis begins during early pregnancy and continues until the third day postpartum.

38. **d.** days 2–4 postpartum
The second stage of lactogenesis occurs between days 2 and 4 postpartum.

39. **d.** initiation of exogenous estrogen
The second stage of lactogenesis is initiated by the delivery of the placenta, a decrease in the progestin concentration, and an increase in the prolactin concentration.

40. **c.** Lactogenesis III
The third stage of lactogenesis occurs between days 7 and 14 postpartum.

41. **a.** Oxytocin
Oxytocin is the hormone responsible for stimulating the contraction of myoepithelial cells; this contraction of cells causes milk ejection, also referred to as the "let-down reflex."

42. **b.** HIV infection
Contraindications to breastfeeding/chestfeeding include infections, such as HIV-positive status, human T-lymphotropic Virus 1, active herpes lesion on the nipple(s) and/or breast(s), varicella infection that developed 5 days prior to birth to 2 days after birth, and the ebola virus.

43. **b.** Mastitis
The patient was exhibiting symptoms of mastitis: erythematous, edematous, wedge-shaped area in the breast, typically unilateral, fever of 101.3°F, and flu-like symptoms.

44. **a.** Raynaud's phenomenon
The patient is exhibiting symptoms of Raynaud's phenomenon: Nipple color changes to purple or blanches, which may be unilateral or bilateral when exposed to cold air. This condition is also associated with severe pain—specifically, a sharp, burning sensation due to the vasospasm of the nipple after breastfeeding/chestfeeding or when the nipples are exposed to cool air.

45. **c.** "The baby's suckling releases a hormone that causes the uterus to contract."
Suckling stimulates the nipple and areola, which signal the hypothalamus to secrete prolactin and oxytocin hormones. Oxytocin stimulates the uterus to contract to facilitate involution.

46. **d.** Reposition the infant to have a better latch.
The nipples may be sore with breastfeeding/chestfeeding but the breastfeeding/chestfeeding patient should not be experiencing pain. Nipple soreness may be due to the malposition of the infant. Pacing the infant in a more supported position for latching may prevent further tissue damage.

47. **b.** mastitis
Given the patient's symptoms of unilateral breast swelling and an erythematous area with a fever, the likely diagnosis is mastitis.

48. **b.** Frequent breastfeeding
To prevent mastitis, breastfeeding/chestfeeding as frequently as the infant desires is recommended.

49. **b.** important antibodies
Although the formula may be prepared with similar nutritional components tailored to the newborn, it lacks the important antibodies that breast milk contains.

Bibliography

Academy of Breastfeeding Medicine. (2018). ABM Protocol #9: Use of galactagogues in initiating or augmenting maternal milk production, second revision 2018. *Breastfeeding Medicine, 13*(5), 307–314. https://doi.org/10.1089/bfm.2018.29092.wjb

American College of Obstetricians and Gynecologists. (2015, reaffirmed 2019). Committee opinion no. 650: Physical activity and exercise during pregnancy and the postpartum period. *Obstetrics and Gynecology, 126,* e135–e142.

American College of Obstetricians and Gynecologists. (2017a, reaffirmed 2019). Committee opinion no. 718: Update on immunization and pregnancy: tetanus, diphtheria, and pertussis vaccination. *Obstetrics and Gynecology, 130,* e153–e157

American College of Obstetricians and Gynecologists. (2017b). Practice bulletin no. 183: Postpartum hemorrhage. *Obstetrics and Gynecology, 130,* e168–e186.

American College of Obstetricians and Gynecologists. (2018a). Committee opinion no. 736: Optimizing postpartum care. *Obstetrics and Gynecology, 131,* e140–e150.

American College of Obstetricians and Gynecologists. (2018c). Committee opinion no. 757: Screening for perinatal depression. *Obstetrics and Gynecology, 132,* e208–e212.

American College of Obstetricians and Gynecologists. (2023). *Practice advisory: COVID-19 vaccination considerations for obstetric–gynecologic care.* https://www.acog.org/clinical/clinical-guidance/practice-advisory/articles/2020/12/covid-19-vaccination-considerations-for-obstetric-gynecologic-care

American Psychiatric Association. (2022). *Diagnostic and statistical manual of mental disorders* (5th ed., text revision). American Psychiatric Publishing.

Association of Women's Health, Obstetric and Neonatal Nurses. (2021). Breastfeeding and the use of human milk. *Nursing for Women's Health, 25*(5), e4–e8. https://doi.org/10.1016/j.nwh.2021.06.005

Berens, P., & Brodribb, W. (2016). Academy of Breastfeeding Medicine clinical protocol #20: Engorgement, revised 2016. *Breastfeeding Medicine, 11*(4), 159–163. https://doi.org/10.1089/bfm.2016.29008.pjb

Berens, P., Eglash, A., Malloy, M., Steube, A. M. & Academy of Breastfeeding Medicine. (2016). ABM clinical protocol# 26: Persistent pain with breastfeeding. *Breastfeeding Medicine*, *11*(2), 46–53.

Blackburn. S. (2017). *Maternal, fetal, & neonatal physiology: A clinical perspective* (5th ed.). Elsevier.

Cunningham, F. G., Leveno, K. J., Dashe, J. S., Hoffman, B. L., Spong, C. Y. & Casey, B. M. (Eds). (2020). *Williams obstetrics* (26th ed.). McGraw-Hill.

Curtis, K. M., Tepper, N. K., Jatlaoui, T. C., Berry-Bibee, E., Horton, L. G., Zapata, L. B. . . . Whiteman, M. K. (2016). U.S. medical eligibility criteria for contraceptive use. *MMWR Recommendations and Reports*, *65*(RR-3), 1–104.

Dagher, R. K., Bruckheim, H. E., Colpe, L. J., Edwards, E., & White, D. B. (2021). Perinatal depression: Challenges and opportunities. *Journal of Women's Health*, *30*(2), 154–159.

Grussu, P., Vicini, B., & Quatraro, R. M. (2021). Sexuality in the perinatal period: A systematic review of reviews and recommendations for practice. *Sexual & Reproductive Healthcare*, *30*, 100668.

Landon, M. B., Galan, H. L., Jauniaux, E. R., Driscoll, D. A., Berghella, V., Grobman, W. A., . . . & Cahill, A. G. (2020). *Obstetrics: Normal and Problem Pregnancies E-Book*. Elsevier Health Sciences.

Mitchell, K. B., Johnson, H. M., Rodríguez, J. M., Eglash, A., Scherzinger, C., Zakarija-Grkovic, I., Cash, K. W., Berens, P., Miller, B., & Academy of Breastfeeding Medicine (2022). Academy of Breastfeeding Medicine clinical protocol #36: The mastitis spectrum, revised 2022. *Breastfeeding Medicine*, *17*(5), 360–376. https://doi.org/10.1089/bfm .2022.29207.kbm

Nutaitis, A. C., Meckes, N. A., Madsen, A. M., Toal, C. T., Menhaji, K., Carter-Brooks, C. M., Propst, K. A., & Hickman, L. C. (2022, August 3). Postpartum urinary retention: An expert review. *American journal of obstetrics and gynecology*, *228*(1), 14–21. https://doi.org/10.1016/j .ajog.2022.07.060

Phillippi, J. & Kantrowitz-Gordon, I. (Eds.). (2025). *Varney's midwifery* (7th ed.). Jones & Bartlett Learning.

CHAPTER 10

Midwifery Care of the Newborn

Melicia Escobar

Physiologic Transition to Extrauterine Life

- Immediate extrauterine transition—immediate transition from intrauterine to extrauterine life depends on changes in four major areas: respiration, circulation, thermoregulation, and glucose regulation
- Respiratory changes
  1. Must immediately begin respiration upon delivery
  2. Factors in the initiation of respiration
     a. Biochemical—relative hypoxia at the end of labor
     b. Physical stimuli—cold, gravity, pain, light, noise
     c. Recoil from pressure on the thorax while passing through the vagina
  3. Sustained respiration depends on a coordinated response of the following:
     a. Central nervous system (CNS) respiratory center
     b. Aortic and carotid chemoreceptors
     c. Thoracic mechanoreceptors
     d. Diaphragm and respiratory muscles
  4. Initial breathing serves the following purposes:
     a. Assist in conversion from fetal to extrauterine circulation
     b. Clear lungs of fluid
     c. Establish lung volume and expand alveoli
  5. Characteristics of normal newborn respiration
     a. Respiratory rate 30–60 breaths per minute
     b. Irregular/fluctuating pattern
     c. Diaphragmatic and abdominal breathing
     d. Obligate nose breathing
     e. Absence of nasal flaring, grunting, and retractions
- Circulatory changes
  1. Transition from fetal to adult circulation begins with the clamping of the umbilical cord and continues throughout the first weeks of life
  2. Characteristics of fetal circulation
     a. Low-pressure system, including placenta (low-resistance circuit)
     b. Minimal circulation to lungs; bypassed via foramen ovale and ductus arteriosus
     c. Foramen ovale favors the circulation of the most oxygen-rich blood to the brain
  3. Transition from fetal to neonatal circulation
     a. Increased systemic resistance due to loss of placental circuit
     b. Increased pressure in the left atrium causes functional closure of the foramen ovale
     c. Initial respiration opens pulmonary vasculature, favoring circulation to the lungs
     d. Increased oxygenation of circulating blood causes constriction and functional closure of ductus arteriosus
     e. Absence of placental circulation closes ductus venosus
- Thermoregulation
  1. Mechanisms of neonatal heat loss. See **Table 10-1**.
     a. Convection
     b. Conduction
     c. Radiation
     d. Evaporation
  2. Neonate creates heat in three ways:
     a. Shivering (inefficient)
     b. Muscle activity (limited benefit)
     c. Thermogenesis by metabolism of brown adipose tissue (BAT)
        (1) BAT stores are decreased in preterm and growth-restricted fetuses
        (2) Hypoglycemia decreases the efficiency of BAT metabolism
  3. Consequences of cold stress
     a. Increased oxygen consumption, leading to relative hypoxia and acidosis
     b. Metabolism of BAT and release of fatty acids decreases pH

Table 10-1 Examples of Neonatal Heat Loss

Convection	Cool draft of air from an open window or fan passes over neonate causing transfer of heat from the baby to the surrounding air. Think: Solid→ Air
Conduction	A naked newborn is placed on a cool scale causing heat to transfer to the scale across the temperature gradient. Think: Direct contact; Solid→ Solid
Radiation	A naked newborn is near closed windows in the winter or poorly insulated walls and loses heat across the temperature gradient. Think: Indirect contact; Solid→ Solid
Evaporation	A newborn covered in amniotic fluid which transfers heat from the baby as it evaporates. Think: Fluid→ Air

Thermoregulation is described in Bell, T. & Reiss, P.J. (2024). Anatomy and physiology of the newborn. In J. Phillippi, J. & I. Kantrowitz-Gordon (Eds.), *Varney's midwifery* (7th ed., p. 1516). Jones and Bartlett Publishers.

   c. Increased use of glucose, depletion of glycogen stores, and hypoglycemia

   d. Worsening hypoglycemia and acidosis may result in respiratory distress

  4. Management

   a. Skin-to-skin contact on the parent's chest or abdomen with a blanket over both

   b. Prewarm blankets and resuscitation area

   c. Dry the newborn immediately and replace wet blankets

   d. Regulate room temperature and minimize exposure to air convection

   e. Postpone newborn bath at least 2 hours

   f. Keep newborn warm and wrapped

- Glucose regulation
  1. Glycogen stores
   a. Predominantly in liver
   b. Accumulated in the third trimester
  2. Risk factors for neonatal hypoglycemia
  3. Glucose regulation in the healthy neonate
   a. There is a lack of consensus between national pediatric organizations regarding blood glucose levels in the screening and treatment of neonatal hypoglycemia. (See **Table 10-2**, Neonatal Hypoglycemia Guidelines.)
   b. Normal physiologic decrease in blood glucose appears to be essential to stimulate physiologic processes promoting glucose production
    (1) Lowest at 1–1.5 to 5 hours after birth
    (2) Stabilizes at 3–4 hours after birth
    (3) The American Academy of Pediatrics (AAP) and the Pediatric Endocrine Society (PES) offer guidelines for the first 48 hours after birth and thereafter
    (4) AAP and PES underscore the need to measure glucose levels as soon as possible in symptomatic infants

    c. Mean glucose levels from 4 to 72 hours are 60 to 70 mg/dL

    d. Sources and mechanisms of glucose maintenance
     (1) Intake of human milk or formula
     (2) Glycogenolysis (use of glycogen stores)
     (3) Gluconeogenesis (production of glucose from free fatty acids), glycerol, and amino acids

  4. Signs and symptoms of hypoglycemia
   a. Weak cry
   b. Jitteriness
   c. Cyanosis
   d. Apnea
   e. Lethargy
   f. Poor feeding

  5. Management
   a. Encourage feeding as soon as possible
   b. Observe for signs/symptoms of hypoglycemia
   c. Assess glucose levels if signs/symptoms or risk factors are present; no recommendation for universal newborn glucose screening for asymptomatic infants without risk factors
   d. Definition and management of neonatal hypoglycemia vary by institution

Ongoing Extrauterine Transition

- Changes in the blood
  1. Red blood cells (RBCs)
   a. Hemoglobin F
    (1) Predominates in fetal circulation
    (2) High affinity for oxygen
    (3) Gradually eliminated in the first month of life
   b. Short RBC life span leads to increased bilirubin and physiologic jaundice
   c. Cord clamping
    (1) Evidence of benefit for infant (particularly, if preterm) with delayed cord clamping (until pulsation stops, mean of approximately 2 minutes) versus immediate cord clamping
    (2) Neutral position on the maternal abdomen is preferable
    (3) Below introitus—theoretically may cause placental transfusion and polycythemia
   d. Normal values
    (1) Hemoglobin
   e. Newborn—13.7 to 20.0 g/dL
   f. Slight rise in the first few days of life due to decreased plasma volume
   g. Mean value at 2 months of age—12.0 g/dL
    (1) Hematocrit—43% to 63%
    (2) RBC count—4.2 to 5.8 million/mm^3
    (3) Reticulocytes—3% to 7%
  2. White blood cells (WBCs) normal value—10,000 to 30,000/mm^3
  3. Platelets
   a. Normal value—150,000 to 350,000/mm^3
   b. Relatively low levels of vitamin K–dependent clotting factors

Table 10-2 Neonatal Hypoglycemia Guidelines

Time Since Birth	0–4 hours	4–24 hours	24–48 hours	>48 hours
AAP (2015)	Asymptomatic neonate screened: ■ <4 hours: should maintain blood glucose >40 mg/dL. ■ 4–24 hours: should maintain blood glucose >45 mg/dL. Symptomatic neonate tested: ■ treat if blood glucose <40 mg/dL.			
PES (Thornton, et al., 2015)	Neonates screened/ tested: ■ <48 hours: should maintain blood glucose >50 mg/dL. Infants unable to maintain this threshold may be at risk for a disorder causing persistent hypoglycemia.			Neonates screened/ tested: ■ >48 hours: should maintain blood glucose >60 mg/dL. Infants at risk of a persistent hypoglycemia syndrome should: ■ have a fast challenge of 6–8 hours ■ maintain blood glucose >70 mg/dL

Data from AAP: American Academy of Pediatrics; PES: Pediatric Endocrine Society. American Academy of Pediatrics. (2011). Clinical report: Postnatal glucose homeostasis in late-preterm and term infants. *Pediatrics, 127*(3), 575–579; Reaffirmed June 2015: (2015). *Pediatrics, 136*(3), e730. https://doi.org/10.1542/peds.2010-3851; [ch10-bib19]; Thompson-Branch, A., & Havranek, T. (2017). Neonatal hypoglycemia. *Pediatrics in review, 38*(4), 147–157. https://doi.org/10.1542/pir.2016-0063

4. Obtaining blood samples
   a. Venous stasis in extremities may lead to false values from heel-stick samples
   b. No longer recommended to use a heel warmer before obtaining a sample (evidence has not shown benefit)
   c. Confirm abnormal results with venipuncture sample
- Changes in the gastrointestinal (GI) system
   1. Relatively mature aspects of the neonatal GI system
      a. Suckling/swallowing
      b. Gag and cough reflexes
   2. Relatively immature aspects of the neonatal GI system
      a. Limited ability to digest fats and proteins
      b. Better absorption of monosaccharides than polysaccharides
      c. Frequent regurgitation due to:
         (1) Incomplete development of cardiac sphincter
         (2) Limited stomach capacity (less than 30 mL)
      d. "Gut closure"
         (1) Maturation process of the intestinal lining and its enzymes and antibodies
         (2) Vulnerability to bacteria, viruses, and allergens until process is complete
         (3) Promoted by breastfeeding/chestfeeding
      e. Large intestine
         (1) Less efficient water conservation than in adult
         (2) Predisposes infant to dehydration
- Changes in the immune system
   1. Natural immunity
      a. Physical and chemical barriers (skin, mucosa, gastric acid)
      b. Phagocytes (neutrophils, monocytes, macrophages)
         (1) Immature phagocytic response
         (2) Relative inability to localize infection

   2. Acquired immunity
      a. Maternal immunoglobulin G (IgG) crosses the placenta, conferring passive immunity to viruses that the pregnant person has encountered
      b. Human milk provides antibodies
      c. Active production of IgG develops slowly throughout childhood as passive immunity diminishes
   3. Immaturity of natural and acquired immune systems predisposes the newborn to infection and sepsis
   4. Protective effect of microbial flora of the vagina (vaginal microbiome) on infant's health (for infants born vaginally); breastfeeding/chestfeeding also helps to establish healthy microbial colonization
- Changes in the renal system
   1. Limited renal circulation
   2. Decreased glomerular filtration rate
   3. Immature tubular function
      a. Relative inability to concentrate urine
      b. Predisposition to fluid and electrolyte imbalances

Immediate Care and Assessment of the Healthy Newborn

- Assessment prior to birth of pertinent maternal history
   1. Genetic history
      a. Family history of structural or metabolic defects
      b. History of genetic syndromes
   2. Maternal elements
      a. Social determinants/demographic factors
         (1) Age <16 years or >35 years
         (2) Overweight or underweight prior to pregnancy
         (3) Education <11 years

(4) Family history of inherited disorders
b. Medical factors
  (1) Cardiac disease
  (2) Pulmonary disease
  (3) Renal disease
  (4) GI disease
  (5) Endocrine disorders, particularly diabetes or thyroid disease
  (6) Chronic hypertension
  (7) Hemoglobinopathies
  (8) Seizures or other neurologic disorders
c. History of present pregnancy/intrapartum factors
  (1) Limited or no prenatal care
  (2) Rh sensitization
  (3) Fetus large or SGA
  (4) Premature labor or delivery
  (5) Hypertensive disorders of pregnancy
  (6) Multiple gestation
  (7) Polyhydramnios
  (8) Premature or prolonged rupture of membranes/chorioamnionitis
  (9) Antepartum bleeding
  (10) Abnormal presentation
  (11) Postmaturity
  (12) Abnormal results in fetal testing
  (13) Anemia
  (14) Meconium staining of amniotic fluid
  (15) Abnormal or indeterminate fetal heart rate (FHR) tracing
  (16) Administration of opioids to the birthing person shortly prior to birth
d. Social determinants/psychosocial history
  (1) Financial, housing, or social resources
  (2) Minority status
  (3) Nutritional status/malnutrition
    (a) Pre-pregnant body mass index (BMI)
    (b) Weight gain during pregnancy
  (4) Parental occupation
  (5) Significant relationships, marriage status
  (6) Violence or abuse
  (7) Smoking during pregnancy
  (8) Alcohol use during pregnancy
  (9) Illicit or prescription drug use

- Assessment at birth
1. During and immediately following the birth
  a. Answer these three questions:
    (1) Is the newborn at term gestation?
    (2) Is the tone good?
    (3) Is the baby breathing or crying?
  b. Gross inspection of anatomy
  c. Place the infant on the maternal abdomen skin-to-skin (preferred) or radiant warmer
  d. Can palpate cord to assess heart rate
2. Apgar scoring
  a. Scale—0 to 10
    (1) Heart rate—0 = absent, 1 = <100, 2 = ≥100
    (2) Respiratory effort—0 = absent, 1 = slow/irregular, 2 = strong cry
    (3) Tone—0 = flaccid, 1 = flexion of extremities, 2 = active motion

(4) Reflex irritability—0 = no response, 1 = grimace, 2 = strong cry
(5) Color—0 = general cyanosis, 1 = acrocyanosis, 2 = completely pink
b. Assigned at 1 and 5 minutes; may be assigned at additional 5-minute intervals when prolonged resuscitation efforts are required (traditionally, until score >7)
c. Primary purpose of Apgar score—objective method of quantifying the newborn's condition and response to resuscitation
d. Poor predictor of long-term outcome
e. Poor reflection of acidemia
f. Not used to determine the need for resuscitation, which resuscitation steps are necessary, or when to use them

- Review of neonatal resuscitation
1. Midwives who provide care in the intrapartum setting should be trained and certified in neonatal resuscitation, preparing individually and in the context of a team; the information presented here is a review, not a substitute for training and certification.
2. Approximately 10% of newborns require some assistance to begin breathing at birth; about 1% require extensive resuscitation
3. Evaluation is based on three signs:
  a. Respirations
  b. Heart rate
  c. Color/target preductal peripheral capillary oxygen saturation levels after birth
    (1) One minute: 60% to 65%
    (2) Two minutes: 65% to 70%
    (3) Three minutes: 70% to 75%
    (4) Four minutes: 75% to 80%
    (5) Five minutes: 80% to 85%
    (6) Ten minutes: 85% to 95%
4. ABCs of resuscitation
  a. Establish an open Airway
    (1) Position the infant on back or side with the neck slightly extended
    (2) Suction mouth, nose, and trachea, as indicated
    (3) Insert endotracheal (ET) tube to ensure open airway, if necessary
  b. Initiate Breathing
    (1) Use tactile stimulation to initiate respirations
    (2) Use positive-pressure ventilation (PPV) starting with 21% oxygen (room air) in term newborns; proper inflation and ventilation of the lungs are a priority
  c. Maintain Circulation—stimulate and maintain circulation with chest compressions and/or medications when necessary; a rise in heart rate is an indicator of effective ventilation and resuscitation efforts
5. Overview of resuscitation
  a. Antenatal counseling of the parents of the parents around NRP, team briefing, and equipment check prior to birth should occur.
  b. Initial steps of resuscitation (first 60 seconds, the "golden minute")

(1) Provide warmth

(2) Dry infant; remove wet linen

(3) Provide tactile stimulation

(4) Position airway

(5) Clear secretions, if necessary

  c. Evaluate respirations, heart rate, and color

(1) If apneic or gasping, or if heart rate <100 beats per minute (bpm), initiate PPV with oxygen saturation monitoring within 30–60 seconds, considering the use of a cardiac monitor

(2) If heart rate <60 bpm after 30 seconds of effective PPV, intubate and continue PPV, and initiate chest compressions; increase oxygen to 100% with chest compressions

(3) If heart rate ≥60 bpm, continue PPV without chest compressions

  d. Medications

(1) Initiate medications when heart rate <60 bpm after 45–60 seconds of coordinated chest compressions and PPV

(2) Dosage based on estimated infant weight

(3) Medications include:

    (a) Epinephrine—increases strength and rate of cardiac contractions and causes peripheral vasoconstriction

    (b) Volume expanders—recommended solution is normal saline

    (c) Sodium bicarbonate—rarely used, but may be beneficial in correcting acidosis during prolonged resuscitation

    (d) Naloxone—narcotic antagonist used in case of severe respiratory depression and a history of maternal opioid administration within the last 4 hours; do not use if maternal history of long-term opioid use

6. Newborns with meconium-stained amniotic fluid

  a. If the baby has a normal respiratory effort, normal tone, and heart rate ≥100 bpm, use a cloth to clear secretions from mouth and nose while the infant remains with the parent; may use a bulb syringe when secretions are obstructing breathing or when having difficulty clearing secretions

  b. If the baby is not vigorous, as evidenced by depressed respirations, depressed tone, or heart rate <100 bpm, initiate PPV; routine ET suctioning of meconium is no longer indicated due to lack of evidence to support this practice

7. Resuscitation of preterm infants at <35 weeks' gestation should be initiated with 21%–30% oxygen, titrating to preductal oxygen saturation range for healthy term infants; percentage of oxygen to be delivered based on an algorithm of infant's oxygen saturation (as determined by pulse oximeter) for age (in minutes)

8. Cessation of resuscitation efforts 20 minutes after birth is reasonable with the following considerations:

  a. Optimal resuscitation efforts

  b. Availability of advanced neonatal care

  c. Labor circumstances

  d. Wishes of the parents

Care During the First Hours After Birth

- Transitional period
  1. Time when the infant stabilizes and adjusts to extrauterine life
  2. Three stages
     a. First period of reactivity
     b. Period of unresponsive sleep
     c. Second period of reactivity
  3. May be altered when the infant is significantly stressed in labor and delivery
  4. Preferred management for the first hour of life; some say during the hospital stay
     a. Maintain contact with the mother/birthing parent
     b. Limit or defer examinations and procedures, or perform them unobtrusively
- First period of reactivity
  1. Begins immediately after birth
  2. Lasts approximately 1–2 hours
  3. Assessment findings
     a. Rapid heart rate and respirations—near upper limits of normal
     b. Respiratory rales present, disappearing by 20 minutes of age
     c. Behavior—alert; eyes open; may exhibit startle, cry, and/or exhibit rooting
     d. Bowel sounds usually present 30 minutes after birth; may pass stool
  4. Encourage breastfeeding/chestfeeding during the first period of reactivity
     a. Facilitated by the infant's alert, active state
     b. Ameliorates physiologic drop in blood glucose at 1–1.5 hours after birth
- Period of unresponsive sleep
  1. Lasts from 1 to 4 hours after birth
  2. Assessment findings
     a. Heart rate decreases—usually to less than 140 bpm
     b. Murmur may be present because of incomplete closure of ductus arteriosus
     c. Slower, more regular respirations
     d. Bowel sounds present but diminished
- Second period of reactivity
  1. Lasts from 2 to 8 hours after birth
  2. Assessment findings
     a. Labile heart rate
     b. Rapid changes in color
     c. Respiration—rate less than 60 breaths per minute without rales or rhonchi
  3. Early feeding
     a. Infant may be interested in feeding during the second period of reactivity
     b. Prevention of hypoglycemia
     c. Stimulation of stool passage
     d. Prevention of jaundice
- Bonding and parent–newborn attachment
  1. Definitions vary; generally referring to the process occurring in the time after birth whereby the mother or birthing parent (and/or other family members) form a

unique, lasting relationship with the newborn (refer to Chapter 9, Postpartum and Lactation, for further information)
2. Factors that may influence bonding and attachment
   a. Parental background
      (1) Care that parents received from their parents
      (2) Social/cultural factors
      (3) Couple and family relationships
      (4) Experiences in previous pregnancies
   b. Care practices
      (1) Interventions and assessments before and after birth
      (2) Behavior of healthcare providers
      (3) Care and support received in birthing area
      (4) Institutional rules and policies
   c. Facilitating factors
      (1) Skin-to-skin contact immediately upon birth
      (2) Breastfeeding/chestfeeding
      (3) Visual contact
      (4) Holding, touching, "getting acquainted"
3. Limitations of bonding and attachment theories
   a. Formation of relationships probably evolves out of many experiences rather than a single critical event
   b. Little evidence that early separation has permanent effects on mother–infant or parent–child relationships
   c. May lead to judgmental responses among healthcare providers, or guilt among parents, when bonding expectations are not met

Plan of Care for the First Few Days of Life

- Feeding—see also Chapter 9, Postpartum and Lactation, for more information
  1. Demand feeding
     a. Indicated for both breastfed and bottle-fed infants
     b. Most infants will stop sucking and may fall asleep when full and satisfied
  2. Breastfeeding/Chestfeeding
     a. Breastfed infants average 8–12 feedings per day
     b. Intake is adequate if the infant seems satisfied and wets four to six diapers per day
     c. Frequent assessment, reassurance, and anticipatory guidance are essential for breastfeeding/chestfeeding parents and infants in the first few days of life
     d. Discourage supplementary bottle-feedings to promote the development of maternal and infant breastfeeding/chestfeeding skills and to ensure adequate milk supply
  3. Formula feeding
     a. Formula-fed infants average six to eight feedings per day
     b. Limited stomach capacity
        (1) Infant may take only 20–30 mL of formula at initial feedings
        (2) Most infants should take 60–120 mL formula per feeding by the third day of life
     c. Demonstrate positioning and burping techniques

- Voiding/stooling
  1. Record the time and characteristics of the first passage of urine and stool
  2. Stool will progress from meconium to yellow-green
  3. Absence of voiding for 24 hours is an indication for pediatric evaluation
- Skin
  1. Full baths and use of antibacterial soap are discouraged
  2. "Dry care"—skin is dried and skin folds are wiped clean with gauze
  3. Warm sponge bath late in the first day of life to clear blood and meconium
  4. Discourage the use of skin lotions, powders, creams, oils
- Medications
  1. Gonorrhea/chlamydia prophylaxis
     a. 0.5% erythromycin ophthalmic ointment
     b. Should be deferred until after the first period of reactivity
  2. Vitamin K
     a. Prevention of early vitamin K deficiency bleeding (VKDB)
     b. AAP recommends vitamin K should be given as a single, intramuscular dose of 0.5–1.0 mg to all newborns; in the United States, there is currently no recommendation for oral vitamin K
  3. Hepatitis B vaccination
     a. First dose within 24 hours of birth in medically stable infants weighing $\geq$2,000 g; infant born to a patient with known hepatitis B should receive both the vaccine and hepatitis B immune globulin, delivered at separate anatomic sites, within 12 hours of birth
     b. Second dose at 1–2 months of age
     c. Third dose at 6–18 months (no earlier than 24 weeks of age)
- Health promotion and safety
  1. All caregivers should wash their hands thoroughly before handling the infant
  2. Follow policies/procedures for infant identification
  3. Follow policies/procedures for infant security
  4. Teaching—safety and signs of illness (see following sections on Discharge Teaching and Safety)

Discharge Planning

- Discharge teaching
  1. Breastfeeding/chestfeeding
     a. On demand, at least every 2–5 hours
     b. Average 8–12 feedings every 24 hours
     c. Allow the infant to remain on the breast until signs of satiety demonstrated
     d. Adequate maternal rest and fluid intake
     e. Sore nipples usually indicate incorrect positioning or latch-on
  2. Formula feeding
     a. Use iron-fortified formula
     b. Clean nipples and bottles thoroughly prior to use

c. 1.5–4 oz every 3–4 hours, increasing gradually based on infant cues of hunger/satiety

d. Supplementary water or juice not recommended

3. Voiding/stooling

  a. Bottle-fed infant stools—yellow-green, firm to pasty; straining is normal and not necessarily indicative of constipation

  b. Breastfed infant stools—yellow-gold, loose or liquid, seedy; frequency varies; stooling with each feed or every other day

  c. Typical number of wet and stool diapers in the first 7 days of life

    (1) Day 1 (first 24 hours after birth): more than one wet diaper; one stool (thick, tarry, black)

    (2) Day 2: more than two wet diapers; three stools (thick, tarry, black)

    (3) Day 3: more than five to six disposable diapers, more than six to eight cloth diapers; more than three stools (transition stools to looser dark green to mustard yellow)

    (4) Day 4: more than six wet diapers; more than three stools (bright mustard yellow, soft, may be watery)

    (5) Days 5–7: more than six wet diapers; more than three stools (bright mustard yellow, may be seedy)

4. Physiologic jaundice

  a. Occurs in more than 50% of newborns

  b. Temporary condition, rarely indicative of disease

  c. Usually peaks at 3–4 days of life

  d. Yellowing of the sclera should be evaluated by a pediatric provider

5. Skin

  a. Sponge bath every day or every other day

  b. Tub baths after cord stump falls off

  c. Mild, unscented soap

  d. Lotions, oils, and powders are unnecessary

  e. Dry/peeling skin is normal and resolves spontaneously

  f. Diaper rash may be treated with petroleum jelly and air exposure, but notify the pediatric provider if persistent

6. Cord care

  a. In developed countries, antiseptic solutions no longer typically applied to cord; keep the area dry

  b. Diaper should be fastened below the cord

  c. Avoid immersion of cord stump in water

  d. Cord will usually drop off at approximately 2 weeks

  e. Redness around the cord base, foul odor, or drainage from the cord should be reported to the pediatric provider

7. Safety

  a. Infant car seats for every car ride

  b. Handheld carrier versus body carrier—pros and cons

  c. Bottle propping is dangerous because of choking risk

  d. Avoid handling hot liquids while handling newborn

  e. Avoid exposure to direct sunshine; sunscreens are not necessarily safe for newborns

  f. Install smoke and carbon monoxide detectors

  g. Avoid exposure to cigarette smoke

  h. Safe sleep environment

    (1) Use a firm sleep surface covered by a snug fitted sheet

    (2) Do not use pillows, blankets, sheepskins, or crib bumpers in infant sleep area

    (3) Keep soft objects, toys, loose bedding, and sleep positioners out of the infant's sleep area

    (4) Do not smoke or let anyone smoke around the infant

    (5) Make sure that nothing covers the infant's head

    (6) Always place the infant on his or her back for sleep, for naps, and at night

    (7) Dress the infant in sleep clothing, such as a one-piece sleeper; do not use a blanket

    (8) The infant's sleep area should be near where the parents sleep

    (9) The infant should not sleep in an adult bed, on a couch, or in a chair alone, with parents, or with any other persons

    (10) Instruct all the infant's care providers to follow these recommendations every time the infant is put to sleep

8. Expected infant behavior

  a. Hiccups are common and do not require treatment

  b. Sneezing is normal and does not necessarily indicate illness

9. Signs of illness

  a. Poor feeding, irritability, lethargy, skin rash, cord problems, vomiting, diarrhea, decreased urine output, rectal temperature >100°F, or change in infant's behavior

  b. Emphasize that neonatal infection is not always accompanied by fever

- Maternal psychosocial barriers/considerations to discharge

1. Current substance use
2. Present or historical psychiatric illness
3. Severe illness or physical disability
4. History of abuse or neglect of a previous child
5. Inappropriate behavior
6. Homelessness or inadequate living arrangements

- Physical barriers to discharge

1. Feedings—newborn must demonstrate adequate intake of human milk or formula prior to discharge
2. Prematurity

  a. Any newborn <37 weeks' gestation or <2,500 g should be observed for a minimum of 3 days or in accordance with pediatric/neonatal department policy

  b. Premature infants must demonstrate the ability to maintain normal body temperature outside the incubator for 24 hours prior to discharge

3. Neonatal opioid withdrawal syndrome (NOWS)

  a. Universal toxicology testing of the birthing person at the time of birth is not recommended; informed consent should be promoted due to the complexity of testing processes, the risk of racial biases, and resulting racial inequities.

b. Resulting from chronic perinatal exposure to opioids

c. Assessment of the infants with NOWS should include a thorough assessment of the maternal medical and psycho-social history (i.e., substance and medication use, childhood adversities, trauma, mental health disorders, cultural beliefs, and infectious diseases).

d. Toxicology testing can occur through urine, meconium, and umbilical cord tissue and should be performed only when clinical details are lacking (e.g., limited prenatal care or placental abruption); this may not be necessary where the birthing person is in treatment receiving frequent toxicology testing.

  (1) Referral to child protective services may be indicated if withdrawal symptoms occur or if the newborn's urine toxicology is positive

e. A standard scoring system should be used across patients for diagnosis and treatment.

f. Newborns should be held for observation

g. If medication is required to treat withdrawal, the newborn must be held until the medication is no longer necessary

h. Discharge checklist to include:

  (1) Newborn should be asymptomatic for 24–48 hours

  (2) Parent education about NOWS, newborn care, and safe sleep

  (3) A plan for Hepatitis C testing follow-up

  (4) Pediatric follow-up within 48 hours of discharge

i. Social work evaluation completed with a plan of safe care referrals to early intervention, home visiting nurse, developmental–behavioral health specialist

4. Congenital abnormalities

a. Heart murmurs suspected to be pathologic should be evaluated prior to discharge

b. Dislocated hips should be evaluated by an orthopedic specialist and treatment should begin prior to discharge

c. Abnormal renal findings on prenatal ultrasound should be evaluated prior to discharge

5. Infections

a. Sepsis—screen infants at risk for sepsis with Rubarth Newborn Scale of Sepsis; diagnostic workup is indicated to help establish the diagnosis, although no laboratory test is 100% sensitive and 100% specific; infants determined to be at risk should be treated with antibiotics until blood cultures are negative for 48–72 hours

b. Syphilis—infants with congenital syphilis or infants of pregnant people with untreated syphilis should receive a spinal tap and be treated within 10 days with intramuscular or intravenous penicillin

c. Pneumonia—infants with pneumonia should be held in hospital for 7–14 days for antibiotic treatment

6. Hyperbilirubinemia

a. Physiologic jaundice

  (1) Not visible in first 24 hours

  (2) Rises slowly and peaks at day 3 or 4 of life

  (3) Total bilirubin peaks at <13 mg/dL

  (4) Lab tests reveal predominance of unconjugated (indirect) bilirubin

  (5) Not visible after 10 days

b. Possible pathologic jaundice

  (1) Visible during the first 24 hours

  (2) May rise quickly to >5 mg/dL in 24 hours

  (3) Total bilirubin >13 mg/dL

  (4) Greater amounts of conjugated (direct) bilirubin

  (5) Visible jaundice persists after 1 week

c. Risk factors for developing significant hyperbilirubinemia

  (1) Lower gestational age

  (2) Jaundice within the first 24 hours

  (3) Predischarge bilirubin values close to the phototherapy threshold

  (4) Hemolysis

  (5) Phototherapy before discharge

  (6) Parent or sibling requiring phototherapy

  (7) Family or genetic history of inherited disorders (e.g., glucose-6-phosphate dehydrogenase (G6PD) deficiency)

  (8) Exclusive breastfeeding with poor intake

  (9) Hematoma or bruising (e.g., postvacuum assisted birth)

  (10) Down Syndrome

  (11) Macrosomic infant of a mother who has diabetes

d. Labs—total serum bilirubin (TSB), blood type, Rh, Coombs's test

  (1) Less invasive transcutaneous bilirubin (TcB) may be used to guide the need for TSB; only TSB should be used to determine treatment

e. Phototherapy, if indicated, may be arranged through home healthcare agency

f. Infants with elevated bilirubin but without hemolytic disease may be discharged if outpatient pediatric follow-up can be arranged

- Criteria for early discharge

1. General criteria

a. Following uncomplicated birth, most infants may be discharged 3–24 hours after birth depending on the hospital/birth center policy

b. Joint decision by the midwife, pediatric provider, and family

c. Uncomplicated antepartum, intrapartum, and postpartum course

d. Early discharge increases the importance of patient and family education to assess newborn

e. Adequate support for the postpartum person at home, including home healthcare referral, if necessary

2. Neonatal criteria

a. Uncomplicated vaginal delivery

b. Full-term infant with adequate growth (2,500–4,500 g)

c. Normal findings on neonatal examination

d. May be a minimum of 6-hour hospitalization but at least sufficient time under provider care to demonstrate:

(1) Thermal homeostasis

(2) Ability to feed

e. Normal laboratory results confirmed

3. Maternal criteria

a. Demonstrated ability with the chosen feeding method

b. Demonstrated ability with cord care

c. Demonstrated ability to assess newborn's temperature with a thermometer

d. Verbalizes understanding of signs of newborn well-being and illness

- Discharge evaluation

1. Complete physical examination with emphasis on the following

a. Frequency and duration of breastfeeding/chestfeeding or frequency and amount of bottle-feeding

b. Number of voids/stools

c. Present weight and birth weight

2. Discharge evaluation should be performed in the presence of parents for teaching, answering questions, and providing anticipatory guidance

- Follow-up care

1. Pediatric follow-up should be arranged prior to discharge

2. Factors influencing the time of first pediatric visit

a. Medical condition of the newborn

b. Length of hospital stay

c. Experience of mother and family in caring for newborns

d. Size of newborn

e. Family psychosocial factors

f. Adequacy of newborn feeding

Newborn Assessment

- History—see the section Immediate Care and Assessment of the Healthy Newborn
- Physical examination

1. General

a. Whole

(1) Proportions

(2) Symmetry

(3) Facies

(4) Gestational age (approximate)

b. Skin

(1) Color

(2) Subcutaneous tissue

(3) Imperfections (bands and birthmarks)

(4) Vernix and lanugo

(5) Cysts and masses

c. Neuromuscular

(1) Movements

(2) Responses

(3) Tone (flexor)

2. Head and neck

a. Head

(1) Shape

(2) Circumference

(3) Molding

(4) Swellings

(5) Depressions

b. Fontanels, sutures

(1) Size

(2) Tension

c. Eyes

(1) Size

(2) Separation

(3) Cataracts

d. Ears

(1) Placement

(2) Complexity

(3) Preauricular tags

e. Mouth

(1) Symmetry

(2) Size

(3) Clefts

f. Neck

(1) Swellings

(2) Fistulas

3. Chest

a. Inspect for deformities (nipples, clavicles, sternum)

b. Observe respiratory function in the abdomen

c. Palpate—breast bud size; clavicle for crepitus and/or swelling

4. Lungs and respiration

a. Retractions

b. Grunting

c. Quality of breath sounds

5. Heart and circulation

a. Rate

b. Rhythm

c. Murmurs—may be present for 1–2 days after birth until ductus arteriosus closes

d. Sounds

6. Abdomen

a. Musculature

b. Bowel sounds

c. Cord vessels—number and type

d. Distension

e. Scaphoid shape

f. Masses

g. Liver edge may be palpable at 2–3 cm below right costal margin

h. Normal spleen and kidneys are not easily felt

i. Femoral pulses are felt when the infant is quiet

7. Genitalia and anus

a. Placement

b. Identify ambiguous genitalia

c. Scrotum—size, skin is wrinkled; determine whether testes are descended

d. Phallus—size, placement of urethra

e. Labia—palpate for masses; identify all structures and determine patency of vaginal orifice

f. Anus—determine patency and relative position to other genital structures

8. Musculoskeletal

a. Posture

b. Hands—digits; polydactyly, syndactyly, webbing, overlapping, shape and texture; "fisting"

c. Feet—degree of flexion, shape, position

d. Neck—rotation

e. Joints—normal range of motion (ROM)

f. Long bone fractures—distortion, swelling, crepitus

9. Spine

a. Symmetry

b. Scoliosis

c. Sinuses

- Gestational age assessment

1. Ballard scale (detailed assessment of gestational age)

a. Estimation of gestational age and maturity based on observation and examination; score total for 40-week infant = 40

b. Elements include posture and tone, and characteristics of skin, lanugo, plantar surface, breast tissue, eyes/ears, and genitals

2. Posture and tone—premature infant generally demonstrates extended posture, less tone, and less resistance to flexion of extremities

3. Skin—premature infant has redder/pinker, translucent skin; postmature infant has cracked, wrinkled skin

4. Lanugo is sparse to absent in the postmature or very premature infants and is most abundant in midterm infants (28–30 weeks)

5. Plantar surface

a. Assessed by the length of the foot from the heel to the tip of the great toe in the premature infant

b. Creases appear by 28–30 weeks' gestation and cover the entire surface at term

6. Breast tissue and areola—progressive development throughout gestation

a. Preterm—flat areola with no palpable breast bud

b. Term infant—raised areola with 3- to 4-mm palpable breast bud

7. Eyes/ears

a. Eyelids are fused in very premature neonate

b. More mature infants exhibit more cartilaginous ear tissue that exhibits greater firmness and recoil when flexed

8. Male genitalia—increasing rugation of the scrotum and descent of testes with advancing gestational age

9. Female genitalia—increasing development of labia majora and decreasing prominence of the clitoris and labia minora with advancing gestational age

10. Anterior vascular capsule of ocular lens—more prominent vasculature at early gestational ages

- Measurements

1. Weight

a. Normal weight for a term newborn is 2,501–4,000 g

b. Less-than-normal birth weight—definitions

(1) Extremely low birth weight—less than 1,000 g

(2) Very low birth weight—1,000 to 1,500 g

(3) Low birth weight—1,501 to 2,500 g

c. Usual growth patterns

(1) Infants typically lose 10%–15% of birth weight in the first 3 days of life

(2) Should regain birth weight by 10–14 days of age

(3) Double birth weight by 4–6 months of age

(4) Triple birth weight by 12 months of age

2. Length

a. Most accurately measured by placing the head against a firm surface, extending the legs, then marking the surface

b. Normal length for a term newborn is 48–53 cm

3. Head circumference

a. Measured from the occiput around the head and above the eyebrows

b. Normal head circumference for a term newborn is 33–35 cm

4. Chest circumference

a. Measured under armpits across the nipple line

b. Normal chest circumference is 30–33 cm, and 2–3 cm less than head circumference

5. Be aware of parents' genetic pool (i.e., one or both of small stature)

- Assessment for congenital disabilities

1. Minor malformations are relatively common, but three or more minor malformations on physical examination are suggestive of a major underlying condition

2. Minor malformations

a. Large fontanels

b. Epicanthic eye fold

c. Hair whorls

d. Widow's peak

e. Low posterior hairline

f. Preauricular skin tags or pits

g. Minor ear anomalies—low-set, rotated, protruding

h. Darwinian tubercule—small nodule on the upper helix of the ear

i. Digital anomalies—curved, webbed, or bent fingers

j. Transverse palmar crease

k. Shawl scrotum

l. Redundant umbilicus

m. Widespread or supernumerary nipples

- Neurologic examination

1. Level of alertness

a. Most sensitive of all neurologic functions

b. Varies depending on gestational age, time of last feeding, sleep patterns, recent stimuli, and recent experiences

c. Findings associated with level of alertness

(1) Response to arousal attempts (e.g., gentle shaking, sound, light)

(2) Level and character of motility

2. Neuromotor findings

a. Tone and posture

b. Motility and power

c. Tendon reflexes—brachioradialis, patellar, Achilles

d. Plantar response—flexion or extension of toes

e. Eyes—red reflex, pupillary reflex, doll's eye reflex, blink reflex

3. Assess for normal, absent, diminished, or exaggerated reflexes—abnormal reflexes suggest nervous system depression, spinal lesion, or CNS disorder or lesion

4. Primary neonatal reflexes

a. Palmar grasp
   (1) Newborn grasps object or finger placed on his or her palm
   (2) Typically disappears by 2 months of age
b. Tonic neck response
   (1) Elicited by rotation of the head to one side
   (2) Newborn extends arm on the side to which the head is rotated and flexes the contralateral arm ("fencing posture")
   (3) Typically disappears by 7 months of age
c. Moro reflex
   (1) "Startle" response, evidenced by abduction and extension of arms with hands open and thumb and index finger semi-flexed to form a "C"
   (2) Elicited by jarring examination table, allowing the infant to fall backward onto the examiner's hand, or making a loud noise
   (3) Typically disappears by 6 months of age
d. Placing and stepping ("walking")
   (1) Elicited by holding the infant upright and placing the soles of feet in contact with a flat surface or table edge
   (2) Typically disappears by 4 weeks of age

- Metabolic screening
  1. No federal guidelines; requirements vary from state to state
  2. Metabolic screening tests mandated in most states; the following are examples
     a. Phenylketonuria (PKU)
     b. Biotinidase deficiency
     c. Congenital adrenal hyperplasia
     d. Congenital hypothyroidism
     e. Cystic fibrosis
     f. Galactosemia
     g. Homocystinuria
     h. Branched-chain ketoaciduria
     i. Sickle cell disease
     j. Tyrosinemia
  3. Timing of metabolic screening
     a. Generally, after 24 hours of age—allowing time for feeding to be established and accumulation of toxic metabolites if disease is present
     b. Preferably 48–72 hours of age
     c. Recommended repeat screening at 2- to 4-week pediatric visit
     d. Law may mandate screening before discharge—for early discharge, repeat screening must be done

Primary Care of the Newborn for the First 6 Weeks

- Well-child surveillance
  1. All newborns should have at least two physical examinations before discharge
  2. Well-child visit
     a. Within 3–5 days for early discharged newborns
     b. Within 10–14 days for newborns held 48 hours

c. Purpose—reexamine newborn, review teaching, perform metabolic screening
d. Assessment components
   (1) Review of maternal, perinatal, and newborn history
   (2) Observation of parents and assessment of family adjustment and interactions
   (3) Newborn interval history, including feeding, behavior, voiding/stooling
   (4) Developmental surveillance (e.g., social and verbal language, gross and fine motor skills)
   (5) Physical examination
e. Universal and selective screening (e.g., hearing, BP, vision)
f. Anticipatory guidance with attention to social determinants of health, parent and family well-being and health, newborn/infant care, nutrition, safety
g. Schedule follow-up visits

- Newborn behavior
  1. Sleep–wake states as classified by Brazelton
     a. Quiet sleep
     b. Active sleep
     c. Drowsy
     d. Quiet alert
     e. Active alert
     f. Crying
  2. Alert state
     a. Determine the infant's ability to feed and interact with the environment
     b. Comprises approximately 15% of daytime hours
  3. Crying
     a. May express need for feeding, holding, stimulation, or sleep
     b. May be indicative of pain
     c. Parental responsiveness to crying does not promote "spoiling" of infant—responsiveness is essential to a newborn's development
  4. Sleeping
     a. Infant may exhibit varying respiratory patterns while sleeping, such as decreased depth and rate or periodic breathing (intermittent cessation of breathing for up to 10 seconds)
     b. Normal infants sleep as much as 60% of the time

- Sensory capabilities
  1. Sensory threshold—level of tolerance for stimuli within which the infant can respond appropriately
     a. Infant may become fatigued or stressed when overstimulated; signs of stress and fatigue include:
        (1) Color changes
        (2) Irregular respiration
        (3) Irritability or lethargy
        (4) Vomiting
     b. Varies significantly among individuals; markedly low in premature or neurologically impaired newborns
  2. Visual capabilities
     a. Normal-term infants can visually fix and track objects
     b. Sharp focus limited to a distance of 10–12 inches
     c. Preference for striped patterns and strong contrasts

d. Limited color perception

e. Ability to recognize parents visually and respond to facial expressions within the first few weeks of life

3. Newborns can detect and discriminate odors

4. Taste capabilities

a. Newborns react strongly to variations in taste

b. Preference for sweets and flavors from maternal diet (prenatal and postnatal flavor learning)

5. Hearing is acute, with the ability to localize sounds and a preference for the mother's voice

6. Touch—sensitive to light touch, as demonstrated by reflex responses

- Regulation of behavior

1. Ability to respond appropriately to stimuli and maintain behavioral states

2. Full-term infants should demonstrate a smooth transition between states from sleep to active alertness; consistently abrupt or unpredictable changes are a cause for concern

3. Ability to maintain an active alert state varies among individuals—some infants have difficulty becoming or remaining alert, whereas irritable infants progress rapidly from alertness to crying

4. Overstimulated infants may require timeout, or relative isolation from stimuli and time to recover

5. Organization—ability to integrate physiologic and behavioral systems in response to the environment without disruption in the state or physiologic functions

a. Maintenance of stable vital signs

b. Smooth state transitions

c. Coordination of movements and responses in interacting with the environment

d. Consolable with the ability for self-consolation (frequently characterized by hand-to-mouth movements)

e. Habituation—ability to block out noxious stimuli

- Developmental milestones in the first 6 weeks as measured by Denver II

1. Personal/social skills—spontaneous and responsive smiling, attentiveness to a face

2. Visual tracking—follows dangling object from midline through 45 degrees

3. Spontaneous vocalization

4. Response to the sound of a bell

5. Gross motor—lifting head momentarily and symmetrical body movements

- Psychological tasks of early infancy as defined by Erikson

1. Development of basic trust

a. Birth through 12–18 months

b. Definition—belief that the world is a place where people and things can be relied on and where needs and wishes will be met

c. Essential for the formation of human attachments throughout life

2. Development of differentiation—ability to discriminate between self and other

3. Ability to elicit caregiving is essential to early development

4. Secure attachment depends on caregivers' characteristics

a. Emotional availability

b. Sensitivity and stimulation

c. Appropriate response to infant cues

d. Consistency

5. In the first year of life, securely attached infants venture out and return to their mother/parent

6. Results of insecure attachment

a. Anxious or unable to cope with changes or distance from mother/parent

b. More negative infant behavior

c. Avoidance/detachment

d. Research suggests long-term impairment, including school problems and delinquency

7. Counseling or parenting classes may be helpful when parents/caregivers are experiencing problems in forming a secure attachment

- Circumcision

1. Increased prevalence in the United States during the 1950s

2. Significant role of cultural, religious, and family traditions

3. Medical complications are rare but serious; include bleeding, infection, and inappropriate operative result

4. Controversial impact on sexual and psychological functioning; no clear evidence

5. AAP (2012) has concluded that there is some benefit of reduced sexually transmitted infections (STIs), urinary tract infections (UTIs), and cancer of the penis in men who are circumcised

a. Although AAP concludes that the evidence for health benefits is not strong enough to recommend routine circumcision for all newborns, the benefits are sufficient to ensure access to this procedure for those families who have chosen to have circumcision performed

b. Opponents maintain that modern sanitary conditions and hygienic practices are more important factors underlying those medical conditions that have shown reductions with circumcision

c. It is important to inform the family members of all known risks and benefits so that they may make an informed, conscious decision

6. Provide pain control if family chooses circumcision

7. Care of circumcised infant

a. Apply petroleum jelly gauze strip to prevent adhesion of tissue to diaper

b. Continue to use petroleum jelly on affected tissue until healed

c. Notify care provider if bleeding, exudate, swelling, or inability to void occur

8. Uncircumcised infant

a. Foreskin should separate and become freely mobile by 4–7 years of age

b. Never forcefully retract the foreskin

c. Infant hygiene—"only clean what can be seen"

d. As the child matures, he should be taught to retract the foreskin and clean

- Nonnutritive sucking

1. Thumb sucking and use of pacifiers subject to parent/family preferences and attitudes

2. Common behavior in utero

3. Infant may use nonnutritive sucking to regulate behavior state or self-console
4. Avoid
   a. Use of empty bottle for nonnutritive sucking—promotes ingestion of air and dental caries; may contribute to otitis
   b. Placing pacifier on string around baby's neck
   c. Prolonged use of and serious dependence on pacifiers

Common Variations from Normal Newborn Findings

- Care of the normal newborn during the first 28 days of life falls within the midwifery scope of practice; the midwife must be able to assess normal findings and identify deviations from normal to provide care within the framework of a management plan that includes consultation, collaborative management, and/or referral as indicated
- Jaundice
  1. Incidence—as many as 50% of newborns
  2. Physiologic versus pathologic jaundice
     a. Physiologic jaundice does not occur within the first 24 hours of life
     b. Total serum bilirubin concentrations increasing by >5 mg/dL per day indicate pathologic jaundice
     c. Physiologic jaundice rarely results in total serum bilirubin concentrations >15 mg/dL
     d. Direct serum bilirubin levels >1.5 mg/dL indicate pathologic jaundice
  3. More common and slower to resolve in breastfed infants
  4. Can be detected by blanching the skin of the nose, palms, or soles of feet—if jaundiced, skin blanches yellow
     a. Inspection can identify jaundice but is not accurate in assessing bilirubin levels
     b. Transcutaneous bilirubinometry (TcB) or serum testing
  5. Treatment
     a. Supplementation of breastfed infants with oral glucose water is not helpful and may be harmful
     b. Frequent feeding to stimulate GI elimination
     c. Management online algorithm: Bilitool very useful because treatment levels vary depending on the age (in hours) of the infant and potential risk factors (such as preterm)
        (1) Phototherapy: first-line treatment
        (2) Exchange transfusion may be indicated
     d. Treatment thresholds are lower at earlier ages—24 to 48 hours after birth
- Obstructed lacrimal ducts
  1. Incidence—50% of newborns exhibit excessive tearing and mucoid discharge from the eyes
  2. Treatment
     a. Massage—apply gentle, firm pressure in a circular motion on the lateral aspect of the nose adjacent to the inner canthus of the eye

b. Clear drainage with cotton ball moistened with warm water, proceeding from inner to outer canthus
     c. Repeat treatment three to four times per day
- Dacryocystitis
  1. Definition—acute infection of lacrimal ducts
  2. Presentation—purulent discharge, swelling, tenderness adjacent to the inner canthus of the eye
  3. Treatment
     a. Same hygiene routine as described for obstructed lacrimal ducts
     b. Aseptic technique to prevent cross-contamination
     c. Topical or systemic antibiotics are indicated
- Skin problems
  1. Cradle cap
     a. Definition—dermatitis resulting from accumulation of sebum on the scalp
     b. Presentation—characteristic yellow, crusting patches on the anterior scalp, often in the area of the anterior fontanel
     c. Treatment
        (1) Vigorous cleansing with mild shampoo and washcloth
        (2) Apply baby oil to area 30 minutes prior to shampooing
        (3) Rub the affected area with a dry washcloth gently but firmly to remove crusting
        (4) If severe, antiseborrheic shampoo may be indicated
  2. Diaper dermatitis
     a. Definition—general term for a variety of skin conditions that can occur in the diaper area
     b. Primary—caused by exposure to moisture and friction
     c. Secondary
        (1) Caused by the colonization of the affected area by a pathogen, most commonly *Candida albicans*
        (2) Presentation—fire-engine red erythema, circumscribed pustulovesicular lesions, often with satellite lesions
     d. Treatment
        (1) Change diapers frequently
        (2) Avoid the use of baby wipes
        (3) Rinse the area with tepid water after every voiding; use tepid water and mild soap after stooling
        (4) Clean and dry skin thoroughly
        (5) Allow exposure of skin to air, especially before reapplying diaper
        (6) Some infants are sensitive to irritants in disposable diapers; change brands or use cloth diapers
        (7) For infants with diarrhea, apply zinc oxide ointment to clean, dry skin to provide a barrier
        (8) Severe irritation may be treated with 1% topical hydrocortisone
        (9) Nystatin topical cream, applied at each diaper change, for *Candida albicans* dermatitis
- Thrush
  1. Definition—oral fungal infection usually caused by *Candida albicans*

2. Peak incidence around the second week of life
3. Often occurs after antibiotic therapy
4. Presentation—characteristic white patches on the buccal mucosa, gums, tongue, and/or palate; lesions may be friable
5. May cause feeding difficulty if extensive
6. Treatment
   a. Nystatin suspension orally four times a day for 1 week
   b. Instill one dropper-full into each buccal pocket
   c. "Paint" lesions with a cotton-tipped applicator
   d. Bottle-fed infants—boil nipples after use
   e. Breastfed infants—treat nursing parent's nipples simultaneously with topical antifungal agents (nystatin, miconazole, clotrimazole) or with oral fluconazole, if topical treatment fails

- Regurgitation
  1. Definition—effortless "spitting up" of a small amount of formula or breastmilk
  2. Exacerbated by excessive swallowing of air, resulting from underfeeding or delayed feeding and prolonged crying, improper positioning, sucking on empty formula bottle
  3. Treatment
     a. Normal self-limiting condition; no treatment necessary
     b. May be reduced if the infant is positioned sitting upright at 50- to 60-degree angle for 30 to 60 minutes after feeding

- Colic
  1. Definition—sudden, loud, and/or continuous unexplained crying often accompanied by flushed facies, mild abdominal distention, adduction of legs, or clenched fists
  2. Affects 10% of infants
  3. No proven organic basis; suggested but unproved causative factors may include:
     a. Overfeeding, especially in bottle-fed infants
     b. Allergy to constituents of formula or lactating parent's diet (milk products often suggested)
     c. Anxiety in the primary caregiver or tension in the household; possibly symptomatic rather than etiologic
     d. Immaturity of the digestive system
  4. Treatment
     a. Attempt to identify factors associated with colic episodes for the individual infant
     b. Correct overfeeding
     c. Trial elimination of milk products from lactating parent's diet
        (1) Efficacy is unknown; anecdotally effective in many cases
        (2) If bovine allergens are implicated, a trial longer than 1 week is necessary to clear a lactating person's system
        (3) Maternal calcium supplementation is suggested with this approach
     d. Some infants respond to warmth, wrapping in a blanket, limitation of stimuli, rhythmic soothing motion, gentle repetitive massage, or soft monotonous music

   e. Probably the most important factor is supportive care for parents, including reassurance and respite opportunities
   f. As a last resort for exhausted parents, the infant may be positioned safely and left to cry for limited periods of time

Deviations from Normal

- Danger signs of neonatal morbidity
  1. CNS signs
     a. Lethargy
     b. High-pitched cry
     c. Jitteriness
     d. Abnormal eye movement
     e. Seizure activity
     f. Abnormal fontanel size or bulging fontanels
  2. Respiratory signs
     a. Intermittent cessation of breathing for more than 15 seconds, usually accompanied by bradycardia or cyanosis
     b. Tachypnea
     c. Nasal flaring, expiratory grunting, and/or chest retractions
     d. Persistent rales and/or rhonchi
     e. Asynchronous breathing movements
  3. Cardiovascular signs
     a. Abnormal rate and rhythm
     b. Murmurs
     c. Changes in blood pressure
     d. Marked differential between upper- and lower-extremity blood pressures
     e. Alterations and/or differentials in pulses
     f. Changes in perfusion and skin color
  4. GI signs
     a. Refusal to feed
     b. Absent or uncoordinated feeding reflexes
     c. Vomiting
     d. Abdominal distention
     e. Changes in stool patterns
  5. Genitourinary signs
     a. Hematuria
     b. Absence of urine or failure to pass urine
  6. Metabolic alterations
     a. Hypoglycemia
     b. Hypocalcemia
     c. Hyperbilirubinemia and jaundice, especially jaundice occurring within the first 24 hours of life
  7. Fluid balance alterations
     a. Decreased urine output
     b. Weight loss of 5%–15% in one day
     c. Dry mucous membranes
     d. Sunken fontanels
     e. Poor skin turgor
     f. Increased hematocrit
  8. Temperature instability
- Preterm infants
  1. Definition—infants born before 37 completed weeks of gestation

2. Associated complications
   a. Respiratory complications
   b. Necrotizing enterocolitis
   c. Intraventricular hemorrhage
   d. Hypothermia
   e. Hypoglycemia
   f. Infection
   g. Hyperbilirubinemia
3. Maternal factors associated with prematurity
   a. Obstetric—uterine malformation, multiple gestation, cervical insufficiency, premature rupture of membranes, hypertensive disorders of pregnancy, placenta previa, history of previous preterm birth, isoimmunization
   b. Medical—diabetes, hypertension, UTI, other acute illness
   c. Psychosocial—poor prenatal care, low socioeconomic status, malnutrition, adolescent pregnancy, substance use
- Small for gestational age (SGA) infants
  1. Definition—birth weight <10th percentile
  2. Symmetric growth restriction
     a. Results from early and prolonged insult(s)
     b. Associated with decreased brain size and intellectual disability
     c. Growth restriction continues after birth
  3. Asymmetric growth restriction
     a. Results from insult(s) late in pregnancy
     b. Head circumference is near normal for gestational age
     c. Rapid postnatal growth and development with normal cognitive development
  4. Maternal factors associated with fetal growth restriction
     a. Obstetric—history of infertility, history of abortions, grand multiparity, hypertensive disorders of pregnancy
     b. Medical—heart disease, renal disease, hypertension, sickle cell disease, PKU, diabetes
     c. Psychosocial—malnutrition, low socioeconomic status, extremes of maternal age, poor prenatal care, substance use
- Postterm infants
  1. Definition—born after 42 completed weeks of gestation
  2. Associated complications
     a. Meconium aspiration
        (1) Physical barrier to gas exchange
        (2) Causes chemical irritation and thickening of the alveolar walls
        (3) Vasoconstriction/vasospasm may cause pulmonary hypertension and persistent fetal circulation
     b. Hypoglycemia
     c. Polycythemia
     d. Hypothermia
  3. Associated maternal and fetal factors
     a. Maternal—primigravid, grand multiparity, previous postterm delivery
     b. Fetal—anencephaly, trisomies
- Large for gestational age (LGA) infants
  1. Definition—birth weight >90th percentile; sometimes defined as birth weight >4,000 or 4,500 g

2. Associated complications
   a. Birth injuries, including fractures and intracranial hemorrhage
   b. Hypoglycemia
   c. Polycythemia
   d. Perinatal asphyxia
3. Maternal factors associated with excessive fetal growth
   a. Gestational diabetes
   b. Genetic predisposition
   c. Excessive weight gain during pregnancy
4. Infants born to a pregnant person with diabetes
   a. Gestational diabetes and hyperglycemia more likely to result in excessive fetal growth (macrosomia)
   b. Chronic or severe diabetes with vascular changes more likely to result in growth restriction
   c. Pregestational diabetes associated with congenital anomalies, including CNS anomalies, congenital heart defects, and tracheoesophageal fistula
- Neonatal infection
  1. Signs of infection in the newborn
     a. Often subtle and nonspecific
     b. Early signs—lethargy, refusal to feed, vomiting, temperature instability
     c. May show subtle changes in color—cyanosis, pallor, mottling
     d. May be related to the involved organ system(s)
        (1) CNS infections—jitteriness, seizures
        (2) Pulmonary infections—respiratory distress, apnea
        (3) Intestinal infections—diarrhea
  2. Signs of chronic intrauterine infection
     a. Growth restriction
     b. Microcephaly
     c. Hepatosplenomegaly
  3. Sepsis
     a. Increased susceptibility because of immature immune function
     b. Evaluation includes blood and cerebrospinal fluid (CSF) cultures; complete blood count (CBC) with differential; IgM titer; chest radiograph; toxoplasmosis, rubella, cytomegalovirus (CMV), and herpes screening
  4. Bacterial infections
     a. Group B b-hemolytic *Streptococcus* (GBS)
        (1) Most common pathogen in neonatal infections
        (2) Etiology—maternal colonization, transmitted to the neonate during labor and delivery
        (3) Preterm newborns at the highest risk
        (4) Early-onset GBS disease—develops within the first 24 hours of life; characterized by respiratory involvement; may be fatal
        (5) Late-onset GBS disease—onset usually after the second week of life; characterized by CNS involvement; rarely fatal but may result in permanent neurologic damage
     b. *Listeria*
        (1) Presentation—diffuse papular rash on trunk and pharynx, respiratory distress, cyanosis, sepsis
        (2) Etiology—maternal colonization, transmitted to the neonate during labor and delivery

c. *Escherichia coli*
  (1) Major cause of neonatal meningitis and sepsis
  (2) Etiology—maternal colonization, transmitted to the neonate during labor and delivery
d. *Neisseria gonorrhoeae*
  (1) Pathogenic for ophthalmia neonatorum
  (2) May cause blindness if untreated
  (3) Prophylaxis—administration of silver nitrate or erythromycin ointment to eyes after birth
  (4) May invade joint capsules, causing septic arthritis, although this is rare
e. Tuberculosis
  (1) Congenital disease is rare unless the pregnant person has untreated, advanced disease
  (2) Primarily affects newborn liver when acquired before birth
  (3) Separation of the newborn from mother is unnecessary if the mother has negative chest radiograph and negative sputum culture, and is receiving treatment
5. Viral and protozoal infections
  a. Toxoplasmosis
    (1) Associated with raw meat and infected feces, especially cat
    (2) Pregnant person is often asymptomatic
    (3) Signs of infection in the newborn include microcephaly, cerebral calcifications, chorioretinitis, hepatosplenomegaly, and jaundice
    (4) Treatment limits further disease but does not correct damage to CNS
  b. Syphilis
    (1) Signs of infection in the newborn include intrauterine growth restriction (IUGR), ascites, rhinitis, jaundice, anemia
    (2) Spontaneous abortion, stillbirth, or newborn demise occurs in 40% of cases when the pregnant person is untreated; another 40% of cases result in congenital syphilis
    (3) Congenital syphilis may result in multisystem organ damage and/or death
  c. Rubella
    (1) Infection in utero may result in IUGR, cardiac anomalies, deafness, blindness, and/or intellectual disability
    (2) Effects depend on gestational age at transmission and duration of infection
  d. CMV
    (1) No effective means of treatment or prevention
    (2) Effects of congenital CMV infection—30% incidence of death in infancy; 90% of survivors have CNS, visual, and/or auditory damage
  e. Herpes
    (1) Transmission typically occurs during the intrapartum period; prenatal infection is rare
    (2) Newborns are susceptible to systemic disease, which may involve hepatitis, pneumonia, encephalitis, and/or disseminated intravascular coagulopathy

(3) Primary maternal infection is associated with a 50% newborn mortality rate and high rates of permanent neurologic damage
(4) Recurrent maternal infection rarely results in severe systemic disease
f. Hepatitis B
  (1) Often results in prematurity and low birth weight
  (2) Onset of disease occurs 4–6 weeks after birth; marked by poor feeding, jaundice, and hepatomegaly
  (3) Most infants infected perinatally demonstrate a carrier state without acute disease
g. Chlamydia
  (1) Most common cause of blindness worldwide
  (2) Intrapartum transmission may result in conjunctivitis, pneumonia, and/or otitis media
  (3) Chlamydial conjunctivitis is not prevented by ocular administration of silver nitrate; erythromycin ophthalmic ointment is preferred
h. Human immunodeficiency virus (HIV) and acquired immunodeficiency syndrome (AIDS)
  (1) Prenatal antiretroviral therapy dramatically reduces vertical transmission; cesarean section prior to the start of labor is recommended for all women with a viral load ≥1,000 copies/mL to further reduce the risk of vertical transmission
  (2) Can be transmitted via human milk
  (3) May result in prematurity, growth restriction, and/or microcephaly
  (4) Opportunistic infection usually manifests within the first months of life
i. Zika
  (1) Antenatal prevention—ensure protection from mosquito bites and sexual transmission; avoid travel to areas where prevalent
  (2) Following travel to an area where there is a risk for Zika exposure, testing is recommended for the following: symptomatic pregnant individuals, asymptomatic pregnant individuals with ongoing Zika exposure, and pregnant individuals with ultrasound findings suspicious of congenital Zika infection
  (3) May result in microcephaly, neurologic problems in infants (full extent remains unknown)
  (4) Zika virus testing and additional neurologic workup are recommended for infants with congenital disabilities consistent with congenital Zika syndrome regardless of maternal lab findings if possible exposure, and for infants without associated congenital disabilities if known Zika infection during pregnancy
j. COVID-19
  (1) Universal screening of the birthing person recommended. Antenatal prevention–immunization, masking, breastfeeding; in the birth setting with known COVID-positive patients, negative pressure isolation, limiting the birth team to essential workers, careful

PPE for all team members, and masking for the birthing person

(2) Transmission possible through postpartum transmission (i.e., from an infected parent, family member, or caregiver), intrapartum transmission (i.e., from exposure to infected secretions or feces), or intrauterine transmission (i.e., transplacental; least likely)

(3) Human milk may provide protective antibodies against infection as well as physical distance (preferably with a barrier) between feedings

(4) Neonatal vaccination not currently available

- Plexus injuries
  1. Prognosis is good; 88%–92% of affected infants recover fully within the first year of life
  2. Thought to result from lateral traction on the shoulder or head during delivery; some evidence of intrauterine effect also exists
  3. Erb's palsy
     a. Accounts for 90% of all plexus injuries
     b. Involves upper part of the plexus (C5 through C7, and occasionally C4)
     c. Shoulder and upper arm are affected
     d. Decreased biceps reflex present
     e. When C4 is involved, diaphragmatic dysfunction present
  4. Total palsy
     a. Accounts for 8%–9% of all plexus injuries
     b. Diffuse plexus involvement (C5 to T1)
     c. Upper arm, lower arm, and hand are affected
     d. Biceps and triceps reflexes are decreased
  5. Klumpke paralysis
     a. Accounts for less than 2% of all plexus injuries
     b. Involves C8 to T1
     c. Lower arm and hand are affected
  6. Associated injuries—clavicle fracture, humerus fracture, shoulder dislocation, facial nerve injury
  7. Management usually consists initially of limiting movement of the affected extremity, and then gradual introduction of gentle ROM exercises
- Neonatal fractures
  1. Fracture of the clavicle—not a significant newborn fracture
     a. Most common neonatal fracture
     b. Signs—hematoma, crepitus, asymmetric tone/movement of upper extremities
     c. Sometimes associated with plexus injuries
  2. Fracture of humerus or femur—significant fractures, may be nosocomial
     a. Rare; usually associated with breech deliveries
     b. Ecchymosis, hematoma, or hemorrhage may occur at fracture site
  3. Skull fracture
     a. Rare; may be associated with forceps delivery
     b. Linear fracture—usually benign, resolves without treatment
     c. Depressed fracture—may be associated with seizures and/or permanent neurologic injury
     d. Signs—cephalohematoma, palpable depression in bone

- Infants with hemolytic disease
  1. Definition—destruction of RBCs, resulting in hyperbilirubinemia and jaundice
  2. Causes—maternal antibodies, enzymatic disorders, infections
  3. Rh incompatibility
     a. Occurs when the pregnant person is Rh negative and the fetus is Rh positive
     b. Positive result on direct Coombs's test indicates the presence of maternal antibodies
     c. May necessitate exchange transfusion
  4. ABO incompatibility
     a. Occurs when a pregnant person is serologic type O and the fetus is type A or B; infrequently when a pregnant person is type A and the fetus is type B
     b. Very rare incidence of hydrops or stillbirth
     c. May result in neonatal jaundice; rarely causes severe hemolysis or anemia
- Hyperbilirubinemia and severe jaundice
  1. Associated with many neonatal complications, including hemolytic disease, prematurity, impaired hepatic function, sepsis, metabolic disorders, hematomas, impaired intestinal function, and others
  2. Kernicterus
     a. Encephalopathy caused by deposition of bilirubin in brain cells
     b. Classic signs—lethargy, diminished reflexes, hypotonia, seizures
     c. Contributing factors—prematurity, hypothermia, asphyxia, acidosis, sepsis
     d. Complications—hearing impairment, cerebral palsy, intellectual disability
  3. Phototherapy
     a. Oxidizes unconjugated bilirubin in the skin, rendering it water soluble and facilitating elimination
     b. Precautions
        (1) Protect infant's eyes from high-intensity light
        (2) Monitor fluid status and temperature
- Infants affected by maternal substance use
  1. Fetal alcohol spectrum disorders (FASDs)—alcohol use in pregnancy can cause FASDs in the neonate
     a. FASDs are physical, behavioral, and intellectual disabilities that last a lifetime; as many as 1 in 20 U.S. schoolchildren may have FASD
     b. Fetal/neonatal effects—microcephaly, facial abnormalities, cardiac defects, malformation of joints, failure to thrive, intellectual disability
     c. May result in withdrawal syndrome in the neonate—characterized by irritability, tremors, tachypnea, tachycardia, poor feeding
  2. Cocaine use
     a. Fetal/neonatal effects—prematurity, low birth weight, IUGR, genitourinary abnormalities, seizures, congenital heart disease, irritability, frantic or poor feeding
     b. May result in long-term behavioral impairment
  3. Opiate use
     a. Minimal long-term effects compared to cocaine and alcohol; primarily affects the immediate neonatal period

b. Neonatal opiate withdrawal syndrome (NOWS)
   (1) Onset shortly after birth
   (2) CNS signs—irritability, tremors, high-pitched cry, hyperstimulability, possible seizure activity
   (3) Other signs—tachypnea, tachycardia, poor or disorganized feeding, hyperthermia, vasomotor instability
   (4) Care is primarily supportive, although methadone or buprenorphine may be necessary in infants with severe symptoms
4. Marijuana use
   a. Little or no evidence for teratogenic effects
   b. Possible newborn behavioral effects—fine tremor, prolonged startle response, irritability, poor habituation to visual stimuli
   c. No behavioral effects demonstrated to persist beyond infancy
5. Prescription drugs with a high potential for misuse
   a. Amphetamines
      (1) Fetal/neonatal effects—genitourinary, cardiac, and/or CNS abnormalities; behavioral state disorganization
      (2) May result in long-term learning disabilities
   b. Benzodiazepines—fetal/neonatal effects include hypotonia, hypothermia, low Apgar scores, respiratory depression, poor feeding; possible association with midline cleft defects
- Congenital anomalies
  1. CNS anomalies
     a. Spina bifida occulta
        (1) Absent or incomplete closure of one or more vertebral arches
        (2) Dimple or hair tuft may be present over site
        (3) Often asymptomatic without requiring treatment
     b. Meningocele/myelomeningocele
        (1) Meningocele—extrusion of meninges and CSF through a defect in the vertebral column
        (2) Myelomeningocele—meningocele with extrusion of spinal cord
        (3) Surgical repair is necessary to prevent rupture and infection
        (4) Myelomeningocele results in loss of sensory and motor function below the level of the defect
     c. Anencephaly
        (1) Congenital absence of cranial vault and underlying brain tissue
        (2) Newborn may manifest heart rate and respiration but will die within a few hours after birth
     d. Hydrocephalus
        (1) Abnormal accumulation of CSF in ventricles of the brain
        (2) Signs—increased head circumference, separation of cranial sutures, bulging tense fontanels, high-pitched cry, and downward deviation of eyes ("setting sun sign")
        (3) Surgical treatment involves the placement of a shunt to drain excess fluid
  2. Respiratory anomalies

a. Choanal atresia
   (1) Definition—congenital blockage of posterior nasal passages
   (2) Respiratory distress is evident at birth if both nares are blocked
   (3) Treatment includes respiratory support and surgical repair
b. Diaphragmatic hernia
   (1) Definition—defect of the diaphragm, allowing herniation of abdominal contents into the thoracic cavity and displacement of heart and lung tissue
   (2) Presentation—respiratory distress and scaphoid abdomen apparent at birth
   (3) Treatment is surgical repair
c. Pulmonary hypoplasia/agenesis
   (1) Definition—underdevelopment or absence of one or both lungs
   (2) Strong association with other anomalies
   (3) Rare condition with a high mortality rate
   (4) Presentation—acute respiratory distress with thoracic asymmetry
3. Cardiovascular anomalies
   a. Anomalies resulting in increased pulmonary blood flow
      (1) Atrial septal defect, ventricular septal defect, patent ductus arteriosus, and atrioventricular canal defect
      (2) Surgical repair required
      (3) Prognosis is usually good
   b. Anomalies resulting in decreased pulmonary blood flow
      (1) Tetralogy of Fallot—pulmonary stenosis, ventricular septal defect, overriding aorta, and right ventricular hypertrophy
      (2) Aortic stenosis—narrowing or stricture of the aortic valve, causing resistance to blood flow in the left ventricle, with decreased cardiac output
      (3) Tricuspid atresia—results in no direct communication between right atrium and right ventricle, in turn resulting in hypoplastic right ventricle and enlarged left ventricle
      (4) Coarctation of the aorta—narrowing near the insertion of the ductus arteriosus, resulting in increased pressure proximal to the defect and decreased pressure distal to the obstruction
      (5) Pulmonic stenosis—narrowing at the entrance of the pulmonary artery; results in decreased pulmonary blood flow and right ventricular hypertrophy, which in turn results from resistance to blood flow
      (6) Surgery is generally more complicated
   c. Anomalies resulting in mixed blood flow (saturated and desaturated blood mix within the heart or great arteries)
      (1) Transposition of the great vessels—aorta arises from the right ventricle and the pulmonary artery arises from the left ventricle, resulting in a circulatory bypass of the lungs and circulation of deoxygenated blood to the body

(2) Truncus arteriosus—failure of embryonic structure to divide into aorta and pulmonary artery
4. GI anomalies
  a. Cleft lip and palate
    (1) Definition—incomplete fusion of lip and palate during prenatal development
    (2) May interfere with feeding and weight gain
    (3) Surgical repair usually results in good cosmetic and functional results
  b. Esophageal atresia and tracheoesophageal fistula
    (1) Definition—abnormal development of trachea and esophagus, resulting in "blind pouch" esophagus and/or communication between the two structures
    (2) Presentation—copious drooling, poor feeding with reflux, acute respiratory distress, and cyanosis with feeding
    (3) Repaired surgically, with good prognosis
  c. Pyloric stenosis
    (1) Definition—obstruction of the pylorus (distal opening of the stomach)
    (2) Affects males three to four times more often than females
    (3) Presentation—vomiting, visible gastric peristalsis, constipation
    (4) Repaired surgically, with good prognosis
  d. Omphalocele
    (1) Definition—defect of abdominal wall with herniation of abdominal viscera through the umbilical ring
    (2) Protruding abdominal viscera usually covered by membrane
    (3) Frequently associated with other anomalies
    (4) Repaired surgically; prognosis depends on the extent of lesion and nature and extent of associated anomalies
  e. Gastroschisis
    (1) Definition—defect of the abdominal wall and evisceration of abdominal organs
    (2) Rarely associated with other anomalies
    (3) Management at birth—cover eviscerated organs with sterile gauze moistened with sterile saline solution
    (4) No oral intake until after repair; IV therapy for fluid and electrolyte maintenance
    (5) Repair may require several surgeries; prognosis depends on the extent of the lesion
5. Genitourinary anomalies
  a. Hypospadias
    (1) Definition—in males, the urethral opening is located on the ventral aspect of the penis
    (2) Circumcision contraindicated—foreskin tissue is often used in surgical repair
    (3) Rare in females, with urethral opening located in the vagina
  b. Epispadias
    (1) Definition—congenital opening of the urethra on the dorsum of the penis
    (2) Often associated with other genitourinary anomalies

    (3) Repaired surgically
  c. Ambiguous genitalia
    (1) Definition—anomalies of the external genitalia precluding identification of the newborn's sex
    (2) May be associated with anomalies of the internal genitalia
    (3) Chromosome studies can determine genotypic sex
    (4) Gender identity problems are frequent; reconstructive surgery is controversial
  d. Exstrophy of the bladder
    (1) Definition—exposure of bladder outside the abdominal wall
    (2) Repaired surgically; often complicated by associated genitourinary anomalies
  e. Patent urachus
    (1) Definition—the persistence of fetal opening between the bladder and umbilical cord
    (2) Repaired surgically
6. Musculoskeletal anomalies
  a. Congenital hip dysplasia
    (1) Definition—abnormal development of the acetabulum, resulting in dislocation of the femoral head
    (2) Presentation—asymmetry of gluteal folds, positive Ortolani sign
    (3) Treatment—reduction and stabilization of femoral head into the acetabulum to allow the development of a stable hip capsule
    (4) Stabilization is accomplished using a Frejka pillow or Pavlik harness
  b. Talipes equinovarus
    (1) Definition—congenital deformity of ankle and foot
    (2) Orthopedic treatment involves the application of splints or successive plaster casts to correct the position of the foot and allow normal development
    (3) Success of treatment depends on early treatment; with early treatment, prognosis is good
7. Chromosomal abnormalities
  a. Down syndrome
    (1) Results from extra chromosome at pair 21
    (2) Signs include close-set, slanting eyes; narrow palpebral fissures; flattened nose; large, protuberant tongue; short, thick fingers with incurving of the fifth digit; simian palmar crease; nuchal thickening
    (3) Involves varying degrees of intellectual impairment
    (4) Associated with multiple congenital anomalies, including cardiac and GI tract defects
  b. Trisomies 13 and 18
    (1) Clinically similar to but more severe than Down syndrome
    (2) High mortality rates; poor life expectancy
8. Inborn errors of metabolism
  a. PKU
    (1) Definition—deficiency of phenylalanine hydroxylase, resulting in inability to metabolize phenylalanine

(2) Results in toxic accumulation of abnormal metabolites of phenylalanine, eventually leading to CNS damage

(3) Treatment—dietary restriction of foods high in phenylalanine

(4) Should be identified and treated before 3 weeks of age

b. Galactosemia

(1) Definition—inability to convert galactose to glucose

(2) Results in toxic accumulation of galactose in the bloodstream

(3) Treatment—dietary restriction of foods containing galactose

- Sleep-related infant deaths

1. Definition—a sudden unexpected infant death during an observed or unobserved period of sleep or in a sleep environment; Unexplained sudden infant death in infancy (or SIDS) is a subcategory referring to sudden *unexplained* death of infant between birth and 1 year of age

2. Prevalence—2 out of 1,000 infants

a. Most prevalent between 2 and 4 months of age

b. Rarely occurs before 3 weeks or after 9 months

3. Unknown cause

a. Theory of delayed development of "arousal" and cardiorespiratory control

b. Earlier research had suggested apnea as the cause, but subsequent research has not shown a strong association between apnea and SIDS

c. No evidence that home cardiorespiratory monitoring saves lives

4. Risk factors and associations

a. Sex disparities—SIDS occurs more often in male than female infants

b. Racial disparities resulting from the marginalization of infants and families; experienced most often by Black and American Indian/Alaska Native populations

(1) Low socioeconomic status

(2) Unemployment

(3) Housing instability

(4) Domestic violence

(5) Lack of access to educational resources

c. Premature birth

d. IUGR

e. Young maternal age

f. Short interpregnancy interval

g. Maternal smoking or use of cocaine or opiates

h. More common in cold weather months

i. More common after midnight and before 8:00 a.m.

5. Recommendations

a. "Back to sleep"—place infants in the supine position to sleep

b. Avoid or reduce modifiable risk factors

c. Provide culturally responsive and racially inclusive resources to mitigate racial inequities

d. Infants should sleep on a separate, firm surface, close to the parents' bed

e. Avoid loose bed clothing or other soft objects in the sleep space

f. Offer a pacifier for sleep; may delay until the breast has been established.

g. Avoid overheating and head covering

h. Exclusive feeding of human milk for the first 6 months if possible and desired

i. Awake and supervised "tummy time" is encouraged

j. Education and guidance must be culturally appropriate

Questions

Select the best answer.

1. Which of the following infants is *least* at risk for neonatal hypoglycemia? An infant with perinatal exposure to:
   a. diabetes mellitus
   b. gestational diabetes mellitus
   c. opioid use
   d. perinatal acidemia

2. Which of the following neonatal observations best describes the appearance and behavior of an infant with an overstimulated central nervous system as a result of NOWS?
   a. Color changes, irregular respiration, irritability or lethargy, and vomiting
   b. Habituation to noxious stimuli and attempts to self-console
   c. Lethargy, flaccid tone, pallor, and inability to maintain an alert active state
   d. Tremors, tachycardia, nonnutritive sucking, nasal flaring, and grunting

3. The midwife performs a physical examination on a newborn 2 hours after birth. Which of the following findings indicates a need for pediatric consultation?
   a. Brief, intermittent episodes of apnea
   b. Preauricular skin tag
   c. Respiratory rate of 50 breaths per minute
   d. Yellow blanching of skin

4. The neonate is limp, blue, and not crying. The midwife determines that resuscitation is necessary. According to the American Academy of Pediatrics (AAP) and American Heart Association (AHA) guidelines, which of the following is the appropriate initial step after the infant is placed under a radiant heater?
   a. Clear secretions if needed
   b. Dry the infant, removing wet linen
   c. Evaluate the heart rate
   d. Provide tactile stimulation

5. After the initial steps of neonatal resuscitation, the midwife notes that spontaneous respiration and tone are

normal, the infant is crying vigorously, and the heart rate is 120 bpm. Which of the following are the next *best* steps?
- a. Initiates PPV with 100% oxygen
- b. Facilitate bonding and breastfeeding
- c. Monitor with neonatal heart rate
- d. Provides oxygen for acrocyanosis

6. Once the need for neonatal resuscitation is determined by the midwife, how should the midwife proceed if meconium staining of the amniotic fluid had been noted during labor?
- a. Begin compressions immediately
- b. Initiate positive pressure ventilation
- c. Stimulate the baby vigorously
- d. Suction the trachea on the perineum

7. Which of the following most directly causes the functional closure of the foramen ovale?
- a. Fluid shift across the alveoli
- b. Increased oxygen to the brain
- c. Increased pressure in the left atrium
- d. Persistence of the placenta

8. A primipara is discussing infant feeding with the midwife. Which statement would indicate to the midwife that further teaching is necessary to correct a misunderstanding?
- a. "Because I'm bottle-feeding, I'm going to stick to a regular 2-hour feeding schedule."
- b. "I'm letting my baby nurse until he seems satisfied with every feeding."
- c. "My 5-day-old baby is only taking about 25 mL of formula at each feeding. I'm very worried."
- d. "My baby is suckling well and wetting diapers, so I think he's getting enough milk."

9. The midwife is counseling a patient about prophylaxis for newborn eye infections. Which of the following describes the rationale for prophylaxis most accurately?
- a. Due to the rapid onset of ophthalmia neonatorum, blindness can occur soon after birth.
- b. Erythromycin prevents blindness by treating chlamydial conjunctivitis.
- c. *Neisseria gonorrhoeae* can cause systemic infection starting with the eyes.
- d. Ophthalmia neonatorum can spread to the brain and cause meningitis.

10. The parent of a 1-month-old infant sounds distraught and tells the midwife that the baby "just cries all the time, so hard that she gets red in the face. She's driving me crazy." Upon further questioning, the midwife learns that the baby's temperature, feeding habits, voiding, and stooling appear to be normal despite the baby's behavior. The midwife correctly tells the parent that:
- a. Getting used to the demands of an infant is a normal part of adjusting to parenthood.
- b. The baby lacks stimulation, so the parent should engage her in active play.
- c. The parent should take the baby to the emergency room immediately.
- d. When it gets to be too much, place the baby safely in her crib and take a break.

11. At her 6-month well-child checkup a baby weighs 12 lb compared to a birth weight of 6 lb. The parent says that she seems to breastfeed well, but frequently spits up afterward. Which of the following is the best response to the parent's concern?
- a. Affirm the parent's breastfeeding/chestfeeding technique.
- b. Obtain a consultation with the pediatrician.
- c. Orders metabolic screening to test for PKU.
- d. Supplement breastfeeding/chestfeeding with formula.

12. Which of the following is characteristic of normal newborn behavior states?
- a. Abrupt, unpredictable changes between Brazelton's states
- b. Ease becoming and remaining alert
- c. Irritability and rapid progression from alertness to crying
- d. Need for constant external stimuli

13. The midwife wishes to estimate a newborn's gestational age. Which standard instrument is appropriate?
- a. Denver II
- b. Erb–Duchenne
- c. Erikson
- d. New Ballard

14. How can parents promote the major psychological tasks of early infancy?
- a. Create a variable schedule.
- b. Demonstrate predictable responses.
- c. Consistently ignore a fussy infant.
- d. Limit emotional availability.

15. The midwife's fully informed discussion about circumcision with the infant's parents should acknowledge that:
- a. It may offer some modest benefit in reducing potential UTIs.
- b. There are adverse long-term impacts on sexual functioning.
- c. There are no medical benefits from circumcision.
- d. The risks of circumcision, while rare, are potentially serious.

16. Which of the following describes the etiology of hemolytic disease in the neonate?
- a. Due to maternal antibodies, enzymatic disorders, and infections
- b. In the presence of fetal blood cells in maternal circulation
- c. If the fetus is exposed to severe prenatal maternal anemia
- d. When the maternal blood type is A, and the fetus's blood type is B

17. Which of the following clusters of newborn signs/symptoms may be associated with suspected maternal opiate use?
- a. Irritability, tremors, high-pitched cry, hyperstimulability
- b. Lethargy, diminished reflexes, hypotonia
- c. Microcephaly, facial abnormalities, cardiac defects
- d. Prematurity, low birth weight, genitourinary abnormalities

18. Which of the following assessment findings is consistent with neonatal prematurity?
    a. Abundant lanugo
    b. Increased recoil of ear tissue
    c. Peeling skin
    d. Translucent skin

19. Prominent vasculature of the anterior lens capsule is most suggestive of which condition?
    a. Elevated total serum bilirubin concentration
    b. Gonococcal or chlamydial conjunctivitis
    c. Herpes virus exposure in the intrapartum period
    d. Relatively immature gestational age

20. Which of the following accurately describes a change from fetal to neonatal circulation after birth?
    a. Decreased oxygenation of circulating blood causing constriction of the ductus arteriosus
    b. Decreased pressure in the left atrium facilitating the closure of the foramen ovale
    c. Loss of high-resistance placental circuit resulting in increased systemic vascular resistance
    d. Relatively high pulmonary vascular resistance resulting in increased circulation to the lungs

21. A partner is concerned about the welfare of the baby after birth following the pregnant parent's positive tuberculosis screening result. Which of the following is the most accurate advice the midwife can offer the partner while awaiting results from the patient's chest radiograph and sputum culture?
    a. Congenital tuberculosis is unlikely to be a problem for the newborn because the pregnant parent shows no signs of active disease.
    b. Even if the chest radiograph is negative, there will need to be a period of isolation from the newborn that may interfere with the initiation of breastfeeding.
    c. If the newborn acquired tuberculosis in utero, the most serious risk is for respiratory problems in the neonatal period.
    d. Subclinical tuberculosis infection in the pregnant parent is associated with a number of congenital malformations.

22. Which of the following newborn assessment findings is likely to be related to gestational diabetes?
    a. High-pitched cry
    b. Serum glucose level below 40 mg/dL
    c. Strong Moro reflex
    d. Bradycardia

23. A defect in the vertebral column that results in extrusion of meninges and CSF is best described as:
    a. hydrocephaly
    b. meningocele
    c. myelomeningocele
    d. spina bifida occulta

24. Which of the following conditions is most likely to result in loss of sensory and motor function below the level of the defect?
    a. Hydrocephaly
    b. Meningocele
    c. Myelomeningocele
    d. Spina bifida occulta

25. The midwife notices that the baby, within the first day of life, drools copiously, feeds poorly with excessive reflux, and turns bluish-gray while feeding. Which condition should the midwife suspect?
    a. Gastroschisis
    b. Omphalocele
    c. Pyloric stenosis
    d. Tracheoesophageal malformation

26. Increased oxygen consumption, hypoglycemia, hypoxia, acidosis, and respiratory distress can be caused in the immediate newborn period by:
    a. cold stress in the birthing room
    b. congenital bacterial infections
    c. maternal opioid use
    d. patent ductus arteriosus

27. Relatively mature capabilities of the newborn's GI system include:
    a. ability to digest fats and proteins
    b. absorption of complex sugars
    c. cardiac sphincter tone
    d. suckling, swallowing, and gag reflex

28. At 1 minute of age, the neonate exhibits a strong cry, some flexion of the arms and legs, a heart rate of 136 bpm, and acrocyanosis. The correct 1-minute Apgar score is:
    a. 6
    b. 7
    c. 8
    d. 9

29. At 5 minutes of age, the neonate exhibits slow irregular respirations, some flexion of extremities, a heart rate of 96 bpm, grimace in response to suction, and generalized cyanosis. The correct 5-minute Apgar score is:
    a. 4
    b. 5
    c. 6
    d. 7

30. Which of the following statements accurately represents the correlation between Apgar scores and the physiological status of the newborn?
    a. Is merely an indicator of adaptation
    b. Is predictive of low cord pH
    c. Reflects expansion of the alveoli
    d. Reflects patency of the foramen ovale

31. In the initial examination of a male infant, the midwife notes drainage of urine from the stump of the umbilical cord. The newborn's condition is most likely:
    a. epispadias
    b. exstrophy of the bladder
    c. hypospadias
    d. patent urachus

32. Which of the following correctly describes the primary function of the newborn's first breaths?
    a. Clear the newborn's lungs of fluid
    b. Compress the alveoli.
    c. Decrease ventilatory pressure
    d. Trigger a decrease in blood pH

33. During the transitional period, thermoregulation in the newborn is achieved through:
    a. alkalosis
    b. evaporation
    c. increased muscular activity like shivering
    d. metabolism of brown adipose tissue

34. Which of the following statements is the most accurate patient education about newborn skincare?
    a. Cradle cap is caused by *Candida albicans* and must be treated with a topical antifungal agent.
    b. If dry or peeling skin does not resolve with baby oil, call the pediatrician.
    c. Primary diaper dermatitis can be treated with baby powder and air exposure.
    d. Tub baths should be avoided for the first 2 weeks of life or until the cord stump has fallen off.

35. Which of the following factors would reassure the midwife that a newborn is potentially a candidate for early discharge from the hospital?
    a. Birth weight was 2,625 g at birth and a Ballard score of 25
    b. Metabolic screening scheduled with a pediatrician in 2 days
    c. Serum glucose level of 28 mg/dL at 12 hours after birth
    d. Total serum bilirubin of 16 mg/dL at 12 hours after birth

36. The midwife is examining a baby prior to discharge. She notes that the head circumference is 34 cm, while the chest circumference is 31 cm. The midwife should:
    a. assess for further signs of hydrocephalus
    b. proceed to the next component of the examination
    c. repeat the measurements
    d. suspect diaphragmatic hernia

37. At what point does the evaluation of the newborn begin?
    a. After neonatal resuscitation
    b. At the moment of birth
    c. Before the infant is born
    d. With crowning of the head

38. Which of the following presentations would contribute to a diagnosis of a growth restriction in an infant?
    a. Symmetric head and chest circumference
    b. Birth weight below the 10th percentile
    c. Head circumference above the 45th percentile
    d. Gestational age of 32 weeks at birth

39. A neonate has abundant lanugo. The gestational age is probably:
    a. 24–26 weeks
    b. 26–28 weeks
    c. 32–34 weeks
    d. 36–38 weeks

40. Which of the following is associated with microcephaly?
    a. Fetal alcohol syndrome disorder
    b. Neonatal Zika infection
    c. Prenatal shingles
    d. Prenatally acquired hepatitis B

41. At her 6-week postpartum visit, which of the following is associated with sudden infant death syndrome (SIDS)?
    a. Male babies are more commonly affected by SIDS.
    b. Side-lying positions reduce the risk of SIDS.
    c. SIDS is most common in the late morning.
    d. The risk of SIDS is higher in the summer months.

42. The normal newborn's sensory capacities are most limited in:
    a. color perception
    b. hearing
    c. near-vision focus
    d. taste sensation

43. The organized infant can:
    a. form significant relationships with others throughout life
    b. hear high-pitched sounds and echoes
    c. self-console and return to a stable behavioral state
    d. sleep for 20%–25% of daytime hours

44. Prior to discharge, a breastfeeding postpartum patient is hesitant about consenting to a metabolic screening panel due to pain associated with the heel stick. To engage in shared decision-making, which of the following is the best information a midwife can offer?
    a. Breastfeeding/chestfeeding is protective against metabolic disorders.
    b. Dietary restrictions may prevent the toxic accumulation of metabolites.
    c. Federal law mandates testing for PKU, galactosemia, and cystic fibrosis.
    d. The window for early, noninvasive metabolic screening has passed.

45. Select the correct combination of intrapartum factor and neonatal finding?
    a. Breech presentation: positive truncal incurvation
    b. Forceps delivery: cephalohematoma
    c. Shoulder dystocia: symmetric Moro reflex
    d. Vertex presentation: asymmetry of gluteal folds

46. Visible gastric peristalsis on observation of the abdomen is most suggestive of:
    a. colic
    b. esophageal fistula
    c. gastroschisis
    d. pyloric stenosis

47. Normal newborn respiratory findings include:
    a. diaphragmatic and abdominal breathing
    b. nasal flaring, expiratory grunting, and retractions
    c. respiratory rate of 40–80 breaths per minute
    d. ventilation primarily through the mouth

48. New parents are worried about their baby's sucking between feedings. Which of the following is the best guidance the midwife can offer about nonnutritive sucking?
    a. Can be promoted by giving an empty bottle
    b. Is an example of behavioral self-regulation
    c. Is not known to occur before birth
    d. May prevent dental and facial malformations

49. Which of the following describes the correct initial treatment for a neonate diagnosed with talipes equinovarus?
    a. Neonatal physical therapy
    b. Rest, ice, and elevation
    c. Successive casting
    d. Surgery after the first steps

50. Which of the following cardiac conditions lacks communication between the right-sided atrium and ventricle?
    a. Aortic stenosis
    b. Coarctation of the aorta
    c. Tetralogy of Fallot
    d. Tricuspid atresia

Answers with Rationales

1. **c.** opioid use
   The other choices indicate risk factors for neonatal hypoglycemia. Opioid use is not a risk factor for hypoglycemia.

2. **a.** Color changes, irregular respiration, irritability or lethargy, and vomiting
   Infants may become fatigued or stressed when overstimulated. Color changes, irregular respiration, irritability or lethargy, and vomiting can be signs of such stress.

3. **d.** Yellow blanching of skin
   Jaundice in the first 24 hours of life is a pathologic finding that warrants immediate further evaluation and treatment. A key component of midwifery newborn care is a management plan that includes recognizing and appropriately co-managing/referring abnormal findings.

4. **a.** Clear secretions if needed
   This is the correct sequence of initial steps in neonatal resuscitation, per Neonatal Resuscitation Program (NRP) guidelines.

5. **c.** Monitor with neonatal heart rate
   There is no need for further oxygenation according to NRP. The appearance of acrocyanosis is common in a neonate despite being appropriately oxygenated. Bonding and breastfeeding/chestfeeding can be initiated after post-resuscitation care has been completed.

6. **b.** Initiate positive pressure ventilation
   Care guidelines for further intervention are based on inadequate respiratory effort. PPV should be prioritized in the presence of meconium-stained fluid. Suctioning on the perineum or ET is not recommended.

7. **c.** Increased pressure in the left atrium
   The increased pressure in the left atrium contributes to the closure of the foramen ovale. Preceding this event are pressure changes that occur in neonatal transition causing the expansion of the alveoli with oxygenated air with the first breaths.

8. **a.** "Because I'm bottle-feeding, I'm going to stick to a regular 2-hour feeding schedule."
   Whether breastfed or bottle-fed, infants thrive best when fed on demand in response to cues of hunger.

9. **b.** Erythromycin prevents blindness by treating chlamydial conjunctivitis.
   Erythromycin prevents blindness caused by the presence of chlamydial infections. Blindness is not rapid onset. Eye infections do not become systemic via the ocular route.

10. **d.** When it gets to be too much, place the baby safely in her crib and take a break.
    Colic affects approximately 10% of infants and can be quite frustrating for parents. Sometimes a short break of stepping out on the porch and breathing fresh air (when assured that the baby is safely in his or her crib) can be restorative and calming for the parent.

11. **a.** Affirm the parent's breastfeeding/chestfeeding technique
    Regurgitation is common in infants. The infant is thriving well and gaining weight appropriately.

12. **a.** Abrupt, unpredictable changes between Brazelton's states
    Abrupt, unpredictable changes between Brazelton's sleep–wake states are not characteristic of normal newborn behavior.

13. **d.** New Ballard
    The New Ballard instrument is the only one of the choices provided that estimates a newborn's gestational age.

14. **b.** Demonstrate predictable responses
    Research suggests that long-term impairment, including school problems and delinquency, can result from insecure attachment in early infancy. A consistent schedule with predictable responses is most effective.

15. **a.** it may offer some modest benefit in reducing potential UTIs.
    It appears that there is some benefit of reduced STIs, UTIs, and cancer of the penis in men who are circumcised, but opponents of this procedure maintain that modern sanitary conditions and hygienic practices are more important factors in reducing the incidence of these diseases in comparison to the benefits from circumcision.

16. **a.** Due to maternal antibodies, enzymatic disorders, and infections
    Hemolytic disease can be caused by maternal antibodies, enzymatic disorders, or infections. The mere presence of fetal blood cells, regardless of blood type or hemoglobin, does not cause hemolytic disease.

17. **a.** Irritability, tremors, high-pitched cry, hyperstimulability
    Irritability, tremors, high-pitched cry, hyperstimulability, tachypnea, tachycardia, disorganized feeding, hyperthermia, and vasomotor instability are all signs of perinatal opioid use.

18. **d.** Translucent skin
    The other answers offer conflicting findings regarding gestational age assessment. This answer lists all the features that are consistent with prematurity.

19. **d.** Relatively immature gestational age
    The vasculature of the anterior capsule of the ocular lens is more prominent with early gestational ages.

20. **d.** Relatively high pulmonary vascular resistance resulting in increased circulation to the lungs
    The placental circuit has low resistance. The opposite is true after birth, when systemic vascular resistance increases with the loss of the placental circuit.

21. **a.** Congenital tuberculosis is unlikely to be a problem for the newborn because the pregnant parent shows no signs of active disease.
    Congenital disease is rare unless the parent has untreated, advanced tuberculosis.

22. **b.** Serum glucose level below 40 mg/dL
    After birth, neonates who have existed in high-glucose environments prenatally, can experience a precipitous drop in serum glucose.

23. **b.** meningocele
    A meningocele is the extrusion of meninges and CSF through the vertebral column.

24. **c.** Myelomeningocele
    Sensory and motor function loss below the level of the defect is noted with a myelomeningocele.

25. **d.** Tracheoesophageal malformation
    Copious drooling, poor feeding with reflux, and acute respiratory distress with feeding are characteristic findings with esophageal atresia and tracheoesophageal fistula.

26. **a.** cold stress in the birthing room
    Cold stress can result in all the consequences listed, thus emphasizing the importance of thermoregulation of the neonate.

27. **d.** suckling, swallowing, and gag reflex
    Suckling, swallowing, and gag reflexes are all relatively mature in the term neonate.

28. **c.** 8
    A perfect score for Apgar is 10. This infant receives only 1 point (out of 2) for color, 1 point (out of 2) for partial flexion of the extremities, 2 points for heart rate (>100), and 2 points each for respiratory effort and reflex irritability (strong cry).

29. **a.** 4
    The neonate receives 0 points for color and only 1 point for each of the other four parameters, for a total of 4.

30. **a.** Is merely an indicator of adaptation
    The Apgar score is useful as a systematic way to assess the newborn's immediate adaptation to extrauterine life. The other statements are inaccurate.

31. **d.** patent urachus.
    A patent urachus is the persistence of a fetal opening between the bladder and the umbilical cord.

32. **a.** Clear the newborn's lungs of fluid
    The first inhalation requires more ventilatory pressure than do later breaths, thus clearing the lungs of fluid.

33. **c.** increased muscular activity like shivering
    Shivering is a method of thermoregulation. Alkalosis does not have a role. Evaporation dysregulates newborn temperature. The infant has a limited supply of BAT, thus limiting the effectiveness of BAT metabolism as a means of thermoregulation.

34. **d.** Tub baths should be avoided for the first 2 weeks of life or until the cord stump has fallen off.
    The infant should receive only sponge baths until the cord stump has fallen off because it is important to keep the area dry.

35. **b.** Metabolic screening scheduled with a pediatrician in 2 days
    Metabolic screening scheduled for day 2 is appropriate for detecting metabolic disorders. Low birth weight with a lower Ballard score indicating a preterm birth, serum glucose below 30 mg/dL, and elevated bilirubin over 15 mg/dL prior to 24 hours are abnormal findings that warrant further monitoring and evaluation.

36. **b.** proceed to the next component of the examination
    The head circumference and chest circumference are normal; thus, the midwife should proceed with the next component of the exam.

37. **c.** Before the infant is born
    The infant's evaluation begins even before birth, considering maternal history, risk factors, fetal testing results, and intrapartum factors.

38. **b.** Birth weight below the 10th percentile
    Growth restriction is characterized by a birth weight below the 10th percentile. Symmetric findings and those above the 45th percentile are within normal limits. Gestational age is inconsequential when considered alone.

39. **b.** 26–28 weeks
    Lanugo is sparse to absent in the postmature or very premature infant and is most abundant in midterm infants (28–30 weeks).

40. **d.** Prenatally acquired hepatitis B
    Hepatitis B often results in prematurity and low birth weight, but not microcephaly.

41. **a.** Male babies are more commonly affected by SIDS.
    While researchers have proposed several theories about the cause of SIDS, the exact cause is unknown. However, we do know that SIDS has associated sex (male), sleep positional (side-lying), temporal (late night/early morning), and seasonal (winter) factors.

42. **a.** color perception
    The normal newborn's sensory capacity is most limited in color perception.

43. **c.** self-console and return to a stable behavioral state
    The organized infant can integrate physiologic and behavioral systems in response to the environment.

44. **b.** Dietary restrictions may prevent toxic accumulation of metabolites.
    PKU results from the absence or deficiency of the enzyme phenylalanine hydroxylase and prevents the correct breakdown of phenylalanine; thus, dietary restrictions may prevent toxic accumulation of metabolites. The health risk is from the resulting accumulation of phenylalanine. Additionally, breast/chestfeeding is contraindicated for infants with galactosemia; it is not preventative. Screening cannot be performed prior to 48 hours as the results may be inaccurate. While the U.S. Department of Health and Human Services does have a recommended universal newborn screening panel for newborns, newborn screening requirements are set by the individual states.

45. **b.** Forceps delivery : cephalohematoma
    Forceps delivery can result in a cephalohematoma due to pressure on the fetal skull. Truncal integration is a normal

finding and not associated with breech. A symmetric Moro reflex is a normal finding; a shoulder dystocia might cause asymmetry. Asymmetry of gluteal folds is usually indicative of congenital hip dislocation and has little to do with vertex presentation.

46. **d.** pyloric stenosis
Visible gastric peristalsis, vomiting, and constipation are common features that present with pyloric stenosis.

47. **a.** diaphragmatic and abdominal breathing
Diaphragmatic and abdominal breathing are normal respiratory findings, whereas the other answer choices are incorrect.

48. **b.** Is an example of behavioral self-regulation

Nonnutritive sucking is an example of a self-regulating behavior for self-consolation. It occurs prior to birth and does not prevent dental or facial malformations.

49. **c.** Successive casting
Talipes equinovarus is a congenital defect of the ankle that is treated with successive casting early in life to correct it. While physical therapy may be indicated, it is not a treatment alone. The other options are not treatments.

50. **d.** Tricuspid atresia
With tricuspid atresia, there is no direct communication between the right atrium and ventricle, meaning there is no tricuspid valve. The other options have their own characteristic cardiac malformations.

Bibliography

American Academy of Pediatrics. (2003, reaffirmed September 2014). Policy statement: Controversies concerning vitamin K and the newborn. *Pediatrics*, 112(1), 191–192.

American Academy of Pediatrics. (2011, reaffirmed June 2015). Clinical report: Postnatal glucose homeostasis in late-preterm and term infants. *Pediatrics*, 127(3), 575–579. https://doi.org/10.1542/peds.2010-3851

American Academy of Pediatrics. (2012). Circumcision policy statement. *Pediatrics*, 130(3), 585–586.

American Academy of Pediatrics. (2021). *Textbook of neonatal resuscitation* (8th ed.). Elk Grove, IL: American Academy of Pediatrics.

Aziz, K., Lee, C. H. C., Escobedo, M. B., Hoover, A. V., Kamath-Rayne, B. D., Kapadia, V. S., Magid, D. J., Niermeyer, S., Schmölzer, G. M., Szyld, E., Weiner, G. M., Wyckoff, M. H., Yamada, N. K., & Zaichkin, J. (2021). Part 5: Neonatal resuscitation 2020 American Heart Association guidelines for cardiopulmonary resuscitation and emergency cardiovascular care. *Pediatrics*, 147(Suppl 1), S160. https://doi.org/10.1542/peds.2020-038505E

Boardman, J., Groves, A., & Ramasethu, J. (2021) *Avery & MacDonald's neonatology: Pathophysiology and management of the newborn* (8th ed.). Wolters Kluwer.

Blackburn, S. T. (2018). *Maternal, fetal, & neonatal physiology: A clinical perspective* (5th ed.). Elsevier.

Centers for Disease Control and Prevention. (2022). *Recommended child and adolescent immunization schedule for ages 18 years or younger—United States, 2022.* Author. https://www.cdc.gov/vaccines/schedules/hcp/imz/child-adolescent.html

Centers for Disease Control and Prevention. (2019). *Dengue and Zika virus testing guidance.* https://www.cdc.gov/zika/hcp/diagnosis-testing/?CDC_AAref_Val=https://www.cdc.gov/zika/hc-providers/testing-guidance.html

Committee on Fetus and Newborn, Committee on Substance Use and Prevention, Patrick, S. W., Barfield, W. D., Poindexter, B. B., Cummings, J., Hand, I., Adams-Chapman, I., Aucott, S. W., Puopolo, K. M., Goldsmith, J. P., Kaufman, D., Martin, C., Mowitz, M., Gonzalez, L., Camenga, D. R., Quigley, J., Ryan, S. A., & Walker-Harding, L. (2020). Neonatal opioid withdrawal syndrome. *Pediatrics*, 146(5), e2020029074. https://doi.org/10.1542/peds.2020-029074

Hagan, J. F., Shaw, J. S., & Duncan, P. M. (2017). *Bright futures.* American Academy of Pediatrics.

Hand, I., Noble, L., & Abrams, S. A. (2022). Vitamin K and the newborn infant. *Pediatrics*, 149(3). https://doi.org/10.1542/peds.2021-056036

Kemper, A. R., Newman, T. B., Slaughter, J. L., Maisels, M. J., Watchko, J. F., Downs, S. M., Grout, R. W., Bundy, D. G., Stark, A. R., Bogen, D. L., Holmes, A. V., Feldman-Winter, L. B., Bhutani, V. K., Brown, S. R., Maradiaga Panayotti, G. M., Okechukwu, K., Rappo, P. D., & Russell, T. L. (2022). Clinical practice guideline revision: Management of hyperbilirubinemia in the newborn infant 35 or more weeks of gestation. *Pediatrics*, 150(3). https://doi.org/10.1542/peds.2022-058859

Kliegman, R. M. & St. Geme, J. (2019). *Nelson textbook of pediatrics* (21st ed.). Elsevier Saunders.

Phillippi, J. & Kantrowitz-Gordon, I. (Eds.). (2025). *Varney's midwifery* (7th ed.). Jones & Bartlett Learning.

Society for Maternal-Fetal Medicine (SMFM), Martins, J. G., Biggio, J. R., & Abuhamad, A. (2020). Society for Maternal-Fetal Medicine consult series #52: Diagnosis and management of fetal growth restriction. *American Journal of Obstetrics and Gynecology*, 223(4), B2–B17. https://doi.org/10.1016/j.ajog.2020.05.010

The Task Force on Sudden Infant Death Syndrome, The Committee on Fetus and Newborn, Moon, R. Y., Carlin, R. F., & Hand, I. (2022). Sleep-related infant deaths: Updated 2022 recommendations for reducing infant deaths in the sleep environment. *Pediatrics*, 150(1). https://doi.org/10.1542/peds.2022-057990

Thornton, P. S., Stanley, C. A., De Leon, D. D., Harris, D., Haymond, M. W., Hussain, K., Levitsky, L. L., Murad, M. H., Rozance, P. J., Simmons, R. A., Sperling, M. A., Weinstein, D. A., White, N. H., Wolfsdorf, J. I., & Pediatric Endocrine Society. (2015). Recommendations from the Pediatric Endocrine Society for evaluation and management of persistent hypoglycemia in neonates, infants, and children. *The Journal of pediatrics*, 167(2), 238–245. https://doi.org/10.1016/j.jpeds.2015.03.057

U.S. Department of Health and Human Services, Office on Women's Health. (2019). *Your guide to breastfeeding.* https://www.womenshealth.gov/breastfeeding

Wambach, K. & Spencer, B. (2021). *Breastfeeding and human lactation* (6th ed.). Jones & Bartlett Learning.

Wyckoff, M. H., Aziz, K., Escobedo, M. B., Kapadia, V. S., Kattwinkel, J., Perlman, J. M., . . . Zaichkin, J. G. (2015). Part 13. Neonatal resuscitation: 2015 American Heart Association guidelines update for cardiopulmonary resuscitation and emergency cardiovascular care. *Circulation*, 132(suppl 2), S543–S560. https://doi.org/10.1542/peds.2015-3373G

CHAPTER 11

Principles of Pharmacology

Beth M. Kelsey

Komkwuan P. Paruchabutr

Pharmacokinetics: The Study of How the Body Processes Drugs

- Absorption
  1. Movement of drug from the site of entry into the systemic circulation
  2. Bioavailability—percentage of active drug that is absorbed and available at the target tissue
  3. Affected by cell membranes, blood flow, drug solubility, pH of the drug, variables related to the gastrointestinal (GI) tract, drug concentration, dosage form, route of administration
- Distribution
  1. Movement of the drug into body fluids and body tissues
  2. Affected by the permeability of capillaries and tissues, systemic circulation, size of the drug molecule, affinity for lipid and aqueous tissues, protein binding, and pH
  3. Plasma protein binding—drugs may attach to proteins (mainly albumin) in the blood; only unbound drug is active; as the free drug is excreted, more of the drug is released from binding to replace what is lost; competition for binding sites by different drugs and hypoalbuminemia can affect the amount of free drug that is available
  4. Blood–brain barrier affects drug distribution—endothelial cells of capillaries surrounding the brain are packed tightly together, which limits passive transport from the blood into cerebral tissue; drug must be highly lipophilic to pass into the brain
  5. Placental barrier affects drug distribution
     a. Several layers of placental tissue separate maternal and fetal circulation, so the placenta is not an absolute barrier to drugs; almost all drugs taken by the mother pass through the placenta to her fetus to some degree, and they reach steady-state levels in the fetus between 50% and 100% of maternal concentration
     b. General determinants of drug transfer across the placenta include lipid solubility, extent of plasma protein binding, and degree of ionization of weak acids and bases
     c. Placenta has enzyme systems that metabolize some drugs, and P-glycoprotein that actively transports some drug substrates away from fetal circulation
  6. Steady state—when the rate of drug elimination equals the rate of drug availability (absorption) (**Figure 11-1**)
  7. Half-life—the time it takes for plasma concentration of a drug to be reduced by 50%; used to determine the time required to reach steady state and dosage interval (**Figure 11-2**)
  8. Volume of distribution—apparent volume in which drug is dissolved; relates to the concentration of drug in the plasma and the amount in the body; may be used to calculate loading dose needed to achieve a desired steady-state drug level immediately
- Metabolism
  1. Chemical inactivation of drug by conversion to a more water-soluble compound (metabolite) that can be excreted from the body
  2. Chemical alterations are produced by microsomal enzymes mainly in the liver
  3. Hepatic first-pass effect—orally administered drug goes from the GI tract through the portal system to the liver before going to the general circulation; some metabolism of the drug may occur as it is taken up by hepatic microsomal enzymes
  4. Drug interactions can affect metabolism by enzyme induction or inhibition

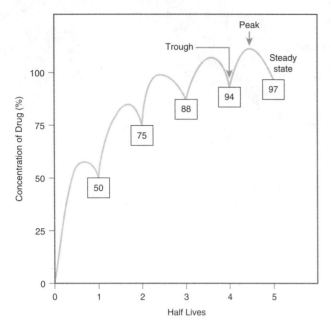

Figure 11-1 Rate of drug elimination.

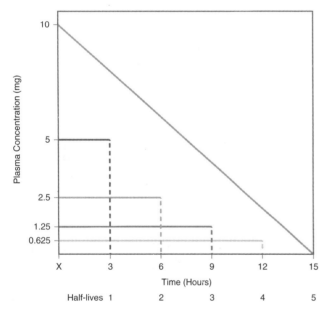

Figure 11-2 Half-life determination.

5. Variation in drug metabolism may be affected by genetics, age, pregnancy, liver disease, diet, alcohol, circadian rhythm
6. Prodrugs—drugs that must be metabolized to become effective (active metabolites); developed to improve stability, increase absorption, or prolong duration of drug activity; that is, valacyclovir is not effective, but its active metabolite, acyclovir, is
• Excretion
1. Removal of drugs from the body via the kidneys, intestines, sweat and salivary glands, lungs, or mammary glands
2. Urinary excretion—the net effect of glomerular filtration, active tubular secretion, and partial reabsorption

3. Enterohepatic recirculation—some fat-soluble drugs may be reabsorbed into the bloodstream from the intestines and returned to the liver
• Pharmacokinetic changes during pregnancy
1. Absorption—not significantly affected
2. Distribution
   a. Increase in plasma volume may result in lower serum levels of the drug
   b. Reduction in plasma proteins (albumin) may result in higher levels of free (unbound) drug
3. Metabolism
   a. Hepatic enzyme systems (e.g., CYP3A4, CYP1A2) are affected by rising levels of estrogen and progesterone; may result in either faster or slower metabolism of some drugs
   b. Blood flow through the liver is not changed significantly, so there is no change in first-pass effects
4. Excretion—increase in glomerular filtration rate (GFR) may result in faster elimination of drugs excreted primarily through the kidneys

Pharmacodynamics: The Study of Mechanism of Drug Action on Living Tissue

• Drug effects produced by:
1. Drug–receptor interaction
2. Drug–enzyme interaction
3. Nonspecific drug interaction
• Drug receptors—cellular protein, enzyme, or membrane that, when bound to a drug, initiates a physiologic response or blocks a response that the receptor normally stimulates
1. Agonist—drug combines with receptor to stimulate a response
2. Antagonist—drug interferes with receptor action or with other drug agonists present
• Drug–response relationship—study of the relationship between the concentration of drug in circulation and the response obtained
1. Affinity—the propensity of a drug to bind itself to a given receptor site
2. Efficacy—ability to initiate biological activity as a result of such binding
• Therapeutic effect
1. All pharmacologic responses have a maximum effect at which no further response is achieved, regardless of drug concentration
2. Therapeutic range (window)—plasma concentration of drug that produces the desired action without toxic effects
3. Therapeutic index (TI)—the ratio of lethal doses in 50% of the population over the median minimum effective dose in 50% of the population; higher TI = safer drug

Pharmacogenomics/ Pharmacogenetics: The Study of Genetic Variations That Influence Drug Metabolism and Drug Response

- Genetic variations account for approximately 15%–30% of interindividual differences in drug responses in general
- Pharmacokinetic processes affected by genetics occur primarily because of polymorphisms that affect the function of CYP450 enzymes, resulting in variations in metabolism of a given drug—poor (slow) metabolizer, intermediate metabolizer, extensive metabolizer, ultra-rapid metabolizer
  1. Poor (slow) metabolizers may have significantly elevated plasma concentrations of a drug and a greater risk of toxicity with the same dose of the drug compared with the other metabolizing rates
  2. Ultra-rapid metabolizers may have difficulty maintaining therapeutic drug levels
  3. Poor (slow) metabolizers may not be able to convert prodrug to active metabolite
  4. Ultra-rapid metabolizers may have increased conversion of prodrug to an active metabolite with an increased risk of toxicity
- Pharmacodynamic processes affected by genetics may occur at the drug receptor level affecting drug response—independent of genetic variations in drug metabolism
  1. Downregulation rather than upregulation of receptors may occur; for example, a person with asthma taking a beta$_2$-agonist to relax muscles and dilate bronchial passages may have the opposite reaction with worsening symptoms
  2. Hypersensitivity drug reactions (e.g., Stevens-Johnson syndrome) may occur because polymorphisms of histocompatibility complex proteins allow some drugs to bind directly, initiating the hypersensitivity reaction
  3. Polymorphic differences in drug receptors are differentially distributed among racial and ethnic groups
- Information on genomic biomarkers is available for some FDA-approved drugs in labeling information. Examples of information include drug exposure and clinical response variability, risk for adverse events, and genotype-specific dosing
- The clinical utility of pharmacogenomic testing is highest when prescribing drugs with a narrow therapeutic window, the risk for adverse drug reactions is high, or the consequences of treatment failure are severe
  1. Goal of pharmacogenomic testing—arrive quickly at an optimal dose with minimal treatment failure or toxicity

Pharmacotherapeutic Considerations

- Medication reconciliation—reduces risks for adverse reactions; unfavorable drug–drug, drug–food, drug–herb interactions; drug prescribing errors
  1. Conduct with any transition in care, when renewing prescriptions, when considering prescribing a new medication
  2. Obtain the most current list of all prescribed medications and determine if taking as indicated
  3. Obtain information on all over-the-counter medications and herbal products used
  4. Document medication list in the client record and keep up-to-date
- Side effects—predictable physiologic responses unrelated to the desired drug effect, natural consequence of chemical or hormonal reactions that take place between the drug and the body, may be dose-dependent, usually resolve on their own, examples are breast tenderness and nausea with combination oral contraceptives
- Adverse drug reactions (ADRs)—unpredictable, unintended, undesired responses to a drug that occur at dosages normally used; can be mild, moderate, or severe; often require intervention
  1. Examples—hypersensitivity/allergic reactions, anaphylaxis, drug intolerance, thrombocytopenia, hemolytic anemia, renal damage, hepatic toxicity, dermatologic effects
  2. Factors that may increase the risk for ADRs
     a. Characteristics of the drug
     b. Individual characteristics—younger or older age, female (assigned at birth), serious illness, genetic polymorphisms
     c. Route of administration—more likely with intravenous, intramuscular, or topical route than with oral route
- Drug interactions
  1. Modification of an expected drug response due to exposure to another drug or substance at approximately the same time; may be pharmacokinetic or pharmacodynamic
  2. Pharmacokinetic—inhibition of absorption, enzyme inhibition, or induction that increases risk for drug toxicity or results in reduced drug effect, altered renal elimination
  3. Pharmacodynamic—additive if two drugs have similar pharmacodynamic effects; antagonistic if two drugs have opposing pharmacodynamic effects
  4. Drug–food interactions may decrease bioavailability by interfering with absorption; may increase bioavailability by inhibiting enzymatic activity in the intestinal wall
  5. Drug–herb interactions may decrease or increase the bioavailability of a drug
- Drug contraindications
  1. Allergies, medical conditions, concurrent use of another drug, age, pregnancy, lactation may be drug contraindications

2. FDA's (2014b) Pregnancy and Lactation Labeling Rule (PLLR)
    a. Assists in assessing benefits versus risks of a drug for pregnant and lactating individuals
    b. Includes subsections for pregnancy, lactation, and individuals of reproductive potential in the Use in Special Populations section
    c. Pregnancy letter categories (A, B, C, D, X) have been removed
    d. Pregnancy subsection—contact information for pregnancy exposure registry for a drug if available, risk summary, clinical considerations, available human and animal data
    e. Lactation subsection—risk summary, applicable clinical considerations, available human and animal data
    f. Individuals of reproductive potential subsection—included if human or animal study data show potential drug-associated effects on fertility and/or implantation loss
3. Lactation and drugs
    a. Properties of the drug that determine how much of the drug will enter breastmilk—pH, protein binding, liposolubility, and molecular weight
    b. Infant pharmacokinetics have influence—drug metabolism variables, such as gastric acid production, liver function, amount of body fat, renal excretion
- Safety in prescribing
    1. Accurate diagnosis
    2. Assessment for previous ADRs
    3. Identification of subgroups that may be at higher risk for ADRs
    4. Medication reconciliation
    5. Selection of optimal and appropriate pharmacologic agents
    6. Patient education that is developmentally, linguistically, and culturally appropriate
- Patient education
    1. Purpose of drug, mechanism of action, effectiveness
    2. Benefits and risks
    3. Dosage and administration
    4. Major side effects/adverse reactions
    5. Appropriate use of antibiotics to prevent antibiotic resistance
- Pharmacologic considerations for elderly patients
    1. Majority of the elderly have one or more chronic conditions and are taking multiple medications—prescription and over-the-counter (OTC)
    2. Age-related decreases in metabolism and excretion of drugs may result in increased plasma concentrations
    3. Increased risk for ADRs—drug–drug/drug–food/drug–herb interactions, side effects, toxic effects
    4. Common ADRs in the elderly—dizziness, GI symptoms, edema, urinary retention or incontinence, confusion
    5. Other considerations that may lead to problems with use of medications—memory deficit, visual deficit, mobility problems, multiple providers and pharmacies, cost

6. Conduct comprehensive drug assessments—prescription medications, OTC medications, herbals, and dietary supplements
7. Be alert to medications as possible causes of untoward physiological or mental status changes
8. Start with low doses and increase slowly
9. Use American Geriatrics Society Beers Criteria to determine potentially inappropriate medication use in older adults (American Geriatrics Society, 2019)
    a. Lists medications best avoided in older adults in general or older adults with certain diseases or syndromes, and medications that should be prescribed at reduced dosage or with careful monitoring to avoid adverse events
    b. Examples of drugs to avoid when possible with elderly patients because of increased risk for adverse events
        (1) Long-acting nonsteroidal anti-inflammatory drugs (NSAIDs)—increased risk for indigestion, stomach ulcers, GI bleeding
        (2) Benzodiazepines—increased risk for falls and confusion; long half-life
        (3) Drugs with anticholinergic effects (e.g., amitriptyline, dicyclomine, oxybutynin)—increased risk for confusion, constipation, urinary retention, blurred vision, low blood pressure
        (4) Muscle relaxants—increased risk for falls and confusion, constipation, urinary retention
        (5) Certain diabetes medications—sulfonylureas (e.g., glyburide, chlorpropamide); increased risk for hypoglycemia
10. Benefits and risks should always be considered; needed treatment for symptoms and conditions should not be withheld based solely on age

Selected Drug Review

- Metronidazole
    1. Class: bactericide, amebicide, antiprotozoal—nitroimidazole
    2. Indications for use include but are not limited to treatment of:
        a. *Trichomonas vaginalis*
        b. Bacterial vaginosis
        c. Pelvic inflammatory disease (PID), in combination with other antibiotics
        d. Pseudomembranous colitis caused by *Clostridium difficile*
        e. Gastric or peptic ulcer associated with *Helicobacter pylori*
    3. Pharmacokinetics
        a. Absorption and distribution
            (1) Oral route—excellent, bioavailability >80%
            (2) Intravaginal route—absorbed systemically; peak serum concentrations are <2% of levels achieved with oral doses
            (3) Widely distributed throughout body tissues and fluids

(4) Crosses placenta and enters breastmilk

(5) Mean elimination half-life is 8 hours

  b. Metabolism—mostly in the liver

  c. Excretion—mostly through urine, some fecal excretion

4. Pharmacodynamics

  a. Disrupts DNA and protein synthesis of susceptible organisms

  b. Amebicidal, bactericidal, antiprotozoal

  c. Selectivity for anaerobic bacteria

5. Side effects/adverse reactions

  a. More common with oral than vaginal route

  b. GI—nausea, vomiting, dry mouth, metallic taste, anorexia, abdominal cramping

  c. Headache

  d. Hypersensitivity

  e. Mild leukopenia or neutropenia—not persistent after treatment

  f. Peripheral neuropathy—high doses, prolonged use

  g. Seizures—high doses, prolonged use

6. Drug interactions

  a. Disulfiram—acute psychosis and confusion if metronidazole taken within 2 weeks of taking disulfiram

  b. Alcohol (including medications with significant alcohol content)—may cause nausea/vomiting, headache, flushing, abdominal cramps

  c. Warfarin—metronidazole can potentiate action

  d. Cimetidine—can decrease hepatic metabolism of metronidazole and increase serum levels

  e. Phenobarbital/phenytoin—can increase hepatic metabolism of metronidazole, clinical significance uncertain

7. Contraindications/precautions

  a. Hypersensitivity

  b. History of drug-induced hematologic dyscrasias

  c. Hematologic disease

  d. Severe hepatic disease/impairment

  e. Renal impairment/renal failure

  f. Preexisting seizure disorder

8. Use in pregnancy and lactation

  a. Considered safe in all trimesters of pregnancy

  b. Interrupt nursing for 12–24 hours after drug dose to allow excretion of the drug

9. Patient education

  a. Take with food to decrease GI irritation

  b. Avoid alcohol and alcohol-containing substances during and for 48 hours after the last dose; CDC 2021 STI treatment guidelines note this is not necessary, metronidazole does not inhibit acetaldehyde as happens with disulfiram

  c. Chew gum or suck on ice or hard candy to help reduce dry mouth and metallic taste

  d. May cause a darkening of urine

  e. Report any central nervous system (CNS) symptoms

  f. If taking for trichomoniasis, refrain from sex until self and partner treatment is complete

- Fluconazole

1. Class: antifungal—triazole

2. Indications for use include but are not limited to treatment of:

  a. Candidiasis—oropharyngeal, esophageal, vulvovaginal

  b. Fungal meningitis—cryptococcosis, *Candida* species, histoplasmosis

3. Pharmacokinetics

  a. Absorption and distribution

    (1) Rapidly absorbed in the GI tract, bioavailability is >90%

    (2) Widely distributed in body tissues and fluids

    (3) Concentration in vaginal tissue approximately equal to plasma concentrations

    (4) Distribution in breastmilk and across the placenta unknown

    (5) Mean elimination half-life is 30 hours

  b. Metabolism—liver via interaction with CYP450 enzyme system, no first-pass metabolism

  c. Excretion—majority through urine (60%–80%) as unchanged drug

4. Pharmacodynamics

  a. Highly selective inhibitor of fungal CYP450 enzymes

  b. Alters fungal cell membrane function and cell-wall synthesis

  c. Broad spectrum of antifungal activity

  d. Emerging resistance of non-*Candida albicans* species

5. Side effects/adverse reactions

  a. Headache

  b. GI effects—nausea, abdominal pain

6. Drug interactions

  a. Cisapride (Propulsid)—prolonged QT interval

  b. Cyclosporin—nephrotoxicity

  c. Carbamazepine (Tegretol)—increased carbamazepine levels, decreased fluconazole levels

  d. Phenytoin (Dilantin)—nystagmus, ataxia

  e. Sulfonylureas—hypoglycemic reactions

  f. Theophylline—increased theophylline levels

  g. Warfarin—increased warfarin levels

7. Contraindications/precautions

  a. History of heart arrhythmia

  b. Hepatic disease

  c. Renal impairment/renal failure

  d. Hypersensitivity

  e. Multiple drug interactions

  f. Pregnancy

8. Use in pregnancy and lactation

  a. Fluconazole should not be used during pregnancy, there are no adequate or well-controlled studies of use during pregnancy

  b. Recommended treatment for vulvovaginal candidiasis in pregnancy is topical azole for 7 days

  c. Distributed in breastmilk at concentrations similar to those in plasma

  d. Considered compatible with breastfeeding

9. Patient education

  a. Symptoms should start to disappear approximately 24 hours after taking the medication

  b. It may take several days for symptoms to go away completely

c. Notify the provider of all medications because several drug interactions are possible
d. Avoid overuse/unnecessary use of antibiotics

- Acyclovir
  1. Class: antiviral—nucleoside analogue
  2. Indications for use include treatment of:
     a. Herpes simplex
     b. Herpes genitalia
     c. Herpes zoster
     d. Varicella
  3. Pharmacokinetics (oral)
     a. Absorption and distribution
        (1) Poorly absorbed, 10%–30% bioavailability; however, therapeutic levels achieved
        (2) Widely distributed
        (3) Crosses placenta and enters breastmilk
        (4) Mean elimination half-life is 2–3.5 hours
     b. Metabolism—mostly in the liver
     c. Excretion—90% in urine as unchanged drug
  4. Pharmacodynamics
     a. Selectively activated in infected cells
     b. Inhibits viral DNA synthesis
     c. Only effective against rapidly replicating herpes virus
     d. Does not eliminate latent herpes virus
  5. Side effects/adverse reactions
     a. GI effects—nausea/vomiting, diarrhea
     b. Headache
     c. Skin rash
     d. Acute renal failure—rare with oral route
  6. Drug interactions—increased risk for renal toxicity with nephrotoxic drugs
  7. Contraindications/precautions—hypersensitivity, renal or hepatic function impairment
  8. Use in pregnancy and lactation
     a. Acyclovir registry has not found any increase in congenital disabilities in pregnant individuals who use this drug
     b. May be used to treat the first episode of genital herpes or severe recurrent herpes
     c. May consider treatment in late pregnancy to reduce the frequency of recurrences at term
     d. Lactation—use if indicated; some excretion in breastmilk
  9. Patient education
     a. Take with a full glass of water
     b. Space doses evenly
     c. Start at the first sign of a recurrent episode
     d. Additional education for suppressive regimens
  10. Other nucleoside analogues—same indications, mechanism of action, adverse reactions, contraindications/precautions
     a. Famciclovir—converted to active form via first-pass metabolism; better bioavailability
     b. Valacyclovir—prodrug converted to acyclovir; better bioavailability, less frequent dosing
- Alendronate
  1. Class: bone resorption inhibitor—bisphosphonate
  2. Indications for use
     a. Prevention of osteoporosis in postmenopausal individuals
     b. Treatment of osteoporosis in postmenopausal individuals
     c. Treatment of osteoporosis in men
     d. Treatment of glucocorticoid-induced osteoporosis
     e. Treatment of Paget's disease of the bone
  3. Pharmacokinetics
     a. Absorption and distribution
        (1) Reaches maximum concentration in bone at 3–6 months
        (2) Systemic bioavailability is low with little exposure to tissues other than bone
        (3) Bioavailability reduced by 40% when taken with food and by 60% when taken with coffee or orange juice
        (4) Approximately 50% of oral dose binds to the exposed bone surface
        (5) Estimated elimination half-life from bone is >10 years
     b. Metabolism—high affinity for bone; no evidence of metabolism in liver
     c. Excretion—50% of the dose that remains after it binds to bone is excreted unchanged in the urine
  4. Pharmacodynamics
     a. Reduces bone resorption by inhibiting the activity of osteoclasts
     b. No direct effect on bone formation
  5. Side effects/adverse reactions
     a. Local irritation of the upper GI mucosa
     b. Esophagitis, esophageal ulcers, esophageal erosions
     c. Hypocalcemia
     d. Severe and occasionally incapacitating bone, joint, and/or muscle pain
     e. Osteonecrosis of the jaw—more likely with intravenously administered bisphosphonate and generally associated with dental work
     f. Low-impact fractures of the femoral shaft—rare, more common in long-term users
     g. Hypersensitivity reactions
  6. Drug interactions—calcium-, magnesium-, or aluminum-containing antacids likely to reduce the absorption of alendronate if taken at the same time
  7. Contraindications/precautions
     a. Abnormalities of the esophagus that delay esophageal emptying
     b. Inability to stand or sit upright for at least 30 minutes after taking alendronate
     c. Hypocalcemia
     d. Renal impairment
     e. Hypersensitivity
  8. Use in pregnancy and lactation
     a. No well-designed studies of use during pregnancy in humans; small studies and case reports have shown no increase in the rate of congenital disabilities or long-term health concerns
     b. Limited evidence indicates that breastfeeding after cessation of long-term bisphosphonate treatment appears to have no adverse effects on infant
     c. No data available on use during breastfeeding; poorly absorbed, so the amount in breastmilk is likely small

9. Patient education
   a. Take in the morning with 8 ounces of plain water
   b. Do not eat food, drink fluids, or take other medications for at least 30–60 minutes
   c. Remain upright for at least 30–60 minutes
   d. Take at least 2 hours before any calcium supplement or antacids
- Oxybutynin
  1. Class: antimuscarinic anticholinergic
  2. Indications for use—treatment of overactive bladder symptoms, including frequency, urgency, nocturia, urge urinary incontinence
  3. Pharmacokinetics
     a. Absorption and distribution
        (1) Rapid; reaches maximum concentration within 1 hour
        (2) Bioavailability is approximately 6%
        (3) Widely distributed in body tissues
        (4) Mean elimination half-life is 2–3 hours
     b. Metabolism—liver via interaction with CYP3A4 enzyme
     c. Excretion—extensively metabolized in the liver, with less than 0.1% of the dose excreted unchanged in the urine
  4. Pharmacodynamics
     a. Targets M_1 and M_3 receptors to reduce muscarinic action of acetylcholine on smooth muscle
     b. Mild antispasmodic—increases bladder capacity, diminishes the frequency of uninhibited contractions of the detrusor muscle
  5. Side effects/adverse reactions
     a. Systemic anticholinergic side effects—for example, dry mouth, blurred vision, constipation, tachycardia, urinary retention, drowsiness, impaired sweating, confusion—are common reasons for discontinuation
     b. Transdermal patch may decrease serum levels of active metabolite and reduce anticholinergic side effects
     c. Heatstroke in hot climates if sweating is impaired
  6. Drug interactions
     a. Inhibitors of CYP3A4 enzyme may cause increased plasma concentrations of oxybutynin
     b. May enhance the effects of other anticholinergic drugs
     c. May enhance the sedative effects of opioids or other sedation-causing agents
  7. Contraindications/precautions
     a. Hypersensitivity
     b. Uncontrolled narrow-angle glaucoma
     c. Gastric retention
     d. Urinary retention
     e. Concomitant use of other anticholinergic drugs
     f. Esophageal disease
     g. Hepatic or renal impairment
     h. Myasthenia gravis
     i. Cardiac disease
     j. Hypertension
     k. Older adults
     l. Dementia

8. Use in pregnancy and lactation
   a. No evidence of impaired fertility or harm to animal fetuses; safety in pregnant individuals has not been established
   b. Not known if oxybutynin is excreted in breastmilk
9. Patient education
   a. Take with full glass of water at the same time each day
   b. May take with or without food
   c. Avoid becoming overheated or dehydrated during exercise or in hot weather
- Atorvastatin
  1. Class: HMG CoA reductase inhibitor—statin
  2. Indications for use—first-line treatment in reducing low-density lipoprotein (LDL) levels
  3. Pharmacokinetics
     a. Absorption and distribution
        (1) Rapid, maximum plasma concentrations within 1–2 hours
        (2) Low systemic bioavailability of approximately 14% due to extensive first-pass metabolism; a benefit as the liver is the target organ for the drug
        (3) Animal studies show drug crosses the placenta and is present in breastmilk
        (4) Mean elimination half-life is 14 hours
     b. Metabolism—liver via interaction with CYP3A4 enzyme
     c. Excretion—eliminated primarily in bile; does not appear to undergo enterohepatic recirculation; less than 2% eliminated via urine
  4. Pharmacodynamics
     a. Reduces cholesterol production in the liver through inhibition of HMG CoA, an enzyme involved in cholesterol synthesis
     b. Stimulates upregulation of LDL receptors in the liver, which bind the LDL and increase extraction from plasma
     c. Some statins cause a decrease in triglycerides and an increase in high-density lipoprotein (HDL) secondary to LDL reduction
     d. Improves plaque stability while reducing endothelial inflammation
  5. Side effects/adverse reactions
     a. Muscle pain and soreness or muscle cramps—may be resolved with a switch to a different statin
     b. Rhabdomyolysis—rare, skeletal muscle breakdown that may cause renal dysfunction; check creatine kinase level if significant muscle pain or weakness or dark-colored urine
     c. GI effects—abdominal pain, constipation, diarrhea, nausea
     d. Asymptomatic elevations in hepatic aminotransferase activity
  6. Drug interactions
     a. Concurrent use of drugs that increase serum levels of statins increases the risk for myopathy and rhabdomyolysis
     b. CYP3A4 enzyme inhibitors—for example, macrolide antibiotics, selective serotonin reuptake

inhibitors, ketoconazole, protease inhibitors, rifampin, calcium channel blockers, cimetidine, and grapefruit juice (large quantities) increase statin serum levels

  c. Concurrent use with other anti-lipid drugs (e.g., gemfibrozil, niacin) increases risk for myopathy and rhabdomyolysis

  d. Warfarin—possible increased anticoagulant effect

  e. Digoxin—slight increase in digoxin levels

7. Contraindications/precautions

  a. Pregnancy and lactation

  b. Active liver disease with elevated liver enzymes

8. Use in pregnancy and lactation

  a. Totality of evidence to date indicates limited potential for statins to cause malformations and other adverse fetal effects

  b. In 2021, FDA has requested removal of absolute contraindication to use during pregnancy from package labeling

  c. FDA does note that most pregnant individuals should discontinue statins and that individual risks and benefits should be considered

  d. Contraindicated during lactation

9. Patient education

  a. Follow a heart-healthy diet and regular exercise regimen along with taking statin

  b. Report promptly any unexplained muscle pain, tenderness, or weakness, particularly if accompanied by malaise or fever

  c. Report promptly any symptoms that may indicate liver injury, including fatigue, anorexia, right upper abdominal discomfort, dark urine, or jaundice

- Metformin

1. Class: antihyperglycemic, biguanide

2. Indications for use—adjunct to diet and exercise to improve glycemic control in adults with type 2 diabetes mellitus

3. Pharmacokinetics

  a. Absorption and distribution

    (1) Steady-state plasma concentrations reached within 24–48 hours

    (2) Bioavailability is approximately 50%–60%

    (3) Mean elimination half-life is approximately 6 hours

  b. Metabolism—liver via interaction with CYP3A4 enzyme

  c. Excretion—extensively metabolized in the liver, with less than 0.1% of the dose excreted unchanged in the urine

4. Pharmacodynamics

  a. Decreases hepatic glucose production and intestinal absorption of glucose

  b. Improves insulin sensitivity by increasing peripheral uptake and utilization

  c. Insulin secretion remains unchanged

  d. May be used as monotherapy or as a combination therapy

5. Side effects/adverse reactions

  a. GI effects—anorexia, nausea, diarrhea, abdominal bloating

  b. Lactic acidosis—rare but serious, may result in hypothermia, hypotension, resistant bradyarrhythmia, and death

6. Drug interactions

  a. Digoxin, cimetidine, ranitidine, nifedipine, trimethoprim; alcohol may potentiate the effects of metformin

  b. Hypoglycemia may occur when metformin is co-administered with oral sulfonylureas and insulin; unlikely when used as monotherapy

7. Contraindications/precautions

  a. Hypersensitivity

  b. Renal disease or dysfunction

  c. Acute or chronic metabolic acidosis

  d. High risk for lactic acidosis—renal impairment, concomitant use of some drugs (e.g., carbonic anhydrase inhibitors such as topiramate), age 65 years old or greater, having a radiological study with contrast, surgery and other procedures, hypoxic states (e.g., acute congestive heart failure), excessive alcohol intake, and hepatic impairment

8. Use in pregnancy and lactation

  a. There are known risks to the pregnant person and fetus associated with poorly controlled diabetes mellitus in pregnancy

  b. Available data indicate that metformin use in pregnancy does not increase congenital abnormalities and is generally well tolerated

  c. There is insufficient information to determine the effects of metformin on the breastfed infant, and no available information on the effects of metformin on milk production

9. Patient education

  a. Discontinue metformin and notify a healthcare provider immediately if experience unexplained hyperventilation, myalgias, malaise, unusual somnolence, or abdominal pain as may be symptoms of lactic acidosis

  b. Be attentive to risks, symptoms, and treatment of hypoglycemia if also on an oral sulfonylurea or insulin

- Relugolix, estradiol (E2), and norethindrone acetate (NETA)

1. Class: combination of gonadotropin-releasing hormone (GnRH) receptor antagonist, estrogen, and progestin

2. Indications for use

3. Reduction of heavy menstrual bleeding associated with uterine fibroids in premenopausal individuals

  a. Management of moderate to severe pain associated with endometriosis in premenopausal individuals

  b. Limitation of use to 24 months due to the risk of continued bone loss which may not be reversible

4. Pharmacokinetics

  a. Absorption and distribution (relugolix)

    (1) Concentrations reach a steady state within 12 days

    (2) Bioavailability is approximately 62%

    (3) Mean elimination half-life is approximately 61 hours

  b. Metabolism (relugolix)—metabolized primarily by CYP3A

c. Excretion (relugolix)—excreted primarily in feces
5. Pharmacodynamics
  a. Relugolix—GnRH receptor antagonist that competitively binds to pituitary GnRH receptors, thereby reducing the release of luteinizing hormone and follicle-stimulating hormone leading to decreased serum concentrations of estradiol and progesterone and reduced bleeding with uterine fibroids and pain associated with endometriosis
  b. E2 binds to nuclear receptors expressed in estrogen-responsive tissues and may reduce the increase in bone resorption and resultant bone loss that can occur due to a decrease in circulating estrogen concentrations from relugolix alone
  c. NETA acts by binding to nuclear receptors that are expressed in progesterone-responsive tissues and may protect the uterus from potential adverse endometrial effects of unopposed estrogen
6. Side effects/adverse reactions
  a. Vasomotor symptoms
  b. Abnormal uterine bleeding
  c. Decreased sexual desire and arousal
  d. Alopecia
  e. Thromboembolic disorders and vascular events
  f. Decreases in bone mineral density that may not be completely reversible—consider assessment with dual-energy X-ray absorptiometry for baseline
  g. Suicidal thoughts or behavior and mood disorders (including depression)
7. Drug interactions
  a. P-gp inhibitors (e.g., erythromycin) increase the concentration of relugolix and may increase the risk of adverse reactions
  b. Combined P-gp inducers and strong CYP3A inducers (e.g., rifampin) may decrease the therapeutic effect of relugolix
8. Contraindications/precautions
  a. Hypersensitivity to any component
  b. High risk of arterial, venous thrombotic, or thromboembolic disorder
  c. Known osteoporosis
  d. Current or history of breast cancer or other hormone-sensitive malignancies
  e. Known hepatic impairment or disease
  f. Undiagnosed abnormal uterine bleeding
  g. Pregnancy
9. Use in pregnancy and lactation
  a. Based on findings from animal studies and its mechanism of action, relugolix may cause early pregnancy loss
  b. Limited human data in pregnant individuals are insufficient to evaluate for a drug-associated risk of major congenital disabilities, miscarriage, or adverse maternal or fetal outcomes
  c. There are no data on the presence of relugolix or its metabolites in human milk, the effects on the breastfed child, or the effects on milk production
10. Patient education
  a. Report promptly any signs or symptoms of thromboembolic disorders and vascular events

  b. Take supplementary calcium and vitamin D if dietary intake is not adequate
  c. Use effective nonhormonal contraception and discontinue this medication if pregnancy occurs
  d. Report promptly any significant mood changes or suicidal thoughts or behavior

- Tamoxifen
1. Class: selective estrogen receptor modulator (SERM)
2. Indications for use
  a. Treatment of estrogen receptor (ER)–positive breast cancer
  b. Prevention of ER-positive breast cancer for high-risk individuals
3. Pharmacokinetics
  a. Absorption and distribution
    (1) Peak plasma concentrations within 5 hours
    (2) Mean elimination half-life is 5–7 days
  b. Metabolism—this prodrug is metabolized to more active forms by various CYP450 enzymes in the liver
  c. Excretion—primarily in feces
4. Pharmacodynamics
  a. Estrogen-antagonist effects—binds to ERs; prevents estrogen from binding, thereby blocking its action at selected target sites (e.g., breast tissue)
  b. Partial estrogen agonist—acts like estrogen in other sites (e.g., uterus, bone)
5. Side effects/adverse reactions
  a. Venous thromboembolism
  b. Endometrial cancer
  c. Hot flashes
  d. Nausea
  e. Menstrual irregularities
  f. Vaginal dryness
  g. Weight gain
  h. Bone loss in premenopausal individuals
6. Drug interactions
  a. May cause a significant increase in the effect of Coumadin-type anticoagulants
  b. Increased risk for thromboembolic events when cytotoxic agents used in combination with tamoxifen
  c. Anastrozole decreases concentrations of oral tamoxifen by an unspecified interaction mechanism
  d. Strong inhibitors of CYP2D6 may cause lower blood levels of active metabolite
7. Contraindications/precautions
  a. Hypersensitivity to drug
  b. History of thromboembolic event
  c. Pregnancy
8. Use in pregnancy and lactation
  a. No adequate and well-controlled studies of use in pregnant individuals
  b. Small number of reports of vaginal bleeding, spontaneous abortions, congenital disabilities, fetal deaths in pregnant individuals
  c. Has been reported to inhibit lactation
  d. Unknown if the drug is excreted in breastmilk
9. Patient education
  a. Take with or without food

b. Report any signs or symptoms that may indicate blood clot formation

c. Report any unusual vaginal bleeding

- Oxytocin (Pitocin)
  1. Class: Uterotonic; "high alert" medication
  2. Indications for use
     a. Induction of labor
     b. Augmentation of labor
     c. Active management of the third stage of labor
     d. Postpartum hemorrhage treatment
     e. Contraction stress test
  3. Pharmacokinetics
     a. Absorption and distribution
        (1) Intravenous route—excellent, absorbed systemically; immediate onset, duration dependent on duration of administration, subsides within 1 hour once discontinued
        (2) Intramuscular route—good; delayed onset, duration of action is 2–3 hours
        (3) Onset of action is 3–4 minutes
        (4) Reaches steady state within 30–40 minutes
        (5) Mean elimination half-life is 6–10 minutes
        (6) Minimal amounts cross the placenta
     b. Metabolism—occurs rapidly in the kidneys and liver
     c. Excretion—small amounts through urine
  4. Pharmacodynamics
     a. Increases intracellular Ca^{2+}, which promotes motility of uterine muscle
     b. Exerts effect via agonist action; uterotonic effect mediated by receptor function
     c. Receptors on the myometrium are upregulated in pregnancy, peaking in early labor; hence, the response is highly individualized as it depends on both the dose and the receptor concentration
     d. Receptors can be downregulated with prolonged exposure
     e. Has diuretic effects in large quantities
  5. Side effects/adverse reactions
     a. More common with excessive dosage or prolonged exposure
     b. Anaphylaxis
     c. Postpartum hemorrhage
     d. Cardiac arrhythmia
     e. Fatal afibrinogenemia
     f. Nausea
     g. Vomiting
     h. Pelvic hematoma
     i. Subarachnoid hemorrhage
     j. Hypertensive episodes
     k. Uterine rupture
     l. Severe water intoxication leading to convulsions, coma, and/or maternal death—particularly with prolonged exposure
     m. Fetal effects—bradycardia, cardiac arrhythmia, brain damage, fetal death, neonatal seizures, low Apgar scores at 5 minutes, neonatal jaundice, neonatal retinal hemorrhage
  6. Drug interactions
     a. Rare

b. Vasoconstrictor (with caudal block anesthesia)—may cause severe hypertension

c. Cyclopropane anesthesia—may result in hypotension, sinus bradycardia

7. Contraindications/precautions
   a. Hypersensitivity
   b. Uterine tachysystole
   c. Abnormal fetal heart rate pattern
   d. Require fluid restriction
   e. At risk for pulmonary edema
   f. Use caution in patients with a history of previous cesarean section
8. Use in pregnancy and lactation—typically used in the third trimester or later
9. Patient education
   a. May be best used once the cervix is ripe
   b. External (sometimes internal) monitoring of uterine contractions and fetal heart rate is required during the administration of drugs in labor
   c. Low-dose protocols can be used for safe administration
   d. If administered postpartum via IM injection, there may be pain upon administration; injection-related education may be provided
   e. Report any headache, nausea, or muscle cramps

- Nitrous oxide (Nitronox)
  1. Class: inhalant; analgesic, anxiolytic
  2. Indications for use include but are not limited to the management of pain and anxiety for:
     a. Labor
     b. Repair of perineal laceration
     c. Third-stage management if needed
     d. Other procedures: IV placement, catheter placement, vaginal examination, intrauterine device (IUD) insertion
  3. Pharmacokinetics
     a. Absorption and distribution
        (1) Inhalation route—self-administered by the patient; tasteless, odorless gas, mixed with oxygen and inhaled by mask; 50/50 concentration nitrous oxide and oxygen
        (2) Onset of action is 1 minute or less
        (3) Rapid elimination—residual effects resolve within 5 minutes
        (4) Readily crosses the placenta, but quickly eliminated
     b. Metabolism—none; reduced by intestinal bacteria
     c. Excretion—primarily in the lungs; minimal amount diffused through the skin
  4. Pharmacodynamics
     a. Not well understood; noncompetitively inhibits the N-methyl-D-aspartate subtype of excitatory glutamate receptors
     b. Other mechanisms of action hypothesized
  5. Side effects/adverse reactions
     a. Neuroapoptosis—at high, prolonged doses
     b. Loss of consciousness—not common when self-administered
     c. Nausea and vomiting
     d. Megaloblastic anemia—in the presence of vitamin B_{12} deficiency

e. Myocardial risk—at high doses

f. Diffusion hypoxia—at high, prolonged doses, followed by a lack of high-concentration oxygen thereafter

g. Alterations in hypoxic drive—when combined with sedatives or opioids; this risk can be attenuated with instruction to breathe more deeply if necessary

h. Fetal effects—no effect on fetal heart rate or contractions; no negative effects on Apgar scoring, neonatal neurobehavioral scores, or sucking behavior

6. Drug interactions

a. Rare

b. Sedatives or opioids may produce a more pronounced respiratory depression

7. Contraindications/precautions

a. Recent trauma

b. Certain respiratory conditions—chronic obstructive pulmonary disease, pneumothorax, emphysema, pulmonary hypertension

c. Acute alcohol intoxication

d. Acute drug intoxication

e. Reduced level of consciousness

f. Increased intracranial pressure

g. Bowel obstruction

h. Recent vitreoretinal or ear surgery

i. Acute vitamin B_{12} deficiency—safe to use if deficiency resolved

j. Use caution in case of occupational exposure for potential effects on patient's fertility at higher doses; scavenging system required to mitigate

8. Use in pregnancy and lactation—typically used in labor or immediate postpartum; safe

9. Patient education

a. Must be able to self-administer; no training required

b. Promotes physiologic labor and birth

c. To use effectively, breathe deeply and slowly at the start of or just prior to a contraction; stop once the contraction has passed

d. May use as an anxiolytic between contractions

e. Relatively safe analgesic, anxiolytic for use throughout the entire labor, during the third stage, or repair

f. No monitoring (i.e., pulse oximetry) is required

g. Discontinue in the event of maternal or fetal compromise, side effects that persist, or if no longer desired

h. Report nausea, vomiting, vertigo

- Betamethasone (Celestone)

1. Class: corticosteroid

2. Indications for use include, but are not limited to, promoting fetal lung maturity in instances of preterm labor where preterm birth is anticipated (including for those with ruptured membranes and multiple gestation)

3. Pharmacokinetics

a. Absorption and distribution

(1) Intramuscular route—most common route; two 12-mg doses given 24 hours apart, for those at risk for preterm delivery within 7 days

(a) A single initial course and single rescue course (at risk of preterm delivery within 7 days) if the initial course occurred 7–14 days prior AND less than 34 weeks' gestation

(b) A single course is recommended for an anticipated late-preterm delivery (between 34 0/7 and 36 6/7 at risk of delivery within 7 days) in select birthing persons who have not received a previous course of antenatal steroids

(2) Intra-amniotic route—less common

(3) Intravenous route—less common

(4) Greatest benefit at 2–7 days after the initial dose

(5) Biological half-life is >72 hours

(6) Easily crosses the placenta when given IM or IV

b. Metabolism—occurs in the liver

c. Excretion—through the kidneys

4. Pharmacodynamics

a. Promotes lung maturity by stimulating surfactant synthesis

b. Increases compliance of lung tissue

c. Reduces vascular capillaries

d. Lacks mineralocorticoid activity (with short-term use)

e. Relatively weak immunosuppressive activity (with short-term use)

5. Side effects/adverse reactions

a. Maternal

(1) Glucose intolerance with transient hyperglycemia (without diabetes)

(2) Increased insulin requirements (with diabetes)

(3) Increased risk for pulmonary edema; higher if used concurrently with beta-adrenergic drugs for tocolysis or for those with multifetal gestation

b. Fetal—fetal heart rate has a biphasic response; initially, a mild elevation, followed by decreased variability on days 2–3 post-administration

c. Long-term effects on hypothalamic–pituitary axis possible; unclear

6. Drug interactions—rare

7. Contraindications/precautions

a. Serial courses not recommended due to potential maternal and fetal harm

b. May be harmful to certain growth-restricted fetuses

8. Use in pregnancy and lactation—no contraindication; can improve newborn outcomes in the setting of preterm birth

9. Patient education

a. Antenatal corticosteroid therapy is one of the most important treatments for preterm neonates and can significantly reduce the following risks:

(1) Respiratory distress syndrome

(2) Intracranial hemorrhage

(3) Necrotizing colitis

(4) Neonatal death

b. Benefit to the fetus/neonate typically outweighs the maternal risk

- Magnesium sulfate ($MgSO_4$)
  1. Class: anticonvulsant; "high alert" medication
  2. Indications for use
     a. Maternal seizure prophylaxis and treatment with preeclampsia and eclampsia
     b. Fetal neuroprotection with anticipated preterm birth (<32 weeks' gestation)
     c. Short-term (<48 hours) tocolytic
  3. Pharmacokinetics
     a. Absorption and distribution
        (1) Intravenous route—excellent, absorbed systemically; immediate onset, duration depends on duration of administration, subsides within 1–2 hours once discontinued; loading dose of 4–6 g in 100 mL over 20–30 minutes; maintenance dose of 2 g/hour for at least 12–24 hours
        (2) Intramuscular route—not preferable; variability in producing effective concentration levels
        (3) Reaches steady state variably, within 12 hours when given IV
        (4) Crosses the placenta; limited amounts in breastmilk
     b. Metabolism—none
     c. Excretion—through the kidneys
  4. Pharmacodynamics
     a. Mechanism of action poorly understood
     b. Blocks neuromuscular transition; depresses CNS
     c. Acts on vascular smooth muscle, causing vasodilation
  5. Side effects/adverse reactions
     a. Flushing
     b. Palpitations
     c. Feeling of warmth
     d. Lethargy
     e. Muscle weakness
     f. Dizziness
     g. Nausea and vomiting
     h. Respiratory depression
     i. Pulmonary edema
  6. Drug interactions—calcium channel blockers
  7. Contraindications/precautions
     a. Concurrent use with calcium channel blockers
     b. Should not use for longer than 5–7 days due to increased risk of fetal and neonatal bone demineralization and fracture
     c. Toxic effects at serum level >7 mg/dL
     d. Calcium gluconate reverses the effects of toxicity
  8. Use in pregnancy and lactation—typically used in second and third trimesters; may be used postpartum if indicated for preeclampsia or eclampsia
  9. Patient education
     a. Short-term, controlled use is safe in pregnancy where indicated
     b. Urine output and magnesium levels will be monitored
     c. Report difficulty breathing, lethargy, weakness, dizziness, nausea, vomiting, or palpitations
     d. For magnesium levels that are too high, a calcium gluconate injection may be given
     e. Plans to breastfeed should proceed

- RhoGAM
  1. Class: Immune globulin; blood product
  2. Indication for use is prevention of Rh (anti-D) isoimmunization in a mother who is Rh negative
     a. Prophylaxis during pregnancy 26–28 weeks gestation
     b. Birth of a Rh-positive baby
     c. Antepartum hemorrhage (suspected or proven)
     d. Pregnancy loss, termination (spontaneous/induced), threatened termination, and ectopic pregnancy
     e. Transfusion of Rh-positive blood or blood products
     f. External cephalic version
     g. Invasive procedures (i.e., amniocentesis, chorionic villus sampling)
  3. Pharmacokinetics
     a. Absorption and distribution
        (1) Intramuscular route—good; effective up to 12 weeks after administration; available in two doses (50 and 300 mcg); multiple doses may be given as warranted by blood loss
        (2) Maximum concentration within 4 days
        (3) Mean elimination half-life is approximately 30 days
        (4) Crosses placenta only minimally; clinically insignificant
     b. Metabolism—nonspecific
     c. Excretion—via feces and urine
  4. Pharmacodynamics
     a. Mechanism of action is unknown
     b. Creates passive anti-D immunity, which promotes clearance of anti-D–coated fetal red blood cells (RBCs) in maternal circulation
     c. Inhibits maternal immune response to anti-D, which is protective of future pregnancies
     d. Not effective where Rh alloimmunization has occurred
  5. Side effects/adverse reactions
     a. Injection-site reactions
     b. Rash
     c. Low-grade fever
     d. Allergy (rare)
  6. Drug interactions
     a. Rare
     b. May inhibit the efficacy of live vaccines
     c. Theoretical risk of contamination, just as with other blood products
  7. Contraindications/precautions
     a. Rh-positive individuals
     b. Neonates
  8. Use in pregnancy and lactation
     a. Typically used at 26–28 weeks' gestation and postpartum
     b. Can be used throughout pregnancy
     c. If the birth occurs within 3 weeks of the previous dose, the postpartum dose may be withheld pending a normal Kleihauer–Betke test (<15 mL of RBCs) for fetal–maternal hemorrhage

9. Patient education
   a. Necessary to reduce the risk of Rh sensitization
   b. Most common risk is a reaction at the site of injection
   c. Although allergic reaction is rare, report symptoms, such as hives, itching, tightness in the chest, wheezing
   d. Postpone live vaccines, with the exception of rubella or measles/mumps/rubella (MMR) if needed, until 12 weeks after RhoGAM administration
   e. Reevaluate rubella titer 3 months after administration if given postpartum with RhoGAM

- Labetalol
  1. Class: Non-cardioselective beta blocker
  2. Indication for use is to treat chronic maternal hypertension and/or severe maternal hypertension
     a. Primarily one of the preferred antihypertensives in pregnancy
     b. Treatment of maternal chronic hypertension orally
     c. Acute treatment of maternal severe range blood pressures (>160/>110 mm Hg) with slow direct intravenous injection
  3. Pharmacokinetics
     a. Absorption and distribution
        (1) Oral administration—200 to 2,400 mg/day orally in two to three divided doses. Commonly initiated at 100–200 mg twice daily
        (2) IV administration 10–20 mg IV, then 20–80 mg every 10–30 minutes to a maximum cumulative dosage of 300 mg; or constant infusion 1–2 mg/min IV
        (3) Bioavailability—rapid and almost completely absorbed (i.e., 90%–100%) from the GI tract following oral administration
        (4) Undergoes first pass in the liver and/or GI mucosa
        (5) Absolute bioavailability is approximately 25%
        (6) Onset
           (a) Oral—20 minutes to 2 hours
           (b) IV—1 to 2 minutes
        (7) Duration
           (a) Oral—dose dependent; approx. 8–12 hours or 12–24 hours after a single 200 or 300 g dose respectively
           (b) IV—slow direct IV injection effects persist for about 2–4 hours, although may be up to 24 hours in some patients
        (8) Mean elimination half-life is 5.5 or 6–8 hours following IV or oral administration, respectively.
     b. Metabolism
        (1) Oral—liver and possibly GI mucosa
        (2) Undergoes extensive first-pass metabolism in the liver and/or GI mucosa
     c. Excretion—mores so in feces (30%–60%) rather than urine (<5%)
  4. Pharmacodynamics
     a. Mechanism of action: Selectively blocks alpha-1 adrenergic receptors; nonselectively blocks beta-1 and beta-1 adrenergic receptors

5. Side effects/adverse reactions
   a. Potential bronchoconstrictive effects
   b. Symptomatic orthostatic hypotension
   c. Dizziness/lightheadedness
   d. Fatigue
   e. Nausea
   f. Dyspepsia
6. Drug interactions
   a. Calcium-channel blocking agents (e.g., verapamil, diltiazem)
      (1) May augment therapeutic and adverse effects
   b. Cimetidine
      (1) Absolute bioavailability of oral labetalol substantially increased, possibly via enhanced absorption or decreased first-pass hepatic metabolism
   c. Diuretics
      (1) Increased hypotensive effect
   d. Halothane
      (1) Synergistic hypotensive effect
   e. Nitroglycerin
      (1) May augment hypotensive effects and antagonism of reflex tachycardia produced by nitroglycerin
   f. Tricyclic antidepressants
      (1) May increase the incidence of tremors
7. Contraindications/precautions
   a. obstructive airway disease (e.g., bronchial asthma)
   b. preexisting myocardial disease
   c. decompensated cardiac function
   d. heart block
   e. bradycardia
   f. other conditions associated with severe and prolonged hypotension
   g. known hypersensitivity to labetalol or any ingredient in the formulation
8. Use in pregnancy and lactation
   a. May use during pregnancy if the benefit outweighs the risk
   b. Crosses placental barrier
   c. Distributed in breast milk
   d. May cause bradycardia in fetus and newborn
9. Patient education
   a. Patients may experience transient scalp tingling at the initiation of therapy
   b. Notify if having orthostatic symptoms (dizziness, lightheadedness)
   c. Continue therapeutic regimen and notify clinician if discontinuing
   d. Notify the clinician of existing or concomitant therapy, including prescription and OTC drugs
   e. Notify the clinician of any signs of difficulty breathing or signs of cardiac failure

- Hydralazine
  1. Class: vasodilator
  2. Indication for use is to treat acute severe maternal hypertension
  3. Pharmacokinetics
     a. Absorption and distribution

(1) 5 mg IV or IM, then 5–10 mg IV every 20–40 minutes to a maximum cumulative dosage of 20 mg; or constant infusion of 0.5 mg–10 mg/hour

(2) Bioavailability—rapid

(3) Onset—10–20 minutes

(4) Duration

  (a) IV and IM—2–6 hours

(5) Plasma half-life approx. 2–4 hours

 b. Metabolism

  (1) GI mucosa and liver

 c. Excretion—primarily in urine and feces (10%)

4. Pharmacodynamics

 a. Mechanism of action: Exact mechanism of action is not fully understood. Lowers blood pressure by causing peripheral vasodilation by direct relaxation of vascular smooth muscle. Interferes with calcium movements within the vascular smooth muscle. It also increases renin activity in the plasma, leading to the production of angiotensin II, causing stimulation of aldosterone and sodium reabsorption.

5. Side effects / adverse reactions

 a. headache

 b. anorexia

 c. diarrhea

 d. tachycardia

 e. Nausea

 f. Palpitations

 g. Angina pectoris

6. Drug interactions

 a. Beta-blockers

  (1) May augment the hypotensive effect

  (2) Concomitant use may minimize adverse cardiac effects (e.g., tachycardia, precipitation of angina) associated with hydralazine

 b. Diuretics

  (1) May augment hypotension

 c. MAO Inhibitors

  (1) May augment hypotension

7. Contraindications/precautions

 a. Coronary artery disease

 b. Mitral valvular rheumatic heart disease

 c. Hypersensitivity to hydralazine

8. Use in pregnancy and lactation

 a. Avoid during the first two trimesters

 b. Administer in the third trimester if the benefit outweighs the risk to the fetus

 c. Distributed in breast milk

9. Patient education

 a. Potential to impair mental alertness or physical coordination

 b. Notify of continued headache with repeated dosing

- Nifedipine

1. Class: calcium channel blockers

2. Indication for use is to treat maternal chronic hypertension and/or severe maternal hypertension

3. Pharmacokinetics

 a. Absorption and distribution

  (1) For treatment of maternal chronic hypertension: **Extended-release preparation—30–120 mg/day orally. Initiate at 30–60 mg once daily

  (2) For urgent blood pressure control: **Immediate release preparation—10 to 20 mg orally, repeat in 20 minutes if needed; then10–20 mg every 2–6 hours; maximum daily is 180 mg

  (3) Bioavailability

   (a) Immediate release—90% absorbed following ingestion

   (b) Extended release—75% to 89%

  (4) Onset—5 to 10 minutes

  (5) Duration

   (a) Immediate release—peak plasma concentration 0.5–2 hours

   (b) Extended release—2.5 to 6 hours

  (6) Half-life

   (a) Immediate release—2 hours

   (b) Extended release—7 hours

 b. Metabolism

  (1) Liver by CYP isoenzymes and CYP3A

 c. Excretion—metabolites in urine (60%–80%) and feces

4. Pharmacodynamics

 a. Mechanism of action: Inhibits calcium ion influx and transmembrane influx into cardiac and smooth muscles

5. Side effects/adverse reactions

 a. headache

 b. mood changes

 c. diarrhea

 d. tachycardia

 e. Nausea

 f. heartburn

 g. wheezing, dyspnea, cough

 h. nasal congestion

 i. sore throat

 j. flushing

 k. heat sensation

 l. tremor

 m. peripheral edema

6. Drug interactions

 a. Beta-blockers

  (1) May augment hypotension, exacerbate angina, heart failure, and arrhythmia

 b. Alcohol

  (1) Increased nifedipine bioavailability

 c. Anticoagulants

  (1) May increase PT

 d. Antifungals (azoles)

  (1) May increase plasma nifedipine concentrations

 e. Antiretroviral agents

  (1) May increase plasma nifedipine concentrations

 f. Benazepril

  (1) May attenuate the tachycardic effect of nifedipine

 g. St. John's wort

7. Contraindications/precautions
   a. Known hypersensitivity to nifedipine
   b. Excessive hypotension
   c. May increase frequency, duration, and/or severity of angina or acute MI
8. Use in pregnancy and lactation
   a. Use in pregnancy if the benefit outweighs the risk
   b. Has been detected in breast milk and compatible with breastfeeding per American Academy of Pediatrics
9. Patient education
   a. Extended release
      (1) Take on an empty stomach
      (2) Do not crush, chew, or break tablet. Swallow whole

- Tranexamic acid
1. Class: Hemostatics
2. Indication for use is treatment menorrhagia (FDA labeled for oral formulation). Off-label IV use for postpartum hemorrhage (defined as >1,000 mL regardless of delivery route)
3. Pharmacokinetics
   a. Absorption and distribution
      (1) Oral—1.3 g (two 650 mg tablets) 3 times daily for a maximum of 5 days during menstruation
         (a) Do not exceed three doses (six tablets) in a 24-hr period or administer for more than 5 days in a monthly menstrual cycle
      (2) IV (off-label for postpartum hemorrhage)—Loading dose of 1 g (Add 1 g vial to 100 mL NS and give over 10 minutes)
         (a) Second dose of 1 g may be readministered if bleeding continues after 30 minutes or recurs within 24 hours of the first dose
      (3) Bioavailability—Orally approximately 45%
      (4) Onset—2 to 15 minutes
      (5) Duration
         (a) Oral peak plasma concentration approximately 3 hours
      (6) Half-Life
         (a) Oral—11 hours
         (b) IV—2 hours
   b. Metabolism
      (1) Small fraction of the drug is metabolized
   c. Excretion
      (1) Primarily urine
4. Pharmacodynamics
   a. Mechanism of action—acts as an anti-fibrinolytic agent, blocks lysine binding sites of plasmogen, and increases the binding affinity of tranexamic acid to plasminogen and plasmin
      (1) Anti-fibrinolytic that inhibits both plasminogen activation and plasmin activity thereby preventing clot breakdown and limiting the promotion of clot formations

      (2) 6–10 times more potent than aminocaproic acid
5. Side effects/adverse effects
   a. Oral
      (1) Headache
      (2) Sinus and nasal symptoms
      (3) Back pain, musculoskeletal pain, joint pain, muscle cramps
      (4) Abdominal pain
      (5) Anemia
      (6) Fatigue
      (7) Migraine/potential for seizures
   b. IV
      (1) Nausea
      (2) Vomiting
      (3) Diarrhea
      (4) Allergic dermatitis
      (5) Giddiness
      (6) Hypotension
      (7) Thromboembolic events
6. Drug interactions
   a. Factor IX complex and anti-inhibitor coagulant concentrates
      (1) May increase thrombotic risk
   b. Hormonal Contraceptives
      (1) May increase thrombotic risk
   c. Tissue plasminogen activators
      (1) May decrease the efficacy of both drugs
   d. Tretinoin
      (1) May exacerbate procoagulant effects of tretinoin
7. Contraindications/precautions
   a. Patients with acquired defective color vision (due to risk of ocular toxicity)
   b. Subarachnoid hemorrhage—cerebral edema and cerebral infarction may be caused by tranexamic acid
   c. Concomitant use of combination hormonal contraceptives
   d. Hypersensitivity reactions to tranexamic acid
8. Use in pregnancy and lactation
   a. It is not known whether tranexamic acid is associated with adverse maternal or fetal outcomes
   b. Crosses the placenta
   c. Distributed in human milk; however, effects on the breastfed infant or milk production are unknown
9. Patient education
   a. Inform patients that increases the risk of blood clots
   b. Notify clinicians if shortness of breath or tightening of the throat and discontinue medication
   c. May cause dizziness and caution while operating heavy machinery or driving
   d. Notify clinicians of all herbal/dietary supplements
   e. Oral formulation
      (1) Do not chew or break
      (2) Can take with or without food

Questions

Select the best answer.

1. Which of the following pharmacokinetic changes could decrease the effect of a medication?
   a. Decrease in plasma protein binding
   b. Increase in hepatic first-pass effect
   c. Increase in enterohepatic recirculation
   d. Increase in bioavailability

2. The 2015 FDA Pregnancy and Lactation Labeling Rule requires inclusion of:
   a. alternative medication choices when a particular drug is contraindicated during pregnancy
   b. any available data on potential drug-associated effects on an individual's fertility
   c. expanded pregnancy letter category (A, B, C, D, X) information
   d. information on a centralized pregnancy exposure registry for all drugs

3. Plasma protein binding most significantly affects drug:
   a. absorption
   b. distribution
   c. metabolism
   d. excretion

4. The half-life of a drug is used to:
   a. calculate the loading dose needed to achieve immediately the desired steady state
   b. determine the time required to reach steady state and the dosage interval
   c. estimate the therapeutic index
   d. predict the likelihood of an adverse reaction

5. Acyclovir is ineffective in eliminating latent herpes virus because it:
   a. has a short elimination half-life of 3–4 hours
   b. has only a 15%–20% bioavailability
   c. is a prodrug that is converted to active form by first-pass metabolism
   d. is effective only against rapidly replicating herpes virus

6. A patient taking metronidazole and cimetidine at the same time is at increased risk for:
   a. bothersome side effects from metronidazole
   b. decreased effectiveness of cimetidine
   c. renal impairment
   d. a severe disulfiram-type reaction

7. The term used to describe a drug that initiates a physiologic response when it is bound to a drug receptor is:
   a. agonist
   b. antagonist
   c. metabolite
   d. prodrug

8. The term used to describe the propensity of a drug to bind with a specific receptor is:
   a. affinity
   b. bioavailability
   c. efficacy
   d. potency

9. Fluconazole is effective in a one-time dose because it:
   a. is rapidly absorbed in the GI tract
   b. has a bioavailability greater than 90%
   c. is widely distributed into body tissues and fluids
   d. has a mean elimination half-life of 30 hours

10. Which of the following statements regarding pharmacokinetic changes during pregnancy is correct?
    a. First-pass metabolism of drugs is increased during pregnancy because of increased blood flow through the maternal liver.
    b. Drug elimination may be faster because of an increase in the GFR.
    c. Higher levels of drug-protein binding may occur with decreased albumin levels.
    d. Drug absorption may be decreased because of increased plasma volume.

11. Instructions for a patient who is prescribed an oral bisphosphonate should include:
    a. take the medication in the evening at bedtime
    b. take the medication with an antacid to avoid GI irritation
    c. take the medication with 8 ounces of plain water
    d. take the medication with orange juice to enhance its absorption

12. A common side effect of oral oxybutynin is:
    a. dry mouth
    b. nausea
    c. increased sweating
    d. muscle pain

13. Which of the following medications is considered a prodrug that is metabolized to a more active form by enzymes in the liver?
    a. Alendronate
    b. Atorvastatin
    c. Oxybutynin
    d. Tamoxifen

14. Rhabdomyolysis, a rare skeletal muscle breakdown that may cause renal dysfunction, may occur as an adverse reaction to:
    a. atorvastatin
    b. fluconazole
    c. metronidazole
    d. tamoxifen

15. Which of the following statements is correct?
    a. A narrow therapeutic range is desired for reducing the possible toxic effects of a drug.
    b. Drug–drug interactions may increase or decrease the bioavailability of a drug.
    c. Drugs that are highly lipophilic are not likely to pass through the blood–brain barrier.
    d. Unpredictable adverse reactions to a drug may occur because of age, body mass, or sex.

16. The partial estrogen agonist effect of tamoxifen may result in:
    a. increased occurrence of hot flashes
    b. increased risk for endometrial cancer
    c. prevention of estrogen binding to receptors in breast tissue
    d. vaginal dryness

17. The low serum bioavailability of atorvastatin is attributed to its:
    a. extensive hepatic first-pass metabolism
    b. high level of protein binding
    c. minimal enterohepatic recirculation
    d. short elimination half-life of 2–3 hours

18. Effects of oxytocin administration are highly individualized due to:
    a. diuretic effects of the drug on the kidneys
    b. first-pass effects in the liver
    c. the presence of other conflicting medication
    d. variability in upregulation of receptors

19. Oxytocin is effective in the management of postpartum hemorrhage due to its:
    a. diuretic effects
    b. expulsive effects
    c. fibrinolytic effects
    d. uterotonic effects

20. The use of nitrous oxide in labor is contraindicated in an individual with:
    a. a history of vitamin B_{12} deficiency
    b. gestational diabetes
    c. chronic obstructive pulmonary disease
    d. a previously placed epidural

21. Which of the following is necessary for the administration of nitrous oxide?
    a. Ability to self-administer
    b. Availability of pulse oximetry
    c. Previous training on usage
    d. Progression into active labor

22. Management with a single rescue course of betamethasone is appropriate for a pregnant individual presenting for triage with:
    a. cervical insufficiency at 21 6/7 weeks' gestation
    b. premature ruptured membranes with thick meconium at 36 1/7 weeks' gestation
    c. preterm labor at 33 6/7 weeks' gestation who completed a single course within 2 days
    d. regular uterine contractions and dilating cervix at 33 4/7 weeks' gestation

23. For a pregnant person with diabetes and at risk for preterm birth who has completed a single course of betamethasone, which of the following effects should be anticipated?
    a. Elevated blood pressure
    b. Elevated heart rate
    c. Increased insulin dosage
    d. Increased risk of infection

24. Which of the following is a reason to draw and assess a magnesium level in a pregnant person with preeclampsia who is on magnesium sulfate for seizure prophylaxis? The patient reports:
    a. a headache
    b. difficulty breathing
    c. increased appetite
    d. severe urticaria

25. Magnesium sulfate should be discontinued after 5–7 days when used in pregnancy due to which of the following adverse outcomes?
    a. Fetal bone demineralization
    b. Fetal heart rate complications
    c. Maternal hemorrhage
    d. Maternal kidney damage

26. A pregnant person is known to be Rh negative and rubella nonimmune. Prior to discharge in the postpartum period, RhoGAM and the MMR vaccine are given. Which of the following should be included in the plan of care?
    a. File a report with the blood bank
    b. Follow up at 12 weeks
    c. Perform a rubella titer in 3 months
    d. Screen for HIV and hepatitis B

27. A pregnant person who is Rh negative received RhoGAM at 37 weeks after undergoing a successful external cephalic version. The patient had a spontaneous vaginal birth at 38 4/7 weeks' gestation, and the newborn is Rh positive. Of the following, which is the most appropriate next step?
    a. Give 300 mcg of RhoGAM IM.
    b. Perform a Kleihauer–Betke test.
    c. Collect a paternal blood sample.
    d. Advise that no RhoGAM is necessary.

28. Which of the following statements regarding pain management in elderly patients is correct?
    a. Age-related increases in excretion of drugs may require more frequent dosing of pain medications.
    b. Benzodiazepine medications, such as alprazolam, may be a better option than a pain medication.
    c. Elderly patients should never take narcotic medications for pain.
    d. Long-acting NSAIDs may be more likely to cause adverse GI reactions in elderly patients.

29. An individual with a genetic polymorphism, causing the person to be a poor (slow) metabolizer of a specific drug compared with an individual without the polymorphism, may have:
    a. a greater risk of toxicity with the same dose of the drug
    b. difficulty maintaining a therapeutic drug level
    c. increased conversion of a prodrug to the active metabolite
    d. increased risk for hypersensitivity reactions to drugs

30. A 32-year-old patient presents at 36 4/7 weeks' gestation with persistent severe range blood pressures in triage. The patient's prenatal course is complicated by anxiety, moderate persistent asthma, and obesity. An IV is started and lab specimens have been collected. Which antihypertensive would be ordered?
    a. Nifedipine
    b. Lisinopril
    c. Labetalol
    d. Hydralazine

31. A prenatal patient wants to discuss options for pain management in the first stage of labor. The patient desires some medicinal pain management but is concerned with the long-term effects of medications and narcotics on the mother and fetus. What is the recommended therapy for this patient?
    a. Hypnobirthing
    b. Bradley method
    c. Morphine
    d. Nitrous oxide

32. A 42-year-old patient presents to triage status post a precipitous delivery at home and arrives via ambulance. As the patient transfers from the stretcher the placenta spontaneously delivers onto the bed. The patient begins to hemorrhage with an estimated blood loss of 2 L and continues to bleed profusely. The patient has a boggy uterus, and no lacerations were detected. The clinician orders IV access × 2, oxytocin, methylergonovine maleate, carboprost, and misoprostol. Which medication is recommended in conjunction with all the other medications along with your other emergent interventions?
    a. Tranexamic acid
    b. Nitroglycerin
    c. Magnesium sulfate
    d. Fresh frozen plasma

33. Betamethasone treatment is indicated for which scenario?
    a. 22-year-old patient G1P0 at 32 2/7 weeks gestation with regular contractions and a cervical exam revealing 4 cm/75%/-2 with an uncomplicated prenatal course
    b. 31-year-old patient G2P1001 at 36 1/7 weeks gestation with cramping that goes away with hydration for the last 3 days and a cervical exam revealing 0 cm/25%/-3
    c. 40-year-old patient G3P0020 at 37 3/7 weeks' gestation with prenatal course complicated by chronic hypertension with contractions every 2–3 minutes. A cervical exam reveals 5 cm /75%/-2
    d. 24-year-old patient G4P1021 at 39 1/7 weeks' gestation with cramping that is intermittent. The patient feels like her "water broke" 2 hours ago

34. A 19-year-old patient with an uncomplicated pregnancy at 38 3/7 weeks' gestation arrived at the clinic for a prenatal care appointment. An initial blood pressure was 172/108 mmHg, and 15 minutes later, a repeat blood pressure was 176/110 mmHg. The patient notes not feeling well. The clinician calls to transfer the patient to the closest facility for obstetric triage. The ambulance will arrive in approximately 10–15 minutes. The clinician recognizes that this is an acute severe range blood pressure and needs to administer an anti-hypertensive. Which anti-hypertensive is best to order and administer in the clinic?
    a. Oral Labetalol
    b. Oral Nifedipine
    c. IV Hydralazine
    d. Oral Methyldopa

35. The main mechanism of action for relugolix, estradiol, and norethindrone acetate in the treatment of uterine fibroids is:
    a. estradiol binding to receptors expressed in estrogen-responsive tissues
    b. gonadotropin-releasing hormone (GnRH) agonist increasing release of luteinizing hormone and follicle-stimulating hormone
    c. GnRH antagonist competitively binding to pituitary GnRH receptors
    d. norethindrone acetate binding to receptors expressed in progesterone-responsive tissues

36. The use of relugolix, estradiol, and norethindrone acetate for the treatment of fibroids and endometriosis-associated pain is limited to 24 months because more prolonged use places the user at increased risk for:
    a. continued bone loss that may be irreversible
    b. endometrial cancer
    c. infertility
    d. thromboembolic disorders or vascular events

37. Mechanisms of action for metformin include:
    a. delay of absorption of carbohydrates
    b. improvement in insulin sensitivity
    c. increase in insulin secretion
    d. increase in intestinal absorption of glucose

38. Which of the following statements concerning genetic variations that influence drug metabolism and drug response is correct?
    a. Genetic variations account for approximately 5% of interindividual differences in drug responses in general.
    b. Information on genomic biomarkers is not currently available in FDA drug labeling.
    c. Polymorphic differences in drug receptors are evenly distributed among racial and ethnic groups.
    d. A characteristic that makes clinical utility of pharmacogenomic testing high is when consequences of treatment failure are severe.

Answers with Rationales

1. **b.** Increase in hepatic first-pass effect
   Orally administered drugs go from the GI tract through the portal system to the liver before entering the general circulation. Some metabolism (chemical inactivation) of the drug may occur as it is taken up by hepatic microsomal enzymes.

2. **b.** any available data on potential drug-associated effects on an individual's fertility

The 2015 FDA Pregnancy and Lactation Labeling Rule requires the inclusion of a female and male reproductive potential subsection if human or animal study data show potential drug-associated effects on fertility and/or implantation loss.

3. **b.** distribution
   Drugs may attach to proteins (mainly albumin) in the blood (plasma protein binding). Only unbound drugs are

active and able to move out of the blood into body fluids and body tissues (distribution).

4. **b.** determine the time required to reach steady state and the dosage interval
The half-life of a drug is the time it takes for the plasma concentration of the drug to decrease by 50%. It can be used to determine the time required to reach steady state and the dosage interval.

5. **d.** is effective only against rapidly replicating herpes virus
Acyclovir is selectively activated in infected cells and works by inhibiting viral DNA synthesis. Because it is effective only against rapidly replicating herpes virus, it is not effective in eliminating latent herpes virus.

6. **a.** bothersome side effects from metronidazole
Cimetidine can decrease the hepatic metabolism of metronidazole and increase its serum levels.

7. **a.** agonist
One mechanism of drug effect is through drug–receptor interaction. A receptor can be a cellular protein, enzyme, or membrane that, when bound to a drug, initiates a physiologic response or blocks a response that the receptor normally stimulates. The term *agonist* refers to a drug that, when combined with the receptor, stimulates a physiologic response. The term *antagonist* refers to a drug that, when combined with the receptor, blocks the response.

8. **a.** affinity
Affinity is the propensity of a drug to bind itself to a given receptor site. Efficacy is the ability of the drug to initiate biological activity as a result of such binding.

9. **d.** has a mean elimination half-life of 30 hours
The half-life is the time it takes for plasma concentration of a drug to decrease by 50%; it is used to determine both the time required to reach a steady state and the dosage interval. Based on a half-life of 30 hours, the recommended dose of fluconazole for uncomplicated vulvovaginal candidiasis is a 150-mg oral tablet taken in a single dose.

10. **b.** Drug elimination may be faster because of an increase in the GFR.
The GFR begins increasing early in pregnancy, peaks at 9–16 weeks, and plateaus at a rate approximately 50% above the pre-pregnancy rate at 34–36 weeks. An increased GFR can result in faster elimination of some drugs, resulting in a lower serum concentration during pregnancy.

11. **c.** take the medication with 8 ounces of plain water
Instructions for the patient being prescribed an oral bisphosphonate should include taking it with 8 ounces of plain water.

12. **a.** dry mouth
The anticholinergic action of oxybutynin may cause side effects such as dry mouth, constipation, urinary retention, blurred vision, impaired sweating, and drowsiness.

13. **d.** Tamoxifen
Tamoxifen is a prodrug metabolized to a more active form by enzymes in the liver.

14. **a.** atorvastatin
Rhabdomyolysis, a rare skeletal muscle breakdown that may cause renal dysfunction, may occur as an adverse reaction to atorvastatin. Check the creatine kinase level if the patient reports significant muscle pain or weakness or dark-colored urine while taking atorvastatin.

15. **b.** Drug-drug interactions may increase or decrease the bioavailability of a drug.
Drug–drug interactions may induce or inhibit enzyme activity, thereby either increasing or decreasing hepatic metabolism and thus the bioavailability of a drug. These interactions may increase the risk of drug toxicity or reduce the effect of a drug.

16. **b.** increased risk for endometrial cancer
The partial estrogen agonist effect of tamoxifen results in an increased risk for endometrial cancer.

17. **a.** extensive hepatic first-pass metabolism
The low serum bioavailability of atorvastatin is attributed to its extensive hepatic first-pass metabolism. This extensive first-pass metabolism is beneficial because the liver is the target organ for the drug to decrease LDL levels.

18. **d.** variability in upregulation of receptors
The effects of oxytocin vary among individuals because, as an agonist, this drug relies upon upregulated and available oxytocin receptors on the uterine myometrium. Thus, the effect varies from individual to individual and with the timing of labor.

19. **d.** uterotonic effects
The uterotonic effects of oxytocin cause contractility in the myometrium, which limits bleeding from vessels in the endometrium. Thus this agent is a first-line treatment in the management of immediate postpartum hemorrhage.

20. **c.** chronic obstructive pulmonary disease
A pulmonary condition, such as chronic obstructive pulmonary disease, is a contraindication for nitrous oxide because this drug alters the hypoxic drive. As nitrous oxide is delivered with high concentrations of oxygen, this combination weakens the ventilatory response to hypoxia, which is dangerous in someone who is already compromised.

21. **a.** Ability to self-administer
Anyone using nitrous oxide must be able to self-administer the drug, controlling when to place and remove the mask from the face. This allows for greater control and mitigates the risk of adverse effects.

22. **d.** regular uterine contractions and dilating cervix at 33 4/7 weeks' gestation
A single rescue course of betamethasone should be given to only those individuals who are at less than 34 0/7 weeks' gestation and have not had a previous course within the past 7–14 days. Additionally, those patients without a threat of preterm birth within 7 days, are previable, and are at greater than 34 0/7 weeks' gestation do not require a single rescue course.

23. **c.** Increased insulin dosage
A maternal side effect of corticosteroids is increased insulin requirements in those individuals with diabetes. This

point should be included in anticipatory guidance given to patients.

24. **b.** difficulty breathing
Magnesium sulfate can have depressive effects on the maternal CNS. Toxicity can occur if serum magnesium levels are too high (>7 mEq/L). If the patient experiences shortness of breathing, toxicity should be considered and a serum magnesium level drawn, as calcium gluconate may be given as an antidote.

25. **a.** Fetal bone demineralization
Although any risk of using the prescribed dosing of magnesium sulfate in pregnancy and labor is outweighed by the benefits when indicated, utilization beyond 5–7 days may increase the risk of fetal and neonatal bone demineralization and fractures.

26. **c.** Perform a rubella titer in 3 months
Because RhoGAM was given with the MMR vaccine postpartum, the efficacy of the MMR vaccine, which is a live vaccine, may have been inhibited. Therefore, drawing a rubella titer in 3 months is recommended to determine if immunity has been established and if there is a need for a booster.

27. **b.** Perform a Kleihauer–Betke test.
When RhoGAM is given within 3 weeks of birth, postpartum administration may be withheld if the result of a Kleihauer–Betke test rules out fetal–maternal hemorrhage of greater than 15 mL of RBCs.

28. **d.** Long-acting NSAIDs may be more likely to cause adverse GI reactions in elderly patients.
The decrease in protective mucus in the intestinal tract that occurs with aging may put elderly individuals at increased risk for indigestion, stomach ulcers, and GI bleeding with use of long-acting NSAIDs.

29. **a.** a greater risk of toxicity with the same dose of the drug
Individuals with a genetic polymorphism that affects the function of CYP450 enzymes, causing them to be poor (slow) metabolizers of a drug, may have significantly elevated plasma concentrations of the drug and greater risk of toxicity with the same dose of the drug compared to those without the polymorphism. Poor (slow) metabolizers may not be able to convert a prodrug to an active metabolite.

30. **d.** Hydralazine
Hydralazine is the best answer since the patient has IV access. Labetalol is contraindicated since the patient has moderate persistent asthma. Lisinopril is an ACE inhibitor and contraindicated in pregnancy. Nifedipine is not indicated since there is IV access.

31. **d.** Nitrous oxide
Nitrous oxide is an option for this patient since onset is within 1 minute and elimination of residual effects is 5 minutes. Hypnobirthing and the Bradley method are alternative options; however, they are not considered medicinal. Morphine is an IV narcotic with long-lasting effects.

32. **a.** Tranexamic acid
Tranexamic Acid, a hemostatic agent, should be administered 1g IV over 10 minutes for a postpartum hemorrhage. Nitroglycerin and magnesium sulfate are not indicated. Fresh frozen plasma will most likely need to be ordered in addition to other blood products, and the massive transfusion protocol will need to be activated. However, in the present moment, tranexamic acid is indicated.

33. **a.** 22-year-old patient G1P0 at 32 2/7 weeks gestation with regular contractions and a cervical exam revealing 4 cm/75%/-2 with an uncomplicated prenatal course
The patient A is less than 34 weeks and likely to deliver within the next 7 days and, therefore, meets the criteria for initiation of betamethasone treatment. Patient B is late preterm; however, there is no indication that she is in active labor or imminent delivery based on her symptoms and does not meet the criteria presently. Both patients C and D are term and, therefore, do not meet the criteria.

34. **b.** Oral Nifedipine
The patient requires urgent treatment for high blood pressure and does not have IV access. The fastest option would be oral nifedipine since onset is 5–10 minutes, and oral labetalol onset is 20 minutes to 2 hours

35. **c.** GnRH antagonist competitively binding to pituitary GnRH receptors
Relugolix is a GnRH receptor antagonist that competitively binds to pituitary GnRH receptors, thereby reducing the release of luteinizing hormone and follicle-stimulating hormone leading to decreased serum concentrations of estradiol and progesterone and reduced bleeding with uterine fibroids and pain associated with endometriosis.

36. **a.** continued bone loss that may be irreversible
Relugolix, a GnRH antagonist, may increase bone resorption with resultant bone loss that can occur due to a decrease in circulating estrogen concentrations and may not be reversible after discontinuation of the medication.

37. **b.** Improvement in insulin sensitivity
The mechanisms of action for metformin include a decrease in hepatic glucose production and intestinal absorption of glucose and an improvement in insulin sensitivity by increasing peripheral uptake and utilization. Insulin secretion remains unchanged.

38. **d.** A characteristic that makes clinical utility of pharmacogenomic testing high is when consequences of treatment failure are severe
The clinical utility of pharmacogenomic testing is highest when prescribing drugs with a narrow therapeutic window, the risk for adverse drug reactions is high, or the consequences of treatment failure are severe.

Bibliography

American College of Obstetricians and Gynecologists. (2010, reaffirmed 2018). Committee opinion #455: Magnesium sulfate before anticipated preterm birth for neuroprotection. *Obstetrics and Gynecology, 115*(3), 669–671.

American College of Obstetricians and Gynecologists. (2016, reaffirmed 2018). Committee opinion #652: Magnesium sulfate use in obstetrics. *Obstetrics and Gynecology, 127*(1), e52–e53.

American College of Obstetricians and Gynecologists. (2017, reaffirmed 2020). Committee opinion #713: Antenatal corticosteroid therapy for maternal maturation. *Obstetrics and Gynecology, 130*(2), e102–e109.

American College of Obstetricians and Gynecologists. Committee on Practice Bulletins-Obstetrics. (2017). Practice bulletin no. 183: postpartum hemorrhage. *Obstetrics Gynecology, 130*(4), e168–e186.

American College of Obstetricians and Gynecologists. (2019). ACOG practice bulletin no. 203: chronic hypertension in pregnancy. *Obstetrics and Gynecology, 133*(1), e26–e50.

American College of Obstetricians and Gynecologists, Committee on Obstetric Practice, & Society for Maternal-Fetal Medicine. (2021). Medically indicated late-preterm and early-term deliveries: ACOG committee opinion, no. 831. *Obstetrics and Gynecology, 138*(1), e35–e39.

American Geriatrics Society. (2019). Updated AGS Beers Criteria for potentially inappropriate medication use in older adults. *Journal of the American Geriatrics Society, 67*(4), 674–694.

Brucker, M. C. & King, T. (2017). *Pharmacology for women's health* (2nd ed.). Jones & Bartlett Learning.

Collins, S., Fiore, A., Boudreau, J. A., & Hewer, I. (2018). Nitrous oxide for the management of labor analgesia. *American Association of Nurse Anesthetists Journal, 86*(1), 72–80.

Demler, T., & Rhoads, J. (2020). *Pharmacotherapeutics for advanced nursing practice.* Jones & Bartlett Learning.

Drugs.com. (2022). *Acyclovir.* https://www.drugs.com/monograph/acyclovir-systemic.html

Drugs.com. (2022). *Alendronate.* https://www.drugs.com/monograph/alendronate.html

Drugs.com. (2021). *Atorvastatin.* https://www.drugs.com/monograph/atorvastatin.html

Drugs.com. (2022). *Fluconazole.* https://www.drugs.com/mtm/fluconazole.html

Drugs.com (2022). *Hydralazine.* https://www.drugs.com/pro/hydralazine.html

Drugs.com. (2022). *Labetalol.* https://www.drugs.com/monograph/labetalol.html

Drugs.com. (2022). *Metformin.* https://www.drugs.com/pro/metformin.html

Drugs.com. (2022). *Metronidazole.* https://www.drugs.com/monograph/metronidazole-systemic.html

Drugs.com. (2022). *Nifedipine.* https://www.drugs.com/monograph/nifedipine.html

Drugs.com. (2022). *Oxybutynin.* https://www.drugs.com/oxybutynin.html

Drugs.com. (2022). *Tamoxifen.* https://www.drugs.com/monograph/tamoxifen.html

Drugs.com. (2022). *Tranexamic Acid.* https://www.drugs.com/monograph/tranexamic-acid.html

Hyer, S., Balani, J., & Shehata, H. (2018). Metformin in pregnancy: Mechanisms and clinical applications. *International Journal of Molecular Sciences, 19*, 1954:1–13.

Kedrion Biopharma Inc. (2024). *Rho(D) immune globulin (human) prescribing information.* https://www.rhogam.com/pdfs/RhoGAM%20Prescribing%20Information.pdf

Okusanya, B. O., Oladapo, O. T., Long, Q., Lumbiganon, P., Carroli, G., Qureshi, Z. . . . Gülmezoglu, A. M. (2016). Clinical pharmacokinetic properties of magnesium sulphate in women with pre-eclampsia and eclampsia. *British Journal of Obstetrics and Gynecology, 123*(3), 356–366.

Page, K., McCool, W. M., & Guidera, M. (2017). Examination of the pharmacology of oxytocin and guidelines for use in labor. *Journal of Midwifery and Women's Health, 62*(4), 425–433.

U.S. Food and Drug Administration. (2014a). *Pitocin.* https://www.accessdata.fda.gov/drugsatfda_docs/label/2014/018261s031lbl.pdf

U.S. Food and Drug Administration. (2014b). *Pregnancy and lactation labeling (drugs) final rule.* https://www.fda.gov/drugs/labeling-information-drug-products/pregnancy-and-lactation-labeling-drugs-final-rule

U.S. Food and Drug Administration. (2021a). *Relugolix, estradiol, and norethindrone acetate.* https://www.accessdata.fda.gov/drugsatfda_docs/label/2022/214846s002lbl.pdf

U.S. Food and Drug Administration. (2021b). *FDA requests removal of strongest warning against using cholesterol-lowering statins during pregnancy; still advises most pregnant patients should stop taking statins.* https://www.fda.gov/drugs/drug-safety-and-availability/fda-requests-removal-strongest-warning-against-using-cholesterol-lowering-statins-during-pregnancy

Workowski, K., Bachmann, L., Chan, P., et al. (2021). Sexually transmitted infections treatment guidelines, 2021. *MMWR, 70*(RR4), 1–187.

Wysocki, K., & Siebert, D. (2019). Pharmacogenomics in clinical care. *Journal of the American Association of Nurse Practitioners, 31*(8), 443–446.

CHAPTER 12

Professional Practice Issues

Beth M. Kelsey
Kathryn Trotter

Ethical Principles

- Ethics are well-founded standards of right and wrong that prescribe what humans ought to do, usually in terms of rights, obligations, benefits to society, fairness, specific virtues
- Ethical values are affected by moral, philosophical, and individual interpretation
- Ethical principles in health care
  1. Autonomy—individuals have the right to self-determine the course of treatment they find most acceptable and with whom information may be shared
  2. Beneficence—the actions one takes as a healthcare professional should promote good
  3. Nonmaleficence—the actions one takes as a healthcare professional should do no harm
  4. Veracity—the healthcare professional should be truthful when giving individuals information about their healthcare needs
  5. Fidelity—the healthcare professional should keep any promises or commitments made in the therapeutic relationship
  6. Justice—the healthcare professional should advocate for fair and equal treatment for all individuals
- Ethical dilemmas in the provision of health care may occur when principles and values intertwine with some degree of conflict
- MORAL model: decision-making model for ethical dilemmas
  1. *Manage* the dilemma—define issues, consider options, identify players
  2. *Outline* the options—examine all options fully
  3. *Resolve* the dilemma—apply basic ethical principles to each option
  4. *Act* by applying the chosen option
  5. *Look* back and evaluate the entire process

Professional Issues

- Advanced Practice Registered Nurse (APRN)—a registered nurse (RN) who meets the following criteria
  1. Completes an accredited graduate-level program preparing the nurse for one of four recognized APRN roles (certified registered nurse anesthetist [CRNA], certified nurse-midwife [CNM], clinical nurse specialist [CNS], and certified nurse practitioner [CNP] and a population focus
  2. Passes a national certification examination that measures APRN role and population competencies and maintains certification
  3. Possesses advanced clinical knowledge and skills preparing the nurse to provide direct care to patients as well as a component of indirect care
  4. Builds on competencies of the RN by demonstrating greater breadth and depth of knowledge and greater synthesis of data to perform more complex interventions with greater role autonomy
  5. Is educationally prepared to assume responsibility and accountability for health promotion/maintenance, assessment, diagnosis, and management of patient problems, including the use and prescription of pharmacologic and nonpharmacologic interventions
  6. Has clinical experience of sufficient depth and breadth to reflect the intended license
  7. Obtains a license to practice as an APRN in one of the four APRN roles (APRN Consensus Workgroup & National Council of State Boards of Nursing APRN Advisory Committee, 2008)
- The four APRN roles
  1. Certified Nurse Practitioner (CNP)
     a. Definition—a licensed, independent practitioner who provides primary and/or specialty health care

in ambulatory, acute, and long-term care settings for individuals, families, and groups; CNPs practice autonomously and in collaboration with other healthcare professionals to assess, treat, and manage acute episodic and chronic illnesses; CNPs are experts in health promotion and disease prevention (American Association of Nurse Practitioners [AANP], 2022c)

b. Practice
   (1) As a primary care provider (PCP), provides care that is integrated and accessible
   (2) Emphasizes health promotion, disease prevention
   (3) Professionally, practice is autonomous, collaborative, and evidence based
   (4) Functionally, practice is defined by state law, regulations, and clinical privileges
   (5) Diagnoses, treats, and manages health problems
   (6) Teaches and counsels individuals, families, and groups
   (7) Clinical roles include researcher, consultant, and patient advocate
   (8) Professional roles include mentor, educator, researcher, and administrator
   (9) Maintains accountability for the care of patients and decisions reached

c. Core competencies of nurse practitioner practice (National Organization of Nurse Practitioner Faculties [NONPF], 2022)—based on doctorate in nursing practice education
   (1) Knowledge of practice
   (2) Person-centered care
   (3) Population health
   (4) Practice scholarship and translational science
   (5) Quality and safety
   (6) Interprofessional collaboration in practice
   (7) Health systems
   (8) Technology and Information Literacy
   (9) Professional acumen
   (10) Personal and professional leadership

d. Education
   (1) Master's degree, post-master's certificate, or doctorate in nursing practice (DNP)
   (2) Includes extensive clinical experience supervised by qualified preceptors within a population focus
   (3) Curriculum—APRN
      (a) Graduate-level core courses—include foundational curriculum content considered essential for all students pursuing a graduate degree in nursing regardless of functional focus (e.g., nursing theory, organizational and systems leadership, quality improvement and safety, health policy and advocacy, interprofessional collaboration, clinical prevention and population health, ethics, research, legal issues, economics)
      (b) APRN direct care core content—includes advanced health assessment, pathophysiology, pharmacology, clinical diagnosis and management, health promotion, and disease prevention
      (c) Additional courses with content specific to the nurse practitioner population focus—family/individual across the lifespan, adult–gerontology, women's health, neonatal, pediatrics, psychiatric–mental health; includes extensive supervised clinical hours
      (d) Nurse practitioner programs are accredited within schools of nursing by one of the formally recognized accreditation bodies for schools of nursing
   (4) Curriculum—women's health nurse practitioner (WHNP) specific
      (a) National Association of Nurse Practitioners in Women's Health (NPWH, 2020) provides guidelines for WHNP practice and education
      (b) Content—client-centered care; primary care; gynecologic, sexual, reproductive, menopause transition, and post-menopausal health; sexual and reproductive health for men; normal and high-risk antepartum and postpartum health; professional role

e. Certification—WHNP
   (1) To be eligible to take the certification examination offered for the WHNP, a student must have graduated from an accredited master's degree, post-master's certificate, or DNP program in the women's health population focus
   (2) WHNP certification provided by National Certification Corporation (NCC)

f. Certification maintenance—must be renewed every 3 years through one of the following mechanisms
   (1) Professional development certification maintenance program—take the NCC specialty assessment evaluation, which covers topics that reflect major content areas tested on the certification examination; results determine topics and amount of continuing education required (15–50 hours, including 5 hours for taking the assessment)
   (2) Complete 50 continuing education hours covering all core certification knowledge competency areas
   (3) Retake the certification examination

2. Certified Nurse–Midwife (CNM)/Certified Midwife (CM)
   a. All items in this section apply to certified midwives as well as certified nurse–midwives
   b. Definition—licensed, independent healthcare provider who provides a full range of primary healthcare services for women, from adolescence to beyond menopause, including gynecologic health and family planning services; preconception care; care during pregnancy, childbirth, and the

postpartum period; care of the normal newborn during the first 28 days of life; and who provides care for all individuals who seek midwifery care, inclusive of all gender identities and sexual orientations, as well as provide treatment of male partners for sexually transmitted infections (American College of Nurse-Midwives [ACNM], 2021).

c. Practice (ACNM, 2022a)
   (1) As a primary healthcare provider, provides care that is integrated and accessible to individuals and families
   (2) Practice is autonomous or collaborative and evidence based
   (3) Provides health promotion, disease prevention, counseling, and education across the lifespan
   (4) Diagnoses, treats, and manages common health problems
   (5) Focuses on childbearing, newborn care, postpartum care, family planning, gynecologic care and primary care
   (6) Accepts accountability for care provided
   (7) Of the various models of practice, private practice in a midwifery group provides the most autonomy
   (8) Site of practice is in all places where women's health care is needed, including the home

d. Hallmarks of Midwifery (ACNM, 2020)
   (1) Recognition of menarche, pregnancy, birth, and menopause as normal physiologic and developmental processes
   (2) Advocacy of nonintervention in normal processes in the absence of complications
   (3) Incorporation of scientific evidence into clinical practice
   (4) Promotion of person-centered care for all, which respects and is inclusive of diverse histories, backgrounds, and identities
   (5) Removal of barriers for persons seeking midwifery care as partners in health care
   (6) Facilitation of healthy family and interpersonal relationships
   (7) Promotion of continuity of care
   (8) Health promotion, disease prevention, and health education
   (9) Promotion of a public healthcare perspective
   (10) Utilizing an understanding of social determinants of health to provide high-quality care to all persons including those from underserved communities
   (11) Advocacy for informed choice, shared decision-making, and the right to self-determination
   (12) Integration of cultural safety into all care encounters
   (13) Incorporation of evidence-based integrative therapies
   (14) Skillful communication, guidance, and counseling

(15) Acknowledgment of the therapeutic value of human presence
(16) Ability to collaborate with and refer to other members of the interprofessional healthcare team
(17) Ability to provide safe and effective care across settings, including home, birth center, hospital, or any other maternity care service

e. Education (ACNM, 2022b)
   (1) Master's degree, post-master's certificate, or DNP
   (2) Includes extensive clinical experience supervised by qualified preceptors
   (3) Some programs do not require nursing and prepare the graduate as a midwife rather than a nurse–midwife

f. Curriculum—based on ACNM Core Competencies (ACNM, 2020)
   (1) Hallmarks of midwifery—art and science of midwifery
   (2) Midwifery care—professional responsibilities
   (3) Midwifery care—midwifery management process
   (4) Midwifery care—fundamentals
   (5) Midwifery care of cis women and transgender and gender non-binary (TGNB) individuals
   (6) Midwifery care of the newborn

g. Certification
   (1) American Midwifery Certification Board (AMCB) certifies both nurse–midwives (CNMs) and midwives (CMs)
   (2) To be eligible to take the AMCB certification exam, student must graduate from a program accredited by Accreditation Commission on Midwifery Education (ACME)
   (3) ACME accredits both nurse–midwife and midwife programs

h. Certification maintenance—must be renewed every 5 years through one of the following two mechanisms
   (1) Complete three AMCB Certificate Maintenance Modules during the 5-year certification cycle—one in each of the three areas of practice (Antepartum and Primary Care of the Pregnant Woman; Intrapartum, Postpartum, and Newborn; and Gynecology and Primary Care for the Well-Woman); and obtain 20 contact hours (2.0 CEUs) of ACNM or Accreditation Council for Continuing Medical Education (ACCME) Category 1 approved continuing education units; Certificate Maintenance Modules completed cannot count toward the required 20 contact hours (2.0 CEUs); up to 10 contact hours can be earned for precepting nurse–midwifery/midwifery students from an ACME-accredited program
   (2) Take the current AMCB Certification Examination no sooner than the fourth year of the

current 5-year certification cycle and obtain 20 contact hours (2.0 CEUs) of ACNM or AC-CME Category 1 approved continuing education units

    i. CNMs and CMs may expand practice and skills beyond the basic core competencies to include colposcopy, newborn male circumcision, endometrial biopsy, ultrasound, and surgical first assistant (ACNM, 2022c; 2022d; 2022e).

3. Certified Registered Nurse Anesthetist (CRNA) (American Association of Nurse Anesthetists, 2020)

    a. Definition—an advanced practice nurse who provides anesthesia and care for patients before, during, and after surgical procedures in which anesthesia is administered; CRNA provides anesthetics to patients in every care setting and for every type of surgery or procedure

    b. Practice

      (1) Provides preanesthetic preparation and evaluation

      (2) Manages anesthesia induction, maintenance, and emergence

      (3) Provides postanesthesia care

      (4) Provides perianesthetic and clinical support functions

    c. Education

      (1) Master's degree or DNP; as of 2025, DNP will be required

      (2) Curriculum is governed by the Council on Accreditation of Nurse Anesthesia Educational (COA) Programs Standards

      (3) Programs are accredited by COA

      (4) National certification is required through the Council on Certification of Nurse Anesthetists

      (5) Must earn continuing education credits to maintain certification

4. Clinical Nurse Specialist (CNS) (National Association of Clinical Nurse Specialists, 2019)

    a. Definition—APRN with role of integrating care across the health–illness continuum and through three spheres of impact: patient, nurse, system

    b. Practice

      (1) Direct care functions—expert practitioner, role model, patient advocate, and educator

      (2) Indirect care functions—change agent, consultant or resource person, liaison person, and innovator

    c. Education

      (1) Master's degree, post-master's certificate, or DNP; as of 2030, DNP will be required

      (2) Curriculum includes core courses in nursing theory, organizational theory, ethics, legal issues, healthcare delivery and CNS role, and population-focused courses/supervised clinical experience

      (3) CNS programs are accredited within schools of nursing by one of the formally recognized accreditation bodies for schools of nursing

      (4) Certification is available for population foci through the American Nurses' Credentialing Center (ANCC)

- Doctorate in nursing practice

  1. Practice-focused rather than research-focused nursing doctoral degree

  2. Entry into a DNP program may be after completion of a baccalaureate nursing degree (BS to DNP) or master's nursing degree (MS to DNP)

  3. Program length varies depending on BS-to-DNP/MS-to-DNP program type as well as APRN role and population focus

  4. NP population-focused tracks require a minimum of 750 direct patient clinical hours (National Task Force on Quality Nurse Practitioner Education, 2022)

  5. American Association of Colleges of Nursing (2004) position statement called for DNP degree to be required for entry into advanced nursing practice by 2015

  6. Currently, school accrediting bodies, APRN certification agencies, and state nursing boards do not require a DNP degree for advanced practice registered nursing practice

- APRN regulation

  2. Consensus model

    a. Completed by APRN Consensus Work Group and National Council of State Boards of Nursing APRN Advisory Committee in 2008

    b. Purpose—development of a national regulatory model for APRNs with relevant definitions, roles, and titles to be used and population foci

    c. Defines four essential components for regulation (LACE)

      (1) *Licensure*—the granting of authority to practice

      (2) *Accreditation*—formal review and approval by a recognized agency of educational degree programs in nursing

      (3) *Certification*—formal recognition of the knowledge, skills, and experience demonstrated by the achievement of standards identified by the profession

      (4) *Education*—formal preparation of APRNs in graduate-degree granting or postgraduate certificate programs

    d. Four APRN roles—nurse anesthetist, nurse–midwife, clinical nurse specialist, nurse practitioner

    e. Six population foci—family/individual across lifespan, adult–gerontology, neonatal, pediatrics, women's health/gender-focused, psychiatric–mental health

    f. Education, certification, and licensure of individuals must be congruent in terms of role and population focus

    g. APRNs may specialize (e.g., palliative care, critical care) but cannot be certified or licensed solely within a specialty area

    h. Identifies titles to be used by APRN

     i. State boards of nursing should be solely responsible for licensing APRNs

     j. Implementation of the model continues to occur incrementally in states; the target date for full implementation was 2015

3. This section includes regulation components for CMs as well as CNMs and nurse practitioners

  a. Scope of practice

    (1) Definition—legal authority granted to a professional to provide and be reimbursed for services

    (2) Defines what APRNs can do with patients, what can delegate, and when collaboration with others is required

    (3) Scope may differ depending on APRN role—clinical nurse specialist, nurse anesthetist, nurse–midwife, nurse practitioner

    (4) Based on state laws promulgated by the various nurse practice acts and rules and regulations for APRN—varies from state to state

    (5) ACNM (2021) provides a definition and scope of practice statement for CNMs and CMs

  b. Nurse practice acts

    (1) Definition—legislative enactments that define the practice of nursing, give guidance within the scope of practice issues, and set standards for practice; passage through state legislatures makes these acts the law under which nursing is practiced

    (2) Regulated on a state-by-state basis

    (3) Authorizes state boards of nursing to establish statutory authority for the licensure of RNs, including APRNs

    (4) Authorizes state boards of nursing to establish a scope of practice, determine disciplinary actions, and regulate practice via legislative statutes

    (5) Licensure statutes limit practice to individuals with specific qualifications as defined by law

    (6) Registration and certification statutes provide a definition and limit as to who may use title, without restraint of practice

    (7) May authorize prescriptive authority

    (8) Regulations reflect a trend to increase APRN authority and autonomy

  c. Licensure

    (1) Definition—process by which a government agency authorizes individuals to practice a profession or occupation by validating that the individual has attained the required degree of competency as prescribed by law to protect the public welfare

    (2) State law governs the requirement for holding a professional license in the state

    (3) All states require APRN to hold a state RN license; currently, not all states require a separate APRN license

    (4) CNMs are licensed through boards of midwifery, medicine, nursing, nurse–midwifery, or departments of health

    (5) CMs may receive a license to practice in Delaware, Maine, New Jersey, New York, and Rhode Island through Boards of Midwifery, Medicine, Complementary Health Care Providers, or Departments of Health; ACNM encourages recognition of CMs in all states, and therefore, it is expected that more states in the future will have provisions for licensure of CMs (ACNM, 2017)

  d. Full practice authority for nurse practitioners (NPs)

    (1) Definition—the collection of state practice and licensure laws that allow NPs to evaluate patients; diagnose, order, and interpret diagnostic tests; initiate and manage treatments, including prescribing medications under the exclusive license authority of the state board of nursing (AANP, 2022a)

    (2) As of October 2022, 26 states, the District of Columbia, and Guam have full practice authority for NPs; several other states have bills for full practice authority in process at this time (AANP, 2022a).

  e. Certification

    (1) Definition—the formal process by which a private agency or organization certifies (usually by examination) that an individual has met standards as specified by that profession (Tracy & O'Grady, 2019)

    (2) National certification examinations provide a consistent standard that the APRN must meet to demonstrate competency for an advanced level of practice in her or his role

    (3) Midwives take the same certification examination as nurse–midwives to receive the professional designation as CM

    (4) Almost all states require national certification for nurse practitioners and nurse–midwives

    (5) Maintenance of a particular level of competence following initial certification is required

  f. Prescriptive authority

    (1) Definition—legal authority to prescribe medications or devices

    (2) Authority is contained in state nurse or midwifery practice acts or in other statutes; varies from state to state

    (3) May require approval of the state board of medicine, midwifery, public health, or pharmacy

    (4) Requires completion of an advanced pharmacology course and continuing education hours to maintain prescribing status

    (5) May require a collaborative practice agreement and/or written protocols

(6) May obtain federal Drug Enforcement Administration (DEA) registration number, depending on the scope of state law

g. Independent and collaborative management of care

  (1) Independent—care of individuals within the provider's scope of practice, based on knowledge, skills, and competencies

  (2) Consultation—seeks advice or opinion of another member of the healthcare team while the NP/CNM/CM retains primary responsibility for the individual's care

  (3) Collaboration—NP/CNM/CM and physician or other healthcare professional jointly manage the care of an individual with complex or complicated health conditions; the goal is to share authority while providing quality care within each individual's scope of practice

  (4) Referral—process by which the provider directs the client to another healthcare professional for management of a particular problem or aspect of the client's care

h. Hospital privileges

  (1) Definition—authorization granted to a practitioner by the healthcare network or a component of the network to provide specific inpatient care services within defined limits based on the practitioner's qualifications and current competence

  (2) Hospitals may have levels of privileges determining the extent of decision-making permitted by the provider (e.g., review records, admit patients, write orders)

  (3) Often the medical staff governing body decides which other providers may have hospital privileges and at what level based on an application and review process

  (4) ACNM's (2016a) Principles for Credentialing and Privileging of CNMs and CMs

    (a) Bylaws and guidelines of hospitals/ healthcare organizations should reflect the scope of practice of CNMs/ CMs as defined by national standards and state laws. They should address the following:

      ○ A broad definition of medical or professional staff avoiding categories

      ○ Delineation of privileges for CNM/CMs that includes admission, discharge, and expanded scope of practice

      ○ CNM/CM accountability, avoiding requirements that increase vicarious liability

      ○ Consultation with, co-management with, or referral to other licensed physicians, independent practitioners

    (b) Bylaws and guidelines should avoid:

      ○ Requiring physician co-signature on CNM/CM notes or orders in medical record

      ○ Inconsistent requirements for continuous professional practice evaluation among medical or professional staff

    (c) CNM/CMs should be included in the development of such guidelines

i. Standards of practice

  (1) Definition—overarching statements that the nursing profession uses to describe the responsibilities of its members to provide safe and competent care

  (2) APRNs are held to standards of practice promulgated both by the nursing profession and standards determined by professional organizations representing their role and population focus

  (3) AANP's (2022b) *Standards of Practice for Nurse Practitioners*

    (a) Process of care—assessment, diagnosis, development of a comprehensive plan of care, implementation of plan, follow-up, and evaluation of patient status

    (b) Care priorities—patient and family education, facilitation of shared decision-making and participation of the patient and family in healthcare decisions, promotion of optimal health, provision of continually competent care, facilitation of entry into the healthcare system, promotion of a safe environment

    (c) Interprofessional and collaborative responsibilities

    (d) Accurate documentation of patient status and care

    (e) Responsibility as a patient advocate

    (f) Quality assurance and continued competence

    (g) Integral roles of nurse practitioners—for example, mentor, preceptor, educator, researcher, consultant, advocate, leader

    (h) Research as a basis for practice

j. ACNM's (2021) *Definition of Midwifery and Scope of Practice of Certified Nurse–Midwives and Certified Midwives* states that midwifery care:

  (1) Is contextualized care characterized by safety, autonomy, and self-determination fostered by CNM/CM within the clinical care setting provided by qualified practitioners

  (2) Is composed of knowledge, skills, and judgments reflected in practice guidelines that guide both scope and services provided

  (3) Is documented completely and accessibly, evaluated using established quality improvement practices

  (4) May including expanded skills beyond the ACNM core competencies

k. Standards of care
 (1) Definition—also called practice guidelines; define a standard of appropriate care; used in legal decisions about care provided
 (2) Standards of care are evidence based and continuously evolving
 (3) APRNs are responsible for remaining up to date on these standards/guidelines
 (4) Examples of sources of practice standards/guidelines—Agency for Healthcare Research and Quality (AHRQ), National Committee for Quality Assurance (NCQA), The Joint Commission, Medicare, professional medical and nursing specialty organizations

- Reimbursement—third-party payers
 4. Major categories of third-party payers—Medicare, Medicaid, indemnity insurance companies, managed care organizations (MCOs), businesses that contract for certain services
 5. Medicare—federal program that provides health insurance for those who are older than 65 years or disabled; not income dependent; four parts (A, B, C, D)
  a. Part A—hospital insurance
   (1) No fee for enrollment—covered by payroll taxes; cost sharing may include deductibles and coinsurance
   (2) Automatic enrollment at age 65 or if eligible for Social Security disability insurance
   (3) Covers inpatient hospital services, skilled nursing facilities, hospice, home health care
  b. Part B—supplementary medical insurance if eligible for Part A
   (1) Pay monthly premium
   (2) Covers provider services, outpatient coverage, diagnostics, durable medical equipment
   (3) Some preventive services are mandated to be covered with no deductible or copayment
  c. Part C—Medicare Advantage Plan—available through participation in coordinated care or private fee-for-service plans and medical savings accounts, covers the same as Part B
  d. Part D—prescription drug coverage—monthly premium, may include deductible of copayment
  e. APRN qualifications to be a Medicare provider
   (1) Current RN and APRN license to practice in the state in which services rendered
   (2) National certification in an advanced practice nurse role
   (3) Master's degree in nursing
   (4) National Provider Identifier (NPI) number—obtained from Centers for Medicare and Medicaid Services (CMS)
 6. Medicaid—a federal program administered by the states to cover mandated healthcare costs for eligible low-income individuals and families
  a. Pregnant individuals and children younger than 6 years of age with family incomes up to 133% of the federal poverty level
  b. Children younger than age 19 in families whose income is at or below the poverty level

c. Adults with short-term (1 year or less) disability and who qualify on the basis of poverty
d. Other adults without short-term disability or children may qualify on the basis of poverty
e. General elements covered
 (1) Hospital and provider services
 (2) Laboratory and radiologic services
 (3) Nursing home and home healthcare services
 (4) Prenatal and postpartum care
 (5) Preventive services
 (6) Medically necessary transportation
 (7) States may opt to cover additional services
f. Reimbursement—determined by states
 (1) Operates as a vendor payment program with broad discretion in determining methodology at the state level
 (2) Providers must accept Medicaid payment rates as payment in full
  (a) APRNs must apply to state Medicaid agency to be a fee-for-service provider; must apply to the MCO to be included on the provider panel
 (3) Payment to hospitals—based on a predetermined fee schedule for the projected cost of care, APRNs not paid directly for inpatient services
 7. Indemnity (private) insurance companies—insurance company that pays for the medical care of its insured but does not deliver health care
  a. APRN must apply to the insurance company for provider status
  b. APRN must submit billing form to the insurance company for reimbursement
 8. MCO—an insurer that provides both healthcare services and payment for services—health maintenance organization (HMO), preferred provider organization (PPO), point-of-service (POS) plan
  a. Financial arrangements determined prospectively under terms of contract; include prospective pricing, service bundling, price discounts/discounted fees for services to certain populations and for coverage of specific conditions
  b. If an APRN is an employee of a group practice, someone within the group negotiates the terms of the MCO contract for the group
  c. If an APRN is in private practice, the APRN applies to the MCO to be a provider and negotiates the terms of the contract
  d. Not all MCOs currently recognize APRNs as PCPs
- Legal liability
 1. Consent—legal permission given by a patient to undergo particular treatments and/or procedures; informed consent—agreement to do something or to allow something to happen only after all the relevant facts are disclosed
  a. Most states have legislation regarding what types of tests, treatments, or procedures require written informed consent and who is authorized to provide informed consent for a minor, or for an incompetent or incapacitated person

b. Components of a written informed consent—descriptions of procedures and/or treatments and/or tests; potential risks and benefits; alternatives; documentation that the patient is acting voluntarily, has received full disclosure, and is competent to act

c. Refusal of treatment—the inherent right of individuals who are conscious and mentally competent to refuse any form of treatment either personally or through their representative; includes do not resuscitate (DNR) orders, refusal for extraordinary care, and implementation of supportive-care-only guidelines

d. Withdrawal of treatment—the decision to terminate treatment that has been initiated after securing informed consent from a patient or the patient's representative, with the legal basis for the decision and subsequent care as noted in the refusal of treatment

2. Documentation and medical records—general principles
   a. Medical records should be complete and legible
   b. Components of documentation for each client encounter
      (1) Reason for encounter and relevant history, physical examination findings, prior diagnostic test results
      (2) Assessment, clinical impression, or diagnosis
      (3) Plan of care—rationale for ordering diagnostic tests or other services unless easily inferred; treatments justified by assessment; plan for follow-up
      (4) Date and legible name of the care provider
   c. Risk factors should be identified
   d. Past and present diagnoses should be accessible to care provider
   e. Client's progress, response to treatments, changes in treatments, and revisions of diagnosis should be documented
   f. Billing codes (Current Procedural Terminology [CPT] and International Classification of Diseases [ICD]) should be supported by what is documented in the medical record

3. Malpractice—failure of the healthcare professional to exercise the degree of skill and learning commonly applied by the average prudent, reputable member of the profession; falls under tort law
   a. Tort law—a branch of civil law (rather than criminal law) that concerns legal wrongs committed by one person against another; an act that causes harm to body or property and for which the injured party is seeking monetary damages; includes assault, battery, intentional infliction of emotional distress, negligence
   b. Intentional tort—a volitional or willful act, with expressed intent to bring harm to the affected person; forms the foundation for consent for treatment requirements
      (1) Assault—intentional threat by word or act to unlawfully touch or strike a person, coupled

with apparent ability, and causing fear in that person that such an act is imminent
      (2) Battery—actual, intentional, and unlawful touching or striking of another person against the will of the other
      (3) False imprisonment—unlawful restraint or detention against the will of the individual
      (4) Intentional infliction of emotional distress—intentional infliction of emotional or mental distress that results in mental reaction, such as anguish, grief, or fright to another person
   c. Negligence tort—involves an act of negligence; conduct lacking in due care; carelessness; doing something any reasonable, prudent person would not do
      (1) Most malpractice suits are based on negligence
      (2) Requires four elements to be present
         (a) Duty—the responsibility to act in accordance with a standard of care
         (b) Breach of duty—violation or deviation from the standard of care
         (c) Causation—determination of whether the injury is the result of negligence
         (d) Damages—must be actual harm to the person or property
   d. Breach of confidentiality—may be an intentional tort, negligence tort, basis of disciplinary action by state health professional regulation board, or violation of state or federal law

4. Coworker incompetence—a legal obligation exists for a licensed professional to assist, relieve, or report any coworker who, through substandard care or impairment, places the health and welfare of patients at risk; official processes relevant to continued practice are determined through agencies and state boards, based on practice act regulations

5. Health Insurance Portability and Accountability Act (HIPAA)
   a. Purpose of HIPAA privacy rule provisions (implemented in 2003)—ensure that individual's health information is properly protected while allowing the flow of information needed to promote high-quality health care and to protect the public's health and well-being
   b. Definitions
      (1) Covered entity—the privacy rule applies to health plans, healthcare clearinghouses, and any healthcare provider who transmits health information in electronic form in connection with transactions
         (a) Health plan—individual and group plans that provide or pay the cost of medical care
         (b) Healthcare clearinghouse—billing services, community health management systems
         (c) Healthcare provider—institutions (e.g., hospitals, health networks) and direct care providers who electronically transmit health information in connection with transactions for which the U.S.

Department of Health and Human Services (USDHHS) has established privacy standards (e.g., claims, benefit eligibility inquiries, referral authorization requests)

    (2) Protected health information (PHI)—all individually identifiable health information held or transmitted by a covered entity in any form (e.g., electronic, paper, oral); pertains even if the individual is deceased

  c. Required disclosures by covered entities

    (1) To individuals (or their personal representatives) specifically when they request access to or an accounting of disclosures of their PHI

    (2) To the USDHHS when it is undertaking a compliance investigation or enforcement of action

  d. Permitted disclosures by covered entities

    (1) The individual who is the subject of the PHI

    (2) The entity's own treatment, payment, and healthcare operation activities

    (3) Informal permission that clearly gives the individual the opportunity to agree or object and if the healthcare provider exercises professional judgment that the use or disclosure of PHI is determined to be in the best interest of the individual

    (4) Public health interests (e.g., communicable disease reporting, abuse or neglect reporting, serious threat to health or safety)

  e. Notice of privacy practices—each covered entity (with certain exceptions) must provide a notice to all patients of its privacy practices, including individual rights and how to exercise them

  f. Administrative requirements—implement policies and procedures designed to comply with privacy rules; designate privacy official to monitor compliance

  g. Complaint process—informal review may resolve the issue fully without formal investigation; if not, begin investigation; Office for Civil Rights (US Department of Health & Human Services, 2022) enforces the privacy rule with potential monetary penalties and imprisonment depending on intent of violation

6. Risk management plan—demonstrates that the APRN is cognizant of risks, is taking reasonable steps to limit risks, and seeks to provide care consistent with best practice; includes the following practice policies and procedures, among others:

  a. Role and scope of practice

  b. Licensing and certification requirements

  c. Practice guidelines and standards

  d. Health record documentation standards and forms

  e. Informed consent policy and process

  f. Protection of privacy/confidentiality policy and process

  g. Collaborative practice relationships

  h. Provisions of practice coverage

  i. Peer review and outcomes-based evaluation processes

  j. Patient complaint or concern review process

7. Professional liability insurance

  a. Recommended that each clinician carry an individual policy

  b. Types of coverage

    (1) Occurrence—covers the event of malpractice that occurred during the policy period without regard to when the claims are reported; provides protections for each policy period indefinitely; broadest protection available

    (2) Claims made—incident must happen and be reported while the policy is in force; requires the purchase of a tail policy to protect, once the policy period ends

  c. Cost of insurance varies with APRN role and population focus

Public Policy

- Definition—set of actions the government takes resulting in a law or legislation when approaching a problem that affects society as a group rather than on an individual level

  1. Public health policy includes laws or legislation that affect health or healthcare

  2. Public health policy examples—Affordable Care Act, Violence Against Women's Act, universal access to family and medical leave; APRN scope of practice

  3. Cost-quality-access triad provides a framework for health policy at all levels

  4. These components are overlapping and interdependent

Evidence-Based Practice

- Definition—the conscientious, judicious, and explicit use of current best evidence in making decisions about the care of individual patients, incorporating both clinical expertise and patient values

  1. Models for implementing evidence-based practice generally include the following steps:

    a. Identification of a clinical problem or question

    b. Search for the best evidence

    c. Critical appraisal of the strength of evidence

    d. Recommendation for action (change, no change, further study)

    e. Implementation of the change if recommended

    f. Evaluation of change in relationship to desired outcomes

  2. Categories of strength of reviewed evidence from individual research and other sources

    a. Level I (A–D)—meta-analysis or multiple controlled studies

    b. Level II (A–D)—individual experimental study

    c. Level III (A–D)—quasi-experimental study

    d. Level IV (A–D)—nonexperimental study

    e. Level V (A–D)—case report or systematically obtained, verifiable quality, or program evaluation data

    f. Level VI—opinion of respected authorities; this level also includes regulatory or legal opinions

3. Level I is the strongest rating per type of research, but quality for any level can range from A to D and reflects basic scientific credibility of the overall study
   a. A indicates a very well-designed study
   b. D indicates the study has a major flaw that raises serious questions about the believability of the findings
4. Methodologies for research
   a. Quantitative research—formative, objective, systematic study process to describe and test relationships and/or to examine cause-and-effect interactions among variables
   b. Qualitative research—systematic, interactive, subjective approach used to describe life experiences and give them meaning

- Major quantitative research study designs
  1. Descriptive—used to explore and describe phenomena in real-life situations, identify and describe variables within the phenomenon, develop conceptual and operational definitions for variables
  2. Correlational—used for systematic investigation of relationships between two or more variables to explain type (positive or negative) relationships but not to examine cause and effect
  3. Quasi-experimental—conducted to explain relationships, clarify why certain events happen, and examine causality between selected independent and dependent variables; limited control developed to provide an alternative for examining causality in situations not conducive to experimental-level controls
  4. Experimental—provides the greatest amount of control possible to examine probability and causality among selected independent and dependent variables for the purpose of predicting and controlling phenomena
- Research terminology
  1. Reliability—the consistency of the measure obtained in a study, exists in degrees expressed as reliability coefficient, 1.00 = perfect reliability, 0.00 = no reliability
  2. Validity—the extent to which a research tool measures what it is supposed to measure
  3. Statistical significance—an indication that the results from an analysis of sample data are unlikely to have been caused by chance, at a specified level of probability (e.g., significance at the 0.05 level indicates the probability that the result would occur by chance is only 5 times out of 100)
  4. Clinical significance—practical importance of research results in terms of whether they have genuine effects on the daily lives of clients or on healthcare decisions
  5. Generalization—extension of the implications of the findings from the sample studied to a larger population or from the situation studied to a larger situation
  6. Replication—reproducing or repeating a study to determine whether similar findings will be obtained
  7. Ethics in research
     a. Protection of human rights in research
        (1) Self-determination
        (2) Privacy
        (3) Autonomy
        (4) Confidentiality
        (5) Fair treatment
        (6) Protection from discomfort and harm
     b. Components of informed consent for study participants
        (1) Purpose of study
        (2) Role of the participant
        (3) Risks and discomforts
        (4) Benefits
        (5) Alternatives
        (6) Assurance of anonymity and/or confidentiality
        (7) Any compensation for participation
        (8) Explanation that participation is voluntary and the individual can refuse to participate without any penalty
        (9) Option to withdraw
        (10) Offer to answer questions
        (11) Institutional review—committee of researcher's peers examines the study for ethical concerns
  8. Quality improvement (QI)
     a. Definition—systematic, evidence-based, data-driven process used to investigate a procedure, protocol, or policy to determine if it addresses an identified need
     b. Major purposes of QI
        (1) Eliminate errors
        (2) Decrease patient safety–related events—events, incidences, or conditions that could have resulted or did result in harm to a patient
        (3) Improve patient care, satisfaction, safety, and outcomes
        (4) Promote individual, group, and community health
        (5) Increase access to quality care
        (6) Increase productivity and contain costs

Patient Safety

- Patient safety terminology (Agency for Health Research and Quality [AHRQ], 2019)
  1. Adverse event—patient harm that arises as a result of medical care (rather than from the underlying disease)
  2. Preventable adverse events—those due to error or failure to apply an accepted strategy for prevention
  3. Ameliorable adverse events—events that, while not preventable, could have been less harmful if care had been different
  4. Adverse events due to negligence—those due to care that falls below the standards expected of clinicians in the community
  5. Near miss—an unsafe situation that is indistinguishable from a preventable adverse event except for the outcome. Patient does not experience harm (either through luck or early detection)
  6. Error—any act of commission (doing something wrong) or omission (failing to do the right thing) that exposes patients to a potentially hazardous situation

- Causes of adverse events in primary care (AHRQ, 2020)
  1. Inappropriate prescribing and overprescribing
  2. Poor communication and care coordination
  3. Diagnostic errors and delays
- Patient safety principles
  1. Commitment to a culture of safety
  2. Optimal communication among team members including the patient
  3. Minimizing competing demands, interruptions, and distractions when providing care
  4. Reduction in unnecessary variation in treatment plans
  5. Implementation of safe medication practices
- Culture of safety
  1. Supports safety as a first priority for all
  2. Starts at the top of the administration with strong leadership and necessary human and financial resources to achieve patient safety
  3. Recognizes the importance of team function in optimizing individual performance
  4. Fosters open communication; welcomes input from every team member at every level
  5. Ensures that team members know they can report errors and leaders will focus not on blaming providers involved in the error but on systems issues that contributed to the patient safety event
  6. Fosters a learning organization by using root-cause analysis when an adverse event occurs; process used to answer four basic questions
     a. What happened in this case?
     b. What usually happens?
     c. Why did this event occur?
     d. What if anything, can be done to prevent it from happening again?
- Communication
  1. The most common cause of preventable adverse outcomes is communication error (The Joint Commission, 2019)
  2. Dimensions of optimal communication for patient safety
     a. Communication with the patient and family
     b. Communication with all individuals caring for the patient
     c. Availability of information necessary for coordination of care
  3. Communicate health information to patients in a manner that encompasses language needs, individual understanding, and cultural and other communication issues
- Reducing unnecessary variation in treatment plans
  1. Develop/implement evidence-based clinical guidelines and bundles while recognizing the importance of individualized care

  2. Best practices guidelines—improve clinical care processes by identifying steps in diagnosis as well as treatment
  3. Bundle—small, straightforward set of evidence-based practices that when performed collectively and reliably, have proven to improve patient outcomes
  4. Council on Patient Safety in Women's Health Care— a multidisciplinary partnership that, along with the Alliance for Innovation in Maternal Health (AIM), has designed safety bundles to reduce severe maternal morbidity and mortality
  5. When appropriate, the clinician may deviate from a guideline; should document the reason for the alternative plan
- Safe medication practices
  1. Be sure all written medication orders are legible
  2. Use only approved abbreviations
  3. Always use a leading zero for doses less than 1 unit (e.g., 0.1, not .1); never use a trailing zero after a decimal point (e.g., 1 mg, not 1.0 mg)
  4. Utilize electronic medical record (EMR) formats that clarify appropriate dosage/intervals and alert regarding medication conflicts, allergies, and potentially inappropriate use of medications in pregnancy or lactation
  5. Incorporate medication reconciliation in clinical practice—the process of comparing medications a patient is taking (and should be taking) with newly ordered medications to address duplications, omissions, and interactions, and the need to continue current medications
- Interprofessional practice
  1. Definition—intentional collaboration across professions and with care team members, patients, families, communities, and other stakeholders to optimize care, enhance the healthcare experience and strengthen outcomes (AACN, 2021)
  2. Goal—patient care that is safe, timely, effective, efficient, equitable and patient-centered (Institute of Medicine, 2001)
  3. Effective interprofessional collaboration
     a. Includes the patient as a member of the healthcare team
     b. Promotes a climate of respect, dignity, inclusion, civility, and trust among healthcare team members
     c. Utilizes effective communication skills including negotiation, consensus building, and conflict resolution
     d. Includes assuming different roles (e.g., member, leader) within the team to develop and improve person-centered care

Questions

Select the best answer.

1. Which of the following is *not* one of the six population foci for the APRN established by the consensus model for APRN regulation?
   a. Critical care
   b. Neonatal
   c. Pediatrics
   d. Women's health

2. Which of the following statements concerning the doctorate in nursing practice (DNP) is correct?
   a. All state boards of nursing require a DNP degree for APRN practice.
   b. It requires a minimum of 500 hours of supervised clinical experience.
   c. Individuals must already be certified as an APRN before entry into the DNP program.
   d. The DNP curriculum focuses on practice more so than on research.

3. One of the Hallmarks of Midwifery is:
   a. advocacy of regular use of technological interventions
   b. informed choice with provider-driven decision-making
   c. integration of cultural safety into care encounters related to gender only
   d. recognition of women's life phases as normal, developmental processes

4. Prescriptive authority in all states requires that the APRN:
   a. apply to the state medical licensing board
   b. complete specific pharmacologic educational requirements
   c. obtain a DEA registration number
   d. practice under a collaborative agreement with a physician

5. The nongovernmental validation of a nurse practitioner's or nurse–midwife's knowledge and acquired skills in a particular population focus is:
   a. licensure
   b. credentialing
   c. certification
   d. registration

6. The best source of information on APRN-specific requirements for prescriptive authority is:
   a. the federal DEA
   b. professional APRN organizations
   c. state boards of nursing
   d. state boards of pharmacy

7. Safe medication practices include:
   a. Always use a trailing zero after a decimal point (e.g., use 1.0 mg, not 1 mg).
   b. Always use a leading zero for doses less than 1 unit (e.g., use 0.1 mg, not .1 mg).
   c. Create your own abbreviations that you use consistently.
   d. Turn off EMR alerts to avoid overload of information received.

8. Which of the following best describes capitation as a financial strategy?
   a. Predetermined payment for services based on an accepted schedule of fees
   b. Predetermined fees set for usual and customary care
   c. Predetermined payment based on a contractual per-member, per-month rate
   d. Predetermined rates negotiated according to what procedures are utilized to treat a patient

9. The goal of HIPAA is to:
   a. decrease the expenses and, therefore, the costs of healthcare delivery
   b. improve the health system by standardizing the exchange of electronic data
   c. reimburse providers and laboratories in a timely fashion
   d. ensure that every person has ready access to appropriate health care

10. A covered entity under HIPAA includes:
    a. any health provider who transmits any health information electronically
    b. all health care employers
    c. governmental agencies that license healthcare providers
    d. life insurance companies

11. A goal of the privacy rule of HIPAA is to:
    a. provide federal protections for privacy and preserve quality care
    b. ensure that research subjects' privacy is maintained during the study
    c. guarantee that the privacy of patients is protected at any cost
    d. increase the level of confidentiality in Medicaid programs

12. One of the principal differences between Medicare Parts A and B is:
    a. the eligibility criteria
    b. the rate of reimbursement
    c. the monthly premium requirement for Part A
    d. the monthly premium requirement for Part B

13. According to the Joint Commission that is responsible for accrediting U.S. healthcare organizations, the most common cause of preventable adverse outcomes is:
    a. communication error
    b. deviation from an established practice guideline
    c. overprescribing
    d. not having a standard for reprimanding those who make an error

14. The nurse practitioner prescribes a medication that could have caused an adverse outcome for the patient because of a potentially serious interaction with another medication the patient was taking. The patient took one dose of the medication before the nurse practitioner recognized

the error. The patient did not experience any harm. The best term for this event is:
a. adverse event
b. ameliorable adverse event
c. near miss
d. preventable adverse event

15. A national provider identification (NPI) number can be obtained from:
a. the Center for Medicare and Medicaid Services (CMS)
b. the Drug Enforcement Agency (DEA)
c. a managed care organization (MCO)
d. the state board of nursing

16. All states are required to provide Medicaid to:
a. children younger than 19 in families whose income is below the poverty level
b. families eligible for the federal Children's Health Insurance Program (CHIP)
c. individuals with long-term disabilities who have incomes below the poverty level
d. individuals older than 65 years with a chronic medical condition

17. Principles of interprofessional practice involve:
a. avoiding conflict among the healthcare team
b. including the patient as a member of the healthcare team
c. maintaining the physician as the leader of the healthcare team
d. rotating leadership among all members of the healthcare team

18. Keeping one's promises or commitments is called:
a. beneficence
b. fidelity
c. veracity
d. justice

19. To maintain AMCB certification, the midwife must:
a. apply for renewal every 3 years
b. complete three maintenance modules plus 20 contact hours of continuing education every 5 years
c. document at least 1,000 clinical hours as a midwife in the previous 3 years
d. take the certification examination every 5 years

20. During a malpractice hearing, an attorney describes the responsibility "to do no harm." The attorney is defining the ethical principle of:
a. justice
b. veracity
c. fidelity
d. nonmaleficence

21. A nurse practitioner or midwife fails to order a test that is clinically indicated. This omission is best described as:
a. maleficence
b. assault
c. an intentional tort
d. negligence

22. A patient presents with an abnormal test result. The appropriate plan of care is to refer for additional testing, but the facility that performs the test has closed for the day. Rather than sending the patient to have the test performed at the hospital, the nurse practitioner/midwife in the practice orders the patient to report to the testing facility the next morning. During the evening, problems arise and the patient is admitted to the hospital with a negative outcome. This is an example of:
a. an intentional tort
b. a negligence tort
c. an inappropriate cause for a malpractice suit
d. withdrawal of treatment without consent

23. Placing an intrauterine contraceptive device in the uterus of a patient who has an intellectual disability and who is not able to give informed consent may constitute:
a. assault
b. battery
c. intentional tort
d. paternalism

24. An elderly woman enters a nursing home after breaking her hip; she signs DNR orders and a statement that she does not want extraordinary care. This individual is:
a. exercising her right to refuse treatment
b. exercising her right to withdraw treatment
c. acting in a manner that should cause concern about her mental competence
d. lacking information needed to make an informed decision

25. A WHNP receives a call from an attorney, who tells her she is named in a suit related to an obstetric incident that occurred 4 years ago. When she calls the insurance company, the nurse practitioner is told that the policy she had at that time will not cover her because the policy was:
a. a claims-made policy
b. tail insurance only
c. an occurrence policy
d. an HMO policy

26. A small, straightforward set of evidence-based practices that when performed collectively and reliably, have proven to improve patient outcomes is called a(n):
a. algorithm
b. indemnity
c. safety bundle
d. standard of practice

27. Which of the following types of research would receive the strongest rating for the strength of evidence?
a. Case report
b. Experimental study
c. Meta-analysis
d. Quasi-experimental study

28. To maintain NCC certification, the WHNP must:
a. apply for renewal every 5 years
b. complete a specialty assessment evaluation that determines the topics and number of hours of continuing education needed before the next renewal cycle
c. document at least 2,000 clinical hours as a WHNP in the previous 5 years
d. take the certification examination every 5 years

29. Under the consensus model for APRNs, what entity is responsible for licensing APRNs?
    a. Advanced practice professional organizations
    b. Individual state boards of nursing
    c. National certification agencies
    d. National Council of State Boards of Nursing

30. A purpose of qualitative research is to:
    a. describe life experiences and give them meaning
    b. examine cause-and-effect interactions among variables
    c. identify and describe variables within a phenomenon
    d. investigate relationships between two or more variables

31. Which of the following is *not* one of the essential components for the regulation of APRNs described in the consensus model?
    a. Certification
    b. Collaboration
    c. Education
    d. Licensure

32. The research design in which the relationships between two or more variables are explained but cause and effect are not examined is:
    a. correlational
    b. descriptive
    c. experimental
    d. quasi-experimental

33. The A–D category applied to the strength of evidence in research is based on:
    a. the ability to replicate the study with the same findings
    b. the quality of the study's design
    c. a review by a panel of experts
    d. the type of research study design

34. Weighing yourself on the same scale 10 times in a row to see if you weigh the same each time is a measure of:
    a. external validity
    b. generalization
    c. internal validity
    d. reliability

35. The research term used to indicate that results from an analysis of sample data are unlikely to have been caused by chance, at a specified level of probability, is:
    a. clinical significance
    b. reliability
    c. statistical significance
    d. validity

36. The term for the process used when an adverse event occurs to specifically answer the four basic questions (What happened in this case? What usually happens? Why did this event occur? What if anything, can be done to prevent it from happening again?) is:
    a. culture of safety
    b. quality improvement
    c. risk management
    d. root-cause analysis

37. The best place for the APRN to find comprehensive standards of practice related to her or his particular role and population focus is:
    a. a national certification organization
    b. a professional organization representing the role and population focus
    c. the state board of nursing
    d. the school of nursing accreditation body

38. Which of the following hospital regulations would be against the principles for credentialing and privileging of CNMs and CMs established by the ACNM?
    a. Guidelines that ensure the midwife is accountable for the care provided and that avoid placing liability on other healthcare professionals
    b. Mechanisms designated to determine the circumstances under which consultation or management by a physician is required
    c. Mechanisms for recognizing expanded practice procedures distinguished from standard privileges granted to midwives
    d. Requirements for credentialing, privileging, and renewing privileges that focus on the difference in types of care provided by midwives and physicians

39. The Centers for Disease Control and Prevention's Sexually Transmitted Diseases Treatment Guidelines best fit the definition of:
    a. expert opinion
    b. scope of practice parameters
    c. standard of care
    d. standard of practice

40. The term used to indicate that the implications of the findings of a study with a particular population can be extended to a larger population is:
    a. generalization
    b. reliability
    c. replication
    d. validity

Answers with Rationales

1. **a.** Critical care
   The six population foci are family/individual across the lifespan, adult–gerontology, neonatal, pediatrics, women's health, psychiatric–mental health.

2. **d.** The DNP curriculum focuses on practice more so than on research.
   Entry into a DNP program may occur after completion of a baccalaureate nursing degree (BS-DNP) or master's nursing degree (MS-DNP). Programs' clinical experience requirements may vary depending on the APRN role.

State boards of nursing do not currently require a DNP for APRN practice.

3. **d.** recognition of women's life phases as normal, developmental processes
   The Hallmarks of Midwifery include recognition of women's life phases as normal, developmental processes.

4. **b.** complete specific pharmacologic educational requirements
   Individual states may require approval of the state board of medicine, although the majority of states have APRN prescriptive authority in nurse and midwifery practice

acts. Some states, but not all, have a collaborative agreement requirement. DEA registration may be obtained depending on individual state scope of practice laws.

5. **c.** certification

Certification is the formal process by which a private agency or organization certifies (usually by examination) that an individual has met standards as specified by that profession. Almost all states require national certification for nurse practitioners and nurse–midwives.

6. **c.** state boards of nursing

Authority for prescriptive authority is contained in state nurse or midwifery practice acts or in other statutes that vary from state to state. Additional approval may be required from other state boards.

7. **b.** Always use a leading zero for doses less than 1 unit (e.g., use 0.1 mg, not .1 mg).

To reduce medication errors, use a leading zero when writing doses less than 1 unit (use 0.1 mg, not .1 mg), but do not use a trailing zero after a decimal point (use 1 mg, not 1.0 mg).

8. **c.** Predetermined payment based on a contractual per-member, per-month rate

Capitation is a way of paying health care providers or organizations in which they receive a predictable, upfront, set amount of money to cover the predicted cost of all or some of the health care services for a specific patient over a certain period of time (Centers for Medicare & Medicaid Services, n.d.).

9. **b.** improve the health system by standardizing the exchange of electronic data

The purpose of HIPAA is to ensure that an individual's health information is properly protected while allowing the flow of information needed to promote high-quality health care and to protect the public's health and well-being.

10. **a.** any health provider who transmits any health information electronically

HIPAA-covered entities (those to whom the privacy rules apply) include health plans, healthcare clearinghouses, and any healthcare provider who transmits health information in electronic form in connection with transactions. Examples of organizations that do not have to follow the privacy and security rules include life insurers, employers, workers' compensation carriers, most schools and school districts, many state agencies like child protective service agencies, most law enforcement agencies, many municipal offices

11. **a.** provide federal protections for privacy and preserve quality care

For the most part, HIPAA privacy rules apply to all PHI. There are two situations in which a covered entity is required to share PHI and at least four situations in which the covered entity may be permitted to disclose PHI.

12. **d.** the monthly premium requirement for Part B

Medicare Part B is supplementary medical insurance available to individuals for a monthly premium if they are eligible for Medicare Part A. Part B covers provider services, outpatient care, diagnostics, and durable medical equipment.

13. **a.** communication error

Dimensions of optimal communication for patient safety include communication with the patient and family, communication with all individuals caring for the patient, and availability of information necessary for coordination of care.

14. **c.** near miss

An adverse event is one in which patient harm arises as a result of medical care (rather than from the underlying disease). It is a preventable adverse event when it is due to error or failure to apply an accepted strategy for prevention (e.g., medication reconciliation). A near miss is an unsafe situation that is indistinguishable from a preventable adverse event except for the outcome. The patient does not experience harm either through luck or early detection.

15. **a.** the Center for Medicare and Medicaid Services (CMS)

The APRN obtains a national provider identification (NPI) number from CMS.

16. **a.** children younger than 19 in families whose income is below poverty level

States must provide Medicaid coverage to the following groups if they meet specified income-eligibility requirements: pregnant individuals and children younger than age 6, children younger than age 19, adults younger than age 65 without dependent children, and adults with short-term disability.

17. **b.** including the patient as a member of the healthcare team

The goal of interprofessional practice is patient care that is safe, timely, effective, efficient, equitable, and patient-centered. The patient is considered a member of the healthcare team. The team uses communication skills that include negotiation, consensus building, and conflict resolution. Different roles (e.g., member, leader) are assumed within the team as appropriate to develop and improve patient-centered care.

18. **b.** fidelity

Fidelity is the ethical principle of the healthcare professional keeping any promises or commitments made in a therapeutic relationship.

19. **b.** complete three maintenance modules plus 20 contact hours of continuing education every 5 years.

AMCB certification must be renewed every 5 years with completion of three maintenance modules plus 20 contact hours of continuing education or retaking the AMCB certification examination (no sooner than the fourth year of cycle) plus 20 contact hours of continuing education.

20. **d.** nonmaleficence

Nonmaleficence is the ethical principle of the healthcare professional doing no harm in actions taken.

21. **d.** negligence

Negligence is conduct lacking in due care, also called carelessness.

22. **b.** a negligence tort
A negligence tort involves conduct lacking in due care or careless conduct. Most malpractice cases are based on negligence.

23. **b.** battery
Battery is the actual, intentional, and unlawful touching or striking of another person against the will of that person.

24. **a.** exercising her right to refuse treatment
Refusal of treatment is the inherent right of an individual who is conscious and mentally capable of refusing any form of treatment either personally or through the person's legal representative.

25. **a.** a claims-made policy.
With claims-made policies, the incident must happen and be reported while the policy is in force to be covered.

26. **c.** safety bundle
A small, straightforward set of evidence-based practices that when performed collectively and reliably, have proven to improve patient outcomes is called a safety bundle. The Council on Patient Safety in Women's Health Care is a multidisciplinary partnership that, along with the AIM, has designed safety bundles to reduce severe maternal morbidity and mortality.

27. **c.** Meta-analysis
Level I (meta-analysis or multiple controlled studies) is the strongest rating. However, quality may range from A to D, with A indicating a very well-designed study and D indicating the study has a major flaw that raises serious questions about the believability of its findings.

28. **b.** complete a specialty assessment evaluation that determines the topics and number of hours of continuing education needed before the next renewal cycle
NCC certification must be renewed every 3 years with the completion of a specialty assessment evaluation that determines the topics and number of hours of continuing education needed (15–50 hours) before the next renewal cycle *or* completion of 50 continuing education hours covering all core certification knowledge areas *or* retaking the certification examination.

29. **b.** Individual state boards of nursing
Under the consensus model, state boards of nursing are solely responsible for licensing APRNs.

30. **a.** describe life experiences and give them meaning
Qualitative research is defined as a systematic, interactive, subjective approach used to describe life experiences and give them meaning.

31. **b.** Collaboration
The consensus model describes four essential components for regulation of APRNs: *l*icensure, *a*ccreditation, *c*ertification, and *e*ducation (commonly referred to as LACE).

32. **a.** correlational
Correlational research study designs are used for systematic investigation of relationships between two or more variables to explain the type (positive or negative) of relationships, but not to examine cause and effect.

33. **b.** the quality of the study's design.
Categories of strength of evidence from research studies are based on a combination of the research design (Levels I–VI) used (e.g., meta-analysis, experimental) and the quality of the design of the study (Levels A–D), which affects the believability of the findings.

34. **d.** reliability
Reliability represents the consistency of a measure obtained in a study.

35. **c.** statistical significance
Statistical significance is an indication that the results from an analysis of sample data are unlikely to have been caused by chance, at a specified level of probability. For example, significance at the 0.05 level indicates the probability that the result would occur by chance is only 5 times out of 100. Clinical significance is a term used to indicate the practical importance of research results in terms of whether they have genuine effects on the daily lives of clients or on healthcare decisions.

36. **d.** root-cause analysis
A culture of safety promotes a learning organization by using root-cause analysis when an adverse event occurs. This process is used to answer four basic questions: What happened in this case? What usually happens? Why did this event occur? What if anything, can be done to prevent it from happening again?

37. **b.** a professional organization representing the role and population focus
Standards of practice are overarching statements that the nursing profession uses to describe the responsibilities of its members to provide safe and competent care. APRNs are held to standards of practice promulgated by the nursing profession and standards determined by professional organizations representing their role and population focus.

38. **d.** Requirements for credentialing, privileging, and renewing privileges that focus on the difference in types of care provided by midwives and physicians
One of the ACNM principles for credentialing and privileging CNMs and CMs is that requirements for credentialing, privileging, and renewing privileges should be equivalent.

39. **c.** standard of care
Standards of care, also called practice guidelines, are evidence-based, continuously evolving standards of appropriate care. Sources for these standards include entities such as the CDC, AHRQ, and professional medical and nursing specialty organizations.

40. **a.** generalization
Generalization extends the implications of the findings of a study from the sample studied to a large population or from a situation studied to a larger situation.

Bibliography

Advanced Practice Registered Nurse Consensus Work Group & National Council of State Boards of Nursing APRN Advisory Committee. (2008). *Consensus model for APRN regulation: Licensure, accreditation, certification, and education.* https://www.ncsbn.org/public-files/Consensus_Model_for_APRN_Regulation_July_2008.pdf

Agency for Healthcare Research and Quality. (2019) *PS safety network: Patient safety 101.* https://psnet.ahrq.gov/primer/patient-safety-101

Agency for Healthcare Research and Quality. (2020). *PS safety network: Patient safety in primary care.* https://psnet.ahrq.gov/perspective/patient-safety-primary-care

American Association of Colleges of Nursing. (2004). *AACN position statement on the practice doctorate in nursing.* https://www.aacnnursing.org/DNP/Position-Statement

American Association of Colleges of Nursing. (2021). *The essentials: Core competencies for professional nursing education.* https://www.aacnnursing.org/Portals/42/AcademicNursing/pdf/Essentials-2021.pdf

American Association of Nurse Anesthetists. (2020). *Scope of nurse anesthesia practice.* https://www.aana.com/wp-content/uploads/2023/01/scope-of-nurse-anesthesia-practice.pdf

American Association of Nurse Practitioners. (2022a). *Scope of practice for nurse practitioners.* https://www.aanp.org/advocacy/advocacy-resource/position-statements/scope-of-practice-for-nurse-practitioners

American Association of Nurse Practitioners. (2022b). *Issues at a glance: Full practice authority.* https://www.aanp.org/advocacy/advocacy-resource/policy-briefs/issues-full-practice-brief

American Association of Nurse Practitioners. (2022c). *Standards of practice for nurse practitioners.* https://www.aanp.org/advocacy/advocacy-resource/position-statements/standards-of-practice-for-nurse-practitioners.

American College of Nurse–Midwives. (2016a). *Position statement: Principles for credentialing and privileging certified nurse-midwives and certified midwives.* https://www.midwife.org/acnm/files/ACNMLibraryData/UPLOADFILENAME/000000000082/Principles-for-the-Credentialing-PS-FINAL-9-12-16.pdf

American College of Nurse–Midwives. (2017). *Comparison of certified nurse-midwives, certified midwives, certified professional midwives clarifying the distinctions among professional midwifery credentials in the U.S.* https://www.midwife.org/acnm/files/cclibraryfiles/filename/000000007423/45%20Updated%20CNM%20CM%20CPM%20Comparison%20Chart%20October%202017.pdf

American College of Nurse–Midwives. (2020). *ACNM core competencies for basic midwifery practice.* https://www.midwife.org/acnm/files/acnmlibrarydata/uploadfilename/000000000050/ACNMCoreCompetenciesMar2020_final.pdf

American College of Nurse–Midwives. (2021). *Definition of midwifery and scope of practice of certified nurse–midwives and certified midwives.* https://www.midwife.org/acnm/files/acnmlibrarydata/uploadfilename/000000000266/Definition%20Midwifery%20Scope%20of%20Practice_2021.pdf

American College of Nurse–Midwives. (2022a). *Standards for the practice of midwifery.* https://www.midwife.org/acnm/files/acnmlibrarydata/uploadfilename/000000000051/standards_for_practice_of_midwifery_sept_2011.pdf

American College of Nurse–Midwives. (2022b). *Position statement: Mandatory degree requirements for midwives.* https://www.midwife.org/acnm/files/acnmlibrarydata/uploadfilename/000000000076/2022_ps_mandatory-degree-requirements-entry-to-midwifery-practice.pdf

American College of Nurse–Midwives. (2022c). *Expansion of midwifery practice and skills beyond basic core competencies.* http://www.midwife.org/acnm/files/acnmlibrarydata/uploadfilename/000000000066/2022_ps_expansion-of-midwifery-practice-beyond-core-competencies.pdf

American College of Nurse–Midwives. (2022d). *Ultrasound in midwifery practice.* https://www.midwife.org/acnm/files/acnmlibrarydata/uploadfilename/000000000318/Ultrasound-in-Midwifery-Practice-FINAL-11-24-18.pdf

American College of Nurse–Midwives. (2022e). *The certified nurse-midwife/certified midwife as first assistant during surgery.* http://www.midwife.org/acnm/files/ACNMLibraryData/UPLOADFILENAME/000000000270/PS-First-Assist-Revisions-FINAL-Feb%202018.pdf

American College of Nurse–Midwives. (2018). *Position statement: Midwives are primary care providers and leaders of maternity care homes.* https://www.midwife.org/acnm/files/acnmlibrarydata/uploadfilename/000000000273/PS-Midwives-are-Primary-Care-Providers-and-Leaders-of-Maternity-Care-Homes-FINAL-22-MAR-18.pdf

Buppert, C. (2021). *Nurse practitioner's business practice and legal guide* (7th ed.). Jones & Bartlett Learning.

Centers for Medicare & Medicaid Services. (n.d.). *Capitation and Pre-Payment.* https://www.cms.gov/priorities/innovation/key-concepts/capitation-and-pre-payment

Foster, I. R. & Lasser, J. (2011). *Professional ethics in midwifery practice.* Jones & Bartlett Learning.

Grace, P. (2018). *Nursing ethics and professional responsibility in advanced practice* (3rd ed.). Jones & Bartlett Learning.

Gray, J., Grove, S. & Sutherland, S. (2020). *Burns and Grove's the practice of nursing research: Appraisal, synthesis, and generation of evidence* (9th ed.). Saunders Elsevier.

Institute of Medicine. (2001). *Crossing the quality chasm: A new health system for the 21st century.* National Academies Press.

Kilpatrick, S. J., Papile, L., & Macones, G. A. (2017). *Guidelines for perinatal care* (8th ed.). American Academy of Pediatrics Committee on Fetus and Newborn & American College of Obstetricians and Gynecologists Committee on Obstetric Practice. https://doi.org/10.1542/9781610020886

National Association of Clinical Nurse Specialists. (2019). *National Association of Clinical Nurse Specialists statement on clinical nurse specialist practice and education* (3rd ed.). https://nacns.org/professional-resources/practice-and-cns-role/cns-competencies

National Association of Nurse Practitioners in Women's Health. (2020). *The women's health nurse practitioner: Guidelines for practice and education* (8th ed.). National Association of Nurse Practitioners in Women's Health.

National Organization of Nurse Practitioner Faculties. (2022). *Nurse practitioner role core competencies.* https://www.nonpf.org/page/NP_Role_Core_Competencies

National Task Force on Quality Nurse Practitioner Education. (2022). *Standards for quality nurse practitioner education, A report of the national task force on quality nurse practitioner education* (6th ed.). National Organization of Nurse Practitioner Faculties.

Polit, D. & Beck C. (2018). *Essentials of nursing research: Appraising evidence for nursing practice* (9th ed.). Wolters Kluwer.

The Joint Commission. (2023). *Comprehensive accreditation manual.* https://store.jcrinc.com/2023-comprehensive-accreditation-manuals/?ref=GOOGLE&utm_source=google&utm_medium=cpc&utm_campaign=2023JCRManuals&gclid=CjwKCAiAmJGgBhAZEiwA1JZoltFsHfT4iw3EAhBQpYcuwhEBR0HBZvBqAFBo-J8qtVHxvhS32JewLRoCGgkQAvD_BwE

The Joint Commission. (2019). *2019 National patient safety goals.* https://www.jointcommission.org/standards_information/npsgs.aspx

Tracy, M. & O'Grady, E. (2019). *Advanced nursing practice: An integrative approach* (6th ed.). Elsevier Saunders.

U.S. Department of Health and Human Services. (2022). *Summary of the HIPAA privacy rule.* https://www.hhs.gov/hipaa/for-professionals/privacy/laws-regulations/index.html

Index

Note: Boxes, figures, and tables are indicated with *b, f,* and, *t* following the page numbers, respectively.